PROGRESS IN BRAIN RESEARCH

VOLUME 123

PERIPHERAL AND SPINAL MECHANISMS IN THE
NEURAL CONTROL OF MOVEMENT

Other volumes in PROGRESS IN BRAIN RESEARCH

PROGRESS IN BRAIN RESEARCH

VOLUME 123

PERIPHERAL AND SPINAL MECHANISMS IN THE NEURAL CONTROL OF MOVEMENT

EDITED BY

M.D. BINDER

*Department of Physiology and Biophysics, University of Washington School of Medicine,
Box 357290, Seattle, WA 98195-7290, USA*

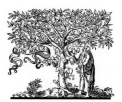

ELSEVIER

AMSTERDAM – LAUSANNE – NEW YORK – OXFORD – SHANNON – SINGAPORE – TOKYO
1999

ELSEVIER SCIENCE B.V.
Sara Burgerhartstraat 25
P.O. Box 211, 1000 AE Amsterdam, The Netherlands

First edition 1999

Library of Congress Cataloging in Publication Data
A catalog record from the Library of Congress has been applied for.

ISBN: 0-444-50288-2
ISBN: 0-444-80104-9 (series)

⊚ The paper used in this publication meets the requirements of ANSI/NISO Z39.48-1992 (Permanence of Paper).
Printed in The Netherlands.

032700/220500 4

v

List of Contributors

I. Bar-Gad, Department of Zoology, Tel Aviv University, Ramat Aviv, Tel Aviv 69978, Israel

P. Bawa, School of Kinesiology, Simon Fraser University, Burnaby, BC, Canada

R. Beer, Rehabilitation Institute of Chicago, Sensory Motor Performance Program, Northwestern University Medical School, 345 East Superior, Chicago, IL 60611, USA

M.D. Binder, Department of Physiology and Biophysics, University of Washington School of Medicine, Box 357290, Seattle, WA 98195–7290, USA

A. M. Brichta, The Neuroscience Group, Discipline of Anatomy, University of Newcastle, Callaghan, NSW 2308, Australia

E. Brustein, University of Montreal, Centre de Recherche en Sciences Neurologiques, Montreal, PQ, Canada

J.T. Buchanan, Department of Biology, Marquette University, 630 N. 15th Street, PO Box 1881, Milwaukee, WI 53201–1881, USA

D.Burke, Prince of Wales Medical Research Institute, Department of Neurology, High Street, Randwick, NSW 2031, Sydney, Australia

R.E. Burke, Laboratory of Neural Control, Bldg. 49, Rm. 3A50, MSC 4455, NINDS, National Institutes of Health, Bethesda, MD 20892–4455, USA

R.A. Burnett, Department of Kinesiology and Applied Physiology, University of Colorado, Boulder, CO 80309–0354, USA

S.L. Butler, Department of Physiology, University of Adelaide, Adelaide SA 5005, Australia

R.J. Callister, Discipline of Anatomy, University of Newcastle, Callaghan NSW 2308, Australia

L.J. Carr, Department of Physiology, University College London, Gower Street, London WC1E 6BT, UK

D.I. Carrasco, Department of Cell Biology, Emory University School of Medicine, Atlanta, GA 30322, USA

M. Catley, Imperial College School of Medicine, Department of Sensorimotor Systems, Division of Neuroscience and Psychological Medicine, Charing Cross Hospital, Fulham Palace Road, London W6 8RF, UK

B.A. Conway, Bioengineering Unit, University of Strathclyde, Glasgow, G4 0NW, Scotland, UK

T.C. Cope, Department of Physiology, Emory University, 1648 Pierce Drive, Atlanta, GA 30322, USA

B.D. Corneil, MRC Group in Sensory-Motor Neuroscience, Department of Physiology, Queens University, Kingston, ON K7L 3N6, Canada

S. Cushing, Department of Physiology, Queens University, Kingston, ON K7L 3N6, Canada

R.D. de Leon, Department of Physiological Science, University of California at Los Angeles, P.O. 951527, Los Angeles, CA 90095–1527, USA

R. Delgado-Lezama, Depto. de Fisiologa, Biofsica y Neurociencias, CINVESTAV, Mexico

J. Dewald, Rehabilitation Institute of Chicago, Sensory Motor Performance Program, Northwestern University Medical School, 345 East Superior, Chicago, IL 60611, USA

R. Donga, Department of Preclinical Sciences, University of Leicester, P.O. Box 138, Leicester LE1 9HN, UK

T. Drew, University of Montreal, Department of Physiology, Centre de Recherche en Sciences Neurologiques, Montreal, PQ, Canada

R. Durbaba, Imperial College School of Medicine, Department of Sensorimotor Systems, Division of Neuroscience and Psychological Medicine, Charing Cross Hospital, London W6 8RF, UK

V.R. Edgerton, Department of Physiological Science, University of California at Los Angeles, P.O. 951527, Los Angeles, CA 90095–1527, USA

P.H. Ellaway, Imperial College School of Medicine, Department of Sensorimotor Systems (Room 10L09), Division of Neuroscience and Psychological Medicine, Charing Cross Hospital, Fulham Palace Road, London W6 8RF, UK

A.W. English, Department of Cell Biology, Emory University School of Medicine, 1648 Pierce Drive, Atlanta, GA 30322, USA

R.M. Enoka, Department of Kinesiology and Applied Physiology, University of Colorado, Boulder, CO 80309–0354, USA

E.E. Fetz, Department of Physiology and Biophysics and Regional Primate Research Center, SJ–40, University of Washington, Seattle, WA 98195, USA

T.W. Ford, Department of Physiology, Royal Free and University College Medical School, Rowland Hill Street, London NW3 2PF, UK

S.C. Gandevia, Prince of Wales Medical Research Institute, Department of Neurology, High Street, Randwick, NSW 2031, Sydney, Australia

J. Gibbs, Department of Physiology, University College London, Gower Street, London WC1E 6BT, UK

M.H. Gladden, Institute of Biomedical and Life Sciences, University of Glasgow, Glasgow G12 8QQ, UK

S.J. Goldberg, Department of Anatomy, Visual Motor Neurosciences Division, Virginia Commonwealth University, College of Medicine, Richmond, VA 23298–0709, USA

B.R. Gooden, Department of Physiology, University of Adelaide, Adelaide SA 5005, Australia

T. Gordon, University of Alberta, Department of Pharmacology, Division of Neuroscience, 525 HMRC, Edmonton, AB T6G 2S2, Canada

A.E. Graves, Department of Kinesiology and Applied Physiology, University of Colorado, Boulder, CO 80309–0354, USA

J.E. Gregory, Department of Physiology, Monash University, Clayton, Victoria 3168, Australia

S. Grillner, Nobel Institute for Neurophysiology, Department of Neuroscience Karolinska Institutet, SE–171 77 Stockholm, Sweden

T.M. Hamm, Division of Neurobiology, Barrow Neurological Institute, St. Joseph's Hospital and Medical Center, Phoenix, AZ 85015, USA

N. Haque, The Royal Hospital for Neuro-disability, London SW15 3SW, UK

L.M. Harrison, Department of Physiology, University College London, Gower Street, London WC1E 6BT, UK

Z. Hasan, College of Health and Human Development Sciences, University of Illinois at Chicago, Chicago, IL 60612 USA

K. Hase, Department of Rehabilitation Medicine, Keio University, Tokyo, Japan

C.J. Heckman, Department of Physiology M211, Northwestern University Medical School, 303 E. Chicago Ave, Chicago, IL 60611, USA

D.M. Halliday, Division of Neuroscience and Biomedical Systems, University of Glasgow, Glasgow G12 8QQ, Scotland UK

G. Holstege, Department of Anatomy and Embryology, University of Groningen, Oostersingel 69, 9713 EZ Groningen, The Netherlands

J. Hounsgaard, University of Copenhagen, Department of Medical Physiology, The Panum Institute, Blegdamsvej 3, DK–2200, Copenhagen N., Denmark

H. Hultborn, University of Copenhagen, Department of Medical Physiology, The Panum Institute, Blegdamsvej 3, DK–2200,Copenhagen N, Denmark

C.M.J.I. Huyghues-Despointes, Department of Neuroscience, University of Florida, Gainesville, FL 32610, USA

E. Jankowska, Department of Physiology, Goteborg University, Medicinaregatan 11, Box 432, SE 405 30 Goteborg, Sweden

W. Jiang, University of Montreal, Centre de Recherche en Sciences Neurologiques, Montreal, PQ, Canada

K.E. Jones, Department of Physiology, University of Manitoba, 730 William Avenue, Winnipeg, MB R3E 3J7, Canada

R.D. Johnson, Department of Physiological Sciences, University of Florida, Gainesville, FL 32610, USA

I. Kagan, Department of Zoology, Tel Aviv University, Ramat Aviv, Tel Aviv 69978, Israel

D. Kernell, Department of Medical Physiology, University of Groningen, Bloemsingel 10, 9712 KZ Groningen, The Netherlands

P.A. Kirkwood, Sobell Department of Neurophysiology, Institute of Neurology, University College London, Queen Square, London WC1N 3BG, UK

K.W. Kornatz, Department of Kinesiology and Applied Physiology, University of Colorado, Boulder, CO 80309–0354, USA

D.H. Laidlaw, Department of Kinesiology and Applied Physiology, University of Colorado, Boulder, CO 80309–0354, USA

R.H. Lee, Department of Physiology M211, Northwestern University Medical School, 303 E. Chicago Ave, Chicago, IL 60611, USA

D.C. Lin, Department of Physiology, Emory University, Atlanta, GA 30322, USA

G.E. Loeb, Department of Biomedical Engineering, University of Southern California, Los Angeles, CA 90089, USA

N.J.S. London, Department of Physiological Science, University of California at Los Angeles, P.O. 951527, Los Angeles, CA 90095–1527, USA

M.J. Mayston, Department of Physiology, University College London, Gower Street, London WC1E 6BT, UK

M.A. Maier, Department of Physiology and Biophysics and Regional Primate Research Center, University of Washington, Seattle, WA 98195, USA

L.M. Mendell, Department of Neurobiology and Behavior, State University of New York at Stony Brook, Stony Brook, New York, 11794–5230, USA

T.S. Miles, Department of Physiology, University of Adelaide, Adelaide SA 5005, Australia

S.H. Moosavi, Imperial College School of Medicine, Department of Sensorimotor Systems, Division of Neuroscience and Psychological Medicine, Charing Cross Hospital, Fulham Palace Road, London W6 8RF, UK

J.B. Munson, Department of Neuroscience, University of Florida, College of Medicine, Gainesville, FL 32610–0244, USA

A. Nardone, Posture and Movement Laboratory, Fondazione Salvatore Maugeri, Medical Center of Veruno (NO), Italy

T.R. Nichols, Department of Physiology, Emory University, Atlanta, GA 30322, USA

M.A. Nordstrom, Department of Physiology, University of Adelaide, Adelaide SA 5005, Australia

S.I. Perlmutter, Department of Physiology and Biophysics and Regional Primate Research Center, University of Washington, Seattle, WA 98195, USA

E.H. Peterson, Neurobiology Program and Department of Biological Sciences, Ohio University, Athens, OH 45701, USA

R.K. Powers, Department of Physiology and Biophysics, University of Washington School of Medicine Box 357290, Seattle, WA 98195–7290, USA

A. Prochazka, University of Alberta, Division of Neuroscience, 507 HMRC, Edmonton, AB T6G 2S2, Canada

W. Proske, Department of Physiology, Monash University, Clayton, Victoria 3168, Australia

Y. Prut, Department of Physiology and Biophysics and Regional Primate Research Center, University of Washington, Seattle, WA 98195, USA

V. F. Raves, University of Alberta, Division of Neuroscience, 507 HMRC, Edmonton, AB T6G 2S2, Canada

F.J.R. Richmond, MRC Group in Sensory-Motor Neuroscience, Department of Physiology, Queens University, Kingston, ON K7L 3N6, Canada

M.C. Ridding, Department of Physiology, University of Adelaide, Adelaide SA 5005, Australia

P.K. Rose, Department of Physiology, Queens University, Kingston, ON K7L 3N6, Canada

J.R. Rosenberg, Division of Neuroscience and Biomedical Systems, University of Glasgow, Glasgow G12 8QQ, Scotland, UK

S. Rossignol, University of Montreal, Centre de Recherche en Sciences Neurologiques, Montreal, PQ, Canada

R.R. Roy, Brain Research Institute, University of California at Los Angeles, P.O. Box 951527, Los Angeles, CA 90095–1527, USA

P. Rudomin, Department of Physiology and Biophysics, Ctr. Inves. y de Estud Avonzados Del Ipn, Ap 14740, Mexico 14 DF, Mexico

W.Z. Rymer, Rehabilitation Institute of Chicago, Sensory Motor Performance Program, Northwestern University Medical School, Room 1406, 345 East Superior, Chicago, IL 60611, USA

S.A. Saywell, Sobell Department of Neurophysiology, Institute of Neurology, University College London, Queen Square, London WC1N 3BG, UK

A.I. Selverston, Institute of Neurobiology, University of Puerto Rico, 201 Blvd. Del Valle, San Juan 00901, Puerto Rico

M. Schieppati, Section of Human Physiology, Department of Experimental Medicine, University of Genoa, Genoa, Italy

M.S. Shall, Department of Physical Therapy, Virginia Commonwealth University, College of Medicine, Richmond, VA 23298–0224, USA

M.L. Shik, Department of Zoology, Tel Aviv University, Ramat Aviv, Tel Aviv 69978, Israel

K. Singh, MRC Group in Sensory-Motor Neuroscience, Queens University, Department of Physiology, Kingston, ON K7L 3N6, Canada

A.J. Sokoloff, Department of Physiology, Emory University, 1648 Pierce Drive, Atlanta, GA 30322, USA

P.S.G. Stein, Department of Biology, Washington University, St. Louis, MO 63130 USA

R.B. Stein, University of Alberta, Division of Neuroscience, 507 HMRC, Edmonton, AB T6G 2S2, Canada

J.A. Stephens, Department of Physiology, University College London, Gower Street, London WC1E 6BT, UK

M.J. Stokes, The Royal Hospital for Neuro-disability, London SW15 3SW, UK

N.J. Strausfeld, University of Arizona, ARL Division of Neurobiology, Tucson, AZ 85721, USA

D.G. Stuart, Department of Physiology, University of Arizona, College of Medicine, Tucson, AZ, 85724 USA

A. Taylor, Imperial College School of Medicine, Department of Sensorimotor Systems, Division of Neuroscience & Psychiatry, Charing Cross Hospital, London W6 8RF, UK

J.S. Thomas, College of Health and Human Development Sciences, University of Illinois at Chicago, Chicago, IL 60612, USA

P.D. Thompson, Department of Medicine, University of Adelaide, Adelaide SA 5005, Australia

T.V. Trank, Division of Neurobiology, Barrow Neurological Institute, St. Joseph's Hospital and Medical Center, Phoenix, AZ 85015, USA

V.V. Turkin, Division of Neurobiology, Barrow Neurological Institute, St. Joseph's Hospital and Medical Center, Phoenix, AZ 85015, USA

N. Tyreman, University of Alberta, Department of Pharmacology, Division of Neuroscience, 525 HMRC, Edmonton, AB T6G 2S2, Canada

P. Wallén, Nobel Institute for Neurophysiology, Department of Neuroscience Karolinska Institutet, SE–171 77 Stockholm, Sweden

A.K. Wise, Department of Physiology, Monash University, Clayton, Victoria 3168, Australia

Preface

This volume of Progress in Brain Research is dedicated to Professor Douglas G. Stuart, whose exemplary career has had a profound influence on both motor control neurobiology and on the scientific lives of his many students and colleagues throughout the world. The chapters in this volume are largely derived from presentations made at a Society for Neuroscience Satellite Symposium held in Doug's honor from November 4–6, 1998 at the University of Arizona in Tucson. The meeting was attended by more than 200 scientists, representing 18 different countries.

Douglas Gordon Stuart was born in Casino, New South Wales, Australia on October 5, 1931. He was educated at Sydney Teachers' College, Michigan State University, and UCLA, where he earned a Ph.D in physiology and neuroscience in 1961. His professional career includes appointments at the Long Beach Veterans' Administration Hospital (1961–65), UCLA (1961–65), UC Davis (1965–67), the University of Arizona (1967–), where he presently holds a Regents' Professorship.

Doug has made important contributions to several different areas in motor control research and has published more than 100 experimental papers in peer-reviewed journals. His papers are distinguished by their rigor and exceptional scholarship. Doug was among the first physiologists to question the notion that sensory input from muscle spindles alone controls the frequency of rhythmic movements. Using shivering and other forms of tremor in cats and humans, he and his colleagues showed that these rhythmic movements are dependent on interactions between rhythm-generating CNS mechanisms and the visco-elastic properties of the limb, in addition to sensory feedback.

Later, Doug and his colleagues made quantitative comparisons of the responsiveness of muscle spindles and Golgi tendon organs to sinusoidal muscle stretches and were the first to describe the contractile effects of fast- and slow-twitch motor units on the firing patterns of the tendon organs. They subsequently analyzed the relationship between the forces generated by single motor units and muscle receptor discharge patterns. Doug and his colleagues also used spike-triggered averaging to uncover the excitatory, mono-synaptic connections between muscle spindle group II afferents and their homonymous and synergist motoneurons. This surprising finding led to an extensive re-evaluation of the roles of muscle spindles and other proprioceptors in the reflex control of muscle activity.

Among Doug's most important and lasting contributions to motor control was the cinematographic analysis of cat hindlimb joint angles and muscle lengths during locomotion that he and his colleagues made in the early 1970s. This work was motivated by his interest in simulating natural-movement conditions for his studies of muscle receptor and motor unit mechanical properties. However, in addition to providing the data he needed, Doug also gave the field its definitive analysis of the step cycle, which turned out to be crucial for testing a number of key hypotheses on reflexes, pattern generation, and muscle receptor function.

Another of Doug's long-standing interests is muscle fatigue. Again, he has made important contributions to this area by demonstrating that the association between the electromyogram and force during fatiguing contractions varies both in different muscles and with different types of muscle activation. He and his colleagues also revealed how subtle alterations in the pattern of motor unit activation can reduce and delay fatigue.

Most recently, Doug's laboratory has focused its attention on the electrical properties of motoneurons and interneurons in the turtle spinal cord. The goal of these studies is to describe how the intrinsic properties of identified neurons in the cord shape the input–output functions of spinal circuits. There is every reason to expect that this new avenue will again yield exciting new data and insights.

Despite the importance of Doug's original experimental work, his more than 70 book chapters, reviews and contributions to symposia volumes have had an even greater impact on the field. In these papers, he has provided critical reviews and elaborated new, synthetic hypotheses. Further, Doug has boldly directed challenges to his colleagues, even outlining the experimental projects they should undertake to resolve differences in their findings.

Outside of his laboratory, Doug's efforts as a champion for the field of motor control are legend. He has organized numerous national and international meetings and worked tirelessly to build interdisciplinary ties between biologists, clinicians, engineers, exercise physiologists and physical therapists. Moreover, he has been an exceptional mentor and role model, effectively 'raising' an entire generation of motor control scientists.

Marc D. Binder

Contents

xv

IX. Control of movement studied in man

SECTION I

Perspectives

M.D. Binder (Ed.)
Progress in Brain Research, Vol 123
© 1999 Elsevier Science BV. All rights reserved.

CHAPTER 1

The segmental motor system – advances, issues, and possibilities

Douglas G. Stuart*

Department of Physiology, College of Medicine, The University of Arizona, Tucson, AZ 85724, USA

DEDICATION

This article is dedicated to members of the post-WWII Moscow Motor Control School: the late Nicolai Bernstein, Israel Gelfand and Michael Tsetlin; Bernstein's student, Victor Gurfinkel; Ludmila Kudina and Raisa Person; Yuri Arshavsky, Michael Berkinblit, Tatiana Deliagina, Anatole Feldman, Olga Fookson, Sergei Kashin, Yakov Kots, Andrey Kulagin, Mark Lipshits, Micha Mirsky, Grigori Orlovsky, Yuri Panchin, Galina Pavlova, Konstantin Popov, Lyubov' Popova, Ivan Rodionov, the late Fyodor Severin, and Mark Shik; and, their many colleagues and trainees, including Yuri Levik and Mark Latash. Working under far-from-optimal circumstances, this group's accomplishments and emphasis on interactions between invertebrate and vertebrate neuroscientists, life- and physical scientists, and basic and clinical scientists, have been an inspiration to those of us who have attempted to emulate their interdisciplinary efforts in our own institutions' research and training programs in motor control neurobiology.

Introduction

The majority of topics addressed in this volume, and its preceding international conference (Binder et al., 1998), can be considered under the rubric of the segmental motor system. This term has proven to be useful in both invertebrate and vertebrate motor control neuroscience for summarizing work

*Corresponding author. Tel.: (520) 626–7103; Fax: (520) 626–2383; e-mail: dgstuart@u.arizona.edu

on: (1) the properties and central actions of posture- and movement-related sensory feedback from the body's somatic structures; (2) interneuron (IN) and motoneuron (MN) discharge properties, MN recruitment properties, and the associations between MN, muscle fiber (MF), and motor unit (MU) properties for the graded development of muscle force; and (3) segmental pattern generation for the elaboration of intrinsic/rhythmic and learned/skillful movements. Each of these areas is being addressed currently from the molecular/

4

cellular to the behavioral level of analysis in a wide variety of invertebrate and vertebrate species. Each has a particular attraction for life- and physical scientists, including roboticists, and each, in time, can provide a seamless integration between fundamental and applied clinical science. In all of the above instances, and irrespective of the level of analysis, the functional outcome is the elaboration of a posture and/or a movement. It is possible for all these reasons that the field of segmental motor research is so alive and well at the close of the 20th century. With this in mind, it is exciting to contemplate what the next generation of segmental motor neuroscientists might discover in the 21st century.

In what follows, I have attempted to capture the spirit of this field, as exemplified in this volume and its preceding symposium, by extolling recent advances, raising current issues, and pointing out future possibilities, at least for the immediate future. These topics are considered in a manner similar to the tripartite division above, even though their operation is highly integrated (chapter by Loeb [36], this volume). My strategy is useful in an historical sense, however, because, in any single decade or two, the areas of particular emphasis wax and wane as dependent on advances in techniques and technologies. For example, in this volume there is less emphasis on the first area, and more on the latter two, the reverse of the segmental motor field of the 1950s–1970s (Stuart and McDonagh, 1998). Some brief remarks are made about suprasegmental, descending command signals, because this area, which is currently profiting from new technical developments, was addressed, in part, in the 1998 conference, and in some of the chapters that follow in this volume.

I have shown how the chapters of the present volume, and some posters at its preceding conference, relate to the current state-of-the-play. What was presented and discussed in Tucson on November 4–6, 1998 also illustrates this timeliness. In my opinion, the present monograph is in the best traditions of the field of segmental motor neuroscience. It has continued to make optimal use of the contents of several post–1960s' international symposium volumes and journal compilations (from Barker [1962] to Stein et al. [1997], Binder and Mendell [1990], Kiehn et al. [1998], Jabre and Binder [1999], and the present volume). This is particularly true for interdisciplinary training programs in motor control (see also chapter by P. Stein [23]).

Finally, I make no apologies for using this chapter as a bully pulpit for expounding on selected issues that are dear to me because they are relevant to the operation of an interdisciplinary training program in movement neuroscience. One primary goal of such programs should be to emphasize a broad perspective and interest in movement neuroscience, from the molecular/cellular to the behavioral level of analysis (Bunge, 1989). Another guiding principle, which is often underemphasized at international conferences, is to truly *mentor* trainees, network them with senior scientists, and extol their work. They are, after all, the next generation of segmental motor neuroscientists!

Properties and central actions of muscle and other limb receptors

Sensory receptors

Advances in the understanding of the properties of the muscle spindle, the Golgi tendon organ, and other mammalian muscle receptors (Stuart and McDonagh, 1997a) are best appreciated by first considering Matthew's (1972) timeless monograph, and then following subsequent advances by reference to Taylor and Prochazka (1981), Taylor et al. (1995), and Proske (1999). This progress has included work on both freely moving animals (Prochazka, 1996) and, for more limited movements, humans (Gandevia and Burke, 1992; Proske, 1999). In retrospect, it is remarkable how much post-WWII effort was directed to unraveling the structure-function relationships of the muscle spindle, but it must be remembered that this structure has an anatomical complexity that approaches that of the eye (Hasan and Stuart, 1984).

It is sobering to reflect that much is still to be learned about the functional significance of the muscle spindle's complex structure (Taylor et al., 1995) and their axons and other sensory receptors' axons (chapter by D. Burke and Gandevia [39]).

For example, what is the association between the consistent gamma innervation of the spindles of birds and mammals, and the beta innervation possessed by some but not all of these receptors? There is still no model that can accommodate the receptor's afferent discharge during a full array of muscle-length perturbations. Furthermore, no current model can predict the nature of fusimotor innervation on the basis of changes in muscle length and afferent discharge, particularly during natural movements (cf. however, Prochazka and Gorassini, 1998). For the latter, it is still not clear why both spindles (length detectors) and tendon organs (force detectors) are necessary. Perhaps the presence of both enables the CNS to distinguish between internal changes (e.g. as brought on by fatigue) and external impediments, like inertia (Hasan and Stuart, 1984). Further experimentation (chapters by Prochazka [11], Proske et al. [12], 1999) and discussion along these lines is both important and necessary as a prelude to further experimentation. Nonetheless, our current understanding of the transducing properties of muscle spindles and tendon organs is relatively more advanced than it is for the higher-threshold mechanoreceptors. These, too, play an important role in segmental motor control (e.g. Cleland and Rymer, 1990), particularly during bouts of exercise when muscle fatigue becomes a factor (Stuart and Callister, 1993; Garland and Kaufman, 1995; Windhorst, 1995). More work on relatively high-threshold mechanoreceptive and ergoreceptive muscle, joint and ligamentous receptors would be helpful at this stage. Such progress is apparent in the allied field of the properties of somatosensory receptors, including nociceptors, and their central involvement in autonomic functions (Sato et al., 1997), and in the perception of pain (Mense, 1993; Schmidt, 1996).

The above effort has been largely on mammalian mechanoreceptors. An all-encompassing monograph equivalent to that of Matthews (1972) on mammalian muscle receptors has not been forthcoming for non-mammalian and invertebrate receptors, so a fruitful field for future enquiry is the extent to which proprioceptors have been subject to evolutionary conservation in both invertebrates and vertebrates, along the lines already discussed for motor control mechanisms in general (e.g. Fetcho, 1992; Pearson, 1993; Callister et al., 1995). For further recent reading on this intriguing topic, the reader is directed, in order, to: Clarac, 1982; Blackshaw, 1993; Gillespie, 1996; Dickinson et al., 1997; Keil, 1997; Watson and Mire, 1999.

There are relatively few technical impediments for advancing understanding of high-threshold mechanoreceptors in surgically reduced animals and in in vitro preparations. For the low-threshold spindles and tendon organs, however, the technology has been at a standstill for almost two decades for further work on freely moving animals. Similarly, for work on conscious humans, the possibility is still remote that a technical advance will shortly enable unitary recordings to be made during learned and unexpected movements of relative freedom and forcefulness. The current emphasis in human studies on behavioral psychophysics (e.g. Kakuda et al., 1997) is well warranted, however, particularly if it can advance along the lines already being applied to the study of precision grip (Flanagan et al., 1999).

Segmental actions of mechanosensory input

In my view, it would be helpful if modern textbooks began their discourse on the central segmental actions of peripheral sensory input onto mammalian MNs and INs by emphasizing the functional significance of Lundberg's (1969) focus on the critical role of segmental ventral-horn INs (Stuart et al., 1999). His work has continually emphasized that interneurons are the primary site of integration (convergence) of descending command signals and sensory feedback. He has also provided us with a major conceptual leap, the concept of alternative reflex pathways: i.e. the pathway chosen by the CNS depending on the phase and intent of a movement (Jankowska and Lundberg, 1981; chapter by Jankowska and Gladden [13]). The mammalian textbook focus is still heavily weighted toward results obtained in anesthetized cat preparations: e.g. the inhibitory action of Ib input from tendon organs onto homonymous MNs. For extensor MNs, however, this pathway is an excitatory one during locomotion (Prochazka, 1996), and it has been studied in detail in unanesthetized decerebrate cats that were spin-alized and chemo-stimulated with nialamide and L-DOPA (Conway et al., 1987; see also McCrea, 1998). This problem is exacerbated by textbooks' initial discourse on such central actions being presented prior to introducing the topic of spinal pattern generation and central pattern generators (CPGs; see below). For over 25 years, CPGs have been particularly revealing about phase-dependent reflex reversals during the elaboration of stepping (Grillner, 1975), this being the predominant princi-ple to emerge from consideration of the segmental actions of mechanosensory input.

Since Lundberg's 1969 article, there has been: (1) a progressive elaboration of his (and Jankow-ska's) ideas and experimental strategies for unraveling spinal cord circuitry in the adult cat (Baldissera et al., 1981; Burke, 1985; McCrea, 1992, 1998); (2) virtuoso work on the identification and functional morphology of segmental INs in cats (Jankowska, 1992; Jordan, 1998; Matsuyama and Mori, 1998; chapter by Jankowska and Glad-den [13]) and, now, even the firing patterns of INs during the voluntary movement of non-human primates (chapter by Fetz et al. [28]); and (3) the testing of the applicability of Lundberg's (1969) ideas to human spinal cord circuitry (e.g. Katz and Pierrot-Deseilligny, 1999; chapter by Schieppati and Nardonne [43]). The summary message from this intense effort must become more widely promulgated by textbooks: ". . . During . . . move-ments . . . the brain can selectively open appropriate afferent pathways to MNs such that the MN command signals to the active muscles are appropriate for the task at hand." (Stuart and McDonagh, 1997b).

Despite the exceptional progress in this unu-sually demanding field, which is certainly not for the faint-at-heart, a host of problems await the next generation of segmental motor neuroscientists. Subtle, and sometimes-marked differences exist between the spinal circuitry controlling different muscle systems (e.g. limb, respiratory, head-neck; chapter by Richmond et al. [37]). This dictates that students of motor control keep abreast of findings on segmental control circuitry in both invertebrates and vertebrates ('interphyletic awareness'; Stuart, 1985; see also chapter by P. Stein [23]), in order to

recognize when a finding illustrates a species and/ or particular-system specialization versus a conserved mechanism that can be considered to be a principle (e.g. phase–dependent reflex reversal).

Work on spinal connectivity patterns would also be facilitated if we had a better understanding of how sensory afferent input is actually used during movement. For example, evidence across and within invertebrate and vertebrate species, and involving a wide variety of tasks, now suggests several roles for proprioceptive input (Hasan and Stuart, 1988). Three roles arise from the mechanics of the musculoskeletal system and the need to smooth and stabilize internally generated motor programs: (1) linearization (correction for) non-linear muscle properties; (2) compensation for lever-arm variations; and (3) correction of interjoint interaction effects. Three additional roles arise from interactions between the mechanics of the musculoskeletal system and the physical environ-ment; (4) selection of appropriate responses to unexpected perturbations; (5) selection of appro-priate synergies of response; and (6) assistance to external forces for movements requiring maneuver-ability rather than stability. To date, the near-exclusive focus has been on the spinal con-nectivity patterns associated with two (1, 4) of the above six functions. The key problems about the other four areas are both technical and the lack of a sufficiently widespread appreciation for the con-tinual need to strengthen the interface between cellular neurophysiology and biomechanics (Hasan et al., 1985). This situation is now changing rapidly, however (e.g. Nichols, 1994; chapters by Nichols et al. [32], and Hasan and Thomas [33]).

Since the early 1970s, a problem that has often been voiced by the most sympathetic of supporters of those who toil on the segmental motor system, is that the information on connectivity is becoming so detailed and complex that its ultimate meaning is lost. For example, while the monosynaptic spindle Ia excitation of MNs is derived largely from the homonymous muscle and its synergists, the remain-der of the alternative-pathway, oligo- and polysynaptic excitation and inhibition of MNs is derived from afferents supplying virtually the entire limb. How can sense be made of this ever-increasing wealth of spinal circuitry (McCrea,

1992)? In my opinion, the answer to this important problem will require a new generation of inter-disciplinary segmental motor scientists. From the 1950s to the mid–1980s, much accrued from the application to spinal reflexology of the proportional feedback control used in engineering control systems. Now, the focus is shifting to the application of more complex control system theories: finite state (conditional)-, adaptive (self-organizing)- and predictive networks; and, fuzzy logic. In a partic-ularly readable and widely cited review, Prochazka (1996; chapter by Prochazka [11]) has emphasized that all of these control systems are being used in modern prosthetics research. He has proposed that each may play one or more roles, usually in combination with each other, in the control of multi-jointed movement during the elaboration of varied motor tasks. The marriage of these concepts to Lundberg/Jankowska-inspired alternative spinal cord circuitry (e.g. chapter by Jankowska and Gladden [13]) is a daunting but realizable inter-disciplinary challenge for the immediate future.

Interneurons, motoneurons, motor units, and the size principle

INs have been added deliberately to this subdivi-sion because, at the segmental level of CNS motor control mechanisms, their properties have generally received far too little attention (i.e. in contrast to their segmental connectivity patterns; viz., Jankow-ska, 1992; chapter by Jankowska and Gladden [13]). This situation is on the verge of changing, however, because, as reviewed elsewhere (McDo-nagh et al., 1999b) technical advances are now providing the requisite tools (Jordan, 1998; chapter by Fetz et al. [28])

Most of what follows in this section is focussed on mammals. The properties of single INs and MNs in non-mammalian vertebrates and invertebrates have been studied and discussed intensively, espe-cially with regard to the operation of segmental pattern-generating circuits (see below). Such prop-erties have not generally been considered, however, in relation to the graded development of muscle force (cf., however, the lamprey work of Buchanan, 1993, 1996; chapter by Buchanan [27]). This then is both an issue and a possibility that is readily accomplishable with present-day techniques.

The passive and transitional properties of INs and MNs

Passive

These properties refer to those biophysical parame-ters measured when the cell is in its quiescent (not discharging, resting) state, and devoid of most (if not all) synaptic and neuromodulatory influences. These parameters include the resting potential (V_r), input resistance (R_N), and membrane time constant (τ_m). For MNs, a large database now exists on the association between these parameters and the cell's morphological properties, as exemplified in Rall et al. (1992) and Binder et al. (1996). For now, the main issues and possibilities to be tested with existing technology include further: (1) delineation of the relative efficacy of the expanding number of ion-channels contributing to V_r; (2) measurements on (and wider appreciation of) the effect on V_r of the ever-present leak conductance produced by an imperfect seal of the membrane with the IC microelectrode (Binder et al., 1996), particularly those with an impedance < 10 MΩ) consideration of a long-standing issue, the unusually low R_N of very-high-threshold cat MNs (Kernell and Zwaag-stra, 1981), despite which the differences in R_N across the MN pool gives a reasonably accurate indication of the efficacy of synaptic and IC-injected currents at the MN soma, their functional threshold, and their order of recruitment; and (3) quantification in *a representative numbers of neu-rons* of the effect of neuromodulators on all of the above passive properties.

Another key issue that seems now resolvable is that study of the fundamental features of V_r, R_N, and τ_m is still in its infancy for mammalian INs, the problem being even more obvious for repetitive-discharge parameters (see below).

It is important that irrespective of the level at which they undertake their research (i.e. molecular/cellular to animal behavior) our current and future movement-neuroscience trainees understand the *functional significance* of cellular properties within the segmental motor system. For example, in regard to τ_m, it is my experience that trainees learn and retain from their cellular neuroscience courses that due to a larger R_N (attributable more to differences in specific membrane resistance rather than the cells' total surface area), its value is greater in the smaller type S MNs vs. the larger FR/FF MNs of the cat. Few trainees seem to realize, however, that a synaptic potential in a cell with a longer τ_m has a longer time to impress its effect upon that cell, and that this possibility is highly relevant to the functional operation of the size principle. It behooves the training faculty to emphasize routinely the functional significance of their didactic presentations on molecular/cellular properties for the next generation of movement neuroscientists.

Transitional

The transitional state refers to neuron behavior as it converts from the passive (resting) state to the threshold state for initiation of a single AP. Transitional properties include the rheobase current (I_{Rh}), and the spike and afterhyperpolarization (AHP) components to the rheobase action potential (AP). Fundamental parameters associated with the AHP include the amplitude of both its fast (AHP_{amp-f}) and slow (AHP_{amp-s}) component, and its duration which is usually characterized by either $AHP_{duration}$ (time from V_{Rh} to the termination of the AHP) or $AHP_{half-decay\ time}$ (voltage trajectory from the maximum hyperpolarized potential to the membrane potential [V_m] at 1/2 amplitude from V_{Rh} to this negative potential).

The various issues about transitional properties, including their neuromodulation, and the possibilities to resolve them with existing technology have been well covered in several recent reviews (e.g. Binder et al., 1996) and also by one of our own laboratory group (Hornby, 1997). For this reason, it seems sufficient here to point out four areas of potentially fruitful future experimentation.

INs vs. MNs. Again, it must be emphasized that except for the lamprey (Buchanan, 1993), and some of our own recent work on the turtle (McDonagh et al., 1998a, b, 1999a, b) the vertebrate database is far too sparse on the fundamental properties of INs, and their comparison to those of MNs.

I_{Rh}. Rheobase is defined operationally as the current necessary to displace (reduce) the V_r to the firing level (threshold) for initiation of a single AP, as measured with an IC microelectrode passing depolarizing current. Its values exhibit a 10-fold range across MNs within a single cat SC motor nucleus supplying a single muscle (Zengel et al., 1985), thereby indicating its association with R_N, and systematic variation with MN type. A practical issue about which there is doctrinaire thought is that this parameter captures aspects of cell excitability that are in addition to those accommodated in R_N (Fleshman et al., 1981; Binder et al., 1996). Our group has used this argument in the selection of cluster analysis parameters for the provisional classification of MNs, and MNs vs. INs, on the basis of electrophysiology alone (cf. Zengel et al., 1985; McDonagh et al., 1998a). The evidence supporting this generalization is relatively sparse, however. This issue invites rapid resolution with existing techniques.

AP spike. In our group, Hornby (1997) has argued that at the *coarse-grain* level, the ionic mechanisms of AP spike generation for turtle MNs (Hounsgaard et al., 1988b) are sufficiently similar to those reported for lamprey (Buchanan, 1993) and cat MNs (e.g. Schwindt and Crill, 1984) that the participating conductances can be assembled for a generic vertebrate MN (his Fig. 1; i.e. an extension of the generic mammalian MN summary of Binder et al., 1996; their Table 1.1.) Many would argue, however, that insufficient measurements are available on this issue: e.g. compare published records of the MN's AP-spike for lamprey vs. turtle vs. cat; i.e. Fig. 6 in Buchanan (1993) vs. Fig. 2 in McDonagh et al. (1999a) vs. Fig. 1 in Schwindt and Crill (1984). Interestingly, this issue has not been addressed for the well-known cat S vs. FR vs. FF MNs (Burke, 1981), even though the value of such a comparison has been well established for other cell groups (e.g. Koeber et al., 1988). A comparison of AP-spike characteristics across segmental ventral-horn neuron types and vertebrate species would be helpful at this time.

AHP. Mechanisms for a fast (duration, 2–10 ms) and slow (10–1000 ms) component of the AHP have been described in cat MNs (Gustafsson and Pinter, 1985), and also observed in turtle MNs (Hounsgaard et al., 1988b). 'Slow' here refers to a component of the AHP sometimes termed 'medium' by others (e.g. Binder et al., 1996) in order to distinguish it from a *very slow* component. As reviewed by Sah (1996), the AHP has been shown to last several seconds in different neuron types and vertebrate species, including mammals (e.g. hippocampal, olfactory lobe, and neocortical neurons; vagal brainstem MNs; peripheral sensory and autonomic ganglia neurons). Because our and Hounsgaard's laboratory have not observed this very slow component in turtle MNs (Hounsgaard et al., 1988b; McDonagh et al., 1998a), and because it has not been emphasized by Buchanan (1993; his Fig. 6) for lamprey MNs, we have retained use of the term 'slow' (viz. Gustafsson and Pinter, 1985; Kiehn et al., 1997) for the AHP component(s) that blend with the clear-cut fast (2–10 ms) AHP component, and which last for 10–1000 ms thereafter.

There are three major, closely related issues on the AHP at this time: (1) the challenge to the doctrinaire position on a close association between the AHP and firing rate (McDonagh et al., 1999a, b) across cell types and species in anesthetized preparations, with full recognition that the original work on anesthetized cats (Kernell, 1965) provided a new opening in the cellular neuroscience of MNs; (2) general acceptance of the finding that neuromodulation in unanesthetized preparations can profoundly reduce the AHP, to disassociate quite clearly its parameters from the firing rates attained (Brownstone et al., 1992; see also below); and (3) general recognition that INs can exhibit a larger AHP than MNs both at rheobase (Buchanan, 1993; his Fig. 6; McDonagh et al., 1999a; their Fig. 2), and during relatively slow firing rates (McDonagh et al., 1998a; their Fig. 1; see also Hounsgaard and Kjaerulff, 1992), and yet attain much higher firing rates than MNs in response to stronger stimulation.

Clearly, an area of fruitful research for the immediate future in a variety of preparations and vertebrate species concerns the mechanisms underlying the AHP of INs vs. MNs during the progression from rheobase to peak firing rate.

The active properties of INs and MNs

The field of segmental motor neuroscience owes much to Kernell for his over–35-year emphasis on the mechanisms and functional significance of the repetitive firing properties of cat hindlimb MNs (Granit et al. [1963] to chapter by Kernell [2]). These properties are captured by: the stimulus current (I)-spike frequency (f) relationship (Granit et al., 1963), and by spike-frequency adaptation (Kernell and Monster, 1982). Both are subject to substantial neuromodulation by synaptic input from repetitively firing INs and other neuromodulatory sources (Binder et al., 1996). The firing-rate properties of ventral-horn INs, and their behavior during the elaboration of posture and movement, are as central to the operation of the segmental motor system as are the analogous properties and performance of MNs.

Recently, we summarized many of the gaps in our present-day understanding of the firing-rate properties of lamina VII–IX INs vs. those of the MNs they innervate in the lamprey vs. turtle vs. cat. This summary covered information from the behavior of membrane ion channels when the cells are under near-resting (passive) conditions, to the cells' activity level during the elaboration of movement (McDonagh et al., 1999b). We focused on properties associated with the I-f relation, and drew attention to the recent Powers et al. (1999) review wherein the current state-of-the-play on the spike-frequency adaptation of mammalian MNs was elegantly summarized. We did not address the state-dependence (e.g. anesthetized vs. conscious; type of task; phase of movement) of repetitive firing as exemplified in the work of Brownstone et al. (1992), the reviews of Binder et al. (1996) and Hornby (1997), and several reports in Stein et al. (1997) and Kiehn et al. (1998). On the basis of selected reports covered in these various reviews, several issues stand out for general consideration by segmental motor neuroscientists. These are summarized below.

INs vs. MNs: cellular properties

For the comparison of IN vs. MN properties, and particularly the repetitive-firing ones, which are of the most functional importance, information is relatively lacking for the cat vs. non-mammalian species like the lamprey and turtle. For example, since the early 1950's advent of IC recording in the mammalian SC there has been *only one* published measurement on the I-f relation of a γ-MN (Westbury, 1981) and *only one* on a ventral-horn IN, it being a Renshaw cell (Hultborn and Pierrot-Deseilligny, 1979). The reverse situation holds for spike-frequency adaptation, with virtually all of what is known being for the cat or rat rather than non-mammalian species. Again, the focus has been on MNs, with the Powers et al. (1999) recent review emphasizing the multiple mechanisms available to them as their firing rate slows in response to sustained, constant-strength stimulation. The mechanisms he has reviewed are also of direct relevance to non-mammalian MNs and to INs, but very little information is available on them, except for the turtle. In this species, we have recent evidence that the mechanisms of spike-frequency adaptation are both quantitatively and qualitatively different for INs vs. MNs (McDonagh et al., 1999a), a finding that warrants further substantial investigation in the same and other vertebrate species.

For all the vertebrate species, the sample sizes for repetitively firing neurons is still quite small for MNs, let alone INs. For non-mammalian animals, little information is available on the sub-classification of ventral horn INs, the current 'gold standard' being the lamprey results of Buchanan (1993, 1996). Nonetheless, the most severe deficit is information about mammalian ventral-horn INs. This deficiency in the IN literature may soon be overcome, however, because it is now possible to introduce ultra-sharp microelectrodes into small neuronal structures like spinal cord INs (e.g. the thinly myelinated reticulospinal axons of the in vivo mammalian lumbosacral SC (Matsuyama and Mori, 1998; Matsuyama et al., 1999; see also chapter by Kernell [2]). Another possibility is to make use of patch-clamp electrodes, which have recently been applied with much success to mammalian ventral-horn INs in SC slice preparations (e.g. Jonas et al., 1998; Palecek et al., 1999). These studies, however, have focussed their attention on ion-channel mechanisms, rather than the more systems-oriented question of how IN firing rates influence the overall operation of the segmental motor system.

The application of patch-clamp techniques to neonatal rat MNs (Hochman et al., 1994; MacLean et al., 1997, 1998; Hochman and Schmidt, 1998) and mature mouse MNs (Jiang et al., 1999a, b) in SC preparations is proving to be a major advance for the segmental motor neuroscience of the immediate future. With few exceptions (e.g. Araki and DeGroat, 1996; Kiehn et al., 1997), however, when patch-clamp recording has been applied successfully to the SC, it has been restricted to the study of MNs, and, except for Jiang et al. (1999a, b) these have been studied in very young animals (0–14 d-old; e.g. Thurbon et al., 1998). During this developmental period, there is a substantial degree of synaptic and ion-channel remodeling such that extrapolation of patch-clamp data on newborn and neonatal animals to the adult must be approached with caution (Takahashi et al., 1992; Jiang et al., 1999b). By use of infrared differential interference contrast (IR–DIC) technology, it is now possible to identify INs quite accurately (based on their size, position in the targeted lamina, high R_N and low capacitance). Their responses can then be studied to sustained current injection (i.e. as recorded in the current-clamp mode, with the cell held near its V_r; e.g. Edwards et al., 1992; Callister et al., 1999). Furthermore, the morphology of the recorded IN can be assessed by including biocytin in the recording electrode.

The above advances have not yet resulted in neonatal rat or mature mouse studies devoted to the firing-rate properties of spinal INs vs. MNs. A substantial database is emerging, however, on the firing-rate properties of medullary and supramedullary INs implicated in the control of breathing (for review see Rekling and Feldman, 1998). Hopefully, SC workers can now emulate these advances by use of a combined patch-clamp, improved SC-slice viability, and IR-DIC video microscopy approach to advance understanding on the properties of SC INs vs. MNs.

INs vs. MNs: discharge during driven, fictive and near-natural movement

Our recent review of this topic (McDonagh et al., 1999b) was motivated by the hope that published reports on IN vs. MN firing rates during fictive and near-natural movement would give insight into the role played by the AHP in the regulation of firing rate (see above). Both Hounsgaard and Kjaerulff (1992) and our group (McDonagh et al., 1998a, 1999a) have shown that during discharge driven by IC current injection, turtle INs can fire at rates considered high for MNs (>50 Hz) while still generating large-amplitude (>20 mV) AHPs. This finding suggests that the quantitative associations between AHP and firing rate must be substantially different for the two cell types, albeit the INs' higher R_N can contribute to their higher firing-rate values.

The available firing-rate data in studies on fictive and near-natural movement is largely about scratching, stepping, and swimming, movements which are less likely to require the high firing rates which can be presumed to occur during jumping, landing, and rapid defensive withdrawals. Hence, while the available literature provides few examples of IN discharge far in excess of that attained by MNs, this may well occur during ballistic movements. It is likely that a database on this issue is available in the raw records of many laboratories. If there was more focus on the I-f relation of both INs and MNs, and its sub-parameters (e.g. f_{min}, the discharge frequency at the stimulus strength just above that required for repetitive firing; f_{max}, the peak firing rate observed in the I-f relation) during fictive and near-natural movement, then segmental motor neuroscientists could exchange information more systematically.

Associations between MN discharge and force production

Our recent commentary on these associations (McDonagh et al., 1999b) in the turtle vs. cat focussed on the functional significance of f_{min} and f_{max}, as revealed in the activation frequency (same f)- force (F) relation of the innervated muscle or its motor units. A particularly valuable analysis of the associations between the I-f and the f-F relations is that of Heckman and Binder (1991) for a full complement of 'model' MNs comprising the spinal motor nucleus of a cat hindlimb muscle supplying the single motor units of that muscle. Comparisons across vertebrates cannot be made to their analysis, however, because the database is too insufficient on

non-mammalian motor units (see below). For f_{min}, our commentary (see also Binder et al., 1996) emphasized the need for movement neuroscientists to resolve an issue that has arisen in human studies: at f_{min}, do low-threshold (force) motor units generate relatively more of their force than high-threshold (force) units? For f_{max}, our commentary (McDonagh et al., 1999b) emphasized the need for an increased emphasis on the comparative consideration of the association between this parameter, the profile of the I-f relation (e.g. presence of a primary vs. a primary and secondary range of firing) and the profile of the f-F relation. These comparative considerations, too, are restricted severely by the lack of data on the f-F relation of non-mammalian muscle and their motor units.

Neuromodulation, including the ubiquity of plateau potentials and their functional significance

This area has been discussed and reviewed in depth throughout the 1990s (e.g. Kiehn, 1990; Hultborn and Kiehn, 1992; Jordan et al., 1992; Binder et al., 1996; Hornby, 1997; Bennett et al., 1998a, b; Gorassini et al., 1999a, b). It is the dominant theme of two recent symposium volumes (Stein et al., 1997; Kiehn et al., 1998), and it is covered in depth in the present volume (chapters by Heckman and Lee [4], Hultborn [3], Delgado-Lezema and Hounsgaard [5], Selverston [22]). For these reasons, I have directed the following remarks to the wider movement-neuroscience readership with an emphasis on trainees other than those in cellular neuroscience.

Background. The *intrinsic* properties of neurons depend on only those conductances operating when the cells are 'at rest' (i.e. devoid of neuromodulatory and/or synaptic input). In this state, MNs behave essentially passively (i.e. linearly; voltage independent) in response to synaptic input, summing all IC-injected and synaptic currents arithmetically at the trigger zone for the generation of APs (Granit et al., 1966). During the past decade, it has become increasingly apparent that *extrinsically*, several ionic conductances may be modified by different synaptic and neuromodulatory inputs to the MNs and thereby alter the cell's input-output function. Such inputs modify the intrinsic MN properties via metabotropic (G-protein mediated) and ionotropic (ligand-gated ion channel) receptor activation. All movement neuroscientists must recognize that the neuromodulation of suprasegmental INs and segmental INs and MNs is as fundamental to the control of movement as the interplay between central excitation and inhibition, and a key mechanism in task-dependent aspects of the neural control of posture and movement.

Plateau potentials. So-called bistable membrane properties, such as plateau potential (PPs) and rhythmic oscillations (see Wallén and Grillner, 1987; Hornby, 1997; chapter by Grillner and Wallén [26]), provide a means of amplifying and prolonging the effects of excitatory synaptic inputs. At a first approximation, a PP is defined as a sustained (several ms to tens/hundreds of ms) epoch of depolarization in a neuron, due to the voltage-gated activation of a non-inactivating Ca^{2+} conductance. This often occurs in the presence of a monaminergic input to the neuron which causes a decreased K^+ conductance, and hence inability of the neuron to counteract the Ca^{2+} current (Hultborn, 1998; see also Kiehn and Harris-Warrick, 1992). A persistent Na^+ inward current also contributes to this potential in at least the decerebrate cat (Lee and Heckman, 1998c). PPs are ubiquitous in the CNS of invertebrates and vertebrates (Pearson and Ramirez, 1992; Pearson, 1993; Selverston, 1998; chapter by Salverston [22]; Selverston et al., 1998), and have been recorded in as phylogenetically 'new' CNS tissue as slices of rat (Schwindt and Crill, 1999) and even human (Sayer et al., 1993) neocortex.

In invertebrates, PPs were first reported by Russell and Hartline (1978), and in vertebrates, PPs were first recorded IC in cat MNs by Schwindt and Crill (1980) and Hounsgaard et al. (1984). (For an important historical precedent, see Hultborn et al., 1975). Shortly thereafter, they were measured quite precisely in turtle SC slice preparations (Hounsgaard and Kiehn, 1989) subsequent to which there has been an explosion of interest. This is because PPs provide the neuron with a valuable means of increasing its firing rate response to a given increment of depolarizing pressure (Lee and Heck-

man, 1998a). It is well for movement neuroscientists to recognize that in the presence of neuromodulation (as is *inevitable* in voluntary movement), the PP is as fundamental to the operation of a spinal IN or MN as its spike and AHP components. I emphasize this point because even today there is reluctance among selected segmental motor neuroscientists, particularly those working in the field of human motor unit recording, to recognize the ubiquity and functional impact of this evolutionary conserved mechanism.

The term bistable firing was introduced by Hounsgaard et al. (1984, 1988a; see also Conway et al., 1987; Crone et al., 1988) to describe the firing phase in which a MN was exhibiting a PP. The term has confused many because it seems to be a more appropriate term to describe the capacity of the neuron to have two states: i.e. to emit APs either without (conventional firing) or with (PP-firing) plateau potentials. This term should be discarded on etymological grounds alone. Also, it has been shown subsequently that PPs can wax and wane in MNs (Lee and Heckman, 1998a, b), with abrupt changes in state certainly occurring (Eken and Kiehn, 1989; Eken, 1998), but probably as the exception, rather than the rule (Gorassini et al., 1999a, b). Furthermore, it is now known that the PP can appear at very low threshold in both the decerebrate cat (Bennett et al., 1998a) and the conscious human (Kiehn and Eken, 1997; Gorassini et al., 1997, 1998).

The key segmental motor issues concerning the PP for the immediate future include determining: (1) across vertebrate species, the relative contribution to the PP of the non-inactivating Ca^{2+} conductance and a persistent Na^+ inward current (chapters by Heckman and Lee [4], Hultborn [3], Delgado-Lezema and Hounsgaard [5], Selverston [22]); (2) how some INs ($\sim 50\%$) can exhibit PPs in unanesthetized turtle SC slices in the absence of neuromodulation (Hounsgaard and Kjaerulff, 1992; McDonagh et al., 1998a); (3) why, in the presence of neuromodulation, the majority of decerebrate cat MNs do not exhibit full-blown PPs ($\sim 65\%$; largely high threshold; Lee and Heckman, 1998a, b; chapter by Heckman and Lee [4]), and why many turtle SC MNs produce no PP ($\sim 36\%$; not necessarily high-threshold; Hornby et al., 1998); (4) the boundary conditions (in a task sense) for PP firing at low and progressively higher voltage-gated thresholds in SC slices, in vivo cat preparations, and the conscious human; and (5) how to reach consensus among human motor unit researchers about when they are recording motor-unit firing patterns indicative of PP discharge in MNs (cf. Bennett et al., 1998b; Gorassini et al., 1998, 1999a; chapter by Hultborn [3]). Clearly, the PP is an exciting new addition to the 1990s' scene in segmental motor neuroscience!

The I-f relation and a challenge to doctrinaire thought. Many synaptic and neuromodulatory influences, can shift the I-f relation by altering a variety of intrinsic sub- and suprathreshold conductances of MNs (Binder et al., 1993, 1996; Hornby, 1997). Similarly, endogenous neuromodulators have been shown to induce PPs in vertebrate MNs (Hornby, 1997). Presumably, both occur during natural movements. The only full-length report, however, on modulation of the I-f relation during a dynamic motor pattern, is the work of Brownstone et al. (1992). During the controlled (using brainstem stimulation) fictive locomotion of the high decerebrate cat (for background, see Stuart and McDonagh, 1998) Brownstone et al. (1992) made several observations that challenged doctrinaire thought (for detailed review: Brownstone, 1989; Hornby, 1997). For example, they reported that the IC injection of depolarizing current to the test hindlimb MNs during the active phase of their locomotor cycle did not alter the I-f relation in the conventionally predicted way: i.e. there was no further increase in spike-frequency with increasing stimulus strength. This and some other findings led Brownstone et al. (1992) to propose that during fictive locomotion, repetitive firing is not regulated by a linear summation of synaptic input at the trigger zone. Among the alternative mechanisms they proposed, hindsight shows that the most promising one was neuromodulation of the intrinsic conductances responsible for the AHP and the manifestation of PPs.

Hornby (1997) has emphasized that a finding that is consistent with a component of the 1992 Brownstone work has been reported by Schmidt (1994) in his study on NMDA-induced fictive

locomotion in the in vitro neonatal rat. He found that the duration of the AHP of MNs was reduced, but he did not comment on this change's effect on spike-frequency. Conversely, in the same preparation, there is recent claim (Edwards et al., 1997) that during 5-HT/NMDA-induced fictive locomotion, AHP changes were equivocal, whereas MN f/I slopes were always reduced by '. . . about 50%, but were always significantly greater than zero . . .': i.e. never to the extent observed in the Brownstone et al. 1992 report.

Clearly, the modulation of the I-f relation during locomotor-like patterns needs further examination due to the relatively small sample size of the important (albeit controversial) and not sufficiently cited Brownstone et al. (1992) report on decerebrate cat preparations, and the potential discrepancies in neonatal rat preparations between the results of Schmidt (1994) and Edwards et al. (1997). Furthermore, it has become increasingly clear that quantification of modulator-induced effects on the I-f relation is tightly linked to consideration of whether such modulation is accompanied by the generation of PPs. In my opinion, work on these topics will be to the forefront of segmental motor neuroscience for several years to come, and it is to the credit of Brownstone et al. (1992; Brownstone, 1989) that they provided this new opening.

Input-output relations of MNs

Building on the pre-WW II Sherringtonian era captured in Creed et al. (1932; see also Stuart et al., 1999) and its post WWII extension by Lloyd (Patton, 1994), it has obviously been of great importance to quantify how synaptic inputs control MN discharge. When I entered neuroscience in the mid–1950s, there was great excitement about the advances made with the then-newly introduced IC recording electrode. At that time, passive EPSP and IPSPs were being recorded in MNs by Eccles' group in Canberra, Australia (summarized in Andersen and Lundberg, 1997). Now, over 40 years later, segmental motor neuroscientists are studying the passive *and active* (firing-rate) responses of MNs to precisely controlled inputs from single sensory and central axons, and describing their

14

results with functionally realistic models. The latter development owes much to the contributions of Rall and his NIH collaborators, including, in particular, Frank and Burke. For example, trainees should consider the historical impact of the following sequence of five consecutive reports that were seminal in this field: Smith et al. (1967); Nelson and Frank (1967); Burke (1967); Rall (1967); Rall et al. (1967); see also Rall (1992); Rall et al. (1992).

The above advances, current issues and possibilities have been reviewed recently in depth by Binder et al. (1996), and are covered broadly in this volume (chapters by Kirkwood et al. [6], Powers and Binder [7], Rose and Cushing [8]). This has freed me to limit my introduction to this field to some historical and trainee-mentoring comments on two technical developments that have advanced this area, spike-triggered averaging and the functional voltage clamp.

Spike-triggered averaging

This technique is a form of cross-correlation in which the single impulses of a single neuron are used as the trigger signal to an electronic averaging device whose input is the synaptic noise of another single neuron. It was first used in neuroscience by Henneman and Mendell (1968), and it enabled them to provide the first-ever measurements of MN EPSPs attributable to the impulses of single Ia axons. The term (abbreviation, STA), itself, was coined in my laboratory by Anthony Taylor (London, UK) in 1974. Subsequent to Henneman and Mendell (1968), STA was used by: (1) Kirkwood and Sears (1974) for the de novo demonstration (to my group's good-natured chagrin) of similar monosynaptic EPSPs attributable to spindle group II axons (a controversial issue in the mid–1970s; see Binder et al., 1982); (2) our own group (Watt et al., 1976; Stauffer et al., 1976) to describe Ia and spII monosynaptic and oligosynaptic EPSPs and IPSPs, and a probabilistic average indicative of di- and oligosynaptic Ib EPSPs and IPSPs, including in all cases particularly small responses (e.g. <5 μV EPSPs vs. the then-accepted 17 μV ones), all being also controversial findings at that time; and (3) Fetz and Finocchio (1975) and, more precisely, Fetz et al. (1976) to most imaginatively describe the di- and oligosynaptic pathway from the actively discharging motor-cortical neurons of the conscious non-human primate to active forelimb muscle fibers during the elaboration of an operantly controlled movement. STA was also used in the early 1970s (Stein et al., 1972) to determine the twitch force of single motor units during low-force voluntary muscle contractions by humans (for the early history of STA, see Fetz et al, 1979). The above findings have all been confirmed many times, but at the time, our own work was treated with skepticism because it challenged doctrinaire thought. The faculty of training programs must discuss this issue with their trainees. Over the years, I have found it important to provide moral support to emerging scientists who have been ill-prepared for the rough and tumble of scientific dispute. This has been the case even when there is no malicious (albeit sometimes pretentious) intent, let alone when a publication or an extramural grant is imperiled on territorial grounds. An ability to stand up for one's clearly presented ideas, a dual sense of humor and irony (the latter good advice to me personally from Daniel Kernell, Groningen, The Netherlands), self-esteem, a relish for the field of open scientific combat (with dignity and politeness), and an ability to be gracious in, and learn and move on from defeat (viz. Eccles, 1977), are all important, and all must be incorporated into the training of future generations of movement neuroscientists.

Functional voltage clamp

Heckman and Binder (1988) introduced this powerful analytical technique to segmental motor neuroscience after 'surviving' some of the problems outlined above. It provides the means to ". . . measure the total amount of current from a synaptic input system that reaches the soma of a MN under steady-state conditions . . ." (p. 1946). The technique involves IC recording in the current-clamp mode and balancing the voltage displacement due to a synaptic input by the intracellular injection of current (I_N) which returns V_M to its control value. They have termed I_N the *effective* synaptic current because ". . . only that fraction of the current that actually reaches the soma and initial segment of the cell affects its recruitment threshold and firing frequency . . ." (p. 1946). In my opinion, this technique has provided a new opening for quantifying the input-output relations of MNs because its use has resulted in the most unequivocal measurements yet achieved for synaptic currents generated in MNs by sensory feedback and descending synaptic inputs. Subsequent to its initial use (Heckman and Binder, 1988) and subsequent refinement (Lindsay and Binder, 1991) for the measurement of subthreshold (passive) MN responses, the technique was extended by Binder and Powers, and their collaborators, to the study of the synaptic currents driving repetitive (active) MN discharge (Powers et al., 1992; for further developments, see Binder et al., 1996).

The training-program relevancy of the above development is that it was first conceptualized by a Ph.D. trainee, Heckman, who had been initially exposed to movement neuroscience in a particularly successful (but now unhappily defunct) kinesiology program at the University of Washington, wherein Heckman had gained segmental motor experience (Heckman et al., 1984; Hayward et al., 1986) under the 1980–83 mentoring by the late Robert Hutton (1939–91; Berryman, 1992). For an assignment as a first-year Ph.D. student in the department of physiology and biophysics at the same institution, he drew on both his previous kinesiology research experiences and advanced graduate physiology course work to conceptualize the above method (not knowing then that its theoretical, but not experimental, basis was already available; Redman, 1976). According to Heckman, his mentor, Binder, ". . . immediately appreciated the significance of this idea even though my explanation and understanding at that time were less than clear. He had me write a second paper the following summer (1983) to refine the proposed protocols further and we began experiments in the Fall . . ." (personal communication to author from Heckman, 06/25/99). In my opinion, this story illustrates the soundness of the American Ph.D. training system for movement neuroscience, which focuses on drawing its students from as broad a set of backgrounds as possible (e.g. applied mathematics, engineering, exercise science/kinesiology,

physical therapy, physics, psychology, and speech science, in addition to the traditional life sciences and medicine) and providing them with advanced graduate courses, the latter usually emphasizing much give-and-take between professor and trainee. The story also speaks to the essential soundness and value of ". . . putting students and their needs first . . ." (Kennedy, 1997; p. 287). At my own institution, the philosophy is that the program has failed if it does not produce completed trainees with more current research potential than their faculty, just as the institution has failed if it does not recruit more talented assistant professors than professors. Otherwise, how can the wheel of science keep rolling forward?

Properties of motor units

A 'motor unit' is now defined as a full MN (i.e. its cell body, dendrites, and axon) and all of the muscle fibers it supplies (Burke, 1981; chapter by R. Burke [15]). The term was coined by Liddell and Sherrington (1924), who limited it to a MN's axon and the muscle fibers innervated by that axon. The concept was established by several others somewhat earlier, however (see, for example, Lucas, 1905, 1909; Mines, 1913; Lewis, 1984).

Segmental motor neuroscience was advanced considerably by the 1960s–1980s contributions of Burke and his collaborators to the study of the combined morphological, histochemical and physiological properties of mammalian motor units and their interrelationships, including the associations between the neural and muscular portions of the unit. This body of work was assembled with widespread impact in the masterful Burke (1981) review that also addressed the far more limited information available on the motor units of non-mammalian vertebrates, and even lesser information on those of invertebrates. It is not an overstatement to emphasize that Burke's 1981 review will serve to guide work for the foreseeable future on the motor units of invertebrates and non-mammalian vertebrates, and further work on particularly the adaptive properties of mammalian motor units. As such, Burke's work has been a major 20th century contribution to segmental motor neuroscience.

16

The main post WWII 'coarse-grain' advance has been the emphasis on the evolutionary conservation from at least crabs (Rathmayer and Maier, 1987) to the human (Stuart et al., 1984) of three distinct 'types' of muscle fiber and motor unit (one slow-twitch; two fast-twitch), with a fourth type intermediate between the two fast twitch ones often emphasized, the extent of its presence being possibly dependent on the demands of usage. A fifth non-twitch type is also prevalent in invertebrates and non-mammalian vertebrates. The main feature of the above arrangement is that both within and across species, the values of single neural and muscular properties (histochemical, morphological, physiological, and now biochemical; e.g. Nemeth et al., 1986) tend to be distributed in a continuum, but when considered in concert, the types usually become evident. None of the above implies that the single muscles of single species do not have *their own specialization* (e.g. swim bladder muscle of toadfish and shaker muscle of rattlesnake tail; Rome et al., 1996; ankle extensors of the skunk, Van de Graaff et al., 1977; hand muscles of human, Bigland-Ritchie et al., 1998; see also chapters by Callister et al. [21], Goldberg and Shall [20], Richmond et al. [37]). Rather, the great value of the coarse-grain typing terminology is that it has *immediate functional relevance* (e.g. Walmsley et al., 1978; Rome et al., 1988) and it has provided a means of *interdisciplinary communication* (Botterman et al., 1978; McDonagh et al., 1980; chapters by Callister et al. [21], Gordon et al. [17]) that has promoted a collective worldwide interest in motor unit neurobiology.

At even the coarse-grain level, much remains to be learned about the classification and properties of motor units, including (among many others): (1) the characterization and typing of non-twitch non-mammalian units; (2) the relative extent and prevalence of unitary- vs. polyneuronal innervation among non-mammalian motor units, unitary- vs. multiterminal innervation of non-mammalian single muscle fibers, and two types of slow-twitch motor units in both mammalian and non-mammalian species; (3) the developmental mechanisms that dictate a muscle's fiber-type and motor unit composition; (4) resolution of conflicting information on the specific tension of slow-twitch vs. fast-twitch mammalian and non-mammalian units; (5) the comparative and adaptive neurobiology of all of the above; and (6) improved technology to measure the force output of human motor units during voluntary contractions. For references on the above, the movement-neuroscience trainee is referred to Edgerton et al. (1996), and the texts of McComas (1977, 1996) which have set a gold standard in motor control training programs for over two decades.

Size principle

> The amount of excitatory input required to discharge a motoneuron, the energy it transmits as impulses, the number of (muscle) fibers it supplies, the contractile properties of the motor unit it innervates, its main rate of firing and even its rate of protein synthesis are all closely correlated with its size. This set of experimental facts and interrelationships has been called the 'size principle.' (Henneman, 1977; p. 50).

The above topic received little but masterful attention at the 1998 symposium that preceded this volume (see below) which is surprising in retrospect, particularly since Tucson and the University of Arizona were the site of a major conference on the topic only a single decade ago (Binder and Mendell, 1990). Recently, there was an exchange of letters in a major journal on some historical aspects of the size principle (Vilensky and Gilman, 1998; Binder, 1998; Fuglevand, 1998). This exchange requires clarification regarding the relation between fixed and orderly motor unit recruitment, EMG interpretation, and the size principle. This is important because it behooves motor control training programs to emphasize to future generations of segmental motor scientists the significance of the effort that went into the elaboration and world-wide testing of this principle from the late 1950s to the present.

In a recent article on the contributions to movement neuroscience of Sir Charles Sherrington (1857–1952; Stuart et al., 1999), our group emphasized his group's pre-WWII contributions to the understanding of the spinal mechanisms involved in the progressive reflex recruitment of MNs to produce a graded development of muscle force, as discussed in their summing-up, the rightly acclaimed text (Creed et al.,1932). In that book, there is no mention of *fixed* motor unit recruitment. This refers to an invariant order of unit recruitment during voluntary and reflex contractions. It is customary to attribute the initial reports on fixed recruitment to Smith (1934) and Lindsley (1935), but there may have been earlier reports (see below).

In 1938, Denny-Brown (1901–81) and Pennybacker reported an *orderly* (small-before-large) motor unit recruitment pattern, there being no further such reports in the 1930s (see Seyffarth, 1940). In their 1938 report Denny-Brown and Pennybacker (1938) cited Liddell and Sherrington (1923) and Sherrington (1929) for their earlier work on fixed recruitment. Surprisingly, this was an error. Neither paper mentioned fixed recruitment order! Subsequently, post-WWII, Denny-Brown *focussed solely on fixed recruitment* in his classical 1949 review on the electromyogram (EMG), and cited the pre-WWII reports of Smith (1934) and Lindsley (1935) on fixed recruitment, with the additional comment that 'others' had observed such recruitment pre-WWII. In my opinion, Denny-Brown was too precise a man and too committed a scientist (Vilensky et al., 1998) to have forgotten about the orderly recruitment observations he reported in 1938 with Pennybacker. Rather, it seems far more likely that with the improvement in EMG technology that followed WWII, he was less certain by 1949 of the validity of the orderly recruitment he had reported in his 1938 paper with Pennybacker. In addition, he may have become concerned about the brief and equivocal nature of his and Pennybacker's (1938) results on orderly recruitment, albeit their historical interest (Stuart and Enoka, 1990), and technical limitations in EMG interpretation at that time. These points deserve emphasis in motor control training programs because it is important that current and future segmental motor scientists appreciate both the technical as well as the academic history of their field (Stuart, 1998).

It remained for Henneman (1915–1996) to firmly establish orderly recruitment using the less-equivocal method of ventral-root-filament recording,

and, *far more importantly*, to add to it his size principle (1957) as an explanation of the underlying mechanisms. Our group and others have provided previous accolades to Henneman for his remarkable size principle contribution (Henneman and Mendell, 1981) to the field of neuroscience and emphasized that a substantial number of issues and possibilities remain for its further refinement (Stuart and Enoka, 1983, 1990; Enoka and Stuart, 1984; Gustaffson and Pinter, 1985; Binder and Mendell, 1990; Young, 1997; see also chapters by Bawa and Jones [19], Carrasco and English [35], Cope and Sokoloff [16], Enoka et al. [34]).

Segmental pattern generation

In my opinion, this area has been the most exciting of the segmental motor areas to follow and participate in these past 40 years because, in contrast to the above two areas, segmental pattern generation has featured since the early 1960s "... the progressive merger of concepts about motor control science, derived from work on both vertebrates and invertebrates ... (*including*) ... an evolutionary conservation of motor control mechanisms that extend from the molecular/cellular level of analysis to the behavioral level of investigation. (Pearson, 1993; Stuart and Callister, 1993)." (Stuart and McDonagh, 1998; p. 22). Such 'interphyletic awareness' (Stuart, 1985; see also Fetcho, 1992; Szekely, 1989; chapter by P. Stein [23]) is also a feature of movement neuroscience in the area of visually guided head-neck movements (Strausfeld, 1997), and olfactory neurobiology (Hildebrand and Shepherd, 1997). Its adoption in other areas of neuroscience is becoming progressively evident (e.g. Ulinsky, 1997).

To introduce the field of segmental pattern generation and the central pattern generator (CPG) for various forms of rhythmic movement, we have recently emphasized (Stuart et al., 1999) that it is helpful to begin with a quote from the preface to a recent volume (Stein et al., 1997), which followed a 1995 symposium (Stein et al., 1995): "... understanding the control of movement requires a multilevel approach ... (*emphasizing*) ... the importance of synthesis and analysis. Reductionist analysis reveals properties of components of the system: specific motor patterns generated by networks, neurons, and neuromolecules (channels, receptors, transmitters, and modulators). Synthesis uses a systems approach regarding the levels of networks and behavior: motor patterns generate movements that are modulated by movement-related sensory feedback. Such a multilevel approach has been reported elsewhere: Bunge (1989) stressed the importance of multilevel approaches in neuroscience; Stein (1995) applied Bunge's perspectives to the neural control of movement; and Getting (1989) emphasized the utilization of reductionist results in the construction of synthetic mathematical models of neuronal networks that generate motor patterns . . . Prior to the 1975 conference (Valley Forge, PA), researchers of vertebrate systems tended to view only vertebrate research as relevant, whereas researchers of invertebrate systems tended to focus only on invertebrate research. The 1975 symposium and its accompanying 1976 volume (i.e. Herman et. al., 1976) revealed common neuron, network, and behavior organizational principles for both vertebrates and invertebrates. That discovery led to a change in the way many investigators and university training programs approached the neural control of movement. The 1985 conference (Stockholm, Sweden) and its 1986 volume (Grillner et al., 1986) offered further support for the view that the nervous system of lower vertebrates share important common features with the nervous system of mammals. Incorporating these previous insights, the 1995 conference (Stein et al., 1995) and its subsequent volume (Stein et al., 1997) add the emerging concept of the current decade: "the modulatory abilities of the neurons that make up a neuronal network confer abilities onto the modulated network that allow it to generate an array of motor patterns responsible for a set of motor behaviors . . ." (paragraphs 3–5 of preface).

The above quotation (see also chapter by P. Stein [23]) captures the excitement of work from the early 1960s onwards, that has shown that for a wide variety of invertebrate and vertebrate species, including the human (Gurfinkel et al., 1998, 1999), IN networks in the brainstem and spinal cord of vertebrates (and their analogues in invertebrates) have the intrinsic capacity (i.e. not dependent upon descending command and sensory feedback signals) to generate rhythmical activation of MNs such as to produce rhythmical movements like chewing, licking, scratching, and locomotion (Arbas et al., 1997; Stein et al., 1997; Kiehn et al., 1998).

Recently, my current colleagues and I have reviewed some of the most significant of the recent advances on spinal pattern generation (Stuart and McDonagh, 1998; Stuart et al., 1999; McDonagh et al., 1999b). They are particularly well covered in the above-cited references and in this volume (Sects. V-VI, and chapters by Hasan and Thomas [33], Nichols et al. [32], R. Stein et al. [41] Schieppati and Nardone [43]). Here, it seems sufficient and important to consider, as *an under-discussed key current issue*, the need for undergraduate and graduate trainees in both all-round and movement neuroscience, to receive a more functional, realistic and up-to-date introduction to segmental motor systems than is currently provided in most textbooks and training programs.

Typically, the current trainee (particularly in mammalian-oriented programs) receives excellent material on the molecular/cellular properties of nerve cells before being introduced to CNS mechanisms, with the latter usually beginning with spinal reflex mechanisms. Usually, trainees consider the latter topic dull and 'old-fashioned'. Certainly, the rote memorization of the alleged hard-wired connections of, for example, the sensory input of spindle Ia, spindle group II, and Golgi tendon organ input, as based on over–40-year-old work on the anesthetized cat is hardly the way to excite such a trainee about the richness and significance of the field of segmental motor neuroscience! Rather, such excitement is readily captured when the initial exposure to CNS mechanisms is to the *genesis of spontaneous rhythmic motor activity*. One such approach was introduced by Getting (1986, 1989). He proposed that trainees learn that the specific circuitry (overall network) required for a given movement (e.g. locomotion) does not appear to have been conserved throughout evolution. Rather the building blocks of their circuits have been conserved, as can be documented didactically in *separate* tables of molecular/cellular, synaptic interaction, and connectivity properties (e.g. plateau potentials, muticomponent synapses, reciprocal inhibition, respectively). The trainee can then learn that each animal species selects properties from each of these tables to 'build' a segmental pattern generator for a particular movement (e.g. locomotion vs. swimming), with the selection process accommodating the *biomechanical properties* of the species under consideration. Depending on the trainee's particular level (in my experience, the above ideas are appropriate for, and well-received by even first-year undergraduates), this introduction to the CNS can include mention of the theory that CNS ganglia (invertebrates) and the brainstem and spinal cord (vertebrates) may indeed contain multiple building blocks, and combine them in different ways to produce CPGs for various movements (e.g. running vs. swimming). Alternatively, or even in parallel, the lower levels of the CNS may contain a 'master' CPG whose subcomponents are weighted in various ways to produce a diversity of rhythmical movements. For more advanced trainees, the fourth building block, neuromodulation (Calabrese, 1998), must also be added, of course.

Once the above concept and an appropriate number of examples of building blocks have been presented, the trainee can then move on to consider the nature of segmental reflex pathways used in the control of movement, with an emphasis on the *concepts* of segmental IN convergence, alternative pathways, and phase-dependent reflex reversal. With the dual concepts of segmental pattern generation and task-dependent segmental reflexes well in hand, the trainee is then ready to move on to the suprasegmental mechanisms involved in the automatic and voluntary control of posture and movement (e.g. chapters by Beer et al. [42], Conway et al. [40], Ellaway et al. [44], Nordstrom et al. [18]).

For the foreseeable future, there are endless advances to be made in our understanding of segmental pattern generation, its suprasegmental command and modulating signals, and the boundary conditions of its modulation by sensory feedback. At the suprasegmental command- and modulation level, new ideas are being formulated, and/or experiments are underway on the: (1) interface between the automatic control of locomotion, and the voluntary control of multi-jointed limb movements (Grillner et al., 1997); (2) the 'readiness' (viz., Bernstein, 1940: Gurfinkel et al., 1999) of reticulospinal axons to convert to signaling motor commands for posture and locomotion (e.g. Selioniv and Shik, 1992; chapter by Bar-Gad et al. [25]); (3) the individuality of the fine architecture of single descending tract axons and the innervation fields of their collaterals' terminations along the length of the spinal neuroaxis (Kuze et al., 1999; Matsuyama et al., 1999); and (4) the dual control of posture and movement (Massion, 1992; Gurfinkel et al., 1999), including, after a several-year hiatus, the ubiquitous but still puzzling precise role of the cerebellum (Mori et al., 1999a, b).

Four aspects of segmental pattern generation seem particularly promising for investigation in the immediate future. Two were mentioned above: how different species select different combinations of cellular, synaptic, and network building blocks to achieve a CPG that accommodates the individual species' biomechanical properties (viz., Full, 1997); and resolving the issue of whether there is a master multiganglionic (invertebrates) or brainstem-spinal cord (vertebrates) CPG for the genesis of rhythmic movements, subcomponents of which are used for separate types of movement, or whether clearly different movements make use of clearly separate CPGs (for review: Dickinson, 1995; Simmers et al., 1995; Calabrese, 1998). A third issue is the task-dependency of CPG operation: i.e. the extent to which a subtle change in the pattern of a rhythmical task requires a modification in the CPG circuitry for the main overall features of the task (Stein and Smith, 1997). Finally, determining the full composition of ganglionic and spinal CPGs for invertebrate and vertebrate locomotion is still as lively and thought-provoking an issue (Pearson and Ramirez, 1997) as it was when raised over 30 years ago by Shik et al. (1966; see also Orlovsky and Shik, 1976).

Clearly, the current and next generation of systems neurobiologists with interdisciplinary expertise in cellular neurophysiology, the biomechanical analysis of movement (Sect. VII), modern morphology/immunohistochemistry, and modeling and simulation have the tools and a wealth of experimental possibilities to continue advancing our understanding of segmental pattern generation and its descending and feedback control, together with the former two areas covered in this article. The giants whose shoulders we students of movement neuroscience currently stand upon, Sir Charles Sherrington (Liddell, 1952; Stuart et al., 1999), Nicolai Bernstein (Latash and Turvey, 1996; Latash, 1998,) and Walter Hess (Wiesendanger, 1997; Stuart, 1998), would be well pleased with this volume and its preceding conference!

Concluding personal remarks

In all ways, it has been a privilege to work in this field these past forty years, and to have experienced: the friendships formed during all-night experiments on in vivo cat preparations in the Sherrington/Eccles-Granit-Lloyd/Lundberg tradition; the cut and thrust, yet camaraderie, of international meetings; the refreshingly unpretentious, informal-yet-rigorous presentations of invertebrate neuroscientists; the collegiality and power of 'interphyletic awareness'; the motivation of applied mathematicians, bioengineers and roboticists; and, the dedication of academic clinicians. Above all, however, has been the satisfaction of helping nurture the ever-continuing emergence of so many talented young interdisciplinary experimentalists and theoreticians. They are moving segmental motor neuroscience forward to a new level of understanding, which, in time, will attain a 'simplicity,' the acquisition of which is an aspiration they share with their mentors, and with generations of previous mentors.

Acknowledgments

I would like to thank the groups that organized and sponsored the November 4–6, 1998, International Conference, *Peripheral and Spinal Mechanisms in the Neural Control of Movement*, The University of Arizona (UA), Tucson, AZ, that preceded this volume. The organizers included: Conference Chair, Dr. Marc Binder; Primary Local Organizer, Dr. Jennifer McDonagh; Print Version of Proceedings, Patricia Pierce; Sponsor Communication, Dr. Mary Williams; Registrar, Lura Hannekamp; Assistant Registrar, Charlotte Garcia; and, Web Site, Robert Reinking. The sponsors included the Muscular Dystrophy Association, and several units of The University of Arizona: the Office of the Vice-President (VP) for Research (VP, Dr. Michael Cusanovich); the Graduate College (Dean, Dr. Thomas Hixon); the College of Medicine (Dean, Dr. James Dalen); the College of Engineering (Dean, Dr. Thomas Peterson); and the Department of Physiology (Chair, Dr. William Dantzler). I would also like to thank Dr. Paul Stein for his input (also supplied many times in the past), and my current collaborators (Drs. Alan Brichta, Robert Callister, George Hornby, Jennifer McDonagh, Patricia Pierce and Robert Reinking) and Drs. Roger Enoka and Ziaul Hasan for reading a draft of this article. The latter two are former UA collaborators who were founding members of the interdisciplinary UA Motor Control Group, together with Drs. Terry Bahill, Thomas Hixon, and Robert Lansing, and three colleagues with a primary appointment at the Barrow Neurological Institute, Phoenix, AZ: Drs. James Bloedel, Alan Gibson, and Thomas Hamm. Preparation of this article was supported, in part, by: USPHS grants NS 20577 and NS 07309, a University of Newcastle (Australia) Visiting Faculty Award (to D.G.S. and Dr. Robert Callister) and, a Visiting Scientist Award from the Okazaki (Japan) National Research Institutes (to D.G.S.; National Institute for Physiological Sciences; host, Prof. Shigemi Mori). The paper's contents are solely the responsibility of the author and do not necessarily represent the views of the awarding agencies.

References

Andersen, P. and Lundberg, A. (1997) John C. Eccles (1903–1997) *Trends Neurosci.*, 20: 324–325.

Araki, I. and De Groat, W.C. (1996) Unitary excitatory synaptic currents in preganglionic neurons mediated by two distinct groups of interneurons in neonatal rat sacral parasympathetic nucleus. *J. Neurophysiol.*, 76: 215–226.

Arbas, E.A., Levine, R.B. and Strausfeld, N.J. (1997) Invertebrate nervous systems. In: W.H. Dantzler (Ed.), *Comparative*

Physiology, Sec. 13, Vol. II, New York: Oxford University Press, pp. 751–852.

Baldissera, F., Hultborn, H. and Ilert, M. (1981) Integration in spinal neuronal systems. In: J.M. Brookhart and V.B. Mountcastle (Eds), *Handbook of Physiology*, Sec. 1, Vol. II, pt 1., *The Nervous System: Motor Control*, Bethesda (MD): American Physiological Society, pp. 509–595.

Barker, D. (Ed.) (1962) *Symposium on Muscle Receptors*, Hong Kong: Hong Kong University Press.

Bennett, D.J., Hultborn, H., Fedirchuk, B. and Gorassini, M. (1998a) Synaptic activation of plateau potentials in hindlimb motoneurons of decerebrate cats. *J. Neurophysiol.*, 80: 2023–2037.

Bennett, D.J., Hultborn, H., Fedirchuk, B. and Gorassini, M. (1998b) Short-term plasticity in hindlimb motoneurons of decerebrate cats. *J. Neurophysiol.*, 80: 2038–2045.

Bernstein, N.A. (1940) Studies of the Biodynamics of Walking, Running and Jumping, Research of the Central Scientific Institute of Physical Culture, Moscow, USSR (In Russian). English translation: H.T.A. Whiting (Ed.), (1984) *Human Motor Actions. Bernstein Reassessed*, Amsterdam: North-Holland, pp. 171–222.

Berryman, J.W. (1992) Robert Stanley Hutton, Sr. *Am. Assoc. Physic. Ed. News*, 13: 11–12.

Bigland-Ritchie, B., Fugelvand, A.J. and Thomas, C.K. (1998) Contractile properties of human motor units: is man a cat? *Neuroscientist*, 4: 240–249.

Binder, M.D. (1998) Henneman's size principle: the right name. Science, 281: 919.

Binder, M.D., Heckman, C.J. and Powers, R.K. (1993) How different afferent inputs control motoneuron discharge and the output of the motoneuron pool. *Curr. Opin. Neurobiol.*, 3: 1028–1034.

Binder, M.D., Heckman, C.J. and Powers, R.K. (1996) The physiological control of motoneuron activity. In: L.B. Rowell and J.T. Shepherd (Eds), *Handbook of Physiology*, Sec. 12, *Exercise: Regulation and Integration of Multiple Systems*, New York: Oxford University Press, pp. 3–53.

Binder, M.D., Houk, J.C., Nichols, T.R., Rymer, W.Z. and Stuart, D.G. (1982). Properties and segmental actions of mammalian muscle receptors: an update. *Fed. Proc.*, 41: 2907–2918.

Binder, M.D., McDonagh, J.C., Reinking, R.M. and Pierce, P.A. (Eds) (1998) Peripheral and spinal mechanisms in the neural control of movement, Proceedings of an international symposium, Tucson, AZ, Nov. 4–6, 1998, Tucson, The University of Arizona. See also http://server.physiol.arizona.edu/SFNTC/Conference/NCM/

Binder, M.D. and Mendell, L.M. (1990) *The Segmental Motor System*, New York: Oxford University Press.

Blackshaw, S.E. (1993) Stretch receptors and body wall muscle in leeches. *Comp. Biochem. Physiol. Comp. Physiol.*, 105: 634–652.

Botterman, B.R., Binder, M.D. and Stuart, D.G. (1978) Functional anatomy of the association between motor units and muscle receptors. *Am. Zool.*, 18: 135–152.

Brownstone, R.M. (1989) On the regulation of repetitive firing in lumbar motoneurones during fictive locomotion in the cat. Ph.D. Thesis, Winnipeg: University of Manitoba.

Brownstone, R.M., Jordan, L.M., Kriellaars, D.J., Noga, B.R. and Shefchyk, S.J. (1992) On the regulation of repetitive firing in lumbar motoneurones during fictive locomotion in the cat. *Exp. Brain. Res.*, 90: 441–455.

Buchanan, J.T. (1993) Electrophysiological properties of identified classes of lamprey spinal neurons. *J. Neurophysiol.*, 70: 2313–2325.

Buchanan, J.T. (1996) Lamprey spinal interneurons and their roles in swimming activity. *Brain Behav. Evol.*, 48: 287–296.

Bunge, M. (1989) From neuron to mind. *News Physiol. Sci.*, 4: 206–209.

Burke, R.E. (1967) Composite nature of the monosynaptic excitatory potential. *J. Neurophysiol.*, 30: 1114–1137.

Burke, R.E. (1981) Motor units: anatomy, physiology and functional organization. In: J.M. Brookhart and V.B. Mountcastle (Eds), *Handbook of Physiology*, Sec. 1, Vol. II, pt 1., *The Nervous System: Motor Control*, Bethesda (MD): American Physiological Society, pp. 345–422.

Burke, R.E. (1985) Integration of sensory information and motor commands in the spinal cord. In: P.S.G. Stein (Ed.), *Motor Control: From Movement Trajectories to Neural Mechanisms. Short Course Syllabus*, Bethesda, MD: Society for Neuroscience, pp. 44–66.

Calabrese, R.L. (1998) Cellular, synaptic, network, and modulatory mechanisms involved in rhythm generation. *Curr. Opin. Neurobiol.*, 8: 710–717.

Callister, R.J., Laidlaw, D.H. and Stuart, D.G. (1995) A commentary on the segmental motor system of the turtle: implications for the study of its cellular mechanisms and interactions. *J. Morphol.*, 225: 213–227.

Callister, R.J., Schofield, P.R. and Sah, P. (1999) The use of murine mutants to study glycine receptor function. *Clin. Exp. Pharmacol. Physiol.*, 26: 929–931.

Clarac, F. (1982) Proprioceptive functions of invertebrates. *J. Physiol. (Paris)*, 78: 665–680. (In French).

Cleland, C.L. and Rymer, W.Z. (1990) Neural mechanisms underlying the clasp-knife reflex in the cat. I. Characteristics of the reflex. *J. Neurophysiol.*, 64: 1303–1318.

Conway, B.A., Hultborn, H. and Kiehn, O. (1987) Proprioceptive input resets central locomotor rhythm in the spinal cat. *Exp. Brain Res.*, 68: 643–656.

Creed, R.S., Denny-Brown, D., Eccles, J.C., Liddell, E.G.T. and Sherrington, C.S. (1932) *Reflex Activity of the Spinal Cord*. Oxford (UK): Clarendon Press.

Crone, C., Hultborn, H., Kiehn, O., Mazieres, L. and Wigstrom, H. (1988) Maintained changes in motoneuronal excitability by short-lasting synaptic inputs in the decerebrate cat. *J. Physiol. (Lond.)*, 405: 321–343.

Denny-Brown, D. (1949) Interpretation of the electromyogram. *Archiv. Neurol. Psychiat.*, 61: 99–128.

Denny-Brown, D. and Pennybacker, J.B. (1938) Fibrillation and fasciculation in muscle. *Brain*, 61: 311–333.

22

Dickinson, M.H., Hannaford, S. and Palka, J. (1997) The evolution of insect wings and their sensory apparatus. *Brain Behav. Evol.*, 50: 13–24.

Dickinson, P.S. (1995) Interactions among neural networks for behavior. *Curr. Opin. Behav.*, 5: 792–798.

Eccles, J.C. (1977) My scientific odyssey. *Ann. Rev. Physiol.*, 39: 1–18.

Edgerton, V.R., Bodine-Fowler, S., Roy, R.R., Ishihara, A. and Hodgson, J.A. (1996) Neuromuscular adaptation. In: L.B. Rowell and J.T. Shepherd (Eds), *Handbook of Physiology*, Sec. 12, *Exercise: Regulation and Integration of Multiple Systems*, New York: Oxford University Press, pp. 54–88.

Edwards, F.A., Gibb, A.J. and Colquhoun, D. (1992) ATP receptor-mediated synaptic currents in the central nervous system. *Nature*, 359: 144–146.

Edwards, R.T., Powers, R.K. and Binder, M.D. (1997) Modulation of the AHP and frequency-current relationship in motoneurons of the isolated neonatal rat spinal cord during locomotor-like activity. *Soc. Neurosci. Abstr.*, 23: 1300.

Eken, T. (1998) Spontaneous electromyographic activity in the adult rat soleus muscle. *J. Neurophysiol*, 80: 365–376.

Eken, T. and Kiehn, O. (1989) Bistable firing properties of soleus motor units in unrestrained rats. *Acta Physiol. Scand.*, 136: 383–394.

Enoka, R.M. and Stuart, D.G. (1984) Henneman's 'size principle': Current issues. *Trends Neurosci.*, 7: 226–228.

Fetcho, J.R. (1992) The spinal motor system in early vertebrates and some of its evolutionary changes. *Brain Behav. Evol.*, 40: 82–97.

Fetz, E.E., Cheney, P.D. and German, D.C. (1976) Corticomotoneuronal connections of precentral cells detected by postspike averages of EMG activity in behaving monkeys. *Brain Res.*, 114: 505–510.

Fetz, E.E. and Finocchio, D.V. (1975) Correlations between activity of motor cortex cells and arm muscles during operantly conditioned response patterns. *Exp. Brain Res.*, 23: 217–240.

Fetz, E.E., Henneman, E., Mendell, L.M., Stein, R.B. and Stuart, D.G. (1979) Properties of single cells in vertebrate motor systems revealed by spike-triggered averaging. In: *Society for Neuroscience, 8th Annual Meeting. Summaries of Symposia.* (BIS Conference Report #49). Los Angeles: UCLA, Brain Information Service/BRI Publications Office, pp.11–32.

Flanagan, J.R., Burstedt, M.K. and Johansson, R.S. (1999) Control of finger tip forces in multidigit manipulation. *J. Neurophysiol.*, 81: 1706–1717.

Fleshman, J.W., Munson, J.B., Sypert, G.W. and Friedman, W.A. (1981) Rheobase, input resistance, and motor-unit type in medial gastrocnemius motoneurons in the cat. *J. Neurophysiol.*, 46: 1326–1338.

Fuglevand, A.J. (1998) Henneman's size principle: the right name? *Science*, 281: 919.

Full, R.J. (1997) Invertebrate locomotor systems. In: W.H. Dantzler (Ed.), *Comparative Physiology*, Sec. 13, Vol. II, New York: Oxford University Press, pp. 853–930.

Gandevia, S.C. and Burke, D. (1992) Does the nervous system depend on kinesthetic information to control limb movements? In: *Controversies in Neuroscience* 1: *Movement Control. Behav. Brain Sci.*, 15: 614–632.

Garland, S.J. and Kaufman, M.P. (1995) Role of muscle afferents in the inhibition of motoneurons during fatigue. *Adv. Exp. Med. Biol.*, 384: 271–278.

Getting, P.A. (1986) Understanding central pattern generators: Insights gained from the study of invertebrates. In: S. Grillner, P.S.G. Stein, D.G., Stuart, H. Forrsberg and R.M. Herman (Eds), *Neurobiology of Vertebrate Locomotion*, New York: Plenum Press, pp. 231–244.

Getting, P.A. (1989) Emerging principles governing the operation of neural networks. *Ann. Rev. Neurosci.*, 12: 185–204.

Gillespie, P.G. (1996) Feeling force: mechanical transduction by vertebrates and invertebrates. *Chem. Biol.*, 3: 223–227.

Gorassini, M.A., Bennett, D.J., Eken, T., Kiehn, O. and Hultborn, H. (1999a) Activation patterns of hindlimb motor units in the awake rat and their relation to motoneuron intrinsic properties. *J. Neurophysiol.*, 82: 709–717).

Gorassini, M.A, Bennett, D.J., Siu, M. and Yang, J. (1997) Reduction in recruitment threshold of human motor units by repeated muscle activation. *Soc. Neurosci. Abstr.*, 23: 2094.

Gorassini, M.A., Bennett, D.J. and Yang, J.F. (1998) Self-sustained firing of human motor units. *Neurosci. Lett.*, 247: 13–16.

Gorassini, M.A., Eken, T., Bennett, D.J., Kiehn, O. and Hultborn, H. (1999b) Activity of hindlimb motor units during locomotion in the awake rat. *J. Neurophysiol.*, In press.

Granit, R., Kernell, D. and Lamarre, Y. (1966) Algebraic summation in synaptic activation of motoneurones firing within the 'primary range' to injected current. *J. Physiol. (Lond.)*, 187: 379–399.

Granit, R., Kernell, D. and Shortess, G.K. (1963) Quantitative aspects of repetitive firing of mammalian motoneurones, caused by injected currents. *J. Physiol. (Lond.)*, 168: 911–931.

Grillner, S. (1975) Locomotion in vertebrates: central mechanisms and reflex interaction. *Physiol Rev.*, 55: 247–304.

Grillner, S., Georgopoulos, A.P. and Jordan, L.M. (1997) Selection and initiation of motor behavior. In: P.S.G. Stein, S. Grillner, A.I. Selverston and D.G. Stuart (Eds), *Neurons, Networks, and Motor Behavior*, Boston: MIT Press, pp. 3–19.

Grillner, S., Stein, P.S.G., Stuart, D.G., Forrsberg, H. and Herman, R.M. (Eds) (1986) *Neurobiology of Vertebrate Locomotion*, New York: Plenum Press.

Gurfinkel, V.S., Ivanenko, Y.P., Levik, Y.S., Kazzenikov, O.V. and Selionov, V.A. (1999) The neural control of posture and locomotion: A lock with two keys. In: G.N. Gantchev, S. Mori, J. Massion (Eds), *Motor Control Today and Tomorrow*, Sofia: Academic Publishing House "Prof. M. Dsinov", pp. 113–123.

Gurfinkel, V.S., Levik, Y.S., Kazzenikov, O.V. and Selionov, V.A. (1998) Locomotor-like movements evoked by leg muscle vibration in humans. *Eur. J. Neurosci.*, 10: 1608–1612.

Gustafsson, B. and Pinter, M.J. (1985) On factors determining orderly recruitment of motor units: a role for intrinsic membrane properties. *Trends Neurosci.*, 8: 431–433.

Hasan, Z., Enoka, R.M. and Stuart, D.G. (1985) The interface between biomechanics and neurophysiology in the study of movement: some recent approaches. In: R.L. Terjung (Ed.), *Exercise and Sports Sciences Reviews*, Vol. 13, New York: MacMillan, pp. 169–234.

Hasan, Z. and Stuart, D.G. (1984) Mammalian muscle receptors. In: R.A. Davidoff (Ed.), *Handbook of the Spinal Cord*, Vols. 2 and 3: *Anatomy and Physiology*, New York: Marcel Dekker, pp. 559–607.

Hasan, Z. and Stuart, D.G. (1988) Animal solutions to problems of movement control: the role of proprioceptors. *Annu. Rev. Neurosci.*, 11: 199–223.

Hayward, L.F., Nielsen, R.P., Heckman, C.J. and Hutton, R.S. (1986) Tendon vibration-induced inhibition of human and cat triceps surae group I reflexes: evidence of selective Ib afferent fiber activation. *Exp. Neurol.*, 94: 333–347.

Heckman, C.J. and Binder, M.D. (1988) Analysis of effective synaptic currents generated by homonymous Ia afferent fibers in motoneurons of the cat. *J. Neurophysiol.*, 60: 1948–1966.

Heckman, C.J. and Binder, M.D. (1991) Computer simulation of the steady-state input-output function of the cat medial gastrocnemius motoneuron pool. *J. Neurophysiol.*, 65: 952–967.

Heckman, C.J., Condon, S.M., Hutton, R.S. and Enoka, R.M. (1984) Can Ib axons be selectively activated by electrical stimuli in human subjects? *Exp. Neurol.*, 86: 576–582.

Henneman, E. (1957) Relation between size of neurons and their susceptibility to discharge. *Science*, 126: 1345–1347.

Henneman, E. (1977) Functional organization of the motoneuron pools: The size principle. *Proc. Int. Union Physiol. Sci.*, 12: 50.

Henneman, E. and Mendell, L.M. (1968) Terminals of single Ia fibers: distribution within a pool of 300 homonymous motor neurons. *Science*, 160: 96–98.

Henneman, E. and Mendell, L.M. (1981) Functional organization of motoneuron pool and its inputs. In: J.M. Brookhart and V.B. Mountcastle (Eds), *Handbook of Physiology*, Sec. 1, Vol. II, pt 1., *The Nervous System: Motor Control*, Bethesda (MD): American Physiological Society, pp. 423–507.

Herman, R.M., Grillner, S., Stein, P.S.G. and Stuart, D.G. (Eds) (1976) *Neural Control of Locomotion*, New York: Plenum Press.

Hildebrand, J.G. and Shepherd, G.M. (1997) Mechanisms of olfactory discrimination: Common principles across phyla. *Annu. Rev. Neurosci.*, 20: 595–631.

Hochman, S., Jordan, L.M. and Schmidt, B.J. (1994) TTX-resistant NMDA receptor-mediated voltage oscillations in mammalian lumber motoneurons. *J. Neurophysiol.*, 72: 2559–2562.

Hochman, S. and Schmidt, B.J. (1998) Whole cell recordings of lumbar motoneurons during locomotor-like activity in the in vitro neonatal rat spinal cord. *J. Neurophysiol.*, 79: 743–752.

Hornby, T.G. (1997) Extrinsic Modulation of the Intrinsic Stimulus Current-Spike Frequency Relationship of Spinal Motoneurons in the Adult Turtle. Unpublished Ph.D preliminary examination proposal, Tucson: The University of Arizona. (See URL: http://server.physiol.arizona.edu/HornbyPrelim.html)

Hornby, T.G., McDonagh, J.C., Reinking, R.M. and Stuart, D.G. (1998) Plateau potential contribution to the stimulus current-spike frequency relation of turtle motoneurons. *Soc. Neurosci. Abstr.*, 24: 914.

Hounsgaard, J., Hultborn, H., Jespersen, B. and Kiehn, O. (1984) Intrinsic membrane properties causing a bistable behaviour of α-motoneurones. *Exp. Brain Res.*, 55: 391–394.

Hounsgaard, J., Hultborn, H., Jespersen, B. and Kiehn, O. (1988a) Bistability of α-motoneurones in the decerebrate cat and in the acute spinal cat after intravenous 5-hydroxytryptophan. *J. Physiol. (Lond.)*, 405: 345–367.

Hounsgaard, J. and Kiehn, O. (1989) Serotonin-induced bistability of turtle motoneurones caused by a nifedipine-sensitive calcium plateau potential. *J. Physiol. (Lond.)*, 414: 265–282.

Hounsgaard, J., Kiehn, O. and Mintz, I. (1988b) Response properties of motoneurones in a slice preparation of the turtle spinal cord. *J. Physiol. (Lond.)*, 398: 575–589.

Hounsgaard, J. and Kjaerulff, O. (1992) Ca^{2+}-mediated plateau potentials in a subpopulation of interneurons in the ventral horn of the turtle spinal cord. *Eur. J. Neurosci.*, 4: 183–188.

Hultborn, H. (1998) The plateau potentials and their role in regulating motoneuronal firing. In: M.D. Binder, J.C. McDonagh, R.M. Reinking and P.A. Pierce (Eds), *Peripheral and Spinal Mechanisms in the Neural Control of Movement*, Proceedings of an international symposium, Tucson, AZ, Nov. 4–6, 1998, Tucson: The University of Arizona, pp. 23

Hultborn, H., and Kiehn, O. 1992. Neuromodulation of vertebrate motor neuron membrane properties. *Curr. Opin. Neurobiol.*, 2: 770–775.

Hultborn, H. and Pierrot-Deseilligny, E. (1979) Input–output relations in the pathway of recurrent inhibition to motoneurones in the cat. *J. Physiol. (Lond.)*, 297: 267–287.

Hultborn, H., Wigstrom, H. and Wangberg, B. (1975) Prolonged activation of soleus motoneurones following a conditioning train in soleus Ia afferents-a case for a reverberating loop? *Neurosci. Lett.*, 1: 147–152.

Jabre, J. and Binder, M.D. (1999) Mechanisms Underlying the Control of Firing in the Healthy and Sick Motoneurone. *J. Physiol. (Paris)*, 93: 1–182.

Jankowska, E. (1992) Interneuronal relay in spinal pathways from proprioceptors. *Prog. Neurobiol.*, 38: 335–378.

Jankowska, E. and Lundberg, A. (1981) Interneurons in the spinal cord. *Trends Neurosci.*, 4: 230–233.

Jiang, Z., Carlin, K.P. and Brownstone, R.M. (1999a) Plateau potentials and wind-up in mouse spinal motoneurons. *Soc. Neurosci. Abstr.*, 25: 1395.

Jiang, Z., Rempel, J., Li, J., Sawchuk, M. and Brownstone, R.M. (1999b) Development of L-type calcium channels and a nifedipine-sensitive motor activity in the postnatal mouse spinal cord. *Eur. J. Neurosci.*, 11: 3481–3487.

Jonas, P., Bischofer, J. and Sandkuhler, J. (1998) Corelease of two fast neurotransmitters at a central synapse. *Science*, 281: 419–424.

Jordan, L.M. (1998) Cholinergic interneurons involved in the control of locomotion. In: M.D. Binder, J.C. McDonagh, R.M. Reinking and P.A. Pierce (Eds), *Peripheral and Spinal Mechanisms in the Neural Control of Movement*, Proceedings of an international symposium, Tucson, AZ, Nov. 4–6, Tucson: The University of Arizona, pp. 33.

Jordan, L.M., Brownstone, R.M. and Noga, B.R. (1992) Control of functional systems in the brainstem and spinal cord. *Curr. Opin. Neurobiol.*, 2: 794–801.

Kakuda, N., Wessberg, J. and Vallbo, A.B. (1997) Is human muscle spindle afference dependent on perceived size of error in visual tracking? *Exp. Brain Res.*, 114: 246–254.

Katz, R. and Pierrot-Deseilligny, E. (1999) Recurrent inhibition in humans. *Prog. Neurobiol.*, 57: 325–355.

Keil, T.A. (1997) Functional morphology of insect mechanoreceptors. *Microsc. Res. Tech.*, 39: 506–531.

Kennedy, D. (1997) *Academic Duty*, Cambridge (MA): Harvard University Press.

Kernell, D. (1965) The limits of firing frequency in cat lumbosacral motoneurones possessing different time course of afterhyperpolarization. *Acta Physiol. Scand.*, 65: 87–100.

Kernell, D., and Monster, A.W. (1982) Time course and properties of late adaptation in spinal motoneurons in the cat. *Exp. Brain. Res.*, 46: 191–196.

Kernell, D. and Zwaagstra, B. (1981) Input conductance, axonal conduction velocity and cell size among hindlimb motoneurons of the cat. *Brain Res.*, 204: 311–326.

Kiehn, O. (1990) Monoaminergic Regulation of Plateau Potentials in Vertebrate Motoneurones: Basic mechanism and Possible Functional Role. Doctoral thesis. Denmark: University of Copenhagen.

Kiehn, O. and Eken, T. (1997) Prolonged firing in motor units: evidence of plateau potentials in human motoneurons? *J. Neurophysiol.*, 78: 3061–3068.

Kiehn, O., and Harris-Warrick, R.M. (1992) Serotonergic stretch receptors induce plateau properties in a crustacean motor neuron by a dual-conductance mechanism. *J. Neurophysiol.*, 68: 485–495.

Kiehn, O., Harris-Warrick, R.M., Jordan, L.M., Hultborn, H. and Kudo, N. (Eds) (1998) Neuronal Mechanisms for Generating Locomotor Activity, *Ann. NY Acad. Sci.*, 860, pp. 1–573.

Kiehn, O., Johnson, B.R. and Raastad, M. (1997) Plateau properties in mammalian spinal interneurons during transmitter-induced locomotor activity. *Neuroscience*, 77: 613–615.

Kirkwood, P.A. and Sears, T.A. (1974) Monosynaptic excitation of motoneurones from secondary endings of muscle spindles. *Nature*, 252: 243–244.

Koeber, H.R., Druzinsky, R.E. and Mendell, L.M. (1988). Properties of somata of dorsal root ganglion cells differ

according to peripheral receptor innervated. *J. Neurophysiol.*, 60: 1584–1596.

Kuze, B., Matsuyama, K., Matsu, T., Miyata, H. and Mori, S. (1999) Segment-specific branching patterns of single vestibulospinal tract axons arising from the lateral vestibular nucleus in the cat: a PHA-L tracing study. *J. Comp. Neurol.*, 414: 80–96.

Latash, M. (Ed.) (1998) *Progress in Motor Control: Bernstein's Traditions in Movement Studies*, Champaign, IL: Human Kinetics.

Latash, M.L. and Turvey, M.T. (1996) *Dexterity and Its Development*, Mahwah, NJ: Lawrence Erlbaum Associates, Publishers.

Lee, R.H. and Heckman, C.J. (1998a) Bistability of spinal motoneurons in vivo: systematic variations in rhythmic firing patterns. *J. Neurophysiol.*, 80: 572–582.

Lee, R.H. and Heckman, C.J. (1998b) Bistability of spinal motoneurons in vivo: systematic variations in persistent inward currents. *J. Neurophysiol.*, 80: 583–593.

Lee, R.H. and Heckman, C.J. (1998c) Role of persistent component of fast sodium channel in rhythmic action potential formation in motoneurons. *Soc. Neurosci. Abstr.*, 24: 1077.

Lewis, D.M. (1984) Mammalian motor units. In: R.A. Davidoff (Ed.), *Handbook of the Spinal Cord*, Vols. 2 and 3: *Anatomy and Physiology*, New York: Marcel Dekker, pp. 269–314.

Liddell, E.G.T. (1952) Charles Scott Sherrington: 1857–1952. In: *Obituary Notices of Fellows of the Royal Society*, Vol. 8, no. 21, London: The Royal Society, pp. 241–270.

Liddell, E.G.T. and Sherrington, C.S. (1923) Recruitment type of reflexes. *Proc. R. Soc. Lond. B Biol. Sci.*, 95: 407–412.

Liddell, E.G.T. and Sherrington, C.S. (1924) Reflexes in response to stretch (Myotatic reflexes) *Proc. R. Soc. Lond. B Biol. Sci.*, 96: 212–242.

Lindsay, A.D. and Binder, M.D. (1991) Distribution of effective synaptic currents underlying recurrent inhibition in cat triceps surae motoneurons. *J. Neurophysiol.*, 65: 168–177.

Lindsley, D.B. (1935) Electrical activity of human motor units during voluntary contraction. *Am. J. Physiol.*, 114: 90–99.

Lucas, K. (1905) On the gradation of contraction in a skeletal muscle fibre. *J. Physiol. (Lond.)*, 33: 125–137.

Lucas, K. (1909) The evolution of animal function. *Science Progress*, 20 cent., London, 3: 472–483.

Lundberg, A. (1969) Convergence of excitatory and inhibitory action on interneurones in the spinal cord. In: M.A.B. Brazier (Ed.), *The Interneuron*, Los Angeles (CA): University of California Press, pp. 231–236.

MacLean, J.N., Cowley, K.C. and Schmidt, B.J. (1998) NMDA receptor-mediated oscillatory activity in the neonatal rat spinal cord is serotonin dependent. *J. Neurophysiol.*, 79: 2804–2808.

MacLean, J.N., Schmidt, B.J. and Hochman, S. (1997) NMDA receptor activation triggers voltage oscillations, plateau potentials and bursting in neonatal rat lumbar motoneurons in vitro. *Eur. J. Neurosci.*, 12: 2702–2711.

Massion, J. (1992) Movement, posture and equilibrium: interaction and coordination. *Prog. Neurobiol.*, 38: 35–56.

Matsuyama, K., Mori, F., Kuze, B. and Mori, S. (1999) Morphology of single pontine reticulospinal axons in the lumbar enlargement of the cat: a study using the anterograde tracer PHA-L. *J. Comp. Neurol.*, 410: 413–430.

Matsuyama, S. and Mori, S. (1998) Lumbar interneurons involved in the generation of fictive locomotion in cats. In: O. Kiehn, R.M. Harris-Warrick, L.M. Jordan, H. Hultborn and N. Kudo (Eds), *Neuronal Mechanisms for Generating Locomotor Activity*, Ann. NY Acad. Sci., 860, pp. 441–443.

Matthews, P.B.C. (1972) *Mammalian Muscle Receptors and Their Central Actions*, London: Arnold.

McComas, A.J. (1977) *Neuromuscular Function and Disorders*, London: Butterworths.

McComas, A.J. (1996) *Skeletal Muscle – Form and Function*, Champaign (IL): Human Kinetics.

McCrea, D.A. (1992) Can sense be made of spinal interneuron circuits? *Behav. Brain Sci.*, 15: 633–643.

McCrea, D.A. (1998) Neuronal basis of afferent-evoked enhancement of locomotor activity. In: O. Kiehn, R.M. Harris-Warrick, L.M. Jordan, H. Hultborn and N. Kudo (Eds), *Neuronal Mechanisms for Generating Locomotor Activity*, Ann. NY Acad. Sci., 860, pp. 216–225.

McDonagh, J.C., Binder, M.D., Reinking, R.M. and Stuart, D.G. (1980) A commentary on muscle unit properties in cat hindlimb muscles. *J. Morphol.*, 166: 217–230.

McDonagh, J.C., Callister, R.J., Brichta, A., Reinking, R.M and Stuart, D.G. (1999b) A commentary on the properties of spinal interneurons vs. motoneurons in vertebrates, and their firing-rate behavior during movement. In: G.N. Gantchev, S. Mori, J. Massion (Eds), *Motor Control Today and Tomorrow*, Sofia: Academic Publishing House "Prof. M. Drinov", pp. 3–31.

McDonagh, J.C., Gorman, R.B., Gilliam, E.E., Hornby, T.G., Reinking, R.M. and Stuart, D.G. (1998a) Properties of spinal motoneurons and interneurons in the adult turtle: Provisional classification by cluster analysis. *J. Comp. Neurol.*, 400: 544–570.

McDonagh, J.C., Gorman, R.B., Gilliam, E.E., Hornby, T.G., Reinking, R.M. and Stuart, D.G. (1999a) Electrophysiological and morphological properties of neurons in the ventral horn of the spinal cord. In: M.D. Binder and J. Jabre (Eds), *Mechanisms Underlying the Control of Firing in the Healthy and Sick Motoneurone*. J. Physiol. (Paris), 93: 3–16.

McDonagh, J.C., Hornby, T.G., Reinking, R.M. and Stuart, D.G. (1998b) Morphological and physiological properties of turtle spinal motoneurons and interneurons. *Soc. Neurosci.*, Abstr., 24: 914.

Mense, S. (1993) Nociception from skeletal muscle in relation to clinical muscle pain. *Pain*, 54: 241–289.

Mines, G.R. (1913) On the summation of contractions. *J. Physiol. (Lond.)*, 169: 1–27.

Mori, S., Matsui, T., Kuze, B., Asanome, K., Nakajima, K. and Matsuyama, K. (1999a) Stimulation of a restricted region in the midline cerebellar white matter evokes coordinated quadrupedal locomotion in the decerebrate cat. *J. Neurophysiol.*, 82: 290–300.

Mori, S., Matsuyama, K., Kuze, B., Mori, F. (1999b). Features of the fastigio-reticulo-spinal system involved in the control of posture and locomotion in the cat. In: G.N. Gantchev, S. Mori, J. Massion (Eds), *Motor Control Today and Tomorrow*, Sofia: Academic Publishing House "Prof. M. Drinov", pp. 31–45.

Nelson, P.G. and Frank, K. (1967) Anamolous rectification in cat spinal motoneurons and effect of polarizing currents on excitatory postsynaptic potential. *J. Neurophysiol.*, 30: 1097–1113.

Nemeth, P.M., Solanki, L., Gordon, D.A., Hamm, T.M., Reinking, R.M. and Stuart, D.G. (1986) Uniformity of metabolic enzymes within individual motor units. *J. Neurosci.*, 6: 892–898.

Nichols, T.R. (1994) A biomechanical perspective on spinal mechanisms of coordinated muscular action: an architecture principle. *Acta Anat.*, 151: 1–13.

Orlovsky, G. and Shik, M.L. (1976) Control of locomotion: A neurophysiological analysis of the cat locomotor system. In: R. Porter (Ed.), *Neurophysiology II*, Vol. 10, *International Review of Neurophysiology*, Baltimore: University Park Press, pp. 291–317.

Palecek, J.I., Abdrachmanova, G., Vlachova, V. and Vyklick, L. Jr. (1999) Properties of NMDA receptors in rat spinal cord motoneurons. *Eur. J. Neurosci.*, 11: 827–836.

Patton, H.D. (1994) David P.C. Lloyd. Biographical Memoirs. *Nat. Acad. Sci.*, 65: 197–209.

Pearson, K.G. (1993) Common principles of motor control in vertebrates and invertebrates. *Annu. Rev. Neurosci.*, 16: 265–297.

Pearson, K.G. and Ramirez, J-M. (1992) Parallels with other invertebrate and vertebrate systems. In: R.M. Harris-Warrick, E. Marder, A.I. Selverston and M. Moulins (Eds), *Dynamic Biological Networks: the Stomatogastric Nervous System*, Cambridge (MA): MIT Press, pp. 263–281.

Pearson, K.G. and Ramirez, J-M. (1997) Sensory modulation of pattern generating circuits. In: P.S.G. Stein, S. Grillner, A.I. Selverston and D.G. Stuart (Eds), *Neurons, Networks, and Motor Behavior*, Cambridge: MIT Press, pp. 225–235.

Powers, R.K., Robinson, F.R., Konodi, M.A. and Binder, M.D. (1992) Effective synaptic current can be estimated from measurement of motoneuron discharge. *J. Neurophysiol.*, 68: 964–968.

Powers, R.K., Sawczuk, A., Musick, J.R. and Binder, M.D. (1999) Multiple mechanisms of spike-frequency adaptation in motoneurones. *J. Physiol. (Paris)*, 93: 101–114.

Prochazka, A. (1996) Proprioceptive feedback and movement regulation. In: L.B. Rowell and J.T. Shepherd (Eds), *Handbook of Physiology*, Sec. 12, *Exercise: Regulation and Integration of Multiple Systems*, New York: Oxford University Press, pp. 89–127.

Prochazka, A. and Gorassini, M.A. (1998) Models of ensemble firing of muscle spindle afferents recorded during normal locomotion in cats. *J. Neurophysiol.*, 507: 277–291.

Proske, U., Wise, A.K. and Gregory, J.E. (1999) The role of muscle receptors in the detection of movements. *Prog. Neurobiol.*, 60: 83–94.

Rall, W. (1967) Distinguishing theoretical synaptic potentials computed for different soma-dendritic distributions of synaptic input. *J. Neurophysiol.*, 30: 1138–1168.

Rall, W. (1992) Path to biophysical insights about dendrites and synaptic function. In: F. Samson and G. Adelman (Eds), *The Neurosciences: Paths of Discovery*, II, Boston: Birkhuser, pp. 214–238.

Rall, W., Burke, R.E., Holmes, W.R., Jack, J.J, Redman, S. and Segev, I. (1992) Matching dendritic neuron models to experimental data. *Physiol. Rev.*, 72 (4 Suppl.): S159–S186.

Rall, W., Burke, R.E., Smith T.G., Nelson, P.G. and Frank, K. (1967) Dendritic location of synapses and possible mechanisms for the monosynaptic EPSPs in motoneurons. *J. Neurophysiol.*, 30: 1169–1193.

Rathmayer, W. and Maier, L. (1987) Muscle fiber types in crabs: studies ion single identified muscle fibers. *Am. Zool.*, 27: 1067–1077.

Redman, R. (1976) A quantitative approach to the integrative function of dendrites. In: R. Porter (Ed), *International Review of Physiology: Neuroscience*, Vol. 10, Baltimore: University Park Press, pp. 1–36.

Rekling, J.C. and Feldman, J.L. (1998) PreBotzinger complex and pacemaker neurons: hypothesized site and kernel for respiratory rhythm generation. *Annu. Rev. Physiol.*, 60: 385–405.

Rome, L.C., Funke, R.P., Alexander, R.M., Lutz, G., Aldridge, H., Scott F. and Freadman, M. (1988) Why animals have different muscle fibre types. *Nature*, 335: 824–827.

Rome, L.C., Syme, D.A., Hollingworth, S., Lindstedt, S.L. and Baylor, S.M. (1996) The whistle and the rattle: the design of sound producing muscles. *Proc. Natl. Acad. Sci. USA*, 93: 8095–8100.

Russell, D.F. and Hartline, D.K. (1978) Bursting neural networks: a reexamination. *Science*, 200: 453–456.

Sah, P. (1996) Ca^{2+}-activated K^+ currents in neurones: Types, physiological roles and modulation. *Trends Neurosci.*, 19: 150–154.

Sato, A., Sato, Y. and Schmidt, R.F. (1997) The impact of somatosensory input on autonomic functions. *Rev. Physiol. Biochem. Pharmacol.*, 130: 1–328.

Sayer, R.J., Brown, A.M., Schwindt, P.C. and Crill, W.E. (1993) Calcium currents in acutley isolated human neocortical neurons. *J. Neurophysiol.*, 69: 1596–1606.

Schmidt, B.J. (1994) Afterhyperpolarization modulation in lumbar motoneurons during locomotor-like rhythmic activity in the neonatal rat spinal cord in vitro. *Exp. Brain. Res.*, 99: 214–222.

Schmidt, R.F. (1996) The articular polymodal nociceptor in health and disease. *Prog. Brain Res.*, 113: 53–81.

Schwindt, P. and Crill, W.E. (1980) Role of a persistent inward current in motoneuron bursting during spinal seizures. *J. Neurophysiol.*, 43: 1296–1318.

Schwindt, P. and Crill, W.E. (1984) Membrane properties of cat spinal motoneurons. In: R.A. Davidoff (Ed.), *Handbook of the Spinal Cord*, New York: Marcel Dekker, pp. 199–242.

Schwindt, P. and Crill, W.E. (1999) Mechanisms underlying burst and regular spiking evoked by dendritic depolarization in layer 5 cortical pyramidal neurons. *J. Neurophysiol.*, 81: 1341–1354.

Selionov, V.A. and Shik, M.L. (1992) Responses of medullary and spinal neurons to simultaneous stimulation of two locomotor points. *Neurophysiology*, 24: 471–481. (In Russian).

Selverston, A.I. (1998) Principles of motor pattern generation derived from invertebrate models. In: M.D. Binder, J.C. McDonagh, R.M. Reinking and P.A. Pierce (Eds), *Peripheral and Spinal Mechanisms in the Neural Control of Movement*, Proceedings of an international symposium, Tucson, AZ, Nov. 4–6, 1998, Tucson, The University of Arizona, pp. 30.

Selverston, A., Elson, R., Rabinovich, M., Huerta, R. and Abarbanel, H. (1998) Basic principles for generating motor output in the stomatogastric ganglion. In: O. Kiehn, R.M. Harris-Warrick, L.M. Jordan, H. Hultborn and N. Kudo (Eds), Neuronal Mechanisms for Generating Locomotor Activity, *Ann. NY Acad. Sci.*, 860, pp. 35–50.

Seyffarth, H. (1940) The behaviour of motor-units in voluntary contraction. *Av Norske Videnskap Akad Oslo. I. Matematisk-Natur Klasse*, 4: 1–63.

Sherrington, C.S. (1929) Some functional problems attaching to convergence. Ferrier lecture, *Proc. R. Soc. Lond. B Biol. Sci.*, 105: 332–362.

Shik, M.L., Orlovsky, G. and Severin, F.V. (1966) Control of walking and running by means of electrical stimulation of the mid-brain. *Biophysics*, 11: 756–765.

Simmers, J., Meyrand, P. and Moulins, M. (1995) Modulation and specification of motor rhythm-generating circuits in crustacea. *J. Physiol. (Paris)*, 89: 195–208.

Smith, O.C. (1934) Action potentials from single motor units in voluntary contraction. *Am. J. Physiol.*, 108: 629–638.

Smith, T.G., Wuerker, R.B. and Frank, K. (1967) Membrane impedance changes during synaptic transmission in cat spinal motoneurons. *J. Neurophysiol.*, 30: 1072–1096.

Stauffer, E.K., Watt, D.G.D., Taylor, A., Reinking, R.M. and Stuart, D.G. (1976) Analysis of muscle receptor connections by spike-triggered averaging: 2. Spindle group II afferents. *J. Neurophysiol.*, 39: 1393–1402.

Stein, P.S.G. (1995) A multi-level approach to motor pattern generation. In: W.R. Ferrell and U. Proske (Eds), *Neural Control of Movement*, New York: Plenum Press, pp. 159–165.

Stein, P.S.G., Grillner, S., Selveston, A. and Stuart, D.G. (Eds) (1995). Neurons, Networks, and Motor Behavior. Proceedings of an International Symposium, Tucson, AZ, Nov. 8–11, 1995. Tucson: The University of Arizona, 87 pp. (See URL: http://server.physiol.arizona.edu/CELL/Department/Conferences.html)

Stein, P.S.G., Grillner, S., Selverston, A.I. and Stuart, D.G. (Eds) (1997) *Neurons, Networks, and Motor Behavior*, Boston (MA): MIT Press.

Stein, P.S.G., McCullough, M.L. and Currie, S.C. (1998) Spinal motor patterns in the turtle. In: O. Kiehn, R.M. Harris-Warrick, L.M. Jordan, H. Hultborn and N. Kudo (Eds), Neuronal Mechanisms for Generating Locomotor Activity, *Ann. NY Acad. Sci.*, 860, pp. 142–154.

Stein, P.S.G. and Smith, J.L. (1997) Neural and biomechanical control strategies for different forms of vertebrate hindlimb motor tasks. In: P.S.G. Stein, S. Grillner, A.I. Selverston and D.G. Stuart (Eds), *Neurons, Networks, and Motor Behavior*, Boston: MIT Press, pp. 61–73.

Stein, R.B., French A.S., Mannard, A. and Yemm, R. (1972) New methods for analysing motor function in man and animals. *Brain. Res.*, 40: 187–192.

Strausfeld, N.J. (1997) Oculomotor control in insects: From muscles to elementary motion detectors. In: P.S.G Stein, S. Grillner, A.I. Selverston and D.G. Stuart (Eds), *Neurons, Networks, and Motor Behavior*, Boston (MA): MIT Press, pp. 277–284.

Stuart, D.G. (1985) Summary and challenges for future work. In: P.S.G. Stein (Org./Ed.), *Motor Control: From Movement Trajectories to Neural Mechanisms, Short Course Syllabus*, Bethesda (MD), Society for Neuroscience, pp. 95–105.

Stuart, D.G. (Ed./Org.). (1998) Paths of Discovery in Motor Control Neurobiology. Graduate colloquium course offered by the Univ. Arizona/Barrow Neurological Institute/Arizona State Univ. Motor Control Group. (See URL: http: //server.physiol.arizona.edu/Physiology/Instruct/695a/695a Syllabus.html)

Stuart, D.G., Binder, M.D. and Enoka, R.M. (1984) Motor unit organization: Application of the quadripartite classification scheme to human muscles. In: P.J. Dyck, P.K. Thomas, E.H. Lambert and R.P. Bunge (Eds), *Peripheral Neuropathy*, Vol. I, Philadelphia: Saunders, pp. 1067–1090.

Stuart, D.G. and Callister, R.J. (1993) Afferent and spinal reflex aspects of muscle fatigue: Issues and speculations. In: A.J. Sargeant and D. Kernell (Ed.), *Neuromuscular Fatigue*, Amsterdam: Royal Netherlands Academy of Arts and Sciences, North-Holland, pp. 169–180.

Stuart, D.G. and Enoka, R.M. (1983) Motoneurons, motor units, and the size principle. In: R.N. Rosenberg and W.D. Willis (Eds), *The Clinical Neurosciences, Neurobiology*. Sec. 5., New York: Churchill Livingstone, pp. 471–517.

Stuart, D.G. and Enoka, R.M. (1990) Hennerman's contributions in historical perspective. In: M.D. Binder and L.M. Mendell (Eds), *The Segmental Motor System*, New York: Oxford University Press, pp. 3–19.

Stuart, D.G. and McDonagh, J.C. (1997a) Muscle receptors, mammalian. In: G. Adelman and B. Smith (Eds), *Encyclopedia of Neuroscience* [CD-ROM also available], Amsterdam: Elsevier Science B.V.

Stuart, D.G. and McDonagh, J.C. (1997b) Muscle receptors, mammalian, spinal actions. In: G. Adelman and B. Smith (Eds), *Encyclopedia of Neuroscience* [CD-ROM also available], Amsterdam, Elsevier Science B.V.

Stuart, D.G. and McDonagh, J.C. (1998) Reflections on a Bernsteinian approach to systems neuroscience: The controlled locomotion of high-decerebrate cats. In: M. Latash (Ed.), *Progress in Motor Control: Bernstein's Traditions in Movement Studies*, Champaign, IL: Human Kinetics, pp. 21–49.

Stuart, D.G., Pierce, P.A., Callister, R.J., Brichta, A.M. and McDonagh, J.C. (1999) Comments on Sir Charles Scott Sherrington's 'Inhibition as a co-ordinative factor'. Nobel Lecture delivered in Stockholm, 12/12/1932, Stockholm, P.A. Norstedt. 1933. In: M.L. Latash and V. Zatsiorsky (Eds), *Classical Papers in Movement Science*, Champaign (IL): Human Kinetics, In press.

Szekely, G. (1989) Ontogeny and morphology of neuronal structures controlling tetrapod locomotion. In: D.B. Wake and G. Roth (Eds), *Complex Organismal Functions: Integration and Evolution in Vertebrates*, New York: Wiley, pp. 117–131.

Takahashi, T., Momiyama, A., Hirai, K., Hishinuma, F. and Akagi, H. (1992) Functional correlation of fetal and adult forms of glycine receptors with developmental changes in inhibitory synaptic receptor channels. *Neuron*, 9: 1155–1161.

Taylor, A., Gladden, M.H. and Durbaba, R. (Eds) (1995) *Alpha and Gamma Motor Systems*, New York: Plenum Press.

Taylor, A. and Prochazka, A. (1981) *Muscle Receptors and Movement*, London: McMillan Publishers.

Thurbon, D., Luscher, H.R., Hofstetter, T. and Redman, S.J. (1998) Passive electrical properties of ventral horn neurones in rat spinal cord slices. *J. Neurophysiol.*, 80: 2485–502.

Ulinsky, P.S. (1997) Vertebrate nervous system. In: W.H. Dantzler (Ed.), *Comparative Physiolog*, Sec. 13, Vol. II, New York: Oxford University Press, pp. 17–53.

Van de Graaff, K.M., Frederick, E.C., Williamson, R.G. and Goslow, G.E. Jr, (1977) Motor unit types of primary ankle extensors of the skunk (Mephitus mephitis). *J. Neurophysiol.*, 40: 1424–1431.

Vilensky, J.A. and Gilman, S (1998) Renaming the 'Henneman Size Principle'. *Science*, 280: 2031.

Vilensky, J.A., Gilman, S. and Dunn, E. (1998) Derek E. Denny-Brown (1901–1981): His life and influence on American neurology. *J. Med. Biograph.*, 6: 73–78.

Wallén, P. and Grillner, S. (1987) N-methyl-D-aspartate receptor-induced, inherent oscillatory activity in neurons active during fictive locomotion in the lamprey. *J. Neurosci.*, 7: 2745–2755.

Walmsley, B., Hodgson, J.A. and Burke, R.E. (1978) Forces produced by medial gastrocnemius and soleus muscles during locomotion in freely moving cats. *J. Neurophysiol.*, 41: 1203–1216.

Watson, G.M. and Mire, P. (1999) A comparison of hair bundle mechanoreceptors in sea anemones and vertebrate systems. *Curr. Top. Dev. Biol.*, 43: 51–84.

Watt, D.G.D., Stauffer, E.K., Taylor, A., Reinking, R.M. and Stuart, D.G. (1976) Analysis of muscle receptor connections by spike-triggered averaging: 1. Spindle primary and tendon organ afferents. *J. Neurophysiol.*, 39: 1375–1392.

Westbury, D.R. (1981) Electrophysiological characteristics of spinal gamma motoneurons in the cat. In: A. Taylor and A. Prochazka (Eds), *Muscle Receptors and Movement*, London, UK: MacMillan, pp. 87–96.

Wiesendanger, M. (1997) Paths of discovery in human motor

control: A short historical perspective. In: M.-C. Hepp-Reymond, G. Marini (Eds), *Perspectives of Motor Behavior and Its Neural Basis*, Basel: S. Karger AG, pp. 103–124.

Windhorst, U. and Boosman, G. (1995) Overview: potential role of segmental motor circuitry in muscle fatigue. *Adv. Exp. Med. Biol.*, 384: 241–258.

Young, R.R. (1997) Elwood Henneman – 1915–1996. *Muscle Nerve*, 20: 133–135.

Zengel, J.E., Reid, S.A., Sypert, G.W. and Munson, J.B. (1985) Membrane electrical properties and predictions of motor-unit type of medial gastrocnemius motoneurons in the cat. *J. Neurophysiol.*, 53: 1323–1344.

Mechanisms underlying repetitive firing in motoneurons

M.D. Binder (Ed.)
Progress in Brain Research, Vol 123

CHAPTER 2

Repetitive impulse firing in motoneurons: facts and perspectives

Daniel Kernell*

Department of Medical Physiology, University of Groningen, Bloemsingel 10, 9712 KZ Groningen, The Netherlands

Introduction

When activating our skeletal muscles, the motoneurons (MNs) practically always deliver more or less prolonged bursts of repetitive firing. We also know that each MN receives thousands of synapses and that hundreds of these have to be more or less simultaneously active for the action potential (AP) threshold to be reached. In maintained synaptic activation, the MNs will be stimulated by relatively steady post-synaptic currents, produced by the summation of many asynchronous post-synaptic events. Hence, a logical way to proceed is to study the input–output relations of MNs by measuring the relation between an activating steady current and AP rate. This is usually done by injecting maintained stimulating currents via an intracellular microelectrode. Control experiments have shown that such injected currents have actions very similar to those often seen for maintained post-synaptic currents ('driving' currents, see below; Granit et al., 1966; Kernell, 1969; Powers and Binder, 1995; Binder et al., 1998).The input–output relations of spinal MNs were initially investigated in anaesthetized animals. Later on it has been found that, in non-anaesthetized animals, the 'base-line' properties seen under anaesthesia are supplemented by additional 'MN-modulating' mechanisms, such as the plateau behavior and other changes of input–

output relations. In this introductory survey, the baseline properties will first be briefly described. Then some comments will be added concerning other aspects, including the 'MN-modulatory' post-synaptic effects (for further details on MN repetitive properties, see reviews: Kernell, 1992; Binder et al., 1993, 1996; Kernell et al., 1999).

Repetitive impulse firing in motoneurons: baseline properties

The f-I relation

As a motoneuron is stimulated by steps of steady current, a higher intensity will typically be needed for producing repetitive firing than for evoking a single AP, i.e. the 'rhythmic threshold current' (R_{thr}) is higher than the rheobase (Granit et al., 1963; Kernell, 1965a). At a current intensity just above R_{thr}, the cell will start a regular rhythmic firing at its characteristic minimum rate (F_{min}). Over a given range of stronger currents, rate increases with current intensity according to the characteristic frequency-current relation of the motoneuron (f-I relation) until the highest possible rate of maintained firing is reached (F_{max}; cf. Kernell, 1965b). In lumbosacral motoneurons of the cat the f-I relation can typically be simplified into mainly two roughly linear ranges, a lower 'primary' range and a higher, less stable and steeper 'secondary' range.

*Corresponding author. Tel.: +31–50–3632660; Fax: +31–50–3632751; e-mail: d.kernell@med.rug.nl

Spike-frequency adaptation

Following the abrupt onset of steady stimulation, frequency declines. The first portion of this decline is rapid and takes place within a few spike intervals up to, sometimes, 0.5–1 s or more. Originally we called this whole first phase the 'initial' adaptation (Granit et al., 1963; Kernell, 1965a). In hypoglossal MNs studied by Sawczuk et al. (1995, 1997) the first brief phase could often be further subdivided into a linear 'initial' and an exponential 'early' period; I will here refer to both these portions as the 'first' phase. Following this first phase there is a second, more gradual phase of decline in rate during, at least, about 0.5–1 min ('late' phase of spike-frequency adaptation; up to 4 min tested, Kernell and Monster, 1982; Spielmann et al., 1993; Sawczuk et al., 1995, 1997).

The two main phases of adaptation have different time relations and they also differ markedly with regard to the behavior of the f-I relation: the slope of this relation (f-I slope) decreases markedly during the first phase but remains constant during the late phase. This illustrates that different mechanisms must be responsible for the two phases of adaptation (for further discussion, see Sawczuk et al., 1997).

MN vs. muscle unit matching

The rhythmic MN characteristics are well adapted to motoneuronal function and some of the properties (e.g. F_{min} and F_{max}) differ systematically between MNs of fast and slower muscle units (review: Kernell, 1992; Kernell et al., 1999). For fast as well as for slower units, the main working range of MNs in maintained firing (i.e. the linear 'primary' range of their f-I relation) corresponds, roughly, to the range of rates needed for an effective grading of muscle force (i.e. the steep portion of the curve relating muscle force to activation rate). The precise manner in which AHPs are matched to muscle speed differs between diffferent hindlimb muscles (Bakels and Kernell, 1993).

Mechanisms of (moto-)neuronal rhythmicity

Theories about the mechanisms for repetitive impulse firing became formulated as soon as sensory and motor unit discharges started to become recorded. Some very general and not mutually exclusive views emerged which are, I think, still useful simplifications for general discussions:

(1) The intervals between the repeated APs might depend on periods of relative refractoriness *following* each one of the APs (Adrian, 1932). Such postspike periods of reduced excitability, gradually changing with time, are produced by the permeability changes associated with long-lasting hyperpolarizing afterpotentials (e.g. in MNs, the postspike afterhyperpolarization, AHP). This seems to be the dominating mechanism for the rhythmicity in spinal MNs. The AHP reflects the fast rise and slow decline of a calcium-dependent potassium-conductance ($g_{K(Ca)}$; e.g. Krnjevic et al., 1978; Wallen et al., 1989; Viana et al., 1993; Safronov and Vogel, 1998). Experimental as well as model studies have indicated that the conductances and currents associated with the AHP are very important for:

(i) the setting of F_{min} (Kernell, 1965b),

(ii) contributing to the MN 'gain', a smaller AHP (smaller $g_{K(Ca)}$) leading to a higher f-I slope (e.g. Hounsgaard and Kiehn, 1989; Wallen et al., 1989; Berger et al., 1992; Viana et al., 1993; see also Fig.1 and corresponding model calculations, e.g. Kernell, 1968),

(iii) causing part of the first phase of adaptation (effect of 'summing' of AHPs; e.g. Kernell, 1972; Kernell and Sjöholm, 1973; Baldissera and Gustafsson, 1974; Sawczuk et al., 1997). It is still uncertain to what an extent the prolonged time course of the AHP reflects a slow time constant for the potassium channel and/or a slow time constant for intracellular Ca^{++} sequestration.

(2) The intervals of a repetitive discharge might depend on the rate of rise of gradually increasing 'active' *prespike* local potentials, presumably generated by voltage-dependent cation-channels with slow kinetics around threshold membrane potential. Such properties are apparently often the dominating mechanisms for rhythmicity in, for instance,

crab axons stimulated with steady current (Hodgkin, 1948). In MNs, similar mechanisms might function in addition to those related to the AHP. Thus, Carp et al. (1991) published recordings suggesting that, in non-anaesthetized adult cats, slowly rising 'active' pre-spike potentials may cause MNs to fire regularly also at intervals longer than the AHPs following single spikes evoked by brief stimuli.

(3) The membrane potential might oscillate also in the absence of spikes; the addition of a sufficient intensity of steady depolarizing current would then cause spikes to appear at the moments of the oscillation peaks. However, in this case a further increase of steady injected current would not necessarily increase the rate of discharge. Although under most experimental circumstances this mechanism does not seem to be of great importance in MNs, it should be kept in mind for special cases, such as the repetitive firing seen during fictive locomotion in decerebrate cats. In this preparation, many MNs seem to discharge with decreased AHPs and, paradoxically, an f-I slope close to zero and with no evidence for the late phase of adaptation (Brownstone et al., 1992; Krawitz et al., 1996). Were the MNs in such cases (partly) discharging on the peaks of relatively synchronized waves of postsynaptic potentials? Or were the APs triggered by waves of rapid intrinsic membrane oscillations (cf. waves at lower rates in intracellular recordings of Hochman and Schmidt, 1998).

For in vitro preparations of the spinal cord, membrane oscillations may be made to appear in single cells by the application of NMDA and serotonin; after pharmacological block of APs, however, such voltage oscillations often seem to occur at rather slow rates as compared to those expected for rhythmic spikes in single cells (neonatal rat MNs, oscillations at about 1.8 Hz; MacLean et al., 1997; adult turtle MNs, illustrated case at about 0.1 Hz, Guertin and Hounsgaard, 1998). Slow intrinsic oscillations may be of importance in connection with the generation of rhythmic movements, such as locomotion.

It should be stressed that this simplified phenomenological dissection of the mechanisms for (moto-)neuronal repetitive firing does not mean to

imply that there are only two or three membrane processes involved in terms of permeabilities or ion channels. Each one of the mechanisms for 'rhythmicity' mentioned above will depend on the joint effects of several ion channels and, besides, other motoneuronal membrane permeabilities may contribute to the overall 'driving' current without being essential for the rhythmicity itself (e.g. plateau currents, see below).

Control of MN firing and MN discharge properties

Short-term effects

There is now much evidence indicating that in the acute context of on-going motor control, the discharge of MNs (and of other central neurons) can be synaptically influenced in two main ways:

(1) by the activity of 'driving' synapses that simply produce depolarizing and hyperpolarizing postsynaptic currents which cause MNs to discharge according to their intrinsic input/output properties for current-to-frequency transduction (i.e. according to their f-I relation). This might be a major function of the majority of synapses, explaining why the effects on repetitive discharges are often about the same for injected and synaptically produced currents (e.g. Granit et al., 1966; Kernell, 1969; Powers and Binder, 1995; Binder et al., 1998).

(2) by the activity of 'MN-modulating' synapses which cause changes to occur in the motoneuronal input/output properties, i.e. the MNs will now react differently to post-synaptic 'driving' currents. Activation of a given set of 'MN-modulating' synapses may produce a combination of various kinds of 'MN-modulation' (see below) plus additional 'driving' currents.

For the vertebrate spinal cord, MN-modulating postsynaptic effects on repetitive firing are now well known for monoaminergic synapses (e.g. serotonin, Hounsgaard et al., 1988; Hounsgaard and Kiehn, 1989; Wallen et al., 1989). It is useful, I think, to subdivide the presently known MN-modulating postsynaptic effects on repetitive discharge behavior into two main subcategories (for a model analysis, see Booth et al., 1997; for further examples of MN-modulation, see Binder et al., 1993, 1996):

(2a) The MN membrane properties may be altered such that low levels of depolarization now evoke persistent currents, typically inward in direction (depolarizing; e.g. Hounsgaard et al., 1988; Hounsgaard and Kiehn, 1989; MacLean et al., 1997; Lee and Heckman, 1998b; Bennett et al., 1998a). Such MN-generated persistent inward currents (PICs) will essentially play the role of 'driving currents' added to those produced by synaptic activity. The increased PIC-conductance may remain constant above a certain threshold of depolarization, or the PIC-activation might, hypothetically, be voltage dependent over a relatively wide range, adding more current for greater degrees of depolarization. In the latter case, the net effect would correspond to an increase of f-I slope; such effects have, however, apparently not yet been determined experimentally.

There is evidence indicating that the generation of PICs

(a) occurs in a time dependent manner (cf. facilitation of plateau potentials by repeated depolarizations, Svirskis and Hounsgaard, 1997; Bennett et al., 1998b);
(b) is different for different portions of the MN membrane (e.g. soma vs. dendrites, Skydsgaard and Hounsgaard, 1996; Booth et al., 1997; Bennett et al., 1998a);
(c) is different for MNs with different motor tasks (e.g. MNs likely to be equipped with fatigue-resistant muscle fibers show better-sustained plateau firing, Lee and Heckman, 1998a).

(2b) The size and, possibly, the time course of the conductances and currents underlying the AHP might become altered. A decreased intensity and/or a faster time course of these currents would increase the f-I slope of the MNs (Fig.1) and, hence, markedly influence the effects of various kinds of synaptic 'drive' onto the same cell. Serotonin is known to decrease the size of AHPs and, consequently, increase the f-I slope (Hounsgaard and Kiehn, 1989; Wallen et al., 1989; Berger et al., 1992).

It should be remembered that the effective intensity of the AHP-current depends on the product between the relevant postspike conductance increase and the 'driving force' for the AHP-current at the threshold for AP initiation, i.e. the difference between the equilibrium potential for the AHP-current and the voltage threshold. Thus, an increased f-I slope would also result from MN-modulating synaptic activity that caused a decrease in the voltage threshold.

A decrease of the time constant for the decline of the AHP-conductance (i.e. making the AHP faster) would not only increase the f-I slope but it would also make the MN fire at higher rates (cf. Fig. 1); such a short-term effect will still have to be demonstrated experimentally. It is, however, interesting to note that human experiments have suggested that the F_{min} of MNs may change depending on their tasks in voluntary motor behavior (i.e. depending on synaptic input; cf. Tax et al., 1989; Vander Linden et al., 1991). Furthermore, the time course of AHPs is known to be influenced by various long-term conditions (see below).

Long-term influences

Both the AHP-properties and those underlying the MN excitability (e.g. input resistance, R_{in}; specific membrane resistance, R_m; etc.) are varying systematically across MN populations, AHPs generally being longer and MN-excitabilities higher (lower current threshold, higher R_{in} and R_m) for MNs of slow-twitch units than for those with faster muscle fibers (review: Kernell, 1992). Also in the adult state, both sets of mechanisms may be manipulated by changing the long-term use and/or environment of the MNs. Thus, the time course of motoneuronal AHPs may change as a result of spinalization and muscle activation (Czéh et al., 1978) or cross-reinnervation (Foehring et al., 1987). Long-term stimulation of the motor nerves has recently been shown to increase both AHP duration and excitability for (some of the) MNs (Munson et al., 1997). Intriguing questions in this context include those concerning the nature of the long-term regulating molecules (role of neurotrophins?).

Future perspectives

Most future perspectives arise, of course, as extrapolations of what is happening now. Thus, it is evident that in the coming years we will learn much more about the ionic bases of the input/output relations of MNs and how these can be influenced by various kinds of 'MN-modulating' synapses (see contributions of Hultborn, Heckman and Hounsgaard in this volume). Besides such crucial enhancements in 'acute' MN understanding, another important and active field of study concerns the ways in which MN properties may be regulated

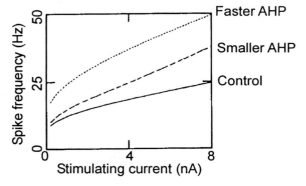

Fig. 1. Schematic illustration of how 'MN-modulating' synapses might influence the input-output relation of a (moto-)neuron via effects on the size or time course of the conductance changes underlying the afterhyperpolarization (AHP-conductance). Relation between spike frequency (Hz) and supra-threshold intensity of injected stimulating current (nA) in a simple neuron model, as shown for a 'Control' case (continuous line) and for two different hypothetical instances of additional synaptic MN-modulation (interrupted lines): 'Smaller AHP' and 'Faster AHP'. In the former case, the postspike AHP-conductance was decreased to half its control value; the f-I slope was then practically doubled. A completely equivalent effect would have been obtained by a 50% decrease of the driving force for the AHP-current (i.e. a decreased difference between the voltage threshold and the equilibrium potential for the AHP-current). In case of the 'Faster AHP', the size of the AHP-conductance was equal to the control value but the time constant for the postspike decline of the AHP-conductance had been decreased to half of the control value. The f-I slope was then doubled and the model fired at higher rates than for the case of decreased AHP amplitude. The calculations were all made for simple threshold-crossing models (Kernell, 1968): each spike had a fixed threshold and was succeeded by an increased potassium conductance that declined with time in a simple exponential manner (time constant of decline in control case: 20 ms).

at longer time-scales. A further example of problems still to be tackled is briefly mentioned below.

Tonic firing properties in MNs: why so vulnerable?

When considering a physiological function, such as the repetitive firing of MNs, one should not forget that, in a pathological context, things might happen which are not simple variations on the normal theme. Motoneurons are generally large but tend, paradoxically, to be vulnerable cells. In a recent in vitro investigation it was noted that hypoglossal MNs had a high vulnerability to the mechanical and metabolic stress associated with the preparation of brain stem slices. Measurements showed that the hypoglossal MNs had a low calcium buffering capacity, and the authors suggested that this contributed to their marked vulnerability (Lips and Keller, 1998).

For MNs of the spinal cord, a slight damage produced by a penetrating microelectrode will cause many of these fairly large neurons to turn 'phasic', i.e. they lose their ability to discharge continuously in response to a steady activating current (Kernell, 1965a). Anecdotal evidence suggests (but does not prove) that this kind of vulnerability might be much more marked for large spinal MNs than for various other kinds of smaller neurons. The loss of 'tonic' firing properties could not be a result of mere depolarization (then the cells would simply start firing) but might be the consequence of something leaking in from the outside. One candidate, again, is calcium. Thus, in diseased MNs, phasic firing properties might conceivably occur if the intracellular mechanisms for calcium buffering and removal were deranged. Calcium is thought to play a role in degenerative MN disease (amyotrophic lateral sclerosis, ALS), and MNs that are susceptible to ALS have less well developed capacities for calcium buffering than is the case for more ALS-resistant MNs (for further information and references, see Appel et al., 1995; Elliott and Snider, 1995; Morrison et al., 1998). Even in the presence of a substantial number of still living MNs, the motor disability of an ALS patient might be considerable if (many of) these MNs had lost their capacity for maintained repetitive firing.

References

Adrian, E.D. (1932) *The mechanism of nervous action.* Oxford University Press, London.

Appel, S.H., Smith, R.G., Alexianu, M., Siklos, L., Engelhardt, J., Colom, L.V. and Stefani, E. (1995) Increased intracellular calcium triggered by immune mechanisms in amyotrophic lateral sclerosis. *Clin. Neurosci.*, 3: 368–374.

Bakels, R. and Kernell, D. (1993) 'Average' but not 'continuous' speed-match between motoneurons and muscle units of rat tibialis anterior. *J. Neurophysiol.*, 70: 1300–1306.

Baldissera, F. and Gustafsson, B. (1974) Firing behaviour of a neurone model based on the afterhyperpolarization conductance time course and algebraical summation. Adaptation and steady state firing. *Acta Physiol. Scand.*, 92: 27–47.

Bennett, D.J., Hultborn, H., Fedirchuk, B. and Gorassini, M. (1998a) Synaptic activation of plateaus in hindlimb motoneurons of decerebrate cats. *J. Neurophysiol.*, 80: 2023–2037.

Bennett, D.J., Hultborn, H., Fedirchuk, B. and Gorassini, M. (1998b) Short-term plasticity in hindlimb motoneurons of decerebrate cats. *J. Neurophysiol.*, 80: 2038–2045.

Berger, A.J., Bayliss, D.A. and Viana, F. (1992) Modulation of neonatal rat hypoglossal motoneuron excitability by serotonin. *Neurosci. Lett.*, 143: 164–168.

Binder, M.D., Heckman, C.J. and Powers, R.K. (1993) How different afferent inputs control motoneuron discharge and the output of the motoneuron pool. *Curr. Opin. Neurobiol.*, 3: 1028–1034.

Binder, M. D., Heckman, C. J. and Powers, R. K. (1996) The physiological control of motoneuron activity. In: *Handbook of Physiology. Exercise. Regulation and Integration of Multiple Systems.* New York: Am. Physiol. Soc., sect. 12, vol. I, p. 3–53.

Binder, M.D., Robinson, F.R. and Powers, R.K. (1998) Distribution of effective synaptic currents in cat triceps surae motoneurons. VI. Contralateral pyramidal tract. *J. Neurophysiol.*, 80: 241–248.

Booth, V., Rinzel, J. and Kiehn, O. (1997) Compartmental model of vertebrate motoneurons for Ca^{2+}-dependent spiking and plateau potentials under pharmacological treatment. *J. Neurophysiol.*, 78: 3371–3385.

Brownstone, R.M., Jordan, L.M., Kriellaars, D.J., Noga, B.R. and Shefchyk, S.J. (1992) On the regulation of repetitive firing in lumbar motoneurones during fictive locomotion in the cat. *Exp. Brain Res.*, 90: 441–455.

Carp, J.S., Powers, R.K. and Rymer, W.Z. (1991) Alterations in motoneuron properties induced by acute dorsal spinal hemisection in the decerebrate cat. *Exp. Brain Res.*, 83: 539–548.

Czéh, G., Gallego, R., Kudo, N. and Kuno, M. (1978) Evidence for the maintenance of motoneurone properties by muscle activity. *J. Physiol. (Lond.)*, 281: 239–252.

Elliott, J.L. and Snider, W.D. (1995) Parvalbumin is a marker of ALS-resistant motor neurons. *Neuroreport*, 6: 449–452.

Foehring, R.C., Sypert, G.W. and Munson, J.B. (1987) Motor-unit properties following cross-reinnervation of cat lateral gastrocnemius and soleus muscles with medial gastrocnemius nerve. II. Influence of muscle on motoneurons. *J. Neurophysiol.*, 57: 1227–1245.

Granit, R., Kernell, D. and Lamarre, Y. (1966) Algebraical summation in synaptic activation of motoneurones firing within the primary range to injected currents. *J. Physiol. (Lond.)*, 187: 379–399.

Granit, R., Kernell, D. and Shortess, G.K. (1963) Quantitative aspects of repetitive firing of mammalian motoneurones, caused by injected currents. *J. Physiol. (Lond.)*, 168: 911–931.

Guertin, P.A. and Hounsgaard J. (1998) Chemical and electrical stimulation induce rhythmic motor activity in an in vitro preparation of the spinal cord from adult turtles. *Neurosci. Lett.*, 245: 5–8.

Hochman, S. and Schmidt,, B.J. (1998) Whole cell recordings of lumbar motoneurons during locomotor-like activity in the In vitro neonatal rat spinal cord. *J. Neurophysiol.*, 79: 743–752.

Hodgkin, A.L. (1948) The local electric changes associated with repetitive action in a non-medullated nerve. *J. Physiol. (Lond.)*, 107: 165–181.

Hounsgaard, J., Hultborn, H., Jespersen, B. and Kiehn, O. (1988) Bistability of α-motoneurones in the decerebrate cat and in the acute spinal cat after intravenous 5-hydroxytryptophan. *J. Physiol. (Lond.)*, 405: 345–367.

Hounsgaard, J. and Kiehn, O. (1989) Serotonin-induced bistability of turtle motoneurones caused by a nifedipine-sensitive calcium plateau potential. *J. Physiol. (Lond.)*, 414: 265–282.

Kernell, D. (1965a) The adaptation and the relation between discharge frequency and current strength of cat lumbosacral motoneurones stimulated by long-lasting injected currents. *Acta Physiol. Scand.*, 65: 65–73.

Kernell, D. (1965b) The limits of firing frequency in cat lumbosacral motoneurones possessing different time course of afterhyperpolarization. *Acta Physiol. Scand.*, 65: 87–100.

Kernell, D. (1968) The repetitive impulse discharge of a simple neurone model compared to that of spinal motoneurones. *Brain Res.*, 11: 685–687.

Kernell, D. (1969) Synaptic conductance changes and the repetitive impulse discharge of spinal motoneurones. *Brain Res.*, 15: 291–294.

Kernell, D. (1972) The early phase of adaptation in repetitive impulse discharges of cat spinal motoneurones. *Brain Res.*, 41: 184–186.

Kernell, D. (1992) Organized variability in the neuromuscular system: a survey of task-related adaptations. *Arch. Ital. Biol.*, 130: 19–66.

Kernell, D., Bakels, R. and Copray, J.C.V.M. (1999) Discharge properties of motoneurones: how are they matched to the properties and use of their muscle units? *J. Physiol. (Paris)*, 93: 87–96.

Kernell, D. and Monster, A.W. (1982) Time course and properties of late adaptation in spinal motoneurones in the cat. *Exp. Brain Res.*, 46: 191–196.

Kernell, D. and Sjöholm, H. (1973) Repetitive impulse firing: comparisons between neurone models based on voltage clamp equations and spinal motoneurones. *Acta Physiol. Scand.*, 87: 40–56.

Krawitz, S., Brownstone, R.M., Noga, B.R. and Jordan, L.M. (1996) Can the nervous system overcome a possible central fatigue process – late adaptation? *Muscle & Nerve*, Suppl. 4: S52.

Krnjevic, K., Puil, E. and Werman, R. (1978) EGTA and motoneuronal after-potentials. *J. Physiol. (Lond.)*, 275: 199–223.

Lee, R.H. and Heckman, C.J. (1998a) Bistability in spinal motoneurons in vivo: systematic variations in rhythmic firing patterns. *J. Neurophysiol.*, 80: 572–582.

Lee, R.H. and Heckman, C.J. (1998b) Bistability in spinal motoneurons in vivo: systematic variations in persistent inward currents. *J. Neurophysiol.*, 80: 583–593.

Lips, M.B. and Keller, B.U. (1998) Endogenous calcium buffering in motoneurones of the nucleus hypoglossus from mouse. *J. Physiol. (Lond.)*, 511: 105–117.

MacLean, J.N., Schmidt, B.J. and Hochman, S. (1997) NMDA receptor activation triggers voltage oscillations, plateau potentials and bursting in neonatal rat lumbar motoneurons in vitro. *Eur. J. Neurosci.*, 9: 2702–2711.

Morrison, B.M., Hof, P.R. and Morrison, J.H. (1998) Determinants of neuronal vulnerability in neurodegenerative diseases. *Ann. Neurol.*, Suppl 1 44: S32–44.

Munson, J.B., Foehring, R.C., Mendell, L.M. and Gordon, T. (1997) Fast-to-slow conversion following chronic low-frequency activation of medial gastrocnemius muscle in cats. II. Motoneuron properties. *J. Neurophysiol.*, 77: 2605–2615.

Powers, R.K. and Binder, M.D. (1995) Effective synaptic current and motoneuron firing rate modulation. *J. Neurophysiol.*, 74: 793–801.

Safronov, B.V. and Vogel, W. (1998) Large conductance Ca^{2+}-activated K^+ channels in the soma of rat motoneurones. *J. Membr. Biol.*, 162: 9–15.

Sawczuk, A., Powers, R.K. and Binder, M.D. (1995) Spike frequency adaptation studied in hypoglossal motoneurons of the rat. *J. Neurophysiol.*, 73: 1799–1810.

Sawczuk, A., Powers, R.K. and Binder, M.D. (1997) Contribution of outward currents to spike-frequency adaptation in hypoglossal motoneurons of the rat. *J. Neurophysiol.*, 78: 2246–2253.

Skydsgaard, M. and Hounsgaard, J. (1996) Multiple actions of iontophoretically applied serotonin on motorneurones in the turtle spinal cord in vitro. *Acta Physiol. Scand.*, 158: 301–310.

Spielmann, J.M., Laouris, Y., Nordstrom, M.A., Robinson, G.A., Reinking, R.M. and Stuart, D.G. (1993) Adaptation of cat motoneurons to sustained and intermittent extracellular activation. *J. Physiol. (Lond.)*, 464: 75–120.

Svirskis, G. and Hounsgaard, J. (1997) Depolarization-induced facilitation of a plateau-generating current in ventral horn neurons in the turtle spinal cord. *J. Neurophysiol.*, 78: 1740–1742.

Tax, A.A.M., Van der Gon, J.J.D., Gielen, C.C.A.M. and Van den Tempel, C.M.M. (1989) Differences in the activation of M biceps brachii in the control of slow isotonic movements and isometric contractions. *Exp. Brain Res.*, 76: 55–63.

Vander Linden, D.W., Kukulka, C.G. and Soderberg, G.L. (1991) The effect of muscle length on motor unit discharge characteristics in human tibialis anterior muscle. *Exp. Brain Res.*, 84: 210–218.

Viana, F., Bayliss, D.A. and Berger, A.J. (1993) Multiple potassium conductances and their role in action potential repolarization and repetitive firing behavior of neonatal rat hypoglossal motoneurons. *J. Neurophysiol.*, 69: 2150–2163.

Wallen, P., Buchanan, J.T., Grillner, S., Hill, R.H., Christenson, J. and Hokfelt, T. (1989) Effects of 5-hydroxytryptamine on the afterhyperpolarization, spike frequency regulation, and oscillatory membrane properties in lamprey spinal cord neurons. *J. Neurophysiol.*, 61: 759–768.

M.D. Binder (Ed.)
Progress in Brain Research, Vol 123
© 1999 Elsevier Science BV. All rights reserved.

CHAPTER 3

Plateau potentials and their role in regulating motoneuronal firing

Hans Hultborn*

Department of Medical Physiology, The Panum Institute, Faculty of Health Sciences, University of Copenhagen, Copenhagen, Denmark

RESULTS

Earlier results and present questions

In 1976 Hultborn et al. described that brief trains of short stretches (vibration) to the triceps surae muscle in the decerebrate cat triggered a sustained increase in the EMG activity in addition to the ordinary short latency (monosynaptic) response. Sometimes this activity slowly fell off, but in many cases the increased EMG activity stayed at a constant level for minutes. In such cases, brief trains of activity in other afferent systems (high threshold afferents or cutaneous afferents) could terminate the motoneuronal discharge at any time (Fig. 1A). Granit and his collaborators (1957) had described a very similar maintained excitability increase (initiated by a few repeated brief muscle pulls) that they ascribed to a 'post-tetanic potentiation'. Hultborn et al. (1976, 1980) suggested that the phenomenon could be due to reverberating activity within closed (inter-)neuronal loops, which could provide a maintained excitatory drive of the motoneurones (Fig. 1A; cf. Forbes, 1929), although intrinsic motoneuronal properties were mentioned as an alternative. Indeed, at the very same time, Schwindt and Crill published a series of articles (Schwindt and Crill, 1980a–c) on a persistent

inward current in motoneurones, which had the properties to maintain motoneuronal activity following a brief excitatory input. The following analysis in the decerebrate unanaesthetized cat (Hounsgaard et al., 1988; Conway et al., 1988) certainly demonstrated that the phenomenon described by Hultborn et al. (1976, 1980) could be explained by intrinsic properties in the individual motoneurone.

Figure 1 B1 shows self-sustained firing in a motoneurone that is initiated and terminated by depolarising and hyperpolarising current pulses respectively. In many cases, when the motoneurones started with a ('spontaneous') steady firing, these pulses could switch the firing frequency between two stable levels (bistable firing). The presence of plateau potentials is best shown following inactivation of the fast sodium spikes (either by a period of heavy depolarization or by injection of the local anaesthetic QX314; see Brownstone et al., 1994, Fig. 1 B2).

When the plateau potentials were present, there was a peculiar frequency acceleration *during* the current pulse (Fig. 1 B3), which had not been described in the classical work on firing adaptation (Granit et al., 1963; Kernell, 1965). Reflecting the activation of the persistant inward current, this firing acceleration had a long delay and slow onset. The initiation of the plateau could also be seen in the response to long-lasting 'triangular' current pulses (Fig. 1 C). At the pulse onset, the membrane

*Corresponding author. Tel.: int. 45-35327461; Fax: int 35327499; e-mail: H.Hultborn@mfi.ku.dk

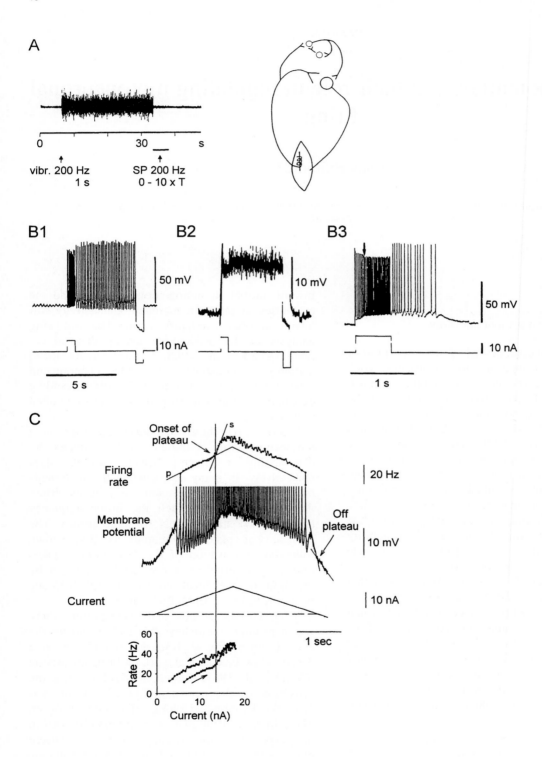

A

vibr. 200 Hz
1 s

SP 200 Hz
0 - 10 x T

B1

B2

50 mV

10 mV

10 nA

5 s

B3

50 mV

10 nA

1 s

C

Onset of
plateau

s

Firing
rate

p

20 Hz

Membrane
potential

Off
plateau

10 mV

Current

10 nA

1 sec

Rate (Hz)

60

40

20

0

0   10   20
Current (nA)

potential increased linearly with the current until firing began, at which point the mean potential transiently dropped due to the afterhyperpolarisation. Then, the membrane potential (and the firing rate) again increased linearly with the current until a critical transition frequency was reached, where the frequency and (potential) increased steeply. This step rise, or jump, in firing frequency indicated the initiation of the plateau (or rather the associated non-inactivating inward currents), since a reduction in injected current after the jump did not bring the firing rate back to that before the jump at matched current levels. This can be seen most clearly by plotting the firing rate against the current amplitude and observing the rate difference at a given current level (Fig. 1 C, bottom graph; referred to as 'counter-clockwise hysteresis').

To summarize, when using classical 'current-clamp' recording conditions the persistant inward current is visualized most directly as a plateau potential after inactivation of the Na^+ spikes. The 'plateau current' is also reflected in the firing pattern as: (1) self-sustained firing, (2) frequency acceleration during constant current injection and (3) a counter-clockwise f/I hysteresis in response to triangular current pulses.

All these signs of plateau properties in the unanaesthetised, decerebrate cat disappears during general anaesthesia, or following spinalisation. This may explain why plateaus were not described in the classical work on motoneurones from the laboratories of Eccles and Granit. The analysis by the Copenhagen group (references below) demon-

strated that the plateau properties were contingent upon an active serotonergic raphe spinal innervation, as injection of the serotonin blocker methysergide was shown to prevent bistable firing behaviour (judged from recordings from the peripheral nerve, Crone et al., 1988). Furthermore, the bistable firing behaviour also disappears following spinalisation, and returns (in the spinal cat) either after injection of the serotonin precursor 5-HTP (which is converted to 5-HT in the terminals; Hounsgaard et al., 1988), the noradrenergic precursor L-DOPA, or the noradrenergic receptor agonist clonidine (Conway et al., 1988). This suggests that both serotonergic and noradrenergic pathways are involved in regulating the plateau properties in motoneurones.

As it is difficult to analyse the ionic basis of the monoamine-dependent plateau potentials under in vivo conditions, Hounsgaard and Kiehn (1989) developed a suitable in vitro preparation of adult turtle spinal cord. In normal medium motoneuronal firing appeared very similar to the classical description of the cat motoneurone. When serotonin was added to the superfusion, the motoneurones displayed plateau properties as described above. Further analysis demonstrated that the 'plateau-current' was at least in part carried by a non-inactivating nifedipine-sensitive Ca^{2+} current (Hounsgaard and Kiehn, 1989). Hounsgaard and Kiehn (1989) originally suggested that the permissive effect by 5-HT was due to removal of an opposing outward current thus 'uncovering' the plateau potentials. Later studies in Hounsgaard's

Fig. 1. Maintained motoneurone activity and plateau potentials. A. Long lasting EMG activity in the soleus muscle following a short train of stretches (vibration, 200 Hz, 1s) to activate muscle spindle Ia afferents. The maintained activity was terminated by a stimulus train (200 Hz) to the cutaneous branches of the superficial peroneal (SP) nerve. Unanaestetized decerebrate cat preparation. (From Hultborn et al. 1976). B. Sustained shifts in excitability triggered by depolarizing and hyperpolarizing currents injected intracellularly. Upper traces are intracellular recordings, lower traces monitor the amount and timing of injected current. B1. Sustained repetitive firing initiated by a short depolarizing current pulse and terminated by a short hyperpolarizing current pulse. B2. In this record the spike-generating mechanism was inactivated. Current pulses now evoked and terminated plateau potentials. B3. Record from another motoneurone demonstrates the frequency acceleration during the rectangular current pulse as a sign of induction of the plateau current. Decerebrate, unanaestetized cat preparation (rearranged from Hounsgaard et al. 1988). C. Firing pattern during injection of triangular current pulses. The figure shows the firing rate (first trace); intracellular recording of the membrane potential and spike activity (second trace); injected current (third trace); graph at bottom shows the frequency plotted against current for the data shown above. A linearly increasing current (ramp) was injected into the cell, while measuring the membrane potential and instantaneous firing frequency. The plateau was considered to be initiated at the point where the frequency and potential jumped steeply (plateau threshold), and a subsequent decrease in current did not reverse this steep jump. In this case the plateau threshold was 27Hz, and remained activated after the cell stopped firing, until the point marked with an arrow. Tops of spikes were clipped. (Modified from Bennet et al. 1998a).

group have demonstrated that the plateau properties are regulated by multiple neuromodulators. As reviewed by Delgado–Lezama and Hounsgaard (Chapter 5 in this volume), the transmitter facilitation of plateau properties involves regulation of several conductances, including an enhancement of the nifedipine sensitive Ca^{2+}-conductance, in addition to the reduction of outward currents. The localization of the plateau current along the soma-dendritic membrane is another question of great functional significance. Using extracellular electrical fields to polarize the dendrites and the soma of the turtle motoneurones differentially (Hounsgaard and Kiehn, 1993) it was shown that the persistent plateau current is mainly localized in distal dendrites.

The preceding summary opens for several questions, which have to be answered before the functional importance of the plateau potentials in motoneurones can be evaluated. First, are the plateau potentials seen in the decerebrate cat and in the in vitro preparation of the turtle spinal cord an 'experimental artefact'? Or are they actually expressed under normal circumstances – in the freely moving animal, and in humans? This question will be further addressed later, and here reference will only be made to the work by Eken and Kiehn (1989) in which bistable firing behaviour was indeed observed from single motor units recorded in unrestrained rats, thus supporting the presence of plateau potentials under normal behaviour. Secondly, given the presence of plateaus, what thresholds do they have in relation to recruitment threshold, or firing rate of the motoneurone? More explicitly, are the plateau potentials initiated only when the greatest efforts are required, (i.e. the very strongest contractions), or are they generated at the recruitment threshold of the motor unit? Thirdly, how large is the plateau current in relation to the currents underlying the classical synaptic excitation and during what kind of motor behaviours are the plateau potentials present?

Activation of the plateau potentials in motoneurones during maintained synaptic input

When the persistent plateau current was induced by intracellular current injection alone (Hounsgaard et

al., 1998), its threshold was typically reached when the firing rate was in the range of 20–50 Hz. In some cells, in particular those innervating slow motor units, the counter-clockwise hysteresis was seen also at very low firing frequencies. The latter results agrees with the observation that a brief period of synaptic excitation could trigger a maintained tonic activity (cf. the EMG recording in Fig. 1A). The possibility that a localised depolarisation of the soma by currents through the recording microelectrode, could make a difference in relation to the more natural distributed input by *synaptic* excitation, was first raised by Hounsgaard et al. (1988). When Hounsgaard and Kiehn (1993; in the turtle) demonstrated that the plateau current mainly originates from the distal dendrites, it was obvious that this problem required further attention. It was on this background that Bennett et al. (1998a) systematically investigated, in triceps surae motoneurones, the threshold of plateau potentials to intracellular current injections during tonic (subthreshold) synaptic excitation and inhibition. In this study the synaptic excitation was evoked by maintained stretch of the triceps surae muscle, and the inhibition by maintained trains of stimulation of the 'antagonist' nerve (reciprocal inhibition). The main finding was that the plateau threshold decreased substantially during synaptic excitation. Of course, as would be expected from simple algebraic summation of inward currents, the synaptic excitation reduced the amount of current needed to initiate firing (recruitment) and to reach plateau threshold. The novel finding was that the intracellular current ramps initiated the plateau at significantly less depolarized membrane potential (as recorded from the soma), or at lower frequencies of firing (Fig. 2) than without tonic synaptic excitation. The reduction in plateau threshold was graded with the amount of excitation; with larger stretches, the plateau threshold was often lowered to near the initial recruitment level. Figure 2 also shows that synaptic inhibition had the opposite effect and increased the plateau threshold. This increase was also graded with the amount of inhibition, and with the largest amounts of inhibition it became virtually impossible to induce the plateau current. When the spikes were blocked with QX 314, it was possible to visualize the same changes in plateau threshold by measuring directly the membrane potential at which they were evoked (seen from the soma) (Bennett et al., 1998a).

Activation of plateau potentials by synaptic excitation without current injections

Under natural circumstances the control of motoneuronal activity solely depends on synaptic excitation and inhibition. Therefore it is important

to determine the plateau threshold with synaptic excitation without additional current injection. As the quantitative effect of synaptic excitation (and inhibition) was graded, one may ask whether plateau potentials can be generated at – or even below – the recruitment level. To answer that question the recruitment of the motoneurone has to be achieved by increasing synaptic excitation without additional current injection through the recording microelectrode. Burke (1968) has shown that activation with constant stretch can only be

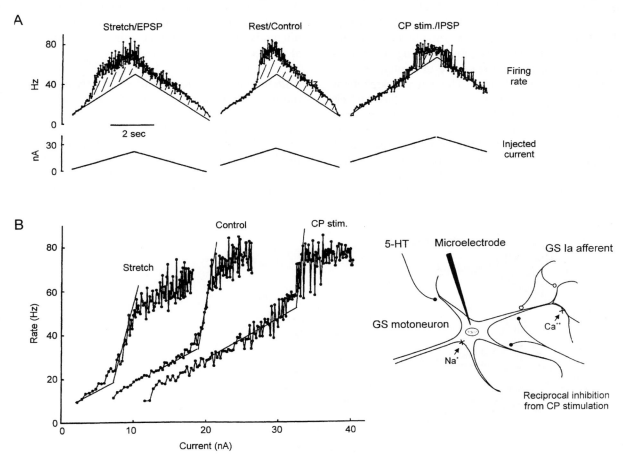

Fig. 2. Influence of tonic synaptic input on plateau threshold in a GS motoneurone. Plateau activation by intracellular current injection was studied with and without a steady (tonic) peripheral synaptic input (Ia afferent excitation, and reciprocal Ia inhibition, cf inset drawing). A. Middle plot, control situation similar to that of Fig. 1C. Left plot, effect of tonic muscle stretch (10 mm) applied throughout the current ramp shown. This tonic synaptic excitation was adjusted to be below the recruitment level (subthreshold) before the current ramp. Right plot, effect of tonic inhibitory nerve stimulation (IPSPs from CP stim. 2T, 100Hz). Hashed regions show contributions of plateau in each case. B. Composite of results from A, showing responses during ascending phase of ramp plotted against current. Note that the plateau threshold frequency is lowered by EPSPs and raised by IPSPs (Modified from Bennett et al. 1998a).

achieved in low threshold ('slow') motoneurones and presently the results are therefore limited to this group.

Sinusoidal muscle stretch was used to increase (decrease) synaptic excitation dynamically – some times paired with different levels of constant *negative* currents to keep the neuron below firing threshold. An example is illustrated in Fig. 3 (Bennett et al., 1998a). When the cell was hyperpolarised sufficiently, it responded phasically to muscle stretch following the typical response pattern of Ia afferents to stretch in paralysed preparations (lowest intracellular recording in Fig. 3A, bias −9nA). When the membrane potential was allowed to depolarise by reducing the hyperpolarising current, the response to stretch became larger and more prolonged. This voltage-dependent amplification and prolongation of the stretch response, indicative of plateau activation, occurred *below* the firing level of the motoneurone This motoneurone was actually recruited at the top of the plateau potential (and occurred already with a bias of −1nA). As seen from the records obtained at different negative bias, the plateau potential

enhanced the synaptic excitation by around 8 mV. The depolarisation caused by the muscle stretch was thus increased at least three-fold, when the negative bias current was reduced enough to permit the plateau potential to develop. Similar plateau activation at, or below, the recruitment level was seen in 12 out 14 motoneurones (Bennett et al., 1998a).

The plateau activation during sinusoidal muscle stretch could often be judged from the firing rate profiles. When the unit was recruited together with the induction of the plateau potential, the firing started abruptly, at a frequency which was significantly above the minimal firing rate (Bennett et al., 1998a).

Plateau potentials in normal motor behaviour as judged from the firing pattern of motor units

In order to evaluate whether plateau potentials are present in intact animals, Eken and Kiehn (1989) used single motor unit recording from freely moving rats. The experimental setup allowed synchronised recording of the EMG-activity and

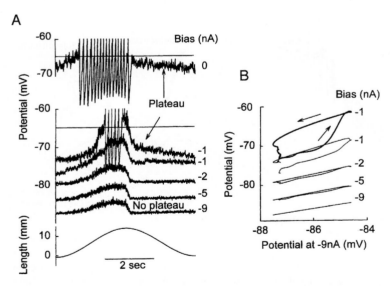

Fig. 3. Stretch activated plateau potentials. A. Response of a soleus motoneuron to sinusoidal muscle stretch with different current bias. Note the amplification and prolongation of the stretch evoked response as the hyperpolarizing bias was reduced. The plateau was tonically activated in the 0nA condition. Firing occurred in this 0nA condition, so it is shown displaced vertically for clarity. B. Input-output properties of the motoneurone. Stretch responses from A plotted against the stretch response obtained at the most hyperpolarized level (− 9nA); the latter was assumed to represent the synaptic input without influence of the plateau current. The arrows indicate the direction of time.(Modified from Bennett et al. 1998a).

the movement, together with afferent nerve stimulation to produce brief periods of synaptic excitation or inhibition. The initial study focused on the firing behaviour of soleus motor units during quiet standing. In this case it was possible to 'reproduce' the bistable firing behaviour seen previously in the cat motoneurones in decerebrate preparations. Abrupt maintained increases in firing frequency (typically from 10 to 20 Hz) were evoked by trains of low threshold afferent stimulation of the homonymous nerve (causing a burst of excitation), while lasting decreases in firing rate (typically from 20 to 10 Hz) were triggered from cutaneous nerves. The frequency jumps could not be graded, but appeared in an 'all-or-none' fashion. Furthermore, they occurred in individual motor units without any change in firing frequency of other simultaneously active units. Therefore, it was suggested that the frequency shifts were related to activation of intrinsic properties of individual motoneurones rather than by long lasting changes in the descending drive. Eken (1998) further investigated the dissociation between activity in different motor units. During tonic muscle activity (quiet standing) individual motor units were recruited in a seemingly random manner, with a 'rotation' of active motor units over time. Again, this behaviour could be explained by 'random' activation/deactivation of plateau potentials in individual low threshold motor units.

Bistable firing with shifts between two stable frequencies may be expected if the Na^+ spike threshold is lower than the plateau threshold, but not if the plateau is induced below the spike threshold (thus before recruitment) (see also Kiehn and Eken, 1998). In the latter case the plateau activation would boast the firing rate at recruitment. It would be expected to see an abrupt jump in frequency to a rate significantly higher than the minimal firing frequency of the unit. Such expectations were supported by the observations on the firing behaviour in intracellularly recorded cat motoneurones in which the plateau potential is activated synaptically just below the recruitment level (Bennett et al., 1998a). With single motor unit recording from unrestrained rats a similar pattern was indeed observed at recruitment by phasic muscle stretch (Gorassini et al., 1999) and during

locomotion (Gorassini et al., 1995 and unpublished).

The firing pattern in human motoneurones has also been investigated for bistable firing during tonic voluntary contractions in combination with short-lasting bursts of vibration (Kiehn and Eken, 1997; Gorassini et al., 1998). Although a bistable firing pattern was never demonstrated, short periods of vibration often recruited new motor units into a 'self-sustained' maintained activity. As this occurred without an increase in firing frequency of other active motor units (simultaneously recorded), it was assumed that the descending drive had remained constant. Once more, these results are thus compatible with the notion that activation of the plateau potentials are actually part of the normal recruitment process.

It is not obvious how one could reconcile the seemingly contradictory findings on the presence of bistable rate shifts in rat soleus motor units during quiet standing (Eken and Kiehn, 1989; indicating a plateau threshold above firing threshold) with the abrupt recruitment but lack of 'bistability' during phasic stretch and walking (Gorassini et al., 1999, indicating a plateau threshold at, or below, firing threshold). One possibility would be that these different conditions are correlated with differences in the dynamic regulation of the plateau properties from descending fiber systems. As reviewed by Jacobs and Fournal (1997), the activity of the descending serotonergic system is strongly correlated to the behavioural situation. It may be intuitively understood that decreasing serotonergic innervation of the motoneurones would cause an increase of plateau threshold, and this has also been formally demonstrated in a compartmental model of vertebrate motoneurones (Booth et al., 1997).

Regulation of plateau properties by preceding activity

L-Ca^{2+} channels have complex properties with two different closed states with a low and high threshold for opening, respectively. There is an equilibrium between these two closed states, with preceding depolarisation increasing the probability for the low threshold state for several seconds. This results in a frequency-dependent facilitation of plateau potentials, which is underlying the 'wind-up' phenomenon in dorsal horn cells (Russo and Hounsgaard, 1996). The same mechanism was later demonstrated in turtle motoneurones (Svirskis and Hounsgaard, 1997). The frequency-dependent facilitation is also seen in cat motoneurones and it contributes significantly in reducing the plateau threshold (Bennett et al., 1998b). Figure 4 A illustrates the f/I relation for a motoneurone with a relatively high initial threshold for plateau activation during triangular ramp current injection. The current ramps were repeated with 3 s intervals. In this example, the first current ramp initiated the

plateau at a threshold frequency of about 35 Hz (open circles), the second at about 25 Hz (filled circles) and the third at 20 Hz (or below, squares). The facilitation was so powerful that the plateau threshold was reached with about 13 nA less than with the first ramp. In the present experimental situation, this facilitation was only induced when the depolarisation approached the plateau threshold and the effect lasted 10–20 s (Bennett et al., 1998b).

The effect of this frequency-dependent facilitation can also been seen in the EMG responses to muscle stretch. Figure 4 B shows inhibition of the

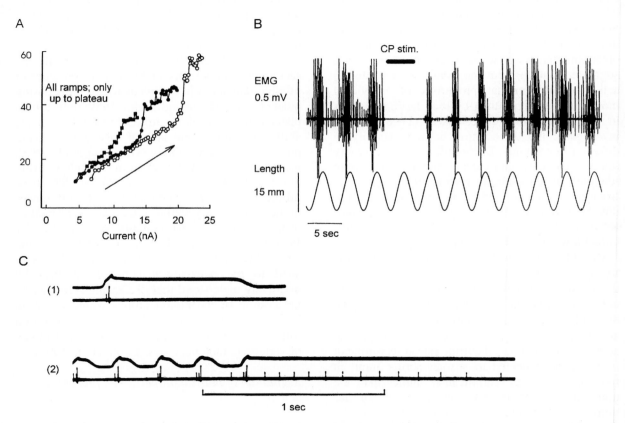

Fig. 4. Frequency dependent facilitation of plateau activation. A. Firing rates plotted against current during 3 successive ramp current injections at 3s intervals (triangular current ramps as in Fig. 1C and Fig. 2). For clarity only responses during the ascending phase of the ramp is shown. The arrow indicates direction of time. Note the overlap in firing in the three cases before the plateau was activated. B. EMG recorded from soleus muscle during continuous sinusoidal stretches of triceps surae. During a period the motoneurone pool was silenced by a long lasting nerve stimulation producing inhibition (CP nerve; 5T, 100Hz, indicated by the bar). Note that the motor unit responses (EMG) to stretch only grew slowly after the pool was silenced. (A-B modified from Bennett et al. 1998b). C. Illustration of a gastrocnemius motoneurone (recorded from a ventral root filament; lower traces) following muscle stretch (monitored in upper traces). Note that repeated stretches were needed to evoke a self-sustained activity (2). (Adapted from Granit et al. 1957).

tonic and phasic activity produced by a sinusoidal muscle stretch by a train of stimuli to the peroneal nerve (Per nerve) which lasted for more than 5 s. Following that pause (during which the frequency-dependent facilitation is supposed to have decayed), it took several cycles to rebuild the previous level of activity. Figure 4 C is illustrating an experiment by Granit et al. (1957) in which a similar build-up of the self-sustained firing in a single motor unit occurs with repeated muscle stretches. As described above, Granit et al. ascribed this to a 'post-tetanic potentiation', thought to occur at pre-motoneuronal level, but in all likelihood their results reflect the post-synaptic mechanism described here.

As described briefly above (and in more detail in the accompanying Chapter 5 by Delgado–Lezama and Hounsgaard, this volume) the plateau properties are controlled by a variety of transmitter systems. Little is known on how these regulatory systems are working under various types of motor activity. One exception is the serotonergic raphespinal projection to motoneurones. In this case chronic recording from single units in the relevant part of the raphe nuclei has revealed a strong relationship to the sleep-awake cycle and the degree of motor activity (Jacobs and Fornal, 1997). Changes from rest, to standing and walking is thus correlated with increasing activity in the raphespinal projection, which would first enable the plateau properties and then further decrease the plateau threshold.

Concluding remarks on the possible significance

In the decerebrate cat, the plateau potentials are readily evoked with intracellular current pulses. With synaptic excitation, they may be initiated at, or below, recruitment threshold. From the work with the classical 'current-clamp' recording, it is obvious that the plateau potentials greatly amplifies the synaptic excitation in the voltage region of the plateau threshold. Recent results using the 'voltage-clamp' technique have further quantified this current (Lee and Heckman, 1998a, b, Heckman and Lee, Chapter 4, this volume). While largely supporting previous conclusions, there are important new results regarding the inward current in differ-

ent types of motoneurones. For instance, even if the current is 'persistent', it shows a decay, which is much more rapid in 'fast' than in 'slow' motoneurones. This is likely to determine the tonic and phasic response properties of these types of motoneurones.

Although the evidence of plateau potentials under normal motor behaviour is circumstantial, it seems hard to find other explanations for the bistable firing of soleus motor units in the quietly sitting rat (Eken and Kiehn, 1989). Assuming that plateau potentials are indeed underlying this behaviour, it seems likely that the firing pattern at recruitment during more phasic movements in rats (Gorassini et al., 1995, 1999) and during voluntary movements in humans (Kiehn and Eken, 1997; Gorassini et al., 1998) reflects induction of plateau potentials at recruitment level, just as demonstrated in the decerebrate cat (Bennett et al., 1998a). During phasic motor activity motor units were often recruited to a high rate of discharge, often with an initial 'doublet' (i.e. > 100 Hz) even with slowly graded synaptic excitation (Gorassini et al., 1999). Such firing patterns have been shown to optimize the speed and amount of force production in the motor unit (Burke et al., 1969; Stein and Parmiggiani, 1979). Further analysis of single motor unit activity in humans during various movements may not only give further evidence for the presence of plateau potentials, but may also contribute to the understanding of how the flexible regulation of the plateau properties is used.

Acknowledgements

Major support has been given by the Danish Medical Research Council, the Novo Nordisk Foundation, the Lundbeck Foundation and the Danish Research Academy.

References

Bennett, D.J., Hultborn, H., Fedirchuk, B. and Gorassini, M. (1998a) Synaptic activation of plateaus in hindlimb motoneurons of decerebrate cats. *J. Neurophysiol.*, 80: 2023–2037.

Bennett, D.J., Hultborn, H., Fedirchuk, B. and Gorassini, M. (1998b) Short-term plasticity in hindlimb motoneurons of decerebrate cats. *J. Neurophysiol.*, 80: 2038–2045.

48

Booth, V., Rinzel, J. and Kiehn, O. (1997) Compartmental model of vertebrate motoneurons for Ca^{2+} spiking and plateau potentials under pharmacological treatment. *J. Neurophysiol.*, 78: 3371–3385.

Brownstone, R.M., Gossard, J.P. and Hultborn, H. (1994) Voltage-dependent excitation of motoneurones from spinal locomotor centres in the cat. *Exp. Brain Res.*, 102: 34–44.

Burke, R.E. (1968) Firing patterns of gastrocnemius motor units in the decerebrate cat. *J. Physiol.(Lond.)*, 196: 631–654.

Burke, R.E., Rudomin, P. and Zajac, F.E. (1969) Catch property in single mammalian motor units. *Science*, 168: 122–124.

Conway, B.A., Hultborn, H., Kiehn, O. and Mintz, I.(1988) Plateau potentials in α-motoneurons induced by intravenous injection of L-DOPA and clonidine in the spinal cat. *J. Physiol.*, 405: 369–384.

Crone, C., Hultborn, H., Kiehn, O., Mazieres, L. and Wigström, H. (1988) Maintained changes in motoneuronal excitability by short-lasting synaptic inputs in the decerebrate cat. *J. Physiol.*, 405: 321–343.

Eken, T. (1998) Spontaneous electromyographic activity in adult rat soleus muscle. *J. Neurophysiol.*, 80: 365–376.

Eken, T. and Kiehn, O. (1989) Bistable firing properties of soleus motor units in unrestrained rats. *Acta Physiol. Scand.*, 136: 383–394.

Forbes, A. (1929) *The Foundations of Experimental Psychology.* Clark University Press, Worcester

Gorassini, M., Bennett, D.J., Kiehn, O., Eken, T. and Hultborn, H. (1999) Activation patterns of hindlimb motor units in the awake rat and their relation to motoneuron intrinsic properties. *J. Neurophysiol.*, 82: 709–717.

Gorassini, M.A., Bennett, D.J. and Yang, J.F. (1998) Self-sustained firing of human motor units. *Neurosci. Lett.*, 247: 13–16.

Gorassini, M., Kiehn, O., Bennett, D.J. and Hultborn, H. (1995) Hindlimb motor unit activity during locomotion in the awake rat. *Soc. Neurosci. Abstr.*, 20: 173.

Granit, R., Kernell, D. and Shortess, G.K. (1963) Quantitative aspects of repetitive firing of mammalian motoneurons, caused by injected currents. *J. Physiol.*, 168: 911–931.

Granit, R, Phillips, C.G., Skoglund, S. and Steg, G. (1957) Differentiation of tonic from phasic alpha ventral horn cells by strech, pinna and crossed extensor reflexes. *J. Neurophysiol.*, 20: 470–481.

Hounsgaard, J., Hultborn, H., Jespersen, B. and Kiehn, O. (1988) Bistability of α-motoneurones in the decerebrate cat and in the acute spinal cat after intravenous 5-hydroxy-tryptophan. *J. Physiol.*, 405: 345–367.

Hounsgaard, J. and Kiehn, O. (1989) Serotonin-induced bistability of turtle motoneurones caused by a nifedipine-sensitive calcium plateau potential. *J. Physiol.*, 414: 265–282.

Hounsgaard, J. and Kiehn, O. (1993) Calcium spikes and calcium plateaux evoked by differential polarization in dendrites of turtle motoneurones in vitro. *J. Physiol.*, 468: 245–259.

Hultborn, H. and Wigström, H. (1980) Motor response with long latency and maintained duration evoked by activity in Ia afferents. In J.E. Desmedt (Ed.), *Spinal and Supraspinal Mechanisms of Voluntary Motor Control and Locomotion.* Progress in Clinical Neurophysiology, Karger, Basel, pp. 99–116.

Hultborn, H., Wigström, H. and Wängberg, B. (1976) Prolonged activation of soleus motoneurones following a conditioning train in soleus Ia afferents – a case for a reverberating loop?, *Neurosci. Lett.*, 1: 147–152.

Jacobs, B.L. and Fornal, C.A. (1997) Serotonin and motor activity. *Curr. Opin. Neurobiol.*, 7: 820–825.

Kernell, D. (1965) The adaptation and the relation between discharge frequency and current strength of cat lumbosacral motoneurones stimulated by long–lasting injected currents. *Acta Physiol. Scand.*, 65: 65–73.

Kiehn, O. and Eken, T. (1997) Prolonged firing in motor units: evidence of plateau potentials in human motoneurons? *J. Neurophysiol.*, 78: 3061–3068.

Kiehn, O. and Eken, T. (1998) Functional role of plateau potentials in vertebrate motor neurons. *Curr. Opin. Neurobiol.*, 8: 746–752.

Lee, R.H. and Heckman, C.J. (1998b) Bistability in spinal motoneurons in vivo: systematic variations in persistent inward currents. *J. Neurophysiol.*, 80: 583–593.

Russo, R.E. and Hounsgaard, J. (1996) Burst–generating neurones in the dorsal horn in an in vitro preparation of the turtle spinal cord. *J. Physiol.*, 493: 55–66.

Schwindt, P.C. and Crill, W.E. (1980a) Role of a persistent inward current in motoneuron bursting during spinal seizures. *J. Neurophysiol.*, 43: 1296–1318.

Schwindt, P.C. and Crill, W.E. (1980b) Properties of a persistent inward current in normal and TEA–injected motoneurons. *J. Neurophysiol.*, 43: 1700–1724.

Schwindt, P.C. and Crill, W.E. (1980c) Effects of barium on cat spinal motoneurons studied by voltage clamp. *J. Neurophysiol.*, 44: 827–846.

Stein, R.B. and Parmiggiani, F. (1979) Optimal motor patterns for activating mammalian muscle. *Brain Res.*, 175: 372–376.

Svirskis, G. and Hounsgaard, J. (1997) Depolarization–induced facilitation of plateau generating currents in ventral horn neurons in the turtle spinal cord. *J. Neurophysiol.*, 78: 1740–1742.

M.D. Binder (Ed.)
Progress in Brain Research, Vol 123
© 1999 Elsevier Science BV. All rights reserved.

CHAPTER 4

Synaptic integration in bistable motoneurons

C.J Heckman* and R.H. Lee

Departments of Physiology and Rehabilitation and Physical Medicine, Northwestern University Medical School, 303 E. Chicago Avenue, Chicago, IL 60611, USA

Introduction

Several types of motoneurons exhibit bistable behavior, in which brief periods of excitation and inhibition can toggle self-sustained firing on and off (Hounsgaard et al., 1988; Hounsgaard and Kiehn, 1989; Rekling and Feldman, 1997; Hsiao et al., 1998; Lee and Heckman, 1998b). In spinal motoneurons in the adult cat, bistable behavior is especially strong, but our recent studies have shown that this bistable behavior varies systematically across the motoneuron pool (Lee and Heckman, 1998b). *Fully bistable* cells can maintain self-sustained firing for many seconds, whereas *partially bistable* cells can generate at most 1–2 s of self-sustained firing. It is important to realize that fully bistable motoneurons tend to have slow axonal conduction velocities and low input conductances. In contrast, partially bistable cells tend to have fast conduction velocities and high input conductances. Thus, fully bistable cells are likely to innervate fatigue resistant muscle fibers and to be either type S or FR in the type classification scheme of Burke and colleagues (1973). Using the single electrode voltage clamp technique, we have also measured the total persistent inward current (I_{PT}) underlying bistable behavior (Lee and Heckman, 1998a). Although I_{PT} is of similar amplitude in fully and partially bistable cells, it tends to slowly decay with time in the partially bistable group while exhibiting little or no decay in fully bistable cells.

*Corresponding author. Tel.: 312–503–2164; Fax: 312–503 5101; e-mail: c-heckman@nwu.edu

In this chapter we first briefly review the evidence that I_{PT} and the plateau potential it generates largely originate in dendritic regions. We then consider the implications of a large and persistent inward current in dendrites for synaptic integration. Finally, we present some guidelines for detecting the signs of plateau potentials in single motor unit firing patterns in human subjects.

Evidence that the total persistent inward current originates at least partly in dendritic regions

Several lines of evidence show that much of I_{PT} originates in dendritic regions. In turtle motoneurons in a slice preparation, Hounsgaard and Kiehn (1993) showed that extracellular electrical fields that hyperpolarized the soma but depolarized the dendrites could evoke sustained plateau potentials. This showed that dendrites were capable of supporting plateaus. Single electrode voltage clamp studies in the spinal motoneurons in the adult cat led to a similar conclusion (Lee and Heckman, 1996). During steady voltage clamp at depolarized holding potentials in the range of -50 to -40 mV, a brief period of excitatory synaptic input generated a sustained tail current (see Fig. 1). The electrode tip was probably in or near the soma, so this tail could not be due to somatic voltage sensitive conductances because their behavior was necessarily held constant by the clamp. Thus the tail current was probably due to a plateau potential in dendritic regions under poor space clamp. A dendritic origin for much of I_{PT} suggests that

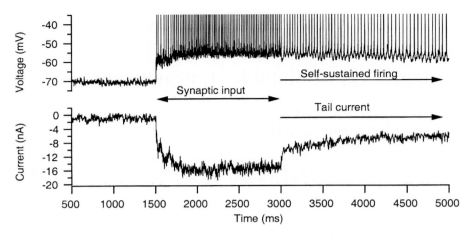

Fig. 1. Bistable behavior in motoneurons is generated by a persistent inward current that originates at least partly in dendritic regions. The upper traces shows self-sustained firing in a medial gastrocnemius motoneuron in response to a 1.5 s period of vibration of the Achilles tendon to activate muscle spindle Ia afferents. In the lower trace, the same input has been applied during steady voltage clamp at about -50 mV. In this case, the Ia input evokes a prolonged tail current. Because the clamp is likely applied at the soma, the tail current is probably due to a plateau potential in dendritic regions under poor space clamp. Data from Lee and Heckman (1996).

synaptic input should be more effective in generating a plateau potential than injected current. Consistent with this, Bennett and colleagues have shown that synaptic activation substantially lowers the frequency of firing for the onset of the plateau (Bennett et al., 1998; see also Hultborn, Chapter 3, in this volume). Thus, there seems little doubt that a considerable portion of I_{PT} originates in dendritic regions.

This does not mean that the soma lacks channels that contribute to I_{PT}. It is clear that the activation of I_{PT} and the consequent plateau potential can be readily affected by current injection in the soma. Perhaps the resolution of this paradox is that much of I_{PT} and its plateau potential originates in the proximal portion of the dendritic tree, as suggested by recent modeling studies (Powers and Binder, personal communication).

Synaptic processing in bistable motoneurons

A large plateau potential in dendritic regions will necessarily have a profound impact on dendritic processing of synaptic input. This will be true even if this plateau is primarily restricted to proximal dendritic regions. It is clear from our voltage clamp studies that the activation of I_{PT} and its plateau potential provides an enormous amplification of synaptic inputs (Lee and Heckman, 1996). During

steady voltage clamp at hyperpolarized membrane potentials (-70 to -90 mV) that prevent activation of the plateau potential, a brief period of tendon vibration to activate muscle spindle Ia afferents produced an average of 4.3 nA of effective synaptic current (standard deviation: 2.4 nA; n = 15). At depolarized holding potentials (-40 to -50 mV), the same input generated about 3.5 times as much current (average: 15.1 nA; standard deviation: 4.9 nA, n = 15). The extra current presumably comes from the dendritic portion of I_{PT}. This is because, just as for the tail current shown in Fig. 1, the clamp holds the behavior of the component of I_{PT} within the soma constant.

What happens to synaptic input when the plateau is already activated? Does the cell become unresponsive to synaptic input? The most functionally relevant answers to these questions are obtained during current clamp conditions when the cell is allowed to generate normal rhythmic firing. Figure 2 shows an example in which tendon vibration was applied repeatedly to evoke a series of brief but steady inputs from muscle spindle Ia afferents to a fully bistable motoneuron. Stable self-sustained firing at about 15 spikes/s is established by the first period of synaptic input, yet each subsequent period of input causes a large increase in firing rate, to about 45 Hz. Thus, by definition, the dendritic

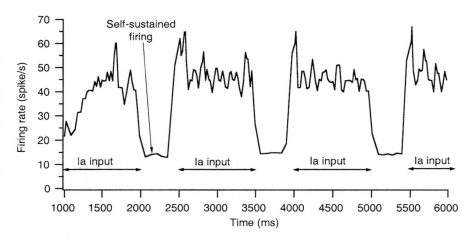

Fig. 2. Synaptic input remains a potent modulator of firing rate even when the cell is already exhibiting self-sustained firing. A series of four periods of Ia input to a motoneuron (evoked by tendon vibration, as in Fig. 1) were applied to a medial gastrocnemius motoneuron. Each period of synaptic input is separated by a short period of self-sustained firing. Note that in each case, the Ia input generates a dramatic increase in firing rate. Unpublished data from Lee and Heckman. Decerebrate cat preparation with exogenous application of the noradrenergic α_1 agonist methoxamine (see Lee and Heckman, 1998b for preparation details).

plateau potential producing the self-sustained firing did not limit the response of the cell to further synaptic inputs. Figure 3 indicates that the cell also remained responsive to injected current. But note the discrepancy in the effectiveness of the synaptic and injected currents. The synaptic input only generated about 5 nA when voltage clamped at a hyperpolarized level yet this modest current

increased firing by 30 spikes/s. To achieve the same level of firing, the injected current had to reach 20 nA. Thus, not only is the cell still responsive to synaptic input during self-sustained firing, the synaptic input actually undergoes tremendous amplification.

The protocols shown in Figs 2 and 3 have been carried out in two other fully bistable cells, each

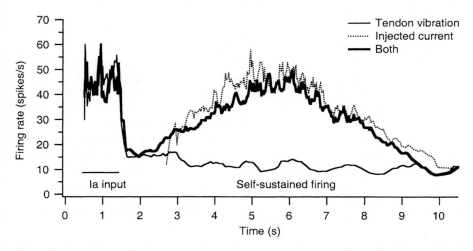

Fig. 3. Comparison of efficacy of synaptic and injected current during self-sustained firing in a fully bistable cell (same cell as in Fig. 2). The thin trace shows the prolonged self-sustained firing evoked by a single 1.5 s period of Ia input from tendon vibration. The dotted line shows the firing pattern in response to a triangular injected current, 20 nA in amplitude. The thick line indicates the firing pattern when the triangular injected current was applied during self-sustained firing.

TABLE 1

Change in firing rate evoked by Ia input during self-sustained firing

Ia input from vibration	Self-sustained firing	Difference	Number of cells	P value for t-test
53 ± 15	21 ± 10	32 ± 11	15	0.000001

Firing rates are expressed in spikes/s and as averages ± standard deviations. The t-test compares average firing during Ia input to that during self-sustained firing.

giving similar results. In addition, a systematic analysis of our previous data strongly supports the existence of potent amplification of synaptic input during self-sustained firing in fully bistable cells. This analysis was done simply by comparing the firing rate during Ia input to that during the subsequent period of self sustained firing that was initiated by the Ia input (data from Lee and Heckman, 1998b). In 15 fully bistable cells, the firing rate during Ia input was ~ 50 spikes/ while during self-sustained the firing rate was ~ 20 spikes/s (see Table 1). Thus, the 30 spikes/s increase in firing produced by Ia input illustrated in Figs. 2 and 3 is a consistent finding in bistable motoneurons. As noted above, measurements of Ia effective synaptic currents at hyperpolarized membrane potentials that avoid plateau activation give values of about 4 nA (Lee and Heckman, 1996). Thus, the average gain during Ia synaptic input during self-sustained firing in bistable motoneurons is 30 spikes/s divided by 4 nA or about 7.5 spikes/s/nA. In contrast, the gain for injected current once the firing acceleration due to plateau onset is complete is only about 1–2 spikes/s/nA (Lee and Heckman, 1998b and see Fig. 4 below).

At least two explanations could account for this amplification of synaptic input during self-sustained firing. First, the plateau potential may make the cell especially sensitive to synaptic noise. Consistent with this, Bennett et. al. (1998) have found that the afterhyperpolarization following a spike becomes smaller once the plateau is activated. However to us, this seems insufficient to explain the potent amplification demonstrated in Figs. 2 and 3. A second, more interesting possibility is that perhaps the plateau potential underlying

self-sustained firing is a stable but partially activated state supported by only a portion of the dendritic tree. In that case, additional dendritic synaptic input would put the rest of the dendritic tree in the 'up' state – i.e. the synaptic input would activate the rest of the plateau generating channels. If this is the case, the primary role of synaptic input to bistable motoneurons would be to control the fraction of the dendritic tree in the 'up' state. The idea that synaptic input controls the extent of a dendritic plateau potential also implies that the plateau should be gradable in amplitude. Our present working hypothesis is that a motoneuron which is already firing in the self-sustained mode still has tremendous gain for small synaptic inputs but saturates in its response somewhere in the moderate amplitude range. This hypothesis must be tested using various amplitudes of synaptic input, because, as shown in Fig. 3, injected current is likely to seriously underestimate the true gain of the bistable motoneuron.

These data are preliminary but suggest an extraordinary picture of synaptic processing in bistable motoneurons. Instead of the more traditional view that dendritic voltage-sensitive conductances merely act to help transfer synaptic current to the soma, in the bistable motoneuron, a relatively small synaptic current acts to control the 'excitability' of the dendritic tree. The potent voltage-sensitive currents that generate the plateau potential in the dendritic tree then provide the main drive for steady rhythmic firing. It is equally important to realize the potency of the dendritic plateau. The 50 spikes/s firing rate produced by the Ia input (see Table (1) is more than enough to generate maximum force levels in type S motor units (Kernell et al., 1983; Botterman et al., 1986). Thus, the dendritic plateau potential completely transforms synaptic processing in fully bistable motoneurons, allowing a modest input to S motor units to generate a maximum output force.

Are motoneurons in the bistable state during normal motor behavior?

Does the unique form of synaptic processing discussed in the previous section contribute to normal motor outflow? Bistable behavior in mammalian motoneurons is dependent on tonic activity in fibers that descend from the brainstem and release the monoamines serotonin and norepinephrine (Hounsgaard et al., 1988; Lee and Heckman, 1998b). The cells in the brainstem nuclei from which monoaminergic fibers in the cord originate are in fact tonically active in the waking state (Aston-Jones et al., 1991; Jacobs and Fornal, 1993). At least some of these cells modulate their firing patterns with movement (Veasey et al., 1997). Jacobs and colleagues (Jacobs and Fornal, 1993) have proposed the general hypothesis that monoaminergic input to the cord during movement acts to enhance motor outflow by increasing the excitability of motoneurons, while suppressing afferent

inflow by presynaptic inhibition of afferents and by actions on interneurons. Hounsgaard and colleagues (Svirskis and Hounsgaard, 1998) have shown that other neuromodulators besides the monoamines can affect plateau potentials and have suggested that motor commands may adjust the characteristics of the plateau potential in motoneurons to match the demands of specific motor tasks. As yet, the nature of this 'matching' process is unclear.

An important first step in understanding normal control of plateau potentials is to recognize when plateau potentials are being utilized in motor behaviors in intact animals or in human subjects.

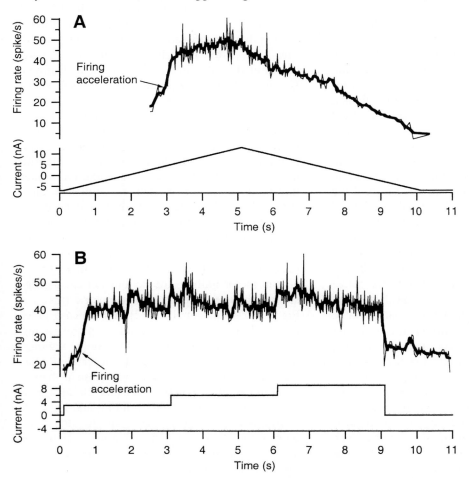

Fig. 4. Firing patterns of a fully bistable cell. Thin lines show instantaneous firing rates. Thick lines showed a smoothed version of the instantaneous rate. A. Firing rate versus time in response to a triangular injected current. B. Firing rate versus time in response to a series of injected current steps. Data from Lee and Heckman (1998b).

Self-sustained firing does occur in humans subjects but is rather difficult to demonstrate (Kiehn and Eken, 1997; Gorassini et al., 1998). Probably, as Bennet et al. (1998) point out, this is because the threshold for activation of the plateau is at or below the recruitment threshold for most motor units. If this is true, we must look to other characteristics of motor unit firing patterns for evidence of plateaus. Figure 4 shows the firing patterns for two different fully bistable motoneurons, with one pattern evoked by a slow triangular shaped injected current and one produced by several long steps of current. This figure provides an interesting guide to the recognition of plateau potentials in human motor unit firing patterns.

Consider first the response to the triangular input in Fig. 4A. In this cell, as in most fully bistable ones, the voltage threshold for I_{PT} is slightly more hyperpolarized than the spike threshold (Lee and Heckman, 1998a). Consequently, right at recruitment there is a strong acceleration in firing rate that gives a high slope of rate vs. time, followed by a transition to a lower slope once I_{PT} is fully activated. In the low slope region, firing rate exhibits more variability than during the acceleration phase. On the descending phase, the firing rate remains linear and firing does not cease until the current has reached a more hyperpolarized level than required for the onset of firing. The lower current for offset than onset of firing rate is probably a consequence of the dendritic origin of much of I_{PT} (Lee and Heckman, 1998a). Thus, a bistable motoneuron exhibits several distinctive characteristics (Hounsgaard et al., 1988; Bennett et al., 1998; Lee and Heckman, 1998b) that could be identified in human motor units during a similar pattern of input: a relatively rapid increase in firing after recruitment, a transition to a lower rate of rise with a high degree of variability as input continues to increase, a linear decrease in firing without changes in slope during the descending phase, and de-recruitment at a lower force than recruitment.

The transition from a high initial slope to a much lower slope is in fact a common feature of motor unit recordings in humans during tasks where isometric force is slowly increased. This phenomenon is sometimes referred to as 'rate limiting' and is especially prevalent in low threshold motoneur-

ons (Heckman and Binder, 1993; Binder et al., 1996). These motoneurons are of course the ones most likely to be type S and consequently most likely to exhibit bistable behavior. Alternative explanations for rate limiting have been advanced, such as a sharp transition in the organization of synaptic input between low and high threshold motoneurons (Heckman and Binder, 1993). However, the onset of a plateau potential appears to provide a simpler explanation (cf. Kiehn and Eken, 1997). In this regard, the time-dependent behavior of the plateau potential could be very helpful in detecting its presence. The acceleration in firing due to the onset of the plateau produces the steep slope during the ascending phase in Fig. 4A. However, an equally rapid increase in firing is observed during a steady step in the cell in Fig. 4B. Thus, the slope of firing vs. time is primarily determined by the time course for the activation of I_{PT} and not by the rate of increase in input (it should be emphasized that this only applies to slow rates of rise – note the slow time scale in Fig. 4A). Thus, if the rate limiting is due to activation of a plateau potential, a transition in slope resembling rate limiting should be apparent following a step-like increase in input that just exceeds the recruitment threshold for the unit. Systematic studies of rate of rise of input on plateau activation are needed to understand its potential role in faster movements.

What about the other characteristics of the firing pattern seen in Fig. 4? In fact, this firing pattern looks almost identical to the firing pattern seen in human motor units in the deltoid muscle during a slow triangular modulation of isometric force (see Fig. 2 of De Luca et al., 1982). In both cases, there is rate limiting on the ascending phase, a high degree of variability in the low slope region, a linear decrease in rate during the descending phase and then a lower level for de-recruitment than for recruitment. It is notable also that DeLuca et al. found less evidence of rate limiting and lower de-recruitment levels in a distal muscle, first dorsal interosseus. This may reflect stronger innervation of proximal vs. distal muscles by the descending monoaminergic systems.

Based on Fig. 4 above, the following criteria can be advanced for detecting whether plateau potentials form a part of normal motor behavior:

(a) Low threshold motor units should exhibit rate limiting whose time course is relatively independent of the rate of rise of isometric muscle force (it should be emphasized that this only applies for the slow part of the range of force modulation, e.g. 5–10% of maximum voluntary force per second or slower).
(b) Firing rate should become somewhat more variable after rate limiting occurs.
(c) There should be no rate limiting during the descending phase of slow force control, but instead firing rate should linearly decrease.
(d) De-recruitment should occur at a lower force level than recruitment.

If a motor unit firing pattern fulfills all four of the above criteria, it seems reasonable to conclude that its motoneuron is exhibiting plateau potential. In addition, based on the presently available evidence in animals, some predictions can be made about the type of tasks in which plateau potentials are most likely to be utilized. Plateau potentials tend to generate sustained firing patterns and it thus seems reasonable to expect that they would be used for motor tasks where steady force generation is needed. Hultborn and colleagues recognized that bistable behavior would be ideal for postural tasks (Hounsgaard et al., 1988). This is because a strong tendency for self-sustained firing in motor units would greatly reduce the proportion of the descending motor command required to maintain a relatively constant force. Two recent studies provide strong support for a role of bistable behavior in postural tasks. Kiehn and Eken (1996) demonstrated that neurotoxic destruction of the monoaminergic input to the rat spinal cord eliminated tonic EMG patterns in the subsequent motor behavior of these animals, forcing them to rely on phasic bursts of activity. In addition, bistable behavior is strongest in motoneurons with slow conduction velocities and low input conductances (Lee and Heckman 1998b). These cells are the most likely to innervate the fatigue resistant muscle units needed for posture. Based on these considerations, the following predictions can be made about the types of muscles and motor tasks in which motor unit firing patterns are most likely to exhibit the four criteria listed above.

(a) Plateau potentials are most likely to occur in low threshold motor units in proximal muscles and least likely to occur in high threshold motor units of distal muscles.
(b) Plateau potentials are most likely to occur in tasks requiring steady stabilization and less likely in tasks where precise and dynamic changes in force are needed.

Conclusions

The predictions in the previous section are obviously of a highly preliminary nature and many questions remain about the role of bistable behaviors in motoneurons in normal motor behaviors. One troubling issue is that firing rates in human subjects tend to be much lower than observed in cat motoneurons in the decerebrate. For example, rate limiting in human subjects generally occurs by about the time firing rate reaches about 15–25 spikes/s, whereas in our data it tended to occur at about 40–50 spikes/s (see Fig. 4). One possible resolution of this discrepancy lies in the threshold of the plateau potential. If this threshold became more hyperpolarized due to synaptic activation or more intense activity in descending monoaminergic fibers, much of the plateau activation would take place in the subthreshold region and the acceleration in firing would take place at lower rates. Alternatively, normal motor behavior simply uses smaller plateau potentials then we have studied in the decerebrate. Smaller plateaus could be achieved by decreasing the monoaminergic drive to motoneurons or by increasing inhibition. The possibility of adjusting the 'degree' of bistability in motoneurons emphasizes the continued need for investigations of synaptic integration in motoneurons across the full spectrum of their electrical behaviors, from the completely non-bistable state seen in anesthetized preparations (e.g. Powers and Binder, 1995) to the fully bistable state in decerebrate preparations with exogeneous monoaminergic agents (e.g. Lee and Heckman, 1996). In the previous section of this chapter, we hypothesized that fully bistable motoneurons have a unique form of dendritic processing of synaptic inputs, where small inputs act to control the excitability of the dendritic tree. An intriguing possibility is that this unique form of synaptic processing is in fact 'normal' for motoneurons in proximal muscles during postural tasks.

Acknowledgments

This work was supported by NIH grants NS34382 and NS28076. We would also like to express our sincere appreciation for the scientific contributions of Dr. Douglas G. Stuart and his colleagues to our understanding of spinal motor control. We also are deeply grateful to Dr. Stuart for his enthusiastic support for the field of spinal motor control in general and for the work in our laboratory.

References

Aston-Jones, G., Shipley, M.T., Chouvet, G., Ennis, M., Bockstaele, E.v., Pieribone, V., Shiekhattar, R., Akaoka, H., Drolet, G., Astier, B., Charlty, P., Valentino, R.J. and Williams, J.T. (1991) Afferent regulation of locus coeruleus neurons: anatomy, physiology and pharmacology. In: C.D. Barnes and O. Pompeiano, (Eds), *Progress in Brain Research*, 88, Elsevier Science Publishers B.V., Amsterdam, 47–75.

Bennett, D.J., Hultborn, H., Fedirchuk, B. and Gorassini, M. (1998) Synaptic activation of plateaus in hindlimb motoneurons of decerebrate cats. *J. Neurophysiol.*, 80: 2023–2037.

Binder, M.D., Heckman, C.J. and Powers, R.K. (1996) The physiological control of motoneuron activity. In: L.B. Rowell and J.T. Shepherd, (Eds), *Handbook of Physiology. Exercise: Regulation and Integration of Multiple Systems.* sect. 12, chapt. 1, Oxford University Press, New York, 1–53.

Botterman, B.R., Iwamoto, G.A. and Gonyea, W.J. (1986) Gradation of isometric tension by different activation rates in motor units of cat flexor carpi radialis muscle. *J. Neurophysiol.*, 56: 494–506.

Burke, R.E. and Tsairis, P. (1973) Anatomy and innervation ratios in motor units of cat gastrocnemius. *J. Physiol.*, 234: 749–765.

De Luca, C.J., LeFever, R.S., McCue, M.P. and Xenakis, A.P. (1982) Behavior of human motor units in different muscles during linearly varying contractions. *J. Physiol. (Lond.)*, 329: 113–128.

Gorassini, M.A., Bennett, D.J. and Yang, J.F. (1998) Self-sustained firing of human motor units. *Neurosci Lett.*, 247: 13–16.

Heckman, C.J. and Binder, M.D. (1993) Computer simulations of motoneuron firing rate modulation. *J. Neurophysiol.*, 69: 1005–1008.

Hounsgaard, J., Hultborn, H., Jespersen, B. and Kiehn, O. (1988) Bistability of α-motoneurones in the decerebrate cat and in the acute spinal cat after intravenous 5-hydroxy-tryptophan. *J. Physiol.*, 405: 345–367.

Hounsgaard, J. and Kiehn, O. (1989) Serotonin-induced bistability of turtle motoneurones caused by a nifedipine-sensitive calcium plateau potential. *J. Physiol.*, 414: 265–282.

Hounsgaard, J. and Kiehn, O. (1993) Calcium spikes and calcium plateaux evoked by differential polarization in dendrites of turtle motoneurones in vitro. *J. Physiol. (Lond.)*, 468: 245–259.

Hsiao, C.F., Del Negro, C.A., Trueblood, P.R. and Chandler, S.H. (1998) Ionic basis for serotonin-induced bistable membrane properties in guinea pig trigeminal motoneurons. *J. Neurophysiol.*, 79: 2847–2856.

Jacobs, B.L. and Fornal, C.A. (1993) 5-HT and motor control: a hypothesis. *Trends Neurosci.*, 16: 346–352.

Kernell, D., Eerbeek, O. and Verhey, B.A. (1983) Relation between isometric force and stimulus rate in cat's hindlimb motor units of different twitch contraction time. *Exp. Brain Res.*, 50: 220–227.

Kiehn, O. and Eken, T. (1997) Prolonged firing in motor units: evidence of plateau potentials in human motoneurons? *J. Neurophysiol.*, 78: 3061–3068.

Kiehn, O., Erdal, J., Eken, T. and Bruhn, T. (1996) Selective depletion of spinal monoamines changes the rate soleus EMG from a tonic to a more phasic pattern. *J. Physiol.*, 492.1: 173–184.

Lee, R.H. and Heckman, C.J. (1996) Influence of voltage-sensitive dendritic conductances on bistable firing and effective synaptic current in cat spinal motoneurons in vivo. *J. Neurophysiol.*, 76: 2107–2110.

Lee, R.H. and Heckman, C.J. (1998a) Bistability in spinal motoneurons in vivo: systematic variations in persistent inward currents. *J. Neurophysiol.*, 80: 583–593.

Lee, R.H. and Heckman, C.J. (1998b) Bistability in spinal motoneurons in vivo: systematic variations in rhythmic firing patterns. *J. Neurophysiol.*, 80: 572–582.

Powers, R.K. and Binder, M.D. (1995) Effective synaptic current and motoneuron firing rate modulation. *J. Neurophysiol.*, 74: 793–801.

Rekling, J.C. and Feldman, J.L. (1997) Calcium-dependent plateau potentials in rostral ambiguus neurons in the newborn mouse brain stem in vitro. *J. Neurophysiol.*, 78: 2483–2492.

Svirskis, G. and Hounsgaard, J. (1998) Transmitter regulation of plateau properties in turtle motoneurons. *J. Neurophysiol.*, 79: 45–50.

Veasey, S.C., Fornal, C.A., Metzler, C.W. and Jacobs, B.L. (1997) Single-unit responses of serotonergic dorsal raphe neurons to specific motor challenges in freely moving cats. *Neuroscience*, 79: 161–169.

M.D. Binder (Ed.)
Progress in Brain Research, Vol 123
© 1999 Elsevier Science BV. All rights reserved.

CHAPTER 5

Adapting motoneurons for motor behavior

Rodolfo Delgado-Lezama[1] and Jorn Hounsgaard[2,*]

[1] *Depto. de Fisiologa, Biofsica y Neurociencias, CINVESTAV, Mexico*
[2] *MFI, Panum Institute, University of Copenhagen Blegdamsvej 3, DK-2200 Copenhagen N., Denmark*

Introduction

Motor commands from the spinal cord to muscle fibers are coded as firing patterns in motor axons. Among all the patterns that motor axons can generate only few ever occur.

In this chapter we will show how the intrinsic properties of motoneurons are specialised and continously fine-tuned to favor these useful patterns over all other impulse patterns.

Motor behavior evolves on time scales of milliseconds and seconds. While rapid changes in activity are easily implemented by changes in synaptic excitation and inhibition of motoneurons, slower changes require increasing levels of processing from the premotor network. This computational burden is relieved by the intrinsic response properties and their regulation in motoneurons.

Defining the firing range

Intrinsic response properties, provided by voltage sensitive ion channels in dendrites and cell bodies of motoneurons, include the ability to fire contineously in response to maintained depolarizing current. The main contributor to this pace-maker property is the slow afterhyperpolarization (AHP) following each spike. The AHP delays repolarization to the firing threshold and allows

*Corresponding author. Tel.: (45) 35 32 75 59; Fax: (45) 35 32 74 99; e-mail: j.hounsgaard@mfi.ku.dk

deinactivation of Na^+ channels. The intrinsic pacemaker properties of motoneurons essentially confine steady state firing to a frequency range from a lower limit of about 5 Hz, just allowing summation of single twitch contractions in muscle fibers, to an upper limit of about 50 Hz resulting in maximal tetanic contraction (Kernell, 1983, 1990). In this way intrinsic pacemaker properties ensure that changes in ionotropic synaptic input to motoneurons also lead to changes in motor activity.

The generation of AHPs is complex, involving several types of ion channels. The hyperpolarizing current is, to a large extent, generated by an SK calcium dependent potassium channel (Barret and Barret, 1976; Schwindt and Crill, 1984; Hounsgaard et al., 1988) which is blocked by apamin. The magnitude and duration of the AHP current is determined by the amount of Ca^{++} entering the cell during each action potential and by the background intracellular Ca^{++} concentration and Ca^{++} sequestering. Each of these elements is regulated. As an example, Ca^{++} influx during spikes is tightly controlled by several outward currents also activated during the spike. Any change in these conductances induces changes in excitability and adaptation pattern and in the relation between stimulus current and firing rate. This is illustrated in Fig. 1A,B by the increased spike duration, increased Ca^{++} influx, increased excitability and increased adaptation induced by reducing the delayed rectifier with TEA. Ca^{++} influx during spikes is also promoted by reducing A-current with 4-aminopyridine and by reducing I_h with Cs^+

(Hounsgaard and Mintz, 1988). On the other hand reducing the AHP with apamin (Fig. 1C,D) has no effect on spike duration but converts the adaptation normally seen at the onset of a depolarizing stimulus current, to an accelerating spike activity during the stimulus and a maintained spike activity which can be terminated by a hyperpolarizing current pulse. This bistable firing pattern in moto-neurons, first described by Schwindt and Crill (1977), is generated by a plateau potential which is mediated by di-hydropyridine sensitive L-type Ca^{++} channels (Hounsgaard and Mintz, 1988; Perrier and Hounsgaard, 1999). These channels do not contribute to the Ca^{++} influx during action potentials and their activation is not followed by an AHP. The generation of plateau potentials in motoneurons is a *latent* property only uncovered after up-regulation of L-type Ca^{++} channels or reduction of the outward current normally activated during depolarization (Hounsgaard and Mintz, 1988; Hounsgaard and Kiehn, 1989; Schwindt and Crill, 1980). The time course of the onset and offset of plateau potentials has a fast, high threshold component and a slow, low threshold, components. The slow component is apparently the result of a voltage sensitive equilibrium between two closed states of L-type Ca^{++} channels, a reluctant state from which the threshold for opening is high and a willing state from which the threshold for opening is low. The time course of the transition between the two states is reflected in the windup of the response to a repeated depolarizing current pulse (Russo and Hounsgaard, 1994, 1996; Svirskis and Hounsgaard, 1997).

Defining the pattern

In the preceding section we saw that the basic intrinsic response properties of motoneurons fav-

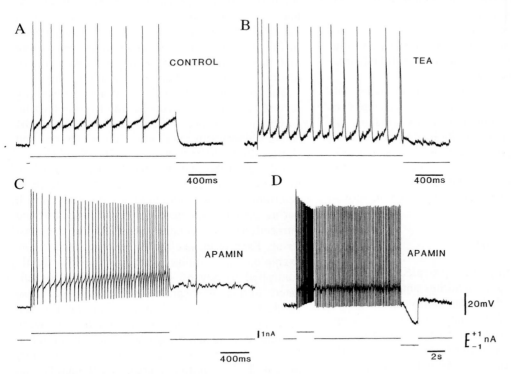

Fig. 1. Change in firing pattern with TEA (A and B) and apamin (C and D). A, the configuration of action potential and firing pattern in normal medium. B, with TEA (1 mM) the action potential is prolonged, the excitability increased, the fast AHP reduced and the slow AHP and adaptation increased. C and D, response of motoneuron after addition of apamin (1 μM) to normal medium. C, initial adaptation of firing frequency followed by acceleration during depolarising pulse from rest. D, with a depolarising bias current a brief depolarising pulse induced a sustained plateau, finally eliminated by a hyperpolarising pulse (from Hounsgaard and Mintz, 1988).

ored maintained firing frequencies within functionally sound boundaries in response to external stimuli. We also saw that a host of voltage sensitive ion channels interacted to produce the response patterns evoked and that small changes in balance between the contributing conductances resulted in markedly changed firing patterns. Such regulatory changes can be induced by metabotropic neurotransmitters. The ability to generate plateau potentials is induced by activation of agonists for 5-HT$_{1A}$ receptors, muscarine receptors, $\alpha 1$ noradrenaline receptors and type I metabotropic glutamate receptors and suppressed by activation of GABA$_B$ receptors (Conway et al., 1988; Hounsgaard and Kiehn, 1989; Lee and Heckman, 1996; Svirskis and Hounsgaard, 1998).

In the unanaesthetized decerebrate cat plateau potentials are probably induced by release of serotonin from terminals of tonically active raphe spinal neurons (Hounsgaard et al., 1988). The mechanisms for receptor induced regulation of plateau properties in motoneurons are not known in any detail. The activation of mGlu, muscarine and GABA$_B$ receptors appear to have direct effects on the voltage sensitivity of L-type Ca^{++} channels (Svirskis and Hounsgaard, 1998). 5-HT reduce the slow AHP (Hounsgaard and Kiehn, 1989) and may also facilitate L-type Ca^{++} channels. Although activation of these metabotropic receptors have converging effects on L-type Ca^{++} channels they also have divergent effects. Figure 2 shows that while 5-HT induce bistablity in motoneurons (Fig. 2A) muscarine induce intrinsic oscillatory activity in response to steady depolarization (Fig. 2B) with a configuration similar to the intrinsic oscillations induced by activation of ionotropic NMDA receptors (Fig. 2C). The three transmitter induced response modes all depend on L-type Ca^{++}

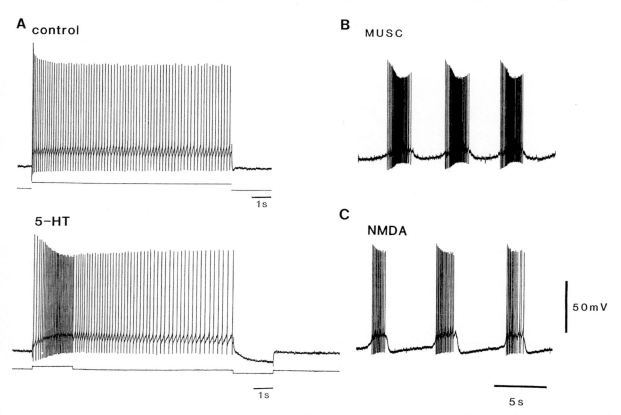

Fig. 2. Response modes of motoneurons induced by A, 5-HT (10 μM) (A); B, muscarine(10 μM) C, NMDA (10 μM) (from A, Hounsgaard and Kiehn, unpublished; B and C, Hounsgaard and Mintz, unpublished.).

channels and are blocked by nifedipine (Guertin and Hounsgaard, 1998, 1999).

Experiments such as those just described show that the intrinsic properties of motoneurons not only favor a functionally relevant range of firing rates but also mediate distinct *intrinsic response patterns* each of which is determined by a particular balance between the different types of voltage sensitive ion channels. Shifts between these modes are defined by the convergent and divergent actions of metabotropic transmitters on particular voltage sensitive ion channels (Nicoll, 1988; Hounsgaard and Midtgaard, 1989). Functionally such state shifts allow the relation between incoming synaptic potentials and motor output pattern to be regulated over a wide range. We suggest that shifts in intrinsic response properties enable motoneurons to be adapted to favor functionally useful response patterns for widely different motor behaviors. We also note that the intrinsic response properties define the time course of responses to synaptic input and often, as in the case of bistability and intrinsic oscillations, dissociate the time scale and dynamics of the output from the time scale and dynamics of the input (Hounsgaard and Midtgaard, 1989; Midtgaard and Hounsgaard, 1989).

Defining recruitment

In the preceeding section we saw that the intrinsic response properties of motoneurons were regulated by metabotropic receptors activated either by bath applied agonists in vitro or by high levels of tonic activity of raphé neurons in the decerebrate cat in vivo. These experiments define the extreme state of modulation when a large fraction of a particular type of metabotropic receptors are activated continuously. In more intact preparations, however, raphé spinal activity may be finely graded with motor behavior (Jacobs and Fornal, 1997). More discrete levels of regulation have been explored in response to brief activation of synaptic afferents (Delgado-Lezama et al., 1997, 1999). In the experiment illustrated in Fig. 3 all ionotropic

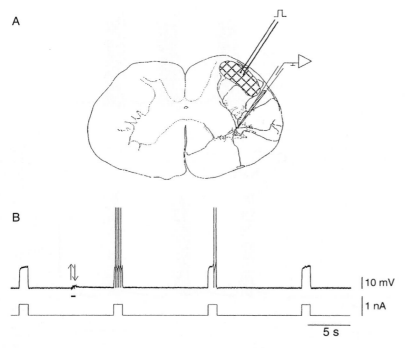

Fig. 3. DLF stimulation increases motoneuronal excitability. A, Schematic representation of the arrangement for recording and stimulation. B, response to depolarising current pulse before and after a brief DLF stimulus train. Synaptic potentials blocked by antagonists for ionotropic receptors. (From Delgado-Lezama et al., 1997).

transmission was blocked so that neither spontaneous nor evoked synaptic potentials occured.
Under these conditions a brief train of impulses in
the dorsolateral funiculus (30 stimuli at 20 Hz)
induced an increased excitability for tens of
seconds (Fig. 3A,B). This increased excitability
was mediated by a facilitation of L-type Ca^{++}

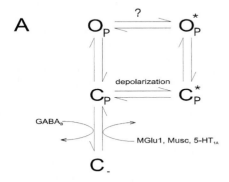

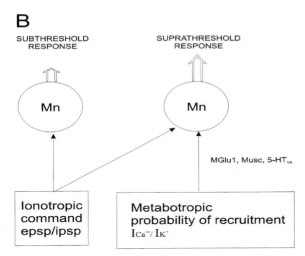

Fig. 4. Summary schemes for the proposed states L-type Ca^{++}
channels in spinal motoneurons as determined by voltage and
metabotropic regulation (A) and of the roles of ionotropic and
metabotropic synaptic transmission (B). A, The equilibrium
between a dormant state in which channel openings are
suppressed (C^-) and the C_P state is controlled by metabotropic
transmitters. Depolarisation induced facilitation controls the
equilibrium between a reluctant, closed state, C_P, and a willing
closed state, C^*_P, from which the open states, O_P and O^*_P, can be
reluctantly or willingly recruited by depolarisation. Transitions
between C^*_P and C^*_P appear to have a time constant of seconds
and provides the slow onset and offset of plateau potentials and
the windup property.

channels since it was blocked by nifedipine. The
facilitation was also blocked by antagonists of the
metabotropic receptors for 5-HT, muscarine and
glutamate whose activation facilitate L-type Ca^{++}
channels. This shows that the regulation originates
from both spinal and supra spinal sources and
involves transmitters with both ionotropic and
metabotropic actions as well as purely modulatory
transmitters.

With brief stimulus trains overt plateau potentials were often absent while the increased
excitability mediated by facilitation of L-type Ca^{++}
channels was readily detectable (Fig. 3A,B). This
led to the suggestion that metabotropic regulation
of L-type Ca^{++} channels was a mechanism for
regulating the recruitment order among motoneurons (Delgado-Lezama et al., 1997).

In contrast to the classical idea that the order of
recruitment in a pool of motoneurons is a fixed
entity defined by the size (input resistance) of
motoneurons more recent data suggest less rigor.
The functionality of the size related recruitment has
been challenged (Gustafsson and Pinter, 1985;
Bigland-Ritchie et al., 1998). It is also clear that the
threshold for recruitment varies for individual
motoneurons. During fictive locomotion the threshold is in general lower than at rest and may vary
during the locomotor cycle (Brownstone et al.,
1992, 1994; Fedirchuk et al., 1998). We suggest
that the threshold for recruitment in motoneurons is
a dynamic property continuously regulated by the
state of the intrinsic response properties, influenced, for instance, by the state of L-type Ca^{++}
channels as determined by the past history of the
cell, windup, and by the sum of converging
metabotropic synaptic transmission. This may
explain how selective recruitment is possible and
reliable although the motor command is widely
distributed in the motor pool. By regulation of the
threshold for recruitment the excitability of some
motoneurons can be upregulated while others are
down-regulated. In this way motor pools can be
prepared for specific motor behavior by enhancing
the probability of recruiting relevant motor neurons, inclusion signal, while decreasing the
probability of recruiting irrelevant motor neurons,
exclusion signal. This may reduce the precision
required from motor commands and thereby the

computational load on the premotor network (Gutman, 1994).

Conclusions

The intrinsic response properties of motoneurons can adapt motoneurons to generate functionally useful output patterns. By the dynamic properties of L-type Ca^{++} channels and their regulation by metabotropic receptors (Fig. 4A) the excitability of motoneurons and the time course of their responses can be regulated over a wide range.

In addition, motor performance may be optimized and refined by supplementing ionotropic motor commands with metabotropic regulation of recruitment order (Fig. 4B).

References

Barrett, E.F. and Barret, J.N. (1976) Separation of two voltage-sensitive potassium currents, and demonstration of a tetrodotoxin-resistant calcium current in frog motoneurones. *J. Physiol. (Lond.)*, 255(3): 737–774.

Bigland-Ritchie, B. and Fuglevand, A. (1998) Contractile Properties of Human Motor Unites: Is man a cat?. *Neuroscientist*, 4.4: 240–249.

Brownstone, R.M., Jordan, L.M., Kriellaars, D.J., Noga, B.R. and Shefchyk, S.J. (1992) On the regulation of repetitive firing in lumbar motoneurones during fictive locomotion in the cat. *Exp. Brain Res.*, 90(3): 441–455.

Brownstone, R.M., Gossard, J.P. and Hultborn, H. (1994) Voltage-dependent excitation of motoneurones from spinal locomotor centres in the cat. *Exp. Brain Res.*, 102(1): 34–44.

Conway, B.A., Hultborn, H., Kiehn, O. and Mintz, I. (1988) Plateau potentials in α-motoneurones induced by intravenous injection of L-dopa and clonidine in the spinal cat. *J. Physiol. (Lond.)*, 405: 369–384.

Delgado-Lezama, R., Perrier, J.F., Nedergaard, S., Svirskis, G. and Hounsgaard, J. (1997) Metabotropic synaptic regulation of intrinsic response properties of spinal motoneurons. *J. Physiol.*, 504.1: 97–102.

Delgado-Lezama, R., Perrier, J.F. and Hounsgaard, J. (1999) Local facilitation of plateau potentials in dendrites of motoneurones by synaptic activation of metabotropic receptors. *J. Physiol.*, 515.1: 203–207.

Fedirchuk, B., McCrea, Dai, Y., Jones, K.E. and Jordan, L.M, (1998) Motoneuron frequency/current relationships during fictive locomotion in the cat. *Soc. Neurosci. Abstr.*, 454.13.

Guertin, P.A. and Hounsgaard, J. (1998) NMDA induced intrinsic voltage oscillations depend on L-type calcium channels by in spinal motoneurons of adult turtles. *J. Neurophysiol.*, 80: 3380–3382.

Guertin, P.A. and Hounsgaard, J. (1999) L-type calcium channels but not N-methyl-D-aspartate receptor channels

mediate rhythmic activity induced by cholinergic agonist in motoneurons from turtle spinal cord slices. *Neuro. Sci. Lett.*, 261, 81–84.

Gustafsson, B. and Pinter, M.J. (1985) On factors determining orderly recruitment of motor units: a role for intrinsic membrane properties. *Trends Neurosci.*, 8: 431–433.

Gutman, A. (1994) Gelfand-Tsetlin principle of minimal afferentation and bistability of dendrites. *Int. J. Neural Syst.*, 5(2): 83–86.

Hounsgaard, J., Hultborn, H., Jespersen, B. and Kiehn, O. (1988) Bistability of alpha-motoneurones in the decerebrate cat and in the acute spinal cat after intravenous 5-hydroxytryptophan. *J. Physiol. (Lond.)*, 405: 345–367.

Hounsgaard, J. and Kiehn, O. (1993) Calcium spikes and calcium plateaux evoked by differential depolarization in dendrites of turtle motoneurones. *J. Physiol.*, 468: 245–259.

Hounsgaard, J. and Midtgaard, J. (1989) Dendrite processing in more ways than one *Trends Neurosci.*, 12(9): 313–315.

Hounsgaard, J. and Mintz, I. (1988) Calcium conductance and firing properties of spinal motoneurones in the turtle. *J. Physiol. (Lond.)*, 398: 591–603.

Hounsgaard, J., Kiehn, O. and Mintz, I. (1988) Response properties of motoneurones in a slice preparation of the turtle spinal cord. *J. Physiol. (Lond.)*, 398: 575–589.

Jacobs, B.L. and Fornal, C.A. (1997) Serotonin and motor activity. *Curr. Opin. Neurobiol.*, 7(6): 820–825.

Kernell, D. (1983) Functional properties of spinal motoneurons and gradation of muscle force. In: J.E. Desmedt (Ed.), *Motor Control in Health and Disease*, Raven Press, New York. pp. 213–226.

Kernell, D. (1990) Spinal motoneurons and their muscle fibers: mechanisms and long-term consequences of common activation patterns. In: M.D. Binder and L.M. Mendell (Eds), *The segmental motor system*, Oxford University Press. pp 36–57.

Lee, R.H. and Heckman, C.J. (1996). Influence of voltage-sensitive dendritic conductances on bistable firing and effective synaptic current in cat spinal motoneurons in vivo. *J. Neurophysiol.*, 76(3): 2107–2110.

Midtgaard, J. and Hounsgaard, J. (1989) Nerve cells as source of time scale and processing density in brain functions. *IJNS*, 1: 89–94.

Nicoll, R.A. (1988) The coupling of neurotransmitter receptors to ion channels in the brain. *Science*, 241(4865): 545–551.

Perrier, J.F. and Hounsgaard, J. (1999) Ca^{2+} activated non-selective cationic (I_{CAN}) current in turtle motoneurons. *J. Neurophysiol.*, 82: 730–735.

Russo, R.E. and Hounsgaard, J. (1994) Short-term plasticity in turtle dorsal horn neurons mediated by L-type Ca^{2+} channels. *Neuroscience*, 61(2): 191–197.

Russo, R.E. and Hounsgaard, J. (1996) Plateau-generating neurones in the dorsal horn in an in vitro preparation of the turtle spinal cord. *J. Physiol. (Lond.)*, 493.1: 39–54.

Schwindt, P. and Crill, W.E. (1977) A persistent negative resistance in cat lumbar motoneurons. *Brain Res.*, 120(1): 173–178.

Schwindt, P.C. and Crill, W.E. (1980) Properties of a persistent inward current in normal and TEA-injected motoneurons. *J. Neurophysiol.*, 43(6): 1700–1724.

Schwindt, P.C. and Crill, W.E. (1984) Membrane properties of cat motoneurons. In: R.A. Davidoff (Ed.), *Handbook of the Spinal Cord*, New York, Basel: Marcel Dekker Inc. pp. 199–242.

Svirskis, G. and Hounsgaard, J. (1997) Depolarization-induced facilitation of a plateau generating current in ventral horn neurons in the turtle spinal cord. *J. Neurophysiol.*, 78: 1740–1742.

Svirskis, G. and Hounsgaard, J. (1998) Transmitter regulation of plateau properties in turtle motoneurons. *J. Neurophysiol.*, 79.1: 45–50.

Input–output functions of motoneurons

M.D. Binder (Ed.)
Progress in Brain Research, Vol 123
© 1999 Elsevier Science BV. All rights reserved.

CHAPTER 6

Assessing the strengths of motoneuron inputs: different anatomical and physiological approaches compared

Peter A. Kirkwood,[1,*] Timothy W. Ford,[1,†] Revers Donga,[1,‡] Shane A. Saywell[1] and Gert Holstege[2]

[1] *Sobell Department of Neurophysiology, Institute of Neurology, University College London, Queen Square, London WC1N 3BG, UK*
[2] *Department of Anatomy and Embryology, University of Groningen, Oostersingel 69, 9713 EZ, Groningen, The Netherlands*

Introduction

The spinal motoneuron is known to be the site of much convergence, in terms of both the total number of axons synapsing on any one neuron and the variety of different sources for these axons. Proving the *existence* of a particular direct connection to motoneurons can be relatively straightforward, anatomically (e.g. VanderHorst et al., 1997) or physiologically (e.g. Kirkwood and Sears, 1980). One need only to ensure that the pre- and postsynaptic elements have been adequately identified and that appropriate criteria have been applied to show a direct connection. Anatomically, double labeling (i.e. labeling of both pre- and postsynaptic elements) would normally be required, ideally in combination with electron microscopy. Physiologically, one should ensure that proper controls in spike-triggered averaging (STA) or cross-correlation experiments are in place

to take account of possible complications arising from oligosynaptic connections or from synchronization with other neurons (Kirkwood, 1979; Kirkwood and Sears, 1980; Davies et al., 1985).

However, assessing the strength of such a set of connections is a rather different matter. In some cases bulk-labeling techniques or electrical stimulation can be used, but often with inputs arising from central sources these methods are not sufficiently selective. Further, in a functional context one may want to know, for *a given motor act*, how much of the motoneuron input comes from a particular source. In such a situation, one needs to assess firstly the strength of individual connections (e.g. the amplitudes of single-fiber EPSPs or the numbers of boutons per afferent fiber per motoneuron) and secondly the numbers and firing rates of such identified active inputs. Since these properties may often vary within a population of neurons, the sampling may also be critical.

In reality, descriptions of inputs are arrived at piecemeal, by a variety of methods, as is the case for the system described in this chapter. The input neurons of interest here are the expiratory bulbospinal neurons (EBSNs) of the caudal ventral respiratory group in the medulla of the cat and are located in the nucleus retroambiguus (NRA). The output neurons are thoracic expiratory motoneurons, which innervate internal intercostal and abdominal muscles. The bulbospinal neurons

*Corresponding author. Tel.: +44(0) 171-837-3611, Ext. 4189; Fax: +44(0) 171-813-3107; e-mail:pkirkwoo@ion.ucl.ac.uk
† Present address: Department of Physiology, Royal Free and University College Medical School, Rowland Hill Street, London NW3 2PF, UK
‡ Present address: Department of Preclinical Sciences, University of Leicester, P.O. Box 138, Leicester LE1 9HN

convey the excitatory expiratory drive from the medullary respiratory central pattern generator to the spinal cord. Their axons almost all cross the midline (at the level of their somata or slightly rostral to it) and descend in the ventral and lateral funiculi, to distribute their drive to thoracic and some lumbar and sacral segments (Monteau and Hilaire, 1991; Iscoe, 1998).

It should be noted that the definition of the neurons, including the motoneurons, as expiratory is an operational one, in terms of their temporal pattern of activation during respiration under anesthesia or decerebration. In the normal life of the animal they are almost certainly multifunctional (Grélot et al., 1996). Even during anesthesia they can be active in other behaviors, particularly those involving raised intra-abdominal pressure, such as vomiting, coughing and vocalization (Iscoe, 1998). Further, on the basis of the projections to and from the NRA, the neurons of this nucleus have been deduced to have yet other functions, notably an important role in mating behavior (VanderHorst and Holstege, 1996; 1997a, b). However, it is not known whether these other functions ascribed to the neurons of the NRA are performed by those which would be classified as EBSNs, or by other neurons. It is unlikely that all NRA neurons are EBSNs and the neurons shown by retrograde labeling to have projections appropriate for the proposed role in mating comprise only a proportion of the total in the NRA (VanderHorst and Holstege, 1995).

The motoneurons we are concerned with, like nearly all motoneurons, must also be considered multifunctional (Iscoe, 1998), though they are synergistically activated by respiratory inputs. They all have their axons in the internal intercostal nerve. This innervates a number of muscles, all of which, except for the parasternal, interchondral muscle, have expiratory actions (Monteau and Hilaire, 1991; Iscoe, 1998). Under the conditions of the experiments described here, these motoneurons all show expiratory activation, though the *degree* to which any one of them is activated varies according to a number of factors, partly explored in this chapter. The parasternal muscles are well known as inspiratory in their activity (Taylor, 1960) and in their actions (De Troyer, 1991). Their motoneurons

were excluded by virtue of their inspiratory activation patterns.

Although this system of neurons is no different from most motor systems, in that it forms a common final path for many motor acts, the respiratory drive gives it a particular advantage by providing it with a readily controlled, continuous, stereotyped behavior under anesthesia. STA or cross-correlation methods may then be used to measure connections under standardized conditions and thereby to assign proportions of the motor drive to the different inputs which are active under those conditions. We have recently returned to investigating this system because we believe that this stereotyped motor behavior, together with its underlying specific pattern of connections, is a useful one in which to study the plasticity of descending fibers following spinal cord injury (Kirkwood and Ford, 1997).

The connections from the EBSNs to the expiratory motoneurons may be monosynaptic or polysynaptic (Kirkwood, 1995; Kirkwood and Road, 1995). Here we are concerned with the monosynaptic component, the estimated strength of which has varied widely between different studies (Iscoe, 1998). The purposes of this chapter are to review the published evidence concerning this connection and to add new data from work in progress. This will illustrate the different approaches which have been used to assess the strength of the connection and will identify some of the reasons why different answers can be obtained. We suggest that the problems of interpretation involved are likely to be common to similar studies in other systems of descending fibers, so the conclusions here should have some general validity.

Methods

The new results described here came from experiments on cats anesthetized with sodium pentobarbitone, paralyzed with gallamine triethiodide (subsequent to surgery) and artificially ventilated with O_2-enriched air and with CO_2 added to produce a brisk respiratory drive. The animals were mounted prone, supported from vertebral clamps and a plate screwed to the skull. They received a thoracic laminectomy and occipital craniotomy. For full details, including care of the preparation, see Kirkwood (1995).

The experiments were of two types, in which the recording procedures and the nerve dissections varied somewhat. The first type was aimed at recording from and intraxonally labeling the thoracic axons of EBSNs, the second at intracellular recording from thoracic motoneurons, with STA from EBSNs. In all experiments, the timing of inspiration, and hence of the central respiratory drive, was defined by efferent discharges recorded from a rostral external intercostal nerve (T5–7). In experiments aimed at bulbospinal axons, no other nerve dissection was needed, though the internal intercostal nerve and a bundle of dorsal ramus nerves from the left side of the segment of interest (T6–10) were usually dissected and used for identification of electrode position for the most medial electrode tracks, via motoneuron antidromic field potentials (Kirkwood et al., 1988). In the intracellular motoneuron experiments, motoneurons were identified by antidromic activation from one of these two nerves or from the external intercostal nerve. These three nerves were usually prepared from two adjacent segments (T5–T8), to allow for recording in either one.

In the bulbospinal axon experiments an array of three fine wire stimulating electrodes (tips at different depths, cathode) with a fourth electrode (anode) 3 mm more rostral was inserted into the left lateral funiculus at the level of the C1 dorsal roots. Axons were penetrated at thoracic levels. The criteria for their identification as EBSN axons were: (a) an incrementing pattern of expiratory discharges (silence in inspiration) and (b) non-synaptic excitation (sharp threshold, lack of temporal summation and relatively constant latency) from one of the C1 electrodes, but *without* collision following a spontaneous impulse. The last criterion is important because ascending expiratory axons, which extended as far as C1, were sometimes encountered (cf. Tanaka and Hirai, 1994). These were identified by the same criteria, but *with* collision. No recording was performed in the medulla. Axons were penetrated in the left lateral, ventral or medial funiculi, using penetrations through the lateral funiculus with glass micro-

electrodes filled with 2% Neurobiotin™ in 1 M KCl (beveled to impedances of 50–150 MΩ) and intra-axonal iontophoretic injections of Neurobiotin were made (+ ve pulses, 22–187 nA min). After a survival time of 2–21 h, the animal was perfused with a phosphate-buffered saline rinse followed by 4% paraformaldehyde, 0.1% glutaraldehyde and 0.2% picric acid in 0.1M phosphate buffer (pH 7.4). The relevant spinal cord segments were removed and post-fixed overnight in the same fixative but without glutaraldehyde and with 25% sucrose. Frozen sections (50 μm, transverse) were cut, processed with avidin-HRP (Sigma)/DAB or ABC Elite (Vector)/DAB, using standard procedures, and counterstained with neutral red.

In the motoneuron experiments, intracellular recordings were made from antidromically identified motoneurons on the left side, using glass microelectrodes broken back to 1.4–1.8 μm external tip diameter and filled with 4 M K$^+$ acetate. Single EBSNs were recorded in the right NRA, 2–3 mm caudal to obex, identified antidromically from electrodes placed in the left ventrolateral funiculus about two segments caudal to the spinal segment used for recording. The criteria for antidromic identification and the calculations of conduction times were as in Kirkwood (1995). STA was performed either on- or off-line (all data was stored on magnetic tape) from the discharges of one or more EBSNs, using at least 1024 sweeps (usually >4096), with the addition of extracellular control averages. Waveforms observed in the averages were only accepted as EPSPs if they fulfilled latency/ rise-time criteria similar to the latency/half-width criteria used for cross-correlation peaks by Kirkwood (1995). In addition to the STA measurements, particular note was made of the form and amplitude of the respiratory drive potentials in the motoneurons (CRDP, Sears, 1964).

Results: anatomy

Previous work

A number of authors have demonstrated projections from the NRA to the thoracic ventral horn, using both retrograde and anterograde labeling techniques. In the cat the locations of intercostal and abdominal muscle motoneurons have been demonstrated using retrograde tracing techniques (Holstege et al., 1987; for other refs, Kirkwood et al., 1988). At the light microscopical level Holstege and Kuypers (1982), using tritiated leucine, were the first to demonstrate direct projections from the caudal medullary ventrolateral tegmental field, including the nucleus retroambiguus, to the intercostal and abdominal motoneuronal cell groups. However, their injections extended into more rostral parts of the NRA, where inspiratory bulbospinal neurons are located (Monteau and Hilaire, 1991), as evidenced by their finding of projections to the phrenic nucleus at C5. Later studies (Feldman et al., 1985; Holstege, 1989) presented more caudal injections and were more relevant to the question here because they avoided the inspiratory neurons. This resulted in an absence of labeled projections to the phrenic nucleus, and presumably therefore also fewer labeled projections from inspiratory neurons to the thoracic motor nuclei.

However, the clearest data have come from a more recent experiment (VanderHorst and Holstege, 1995) in which rather precise injections of wheatgerm-agglutinin horseradish peroxidase (WGA–HRP) in the caudal NRA were combined with an ipsilateral upper cervical hemisection to eliminate the ipsilateral projections from nearby, but more medially located neurons. Figure 1 shows previously unpublished drawings of the pattern of label seen at three different thoracic segments in this experiment.

There is a clear concentration of the label in the contralateral ventral horn, with a similar but weaker ipsilateral distribution. Since the cord was hemisected at C2 (note the exclusively contralateral white matter label) the ipsilateral label must have come from collaterals recrossing the midline. In common with each of the other studies cited above, a feature of this pattern is a very heavy concentration of the label in clumps in the ventrolateral portion of the ventral horn. This is where the lateral group of motoneurons is located, including those innervating internal intercostal and abdominal muscles, which have expiratory actions (Monteau and Hilaire, 1991). This pattern therefore would seem to be evidence for a strong and specific pathway

from the NRA to these motoneurons. However, there are some problems with this interpretation if it is based only on this type of experiment. Firstly, the most ventrolateral part of the ventral horn, which is most strongly labeled in Fig. 1, is also the location of the motoneurons innervating the inspiratory-activated, parasternal muscle (Lipski and Martin-Body, 1987; Kirkwood et al., 1988). Secondly, in these drawings there are similar strong clumps of label ventromedially, which is another location where motoneurons activated in inspiration are found (external intercostal and levator costae, Monteau and Hilaire, 1991). A priori, these motoneurons with inspiratory actions would not be expected to receive connections from EBSNs. Finally, measurements of the terminals of *individual* EBSN axons, both anatomical and physiological, as described below, do not show these strong concentrations. Thus, although the projections demonstrated this way appear strong, whether the connections to motoneurons should or should not be considered as such needs support from other types of measurement.

Present experiments

Seven EBSN axons were considered successfully labeled (injected in segments T6-T10). For all of these, collaterals were identified. A further two EBSN axons were labeled, for which no collaterals were found, but the labeling in each case was faint, so the absence of collaterals for these may be an artifact of the weak staining. The axons were widely distributed in the ventral and lateral funiculi (Fig. 2A), corresponding to the white matter label in Fig.1 or to the physiological measurements of Kirkwood (1995). The initial trajectories of selected collaterals are included in Fig. 2A and look very similar to those in Fig. 1. The measurements described below are based only on collaterals considered to be well stained, i.e. terminating in boutons rather than simply fading out, as was observed for the collaterals most distant from the site of injection or in less well stained examples. An exception to this restriction was made for collaterals crossing the midline. Several collaterals did this (Fig. 2C) and, although a few boutons were seen contralateral to their stem axons, most collaterals became faint once they had crossed the midline and thus this part of their projection is likely to be underestimated in our data.

The extent of individual collaterals varied widely, as seen in Fig. 2. This variation was not an artifact of limited staining, because, for some axons, collaterals more distant from the injection site were longer and more complex than others nearer to it. Collaterals typically branched into a rostrally and a caudally directed process soon after entry into the gray matter. Often the two ran in different parts of the ventral horn, one laterally, one

medially, frequently close to the lateral or medial borders, i.e. within the areas which appeared heavily labeled in Fig. 1. A trajectory running diagonally ventrolateral to dorsomedial (Fig. 2C, cf. Fig. 4E) was also common.

The rostrocaudal spread of individual collaterals was also variable, as was the spacing between collaterals (Fig. 3). It was notable that there were often quite wide gaps between the most distal terminals of adjacent collaterals (5–6 mm in the best stained parts of the axons in Fig. 3) so that many motoneurons must have been out of range of being contacted by a given axon (cf. Shinoda et al.

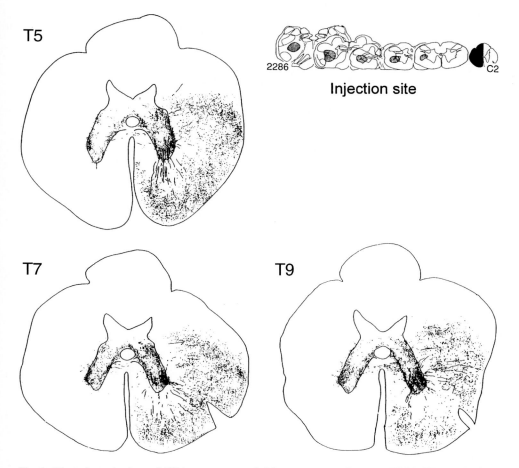

Fig. 1. Thoracic projections of NRA neurons revealed by an anterograde tracer (WGA–HRP). Distributions of the reaction product seen at three different thoracic spinal cord segments in the cat, following injections in the NRA, coupled with an ipsilateral C2 hemisection. The illustrations for each segment represent superimposed drawings of six consecutive collected (1:4) sections. Inset, injection site, centered on the NRA. The projections to the lumbar cord of this cat, labeled from the same injections (case no. 2286), have already been illustrated (VanderHorst and Holstege, 1995).

1986). Another common feature was that the rostrally or caudally running branches (typically rather fine: dia. 0.5–1 μm), could be followed through several 50 μm sections without any branching or terminals visible, before terminating with modest branching and a few boutons. The presence of such fine rostro-caudally running branches was deduced from the distribution of terminal and focal synaptic potentials by Kirkwood (1995).

Individual boutons varied in size and shape. Formal measurements of diameter have not been made, and may be difficult because of uncertainties in staining towards the ends of some collaterals, but our impression is that although some large (up to 2.5 μm) boutons were present most were small (≤ 1 μm). Short chains of boutons *en passant* were frequently seen. Preterminal processes were often very fine, apparently at the limit of resolution of the microscope, as has been reported for other descending axons (e.g. Rouiller et al., 1996). For two axons with well-stained collaterals the ratios of boutons *en passant* to *terminaux* were 116/53 and 448/243. Very few boutons were found close to counterstained neuronal somata. Examples of boutons are illustrated in Fig. 4A–C.

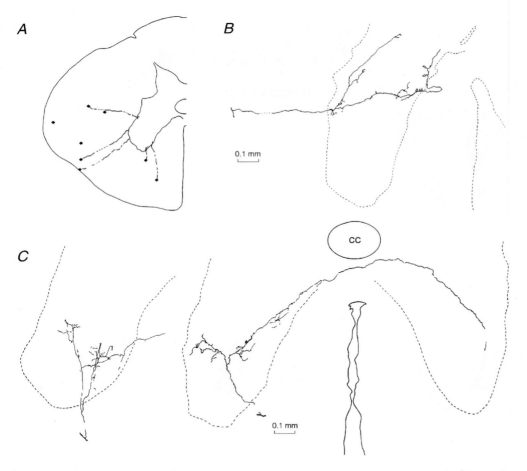

Fig. 2. Features of individual EBSN axons, labeled with Neurobiotin. A, positions of stem axons (♦) plotted onto a typical spinal cord section outline. For five of the axons, the initial trajectory of one of their collaterals is also plotted. B, C, drawings of individual collaterals. The two collaterals shown in C came from the same axon, and are represented by C2 and C3 in Fig. 3A. The collateral in B, is typical in the way it divided into two main branches. The lateral branch was found entirely in the sevens sections (0.35 mm) rostral to the first branch point, the medial branch entirely in the 10 sections (0.5 mm) caudal to that point. CC, central canal.

Although the trajectories of the collateral branches most often ran along the lateral or medial border of the ventral horn, the distributions of terminals for individual collaterals or individual axons was rather more uniform (Fig. 4D–F). There was no indication of clumping, as is apparent in the drawings of Fig. 1. It is also worth noting that the distributions from even individual collaterals, such as in Fig. 4D,E represent the projection of many sections onto one transverse plane. Because of the common rostrocaudal trajectory of many of the branches, in any one transverse section there might often be only a few terminals, located perhaps in one small area. This could be relatively dorsal, ventral, medial or lateral, just as was seen electrophysiologically (see below and Fig. 5).

These results emphasize that the darkfield images from anterograde tracing experiments, including the drawings in Fig. 1, are likely to include a high proportion of label in preterminal collateral branches and thus may correspond more closely to the collateral trajectories than to the distributions of boutons. Although it may be possible in the microscope to distinguish between fibers and terminals, the actual distribution of terminals from these experiments is hard to repre-

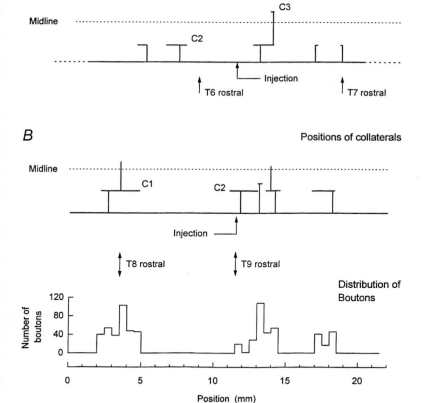

Fig. 3. Longitudinal plots of the collateral organization for two axons. A, axon with the two collaterals (C2, C3) illustrated in Fig. 2C. B, Another axon, also including its corresponding longitudinal distribution of boutons. The collaterals C1 and C2 are the two individual collaterals illustrated in Fig. 4D,E. The diagrams are to scale only along the long axis (scale in B also applies to A). Segmental boundaries were defined as the position of the most rostral dorsal root in each segment. For each collateral, the position of its origin, the total spread of its branches and the position of any crossing branch is illustrated. The extents of the most rostral and the two most caudal collaterals in A may have been underestimated because of faint staining.

sent. It is nevertheless, clear that the areas of termination must cover both the areas containing the motoneuron somata, which also contain their many rostrocaudally running dendrites and the areas containing their dorsally directed dendrites. Like the collaterals, the dorsally directed dendrites have a tendency to be grouped towards the lateral or medial border of the ventral horn (Lipski and Martin-Body, 1987). However these same areas also contain a great many interneurons (Fig. 4G), especially medially (Kirkwood et al., 1988). Moreover, interneurons located medially or more dorsally often have dendrites extending laterally or ventrally (Saywell et al., 1998).

Thus, although on the basis of all the anatomical evidence so far, motoneurons would be considered the most likely targets of the EBSNs, the evidence for this is, strictly speaking, circumstantial. Only the most recent of the anatomical evidence has unequivocally demonstrated, via double-labeling experiments, that the NRA-motoneuronal projections are actually direct and rather numerous. Both in the cat (Boers and Holstege, 1999) and in the monkey (VanderHorst et al., 1999), it has been demonstrated at the ultrastructural level that there are direct, presumed excitatory, projections to the external oblique abdominal muscle motoneurons. Moreover, these direct projections were not diffi-

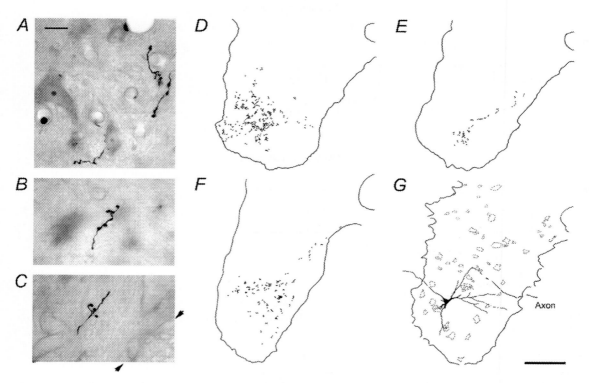

Fig. 4. Features of terminal fields of individual EBSN axons. A–C, photomicrographs of typical terminal arrangements (digitally-assembled montages of images at 3–5 different focal planes, 100× objective). A,B, examples of boutons among the large neurons in lamina IX. C, example of boutons located more dorsomedially in lamina VIII (arrowheads indicate the medial border of the ventral horn. D,E, distributions of boutons in the transverse plane for two individual collaterals of the axon of Fig. 3B, collaterals C1, C2 respectively. F, equivalent distribution of all the boutons labeled for the axon of Fig. 3A. G, partial reconstruction (soma plus proximal dendrites and axon) of an identified interneuron in lamina IX, intracellularly recorded and labeled with Neurobiotin. The interneuron had an early expiratory (decrementing) firing pattern and a descending axon traced for several mm in the contralateral medial funiculus. Dotted cell outlines show the Nissl stained cells or fragments in the same 50 μm section as the main part of the soma. Note that the interneuron is one of the largest cells in this section. Previously unpublished data from Saywell et al. (1998). Calibration in A applies to A–C, 20 μm; calibration in G applies to D–G, 0.2 mm.

cult to find, and the great majority of the terminals observed each had a synaptic contact with a motoneuronal dendrite. These measurements were made on motoneurons in an upper lumbar segment, thus confirming the physiological results of Road and Kirkwood (1993) (cf. Kirkwood and Road, 1995). The light-microscopical appearance of the projections is rather similar at lumbar and thoracic levels, but the electron microscopical measurements have yet to be extended to the thoracic segments.

Results: physiology

Previous work

The existence of direct connections from EBSNs to motoneurons has been known since the preliminary publication of Kirkwood and Sears (1973). Following Mendell and Henneman (1971) and Jankowska and Roberts (1972), this was the first use of STA to demonstrate a previously unknown connection and the first use for a long descending pathway. The result remained unconfirmed until Cohen et al.

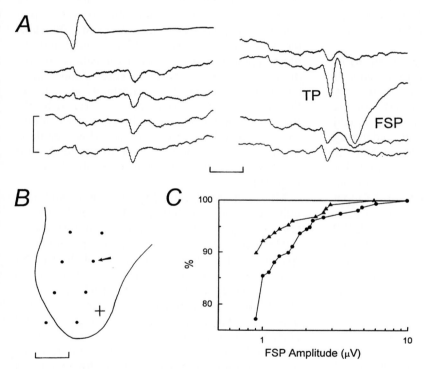

Fig. 5. Spatial factors in the distribution of EBSN terminals. A, systematic sampling of the field potentials recorded using STA from an EBSN: averages made from extracellular recordings via a tungsten electrode at eight sites in the ventral horn (TP, terminal potential; FSP, focal synaptic potential); uppermost trace, trigger spike. B, arrangement of the grid of sites used for the recordings illustrated in A. The grid was positioned with respect to the motoneuron antidromic field potentials; reference point indicated by the cross. Ventral horn outline is schematic. The averages in A are displayed so as to correspond to the arrangement of sites in B, the site with the largest FSP in A being arrowed in B. Calibrations, 5 μV, 1 ms, 2.5 mm. For more details, see Kirkwood (1995), from which A,B were reproduced, with permission. C, cumulative histograms of FSP amplitudes. FSP amplitudes (>1 μV) from each site of a single grid as in B, positioned within the most rostral mm of a segment and/or within the caudal half of a segment were measured from a number of EBSNs. The eight amplitudes from each grid contributed to one or other of the two histograms. Filled circles, rostral sites; filled triangles, caudal sites. Note the log scale on the abscissa. The two curves superimpose well if one of them is shifted on the amplitude axis by a factor of 1.6. The data in C was replotted from the data of Kirkwood (1995), but with the an enlarged sample of EBSNs.

(1985) showed that peaks in cross-correlations between the discharges of EBSNs and thoracic expiratory nerve discharges were common. However, these measurements were uncalibrated, in that it was not known what sizes of EPSPs the peaks in their cross-correlograms represented. Thus, Merrill and Lipski (1987) were able to dismiss these otherwise clear observations, when in an apparently thorough survey of connections by STA, they found only two EPSPs (amplitudes 55, 62 μV) in 57 EBSN/motoneuron pairs. Their result confirmed the existence of the connection but relegated its importance to that of a small variant on an assumed oligosynaptic pathway via respiratory interneurons, which they recorded in the same region. This interpretation, of course, could still be considered consistent with the anatomical data then available, as explained above.

The pendulum swung back again with Kirkwood's (1995) cross-correlation measurements of the direct connections. These results were very similar to those of Cohen et al. (1985), but the peaks in the cross-correlation histograms could now be interpreted in terms of their underlying EPSPs (see Kirkwood and Sears, 1991) and the peaks were carefully screened to be appropriate for a monosynaptic effect in latency and duration. From these measurements the strength of the input was calculated to be more than ten times greater than in Merrill and Lipski (1987), a mean EPSP size of 22 μV instead of 2.05 μV. Taking account of the likely numbers of EBSNs active, this was enough to provide about 10 mV of depolarization to the motoneurons i.e. most of that needed to bring them to threshold.

> The calculations for this last deduction may be made in different ways. Here the basis was EPSP amplitudes, with the assumption of linear addition. A more sophisticated model (Rose and Cushing, Chapter 8, this volume), with assumed unitary conductances (therefore allowing for non-linear addition) suggests that motoneurons need a much larger fraction of their inputs active than was assumed by Kirkwood (1995), especially for a high level of drive. However, for motoneurons close to threshold, non-linear addition of EPSPs is of less consequence and the differences between

the models is much less. The starting point for the expiratory motoneurons has to be the EPSP amplitudes, because these are what were measured or estimated. Moreover, these measurements or estimates were made with the motoneurons in a depolarized or firing state. We do not have figures for the unitary conductances, nor data on the electrotonic properties of these motoneurons. Linear addition of these EPSPs, even in the light of Rose and Cushing's calculations, may therefore still be considered to be a reasonable assumption.

The wide disparity between the cross-correlation results and the STA results of Merrill and Lipski (1987), led Kirkwood (1995) to conclude that two different populations of motoneurons were represented in the two sets of measurements. Which of these two populations should be considered the most representative? As an explanation for the discharge of expiratory motoneurons under these conditions (relatively light barbiturate anesthesia), the motoneurons monosynaptically excited by the EBSNs, as demonstrated in the cross-correlations, would clearly be of most interest. However these motoneurons may be only 10% of the total, so it could be argued that this connection should not be regarded as typical.

Moreover, an additional factor which could have influenced the sampling in Merrill and Lipski's (1987) study also became apparent in Kirkwood's (1995) study. This factor is an inhomogeneity in the spatial distribution of the terminals of the EBSNs within a spinal segment, which was demonstrated by using the extracellular variant of STA (Taylor et al., 1977). This technique reveals terminal potentials (TPs), representing conduction in pre-terminal branches, and focal synaptic potentials (FSPs), representing post-synaptic currents in the terminal regions (Munson and Sypert, 1979). An example is illustrated in Fig. 5A,B, showing how, in any one transverse plane, the FSPs from the EBSNs are found typically within a restricted location. In this case the FSPs with amplitudes > 1 μV appeared at only two (rather dorsomedially located) of eight standardized recording sites in the ventral horn. In Fig. 5C cumulative distributions are shown for FSP amplitudes for a number of EBSNs, measured at eight such standardized sites at either a rostral position in the segment (defined by the dorsal root entry points) or more caudally. The curve for the rostral sites is well to the right of that for the caudal one, demonstrating that FSPs in the rostral region were on average 1.6 times as large as, or more frequent than caudally. A similar pattern was seen for the TPs.

On the assumption that this pattern does not represent restricted impulse conduction in more caudal collaterals (cf. Wall and McMahon, 1994), the result indicates that collateral branches are more common or widespread in the rostral region. Does the effect show up in the anatomical measurements? By bulk labeling methods it has not yet been investigated. In our intra-axonal injection experiments we have of course looked for it. In fact, to verify this result is quite demanding. The typical length of a thoracic segment is 10 mm, but the length of axon *with reliable labeling of collaterals* in our experiments was usually less than ±10 mm from the injection site. Most of our injections were in the rostral part of the segment. Shorter collaterals or fewer terminations further away from the rostral end of the section might then arise artifactually because they were further from the injection site. The only data which will reliably show an uneven distribution of the terminations would be where more distant terminations were more profuse than closer ones. Only two axons were sufficiently well filled to test whether or not terminations were more common in the rostral than the caudal parts of a segment. One of them, injected about 2.7 mm from the rostral end of the segment, did not appear to fit the pattern (Fig. 3A). However, our best filled axon showed a well-filled exuberant collateral in rostral T8, none in mid/caudal T8, but a cluster of collaterals in rostral T9 (Fig. 3B). This one axon thus gives independent anatomical support to the physiological data. In addition, supporting evidence comes from preliminary data from an anterograde labeling study using injections of the lectin, PHA-L into the NRA (Ford et al., 1997).

Present experiments

We are presently repeating the measurements of Merrill and Lipski (1987), but now in the context of the results from Kirkwood (1995). The results to date have all been derived from STA in motoneurons located in the rostral part of the segment. Those of interest had axons in the internal intercostal nerve and showed an expiratory central respiratory drive potential (CRDP, Sears, 1964), i.e. they were more hyperpolarized in inspiration than in expiration. For these motoneurons both of the factors suggested above (i.e. a bias in the connections towards motoneurons in the rostral part of a segment and towards active motoneurons) seem to be important in determining the connectivity.

With regard to the first factor, STA EPSPs (Fig. 6B) were observed in 17/38 EBSN/motoneuron pairs, with a mean amplitude of 58 ± 55 μV (S.D.), i.e. about 10 times stronger than in Merrill and Lipski (1987). We must assume that when we repeat these measurements more caudally in the segment, then we will find much sparser connections, i.e. the reason these connections were not found by Merrill and Lipski is because they did not

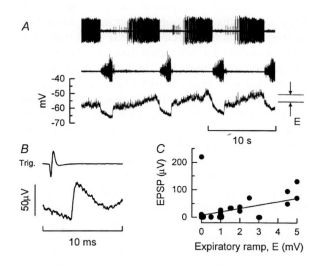

Fig. 6. Relationship between EPSPs from single EBSNs and respiratory drive potentials in expiratory motoneurons. A, example of original recordings: top, EBSN; middle, external intercostal nerve; bottom, motoneuron (E, expiratory ramp). B, STA EPSP from this pair. Trig., trigger spike. C, EPSP amplitude plotted against E. Line, linear regression ($r = 0.42$, $p = 0.009$). Figure reproduced from Ford et al. (1999), with permission.

sample sufficiently rostral within the segment. This being so, then the regional difference in the functional projections of the axons seen in the FSPs will be seen to be reflected in a difference in the connectivity to expiratory motoneurons. Moreover, this difference in connectivity could be large enough to explain the difference between the results of Merrill and Lipski (1987) and the cross-correlation results, though the functional significance of the strong rostral connections would remain obscure.

With regard to the second factor, even within the population of rostrally located motoneurons, the direct connections from the EBSNs seem to be restricted to a certain group. This was demonstrated by relating the amplitudes of the EPSPs (which covered a wide range, 7–220 μV) to the overall level of expiratory excitation in the motoneuron, as shown by the CRDP. The CRDP has two main components, an inhibition during inspiration (Sears, 1964) and an incrementing depolarization during expiration, this latter corresponding to the incrementing discharge of the EBSNs (Fig. 6A). The amplitudes of this ramp also covered a wide range. For many examples it was zero, the CRDP then consisting only of an apparent inhibition during inspiration. When the EPSP amplitude was plotted against the ramp amplitude, a clear positive correlation was seen (Fig. 6C). The slope of this correlation was large enough to suggest that all of the expiratory depolarization in firing motoneurons is derived from this source, as follows. A reasonable estimate for the ramp of excitation in a firing motoneuron (Sears, 1977) would be between 6 and 12 mV (uncertainty is present because there may be a step of depolarization at the start of expiration as well as the ramp component, but that step would not be distinguishable from the termination of the inspiratory inhibition). Only a modest extrapolation of the relationship shown in Fig. 6C is needed to give a mean EPSP amplitude of around 100 μV. The necessary integral of the input of 20 000 such EPSPs per second (Kirkwood, 1995; cf. Sears, 1977; cf. Prochazka et al., 1989) could then be achieved by 200 contralateral EBSNs firing at a typical 100 impulses/s, or even fewer when crossing collaterals are taken into account. This number is thus well below the 400 EBSNs assumed to be present on each side of the medulla by Kirkwood (1995). It follows that the proportionately smaller ramps actually measured could also be derived entirely from the monosynaptic excitation.

The relationship between the EPSP amplitude and the excitatory ramp of the CRDP is remarkably strong. The extrapolated average amplitude of around 100 μV is more than four times larger than predicted from the cross-correlation measurements. One reason for this may be inaccuracies in the assumptions used in predicting this EPSP amplitude from the cross-correlation peaks. However, although an error of a factor of two might not be so much of a surprise (cf. comparisons between different studies in Kirkwood and Sears, 1991), a factor of more than four suggests there could be an additional explanation. It could well be that not all firing expiratory motoneurons receive such strong monosynaptic excitation, and the rostrally located motoneurons with a strong respiratory drive would then be seen as an even more specialized group.

Clearly, further investigations are needed to identify what this group of motoneurons represents, including similar STA measurements in the caudal parts of the segments. One possibility is that motoneuron size or motor unit type might be a factor (Munson, 1990), but the effect would be an extreme example of this phenomenon (no input at all to many motoneurons, a very strong input for a few). It is also interesting that this highly specialized connection, which appears to be solely responsible for the expiratory motoneuron output in these conditions, may nevertheless be quite inappropriate for some other motor acts (Kirkwood and Road, 1995). The restriction of the monosynaptic input to a subgroup of the expiratory motoneurons is also reminiscent of the organization of the inspiratory input to inspiratory thoracic motoneurons, where this input appears to be transmitted via one more synapse to the motoneurons of one group as compared to another (Vaughan and Kirkwood, 1997). A wide variation in the CRDP amplitude between different motoneurons is also present in the inspiratory population, which may be related to spatial factors in the muscle (Kirkwood and Sears, 1978), the spatial factors themselves perhaps having mechanical significance (Wilson and De Troyer, 1993).

Discussion

As is the case for most neural systems, our understanding of the organization of the connections here has come in an iterative fashion. The new anatomical measurements, both from the single fibers and from Fig.1, add to that process. The details of the collaterals confirm many features already reported from physiological measurements (Kirkwood, 1995) and they make more explicit the existence of features which can be deduced only indirectly from the bulk labeling experiments. Among these features are collaterals crossing the midline, though the bulk labeling methods (e.g. Fig. 1) probably give a truer picture of the relative sizes of the projections to the two sides, on account of the fading in the staining for crossing collaterals in the single-axon experiments. Most importantly, the general correspondence between the pattern of the projections from the single axons with that of the bulk labeling confirms that this latter projection is likely to be comprised primarily of the EBSN axons.

However, as argued earlier, the measurements on the single axons also serve to emphasize the indirectness of the conclusions that can be drawn from the bulk labeling with regard to the direct contacts on motoneurons. This indirectness may be regarded as a nicety by some. For instance, in a different context, that of corticospinal connections, Dum and Strick (1996) pointed out that physiological verification of connections to motoneurons usually did follow the demonstration of even relatively weak anatomical projections to lamina IX (cf. Boers and Holstege, 1999; VanderHorst et al. 1997, 1999). However, the situation for the thoracic segments is particularly critical in this regard. Here the motoneurons are not restricted to the columns described by Rexed (1952): motoneurons are found across the whole width of a very narrow ventral horn, locations of motoneurons with inspiratory activation patterns (external intercostal and inter-chondral muscle) and expiratory patterns (internal intercostal and abdominal muscle) overlap almost completely (Lipski and Martin-Body, 1987), and a great many interneurons are also found in the same locations (Kirkwood et al., 1988).

Moreover, although the STA results do confirm that there are some strong connections, a striking aspect of the physiological results is that, considering the whole population of motoneurons within the area of termination defined anatomically, the direct connections are in fact made only to a small minority of these cells. Connections from the EBSNs to one major group, the motoneurons with inspiratory actions, or to motoneurons with axons in the dorsal ramus are very rare (Merrill and Lipski, 1987; Saywell et al., 1999). Even for the expiratory motoneurons in the rostral part of the segment they are present for less than 50% of these cells. These results thus emphasize that in order to make useful statements about the strengths of inputs to motoneurons, quantification becomes essential.

In the corticospinal analogy quoted above, when comparing projections from cortical areas SMA and M1, Dum and Strick (1996), like Rouiller et al. (1996), emphasized the relevance of the *existence* of a direct connection. However, for a proper comparison of the function of the two projections, a quantitative approach, including both physiological and anatomical measurements may be more important (Lemon et al., 1998; cf. discussion in Rouiller et al., 1996). The measurement of single unit connections by STA, as here, is a powerful method that can allow previously unsuspected specificities to show up. The method was first used by Mendell and Henneman (1971) to show the near universal connectivity of muscle spindle afferents to homonymous motoneurons, a result which is often used as a model for other motoneuron inputs. The present results describe the organization of a central input to motoneurons which appears to be rather different, being restricted to a particular group of motoneurons. For these motoneurons, however, this input is clearly of great importance and must be regarded as a very strong one. This example may be the only one to date where the input from only one set of central neurons has been calculated to be sufficient to bring the motoneurons to threshold (but cf. Prochazka et al., 1989). It will be important to determine what the particular group of motoneurons here represents. We suggest that it will be equally important to determine for most other descending pathways whether they are organized in this fashion, with individual inputs being directed to only a subset of motoneurons within a given motor nucleus, or whether they are organized with a more uniform distribution of inputs, like the spindle afferents of Mendell and Henneman (1971).

Acknowledgements

We would like to thank S. Mori, K. Nakajima and K. Matsuyama for their collaboration at the start of the anatomical experiments, J.D. Road and C.W. Vaughan, who each participated in one or two of the physiology experiments, A. Taylor, who kindly allowed us to use his laboratory for some experiments while ours was being rebuilt, L. Levita, for assistance with measurements on the collaterals, and V.G.M. VanderHorst who was largely responsible for producing the data for Fig. 1. The work was supported by the Wellcome Trust and the International Spinal Research Trust.

List of abbreviations

CRDP	Central respiratory drive potential
DAB	Diaminobenzidine
EBSN	Expiratory bulbospinal neuron
EPSP	Excitatory post-synaptic potential
FSP	Focal synaptic potential
HRP	Horseradish peroxidase
NRA	Nucleus retroambiguus
M1	Primary motor area
PHA-L	*Phaseolus vulgaris*-leucoagglutinin
SMA	Supplementary motor area
STA	Spike-triggered averaging
TP	Terminal potential
WGA	Wheatgerm-agglutinin

References

Boers, J. and Holstege, G. (1999) Evidence for direct projections from the nucleus retroambiguous to the motoneurons of the external oblique in the female cat. *Soc. Neurosci.*, Abstracts, 25, 51.3.

Cohen, M.I., Feldman, J.L. and Sommer, D. (1985) Caudal medullary expiratory neuron and internal intercostal nerve discharges in the cat: effects of lung inflation. *J. Physiol.* 368: 147–178.

Davies, J.G.McF., Kirkwood, P.A. and Sears, T.A. (1985) The detection of monosynaptic connexions from inspiratory bulbospinal neurones to inspiratory motoneurones in the cat. *J. Physiol.*, 368: 33–62.

De Troyer, A. (1991) Inspiratory elevation of the ribs in the dog: primary role of the parasternals. *J. Appl. Physiol.*, 70: 1447–1455.

Dum, R.P. and Strick, P.L. (1996) Spinal cord terminations of the medial wall motor areas in macaque monkeys. *J. Neurosci.*, 16: 6513–6525.

Feldman, J.L., Loewy, A.D. and Speck, D.F. (1985) Projections from the ventral respiratory group to phrenic and intercostal motoneurons in cat: an autoradiographic study. *J. Neurosci.*, 5: 1993–2000.

Ford, T.W., Matsuyama, K., Mori, S. and Nakajima, K. (1997) Projections from the nucleus retroambigualis (nRA) to the thoracic spinal cord of the cat studied with the anterograde axonal tracer *Phaseolus vulgaris*-leucoagglutinin (PHA–L). *J. Physiol.*, 505.P: 85P.

Ford, T.W., Saywell, S.A. and Kirkwood, P.A. (1999) Relationship between single-fibre EPSPs and respiratory drive potentials in expiratory motoneurones. *J. Physiol.*, 519.P, 69P.

Grélot, L., Milano, S., Gestreau, C. and Bianchi, A.L. (1996) Are medullary respiratory neurones multipurpose neurones? In: H. Bostock, P.A. Kirkwood and A.H. Pullen (Eds), *The Neurobiology of Disease: Contributions from Neuroscience to Clinical Neurology*, Cambridge University Press, Cambridge, pp. 299–308.

Holstege, G. (1989) Anatomical study of the final common pathway for vocalization in the cat. *J. Compara. Neurol.*, 284: 242–252.

Holstege, G. and Kuypers, H.G.J.M. (1982) The anatomy of brain stem pathways to the spinal cord in the cat. A labeled amino acid tracing study. In: H.G.J.M. Kuypers and G.F. Martin (Eds), *Descending Pathways to the Spinal Cord, Progress in Brain Research*, Vol. 57, Elsevier, Amsterdam, pp. 145–175

Holstege, G. van Neerven, J. and Evertse, F. (1987) Spinal cord location of the motoneurons innervating the abdominal, cutaneous maximus, latissimus dorsi and longissimus dorsi muscles in the cat. *Exp. Brain Res.*, 67: 179–194.

Iscoe, S. (1998) Control of abdominal muscles. *Prog. Neurobiol.*, 56: 433–506.

Jankowska, E. and Roberts, W. J. (1972) Synaptic actions of interneurones mediating reciprocal Ia inhibition of motoneurones *J. Physiol.*, 222: 623–642.

Kirkwood, P.A. (1979) On the use and interpretation of cross-correlation measurements in the mammalian central nervous system. *J. Neurosci. Methods*, 1: 107–132.

Kirkwood, P.A. (1995) Synaptic excitation in the thoracic spinal cord from expiratory bulbospinal neurones in the cat. *J. Physiol.*, 484: 201–225.

Kirkwood, P.A. and Ford, T.W. (1997) Plasticity in functional projections of expiratory bulbospinal neurones in the cat. *J. Physiol.*, 504.P: 28–29S.

Kirkwood, P.A., Munson, J.B., Sears, T.A. and Westgaard, R.H. (1988) Respiratory interneurones in the thoracic spinal cord of the cat. *J. Physiol.*, 395: 161–192.

Kirkwood, P.A. and Road, J.D. (1995) On the functional significance of long monosynaptic descending pathways to spinal motoneurones. In: A. Taylor, M.H. Gladden and R. Durbaba (Eds), *Alpha and Gamma Motor Systems*, Plenum Press, London, pp. 589–592.

Kirkwood, P.A. and Sears, T.A. (1973) Monosynaptic excitation of thoracic expiratory motoneurones from lateral respiratory neurones in the medulla of the cat. *J. Physiol.*, 234: 87–89P.

Kirkwood, P.A. and Sears, T.A. (1978) The synaptic connexions to intercostal motoneurones as revealed by the average common excitation potential. *J. Physiol.*, 275: 103–134.

Kirkwood, P.A. and Sears. T.A. (1980) The measurement of synaptic connections in the mammalian central nervous system by means of spike triggered averaging. In: J.E. Desmedt (Ed.), *Spinal and Supraspinal Mechanisms of Voluntary Motor Control and Locomotion, Progress in Clinical Neurophysiology*, Vol. 8, Karger, Basel, pp. 44–71.

Kirkwood, P.A. and Sears, T.A. (1991) Cross-correlation analyses of motoneurone inputs in a coordinated motor act. In: J. Krüger (Ed.), *Neuronal Cooperativity*, Springer-Verlag, Berlin, pp. 225–248.

Lemon, R.N., Baker, S.N., Davis, J.A., Kirkwood, P.A., Maier, M.A. and Yang, H.-S. (1998) The importance of the corticomotoneuronal system for control of grasp. In: *Sensory Guidance of Movement, Novartis Foundation Symposium 218*, Wiley, Chichester, pp. 202–218.

Lipski, J. and Martin-Body, R.L. (1987) Morphological properties of respiratory intercostal motoneurons in cats as revealed by intracellular injection of horseradish peroxidase. *J. Compara. Neurol.*, 260: 423–434.

Mendell, L. M. and Henneman, E. (1971) Terminals of single Ia fibers: location, density and distribution within a pool of 300 homonymous motoneurons. *J. Neurophysiol.*, 34: 171–187.

Merrill, E.G. and Lipski, J. (1987) Inputs to intercostal motoneurons from ventrolateral medullary respiratory neurons in the cat. *J. Neurophysiol.*, 57: 1837–1853.

Monteau, R. and Hilaire, G. (1991) Spinal respiratory motoneurons. *Prog. Neurobiol.*, 37: 83–141.

Munson, J.B. (1990) Synaptic inputs to type-identified motor units. In: M.D. Binder and L.M. Mendell (Eds), *The Segmental Motor System*, Oxford University Press, New York, pp. 291–307.

Munson, J.B. and Sypert, G.W. (1979) Properties of single central Ia fibres projecting to motoneurones. *J. Physiol.*, 296: 315–328.

Prochazka, A., Hulliger, M., Trend P., Llewellyn M. and Dürmüller, N. (1989) Muscle afferent contribution to control of paw shakes in normal cats. *J. Neurophysiol.*, 61: 550–562

Rexed, B. (1952) A cytoarchitectonic organization of the spinal cord in the cat. *J. Compara. Neurol.*, 96: 415–495.

Road, J.D. and Kirkwood, P.A. (1993) Distribution of monosynaptic connections from expiratory bulbospinal neurones to motoneurones of different expiratory muscles in the cat. Abstracts XXXIII International Congress of Physiological Sciences: 141.39/P.

Rouiller, E.M., Moret, V., Tanné, J. and Boussaoud, D. (1996) Evidence for direct connections between the hand region of the supplementary motor area and cervical motoneurons in the macaque monkey. *Eur. J. Neurosci.*, 8: 1055–1059.

Saywell, S.A., Ford, T.W. and Kirkwood, P.A. (1998) Morphology and projections of thoracic interneurones. *J. Physiol.*, 509.P: 170P.

Saywell, S.A., Ford, T.W. and Kirkwood, P.A. (1999) Reinvestigation of connections from expiratory bulbospinal neurones to thoracic motoneurones. *J. Physiol.*, 518.P, 68P.

Sears, T.A. (1964) The slow potentials of thoracic respiratory motoneurones and their relation to breathing. *J. Physiol.*, 175: 404–424.

Sears, T.A. (1977) The respiratory motoneuron and apneusis. Federation Proceedings 36: 2412–2420.

Shinoda, Y, Yamaguchi, T. and Futami, T. (1986) Multiple axon collaterals of single corticospinal axons in the cat spinal cord. *J. Neurophysiol.*, 55: 425–448.

Tanaka, Y. and Hirai, N. (1994) Physiological studies of thoracic spinocerebellar tract neurons in relation to respiratory movement. *Neurosci. Res.*, 19: 317–326.

Taylor, A. (1960) The contribution of the intercostal muscles to the effort of respiration in man. *J. Physiol.*, 151: 390–402.

Taylor, A., Stephens, J.A., Somjen, G., Appenteng, K. and O'Donovan, M.J. (1977) Extracellular spike-triggered averaging for plotting synaptic projections. *Brain Res.*, 140: 344–448.

VanderHorst, V.G.M. and Holstege, G. (1995) Caudal medullary pathways to lumbosacral motoneuronal cell groups in the cat: evidence for direct projections possibly representing the final common pathway for lordosis. *J. Compara. Neurol.*, 359: 457–475.

VanderHorst, V.G.M. and Holstege, G. (1996) A concept for the final common pathway of vocalization and lordosis behavior in the cat. In: G. Holstege, R. Bandler and C.B. Saper (Eds), *The Emotional Motor System, Progress in Brain Research*, Vol. 107, Elsevier, Amsterdam, pp. 327–341.

VanderHorst, V.G.M. and Holstege, G. (1997a) Estrogen induces axonal outgrowth in the nucleus retroambiguus-lumbosacral motoneuronal pathway in the adult female cat. *J. Neurosci.*, 17: 1122–1136.

VanderHorst, V.G.M. and Holstege, G. (1997b) Nucleus retroambiguus projections to lumbosacral motoneuronal cell groups in the male cat. *J. Compara. Neurol.*, 382: 77–88.

VanderHorst, V.G.M., de Werd, H. and Holstege, G. (1997) Evidence for monosynaptic projections from the nucleus retroambiguus to hindlimb motoneurons in the cat. *Neurosci. Lett.*, 224: 33–36.

VanderHorst, V.G.J.M., Terasawa, E., Ralston, H.J., and Holstege, G. (1999) Monosynaptic projections from the

82

nucleus retroambiguus to motoneurons supplying the abdominal wall, axial, hindlimb, and pelvic floor in the female rhesus monkey. *J. Compara. Neurol.,*, submitted.

Vaughan, C.W. and Kirkwood, P.A. (1997) Evidence from motoneurone synchronization for disynaptic pathways in the control of inspiratory motoneurones in the cat. *J. Physiol.*, 503: 673–691.

Wall, P.D. and McMahon, S.B. (1994) Long range afferents in rat spinal cord. 3. Failure of impulse transmission in axons and relief of the failure after rhizotomy of dorsal roots. *Philosoph. Trans. Roy. Soc. Lond.*, Series B 343: 211–223.

Wilson, T.A. and De Troyer, A. (1993) Respiratory effect of the intercostal muscles in the dog. *J. Appl. Physiol.*, 75: 2636–2645.

M.D. Binder (Ed.)
Progress in Brain Research, Vol 123

CHAPTER 7

Models of spike encoding and their use in the interpretation of motor unit recordings in man

Randall K. Powers* and Marc D. Binder

Department of Physiology & Biophysics, University of Washington School of Medicine, Seattle, WA 98195, USA

Introduction

Recordings of motor unit activity in human subjects have provided a wealth of information about how the reflex and descending control of motoneurons change as a function of task, during fatigue and following injury. Our understanding of the organization of synaptic inputs to human motoneurons has been largely derived from measurements of the effects of activating a set of peripheral or descending fibers on the discharge probability of one or more motoneurons. The effects of a specific source of synaptic input on motoneuron behavior are assessed by compiling a peri-stimulus time histogram (PSTH; review in Kirkwood, 1979), which measures the probability of discharge of an individual motoneuron as a function of time from the stimulus, or by measuring the change in the discharge of a population of motoneurons, as reflected in the mean level of rectified electromyographic activity (EMG).

The magnitude and time course of a stimulus-evoked change in firing probability of a motor unit or a population of motor units is thought to reflect the size and shape of the underlying synaptic potential. Thus, changes in the response of a motoneuron to a given stimulus are generally assumed to reflect some alteration in the efficacy of presynaptic circuitry, i.e. either changes in pre-

*Corresponding author. Tel.: 206–685–2633; Fax: 206–685–0619; e-mail: rkpowers@u.washington.edu

synaptic inhibition in the case of a monosynaptic pathway (e.g. Stein and Capaday, 1988) or some modification in interneuronal excitability in the case of polysynaptic pathways (e.g. Pol et al., 1998). Although presynaptic factors are undoubtedly important, changes in motoneuron responsiveness may also play a role. As pointed out by Kirkwood and colleagues (Chapter 6, this volume) motoneuron responsiveness depends upon the characteristics of the background synaptic noise. Furthermore, motoneuron responsiveness is under neuromodulatory control (see Hultborn, Chapter 3; Heckman and Lee, Chapter 4; and Delgado-Lezama and Hounsgaard, Chapter 5, this volume).

The focus of this chapter is on postsynaptic mechanisms affecting the relation between synaptic inputs and their effects on firing rate. Figure 1 is a schematic representation of the transformation of an excitatory synaptic input into a change in motoneuron firing probability. Three different locations within the motoneuron that influence this transformation are highlighted: (1) the dendrites, (2) the soma and (3) the initial segment and axon hillock. Evoked or spontaneous activity in excitatory presynaptic fibers leads to transmitter release from their terminals (symbolized by the open triangle contacting the dendritic cable), and a portion of the current flowing through the ligand-gated channels reaches the soma. Spread of the current from the soma to the adjacent spike initiation zone (presumed to be the initial segment or axon hillock, cf. (Coombs et al., 1957)) increases the probability of spike initiation, which is reflected as a peak in the PSTH (Fetz and Gustafsson, 1983; Gustafsson and McCrea, 1984; Cope et al., 1987).

The vast majority of synaptic contacts are made upon on the dendrites, as they account for over 90% of the surface area of motoneurons (Rose et al., 1985; Bras et al., 1987; Cullheim et al., 1987). Thus, factors that affect the transfer of synaptic current from a dendritic site to the soma will clearly alter the effect of the synaptic input on motoneuron discharge behavior. For example, the local voltage change produced by a synaptic input may activate voltage-sensitive channels on the dendrites that could either amplify or reduce the amount of synaptic current reaching the soma (e.g. (Bernander et al., 1994; Schwindt and Crill, 1995; Lee and Heckman, 1996; Bennett et al., 1998), and Hultborn, Chapter 3, and Heckman and Lee, Chapter 4, this volume). Ongoing synaptic activity will also affect the transfer of current from the stimulated synapse to the soma by altering membrane conductance as well as the driving force for current flow (e.g. Rall, 1967; Jack et al., 1975, and Rose

Effects of Synaptic Events on Motoneuron Discharge

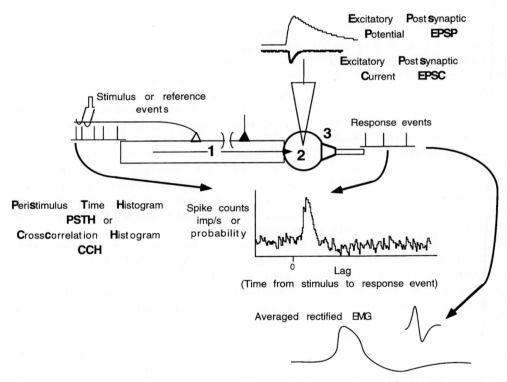

Fig. 1. Schematic illustration of the effects of a synaptic input on motoneuron firing probability. Evoked or spontaneous activity in excitatory presynaptic afferents leads to transmitter release from the synaptic terminals (open triangle) onto the motoneuron dendrites (1), and a portion of the synaptic current flows toward the soma (2). An intracellular electrode in the soma will record an associated excitatory postsynaptic current (EPSC) under voltage-clamp conditions or an excitatory postsynaptic potential (EPSP) under current-clamp conditions. The electrotonic spread of the synaptic potential to the adjacent spike trigger zone (3) influences the probability of spike occurrence. The change in firing probability can be quantified by compiling a post-stimulus time histogram (PSTH) or cross-correlation histogram (CCH) between the times of discharge in one or more afferent fibers and the times of motoneuron spikes. If the activity of a population of motoneurons is recorded with EMG electrodes on the surface of the muscle, stimulus-evoked changes in the average rectified EMG appear as a filtered version of the PSTH profile.

and Cushing, Chapter 8, this volume). Our ability to predict the actual contribution that each of these dendritic mechanisms makes is limited by the paucity of direct data on the membrane properties of motoneuron dendrites. The lack of data arises in part from the fact that motoneuron dendrites branch profusely and decrease in diameter at increasing distances from the soma (Rall et al., 1992). These anatomical features make patch recordings from distal dendrites difficult to obtain. Fortunately, easily obtained somatic recordings provide a functionally important measure of the net current available to affect spike initiation in the nearby initial segment.

The synaptic current reaching the soma can be recorded by an intrasomatic electrode as an excitatory postsynaptic current (EPSC) under voltage-clamp conditions or an excitatory post-synaptic potential (EPSP) under current clamp conditions. The electrotonic spread of the EPSP to the nearby spike initiation zone then determines its effect on firing probability. During repetitive discharge, the spike-triggering efficacy of an EPSP will depend upon when it occurs within the motoneuron's interspike interval, since the difference between the somatic membrane potential and the threshold potential for spike initiation varies during this interval (Calvin, 1974; Powers and Binder, 1996). The average effect of an EPSP on motoneuron discharge is reflected in the peak in the PSTH, and a filtered version of the effects of the stimulus on many motoneurons can be recorded as a change in mean rectified surface EMG following the stimulus. However, the net change in EMG bears a complex relation to the changes in the timing of action potentials in individual motor units (Miles and Turker, 1987), so that the most straight-forward way of estimating the time course of synaptic potentials (PSPs) is through the analysis of PSTH features.

Previous models of the relation between the features of synaptic potentials and peristimulus-time histograms

Previous models of this PSP-to-PSTH transform have been based either on direct comparisons of synaptic potentials and PSTHs recorded in the same motoneurons of experimental animals or on simplified models of the interspike somatic voltage trajectory of tonically-discharging motoneurons. Based on direct PSP and PSTH comparisons, three different linear models have been proposed to account for the relation between the time course of the PSP and its effects on firing probability: the PSTH has been approximated as a scaled version of the PSP (Moore et al., 1970), the PSP derivative (Knox, 1974; Fetz and Gustafsson, 1983) or a linear combination of the two (Kirkwood and Sears, 1978). The degree to which the PSTH peak resembles the PSP, its derivative, or a combination of the two depends upon the experimental conditions in general and upon the ratio of the amplitude of the PSP to that of the background noise in particular (Fetz and Gustafsson, 1983; Gustafsson and McCrea, 1984; Cope et al., 1987). Although most PSTHs can be fit with a scaled version of the PSP and its derivative (Gustafsson and McCrea, 1984), the values of the scaling constants vary widely among different motoneurons (Gustafsson and McCrea, 1984), and even for different PSPs recorded in the same motoneurons (Poliakov et al., 1997).

Threshold-crossing models of motoneuron discharge are based on the observation that during repetitive discharge, the interspike voltage trajectories of cat lumbar motoneurons are fairly stereotyped. This was first reported by Calvin and Stevens (Calvin and Stevens, 1968), who noted that after an initial hyperpolarization, membrane potential rises linearly to the next spike, and that the slope of this voltage ramp (i.e. the 'ramp slope') shows relatively little variation. Schwindt and Calvin (1972) studied interspike voltage trajectories in a more systematic fashion and noted that over most of the primary range of discharge, the ramp slope was invariant, except at the very lowest discharge rates. A number of investigators used these data to interpret the effects of synaptic inputs on the discharge of human motoneurons by representing the interspike trajectory as an initial post-spike decrease in membrane potential followed by a linear rise to firing threshold (e.g. Ashby and Zilm, 1982b; Fetz and Gustafsson, 1983; Nordstrom et al., 1992). With these models, spikes are advanced by an EPSP whenever the rising phase of the EPSP exceeds the difference between the instantaneous membrane potential and the spike threshold. The advantage of such models is that quantitative predictions of the relationships between EPSP and PSTH parameters can be made from simple geometrical considerations (Fetz and Gustafsson, 1983; Nordstrom et al., 1992). However, errors in estimates based on these models may arise from the omission of key biophysical features of real motoneurons, such as interspike variations in conductance, variation in the voltage threshold for spike initiation, and the extent to which the interspike membrane potential trajectory deviates from a straight line.

Motoneuron action potentials are followed by an afterhyperpolarization (AHP) produced by a calcium-activated potassium conductance (review in Binder et al., 1996). The AHP is associated with measurable changes in membrane conductance. The AHP conductance reaches a maximal value shortly after the spike at a value of about twice the resting membrane conductance, after which it declines roughly exponentially (Baldissera and Gustafsson, 1974). During repetitive discharge, the variations in conductance that occur between spikes can be partly attributed to the AHP conductance (Mauritz et al., 1974), but may also include a paradoxical decrease in membrane conductance toward the end of the interspike interval (Schwindt and Calvin, 1973). This latter feature is thought to reflect the activation of a persistent inward current (Schwindt and Crill, 1982). As a result of these variations in conductance, the amplitude and time course of PSPs will vary depending upon when they occur within the interspike interval. Although these variations in conductance are likely to affect the spike-triggering efficacy of PSPs, threshold-crossing models typically assume that membrane conductance remains fixed at its resting value.

Calvin and Stevens (1968) noted that the voltage threshold for spike initiation may also vary during the interspike interval, and this possibility has also been acknowledged in a number of theoretical studies of motoneuron discharge (e.g. Ashby and Zilm, 1982b; Fetz and Gustafsson, 1983). However, this variation in threshold is also not generally incorporated into threshold-crossing models. The threshold for spike initiation is likely to reflect the

state of voltage-dependent channels in the soma and initial segment and so would be expected to vary as a function of the recent history of membrane voltage. The top two panels of Fig. 2 show that this is in fact the case. The right panel shows the effects of injecting brief, 'just-threshold' current pulses at different points within the interspike interval. It is clear that the voltage-threshold for spike initiation is not constant, but in fact follows the time course of the interspike membrane potential trajectory, reaching a minimum early in the interval and then rising to its final value (Powers and Binder, 1996). The left panel shows the effects of adding a hyperpolarizing current pulse prior to a just-threshold depolarizing pulse. Spike threshold is decreased following membrane hyperpolarization, again showing that the threshold is dependent on the recent time course of the somatic membrane potential.

Another potential problem with simple threshold-crossing models is that a linear representation of the interspike voltage trajectory may not be appropriate at low discharge rates. As Matthews (1996) has recently suggested, the responses of cat motoneurons to steps of injected current may not be an appropriate model for human motoneuron discharge. In response to steps of injected current, motoneurons begin to fire very regularly once a threshold current is reached, and the mean interspike interval (ISI) at this minimum rate is approximately equal to the duration of the post-spike afterhyperpolarization (AHP) measured at rest (Kernell, 1965, 1979). In contrast, when human motor units are discharging near their minimum rates, the ISIs are quite variable: the ISI histograms are positively skewed with an exponential tail of long intervals (see Matthews, 1996 and references therein). Matthews (1996) has proposed that these long intervals arise when the AHP following the preceding spike is completed and the motoneuron is randomly excited by synaptic noise. If this were true, then the last part of the interspike interval trajectory should often exhibit an exponential, rather than a linear rise to threshold. The bottom panel of Fig. 2 is a schematic representation of an interspike trajectory for a motoneuron firing at a low rate (lower trace) along with the time course of the voltage threshold (dotted line). The solid oblique and horizontal lines illustrate a linear approximation to the voltage trajectory together with an assumed constant voltage threshold. The difference between the membrane potential and threshold (i.e. the 'distance to threshold') at a given point within the interspike interval is indicated by the bold double arrow for the linear trajectory and constant threshold, and by the thin double arrow for the curved trajectory and variable threshold. Clearly, the distance to threshold and therefore the spike-triggering efficacy of an EPSP are very different in the two representations.

A more realistic approximation of motoneuron behavior can be obtained by modifying a threshold-crossing model to include interspike variations in spike threshold and membrane conductance (Powers and Binder, 1996). More elaborate motoneuron models can be developed based on a compartmental representation of the initial segment, soma and dendrites, together with Hodgkin–Huxley (Hodgkin and Huxley, 1952) representations of the spike

conductances (Traub, 1977; Traub and Llinas, 1977; Jones and Bawa, 1997). One such model has recently been used to simulate the experimentally-observed relation between the effect of an excitatory input on firing probability and the background discharge rate of the motoneuron (Jones and Bawa, 1997). However, given the present level of uncertainty concerning the properties and spatial distribution of ion channels in motoneurons (Binder et al., 1996), the advantages of multi-compartmental models may be outweighed by their added complexity and the lack of constraints on model parameter values.

Using injected current transients to mimic synaptic potentials and their effects on motoneuron discharge

Our approach to understanding the relation between synaptic potentials and their effect on motoneuron discharge has been to develop an empirically-based model of roughly the same order

Variations in Spike Threshold

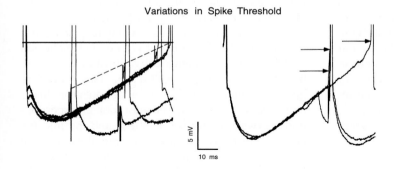

Changes in Interspike Voltage Trajectory at Low Firing Rates

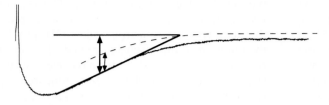

Fig. 2. Variations in spike threshold and interspike voltage trajectory. Upper left panel: superimposed interspike interval voltage trajectories with superimposed just threshold injected current pulses. The solid horizontal line shows the voltage threshold for spike initiation in the absence of superimposed current pulses. Current pulses during the interspike interval evoke spikes at a lower voltage level, suggesting a time course of spike threshold variation indicated by the dashed line (adapted from Figure 5A of Powers and Binder, 1996). Upper right panel: the threshold for spike initiation by a depolarizing current pulse can be lowered by a preceeding hyperpolarizing pulse. Lower panel: Schematic illustration of the interspike membrane voltage and spike threshold trajectories for a motoneuron firing at a low rate. The distance to threshold at a given point in the interspike interval (thin double arrow) is different than that predicted from a linear approximation to the membrane trajectory and a constant spike threshold (bold double arrow).

of complexity as previous models. Like many of its predecessors, our model is based on direct comparisons of PSPs and PSTHs recorded from the same cells. However, we have been able to obviate the need to pool data derived from many different cells that has limited the accuracy of previous models (e.g. Fetz and Gustafsson 1983; Gustafsson and McCrea 1984; Cope et al., 1987). To do so, we have used currents injected through a microelectrode to mimic synaptic potentials (cf. Reyes and Fetz, 1993; Powers and Binder, 1996), allowing precise experimental control over the time course and amplitude of the simulated synaptic inputs and background synaptic noise. Figure 3 shows the basic features of our experimental protocol. We use long steps of injected current to elicit repetitive discharge in both cat lumbar motoneurons recorded in vivo and rat hypoglossal motoneurons recorded in vitro. We superimpose two types of waveforms onto the current step: the first is composed of one or more Poisson trains of injected current transients. Each current transient ($c_k(t)$) is described by an alpha function (Rall, 1967): $c_k(t) = a_k(t/\tau_k)$ exp $(1 - t/\tau_k)$. The rise time (τ_k) and amplitude (a_k) can be varied to mimic the synaptic currents underlying a wide variety of PSP sizes and shapes. The second type of waveform is a random noise process whose amplitude and frequency content can be varied to mimic various types of background synaptic noise. Finally, prior to and following the current step we inject a series of brief, hyperpolarizing current pulses.

We can use the responses of the motoneurons to these stimuli to investigate the relation between our simulated synaptic potentials and their effects on discharge probability. The average voltage response to the hyperpolarizing current pulses is used to calculate the passive impulse response of the neuron, which is the voltage response to a 1 nA current pulse with a width equal to our sampling interval of 100 μs. It is typically well fit by the sum of two negative exponential functions of time. By convolving an individual current transient that simulates a synaptic current with this impulse response we obtain an estimate of the change in voltage it produces, i.e. our simulated EPSPs and IPSPs. As indicated schematically at the top of Fig. 3, the continuous convolution integral can be

approximated by treating the current-transient as a sequence of current pulses 100 μs apart, multiplying the passive impulse response to each pulse by the pulse amplitude, and adding up the result. Finally, since we know the times at which both the motoneuron spikes and the current transients occur, we can use this information to calculate a PSTH. If several trains of current transients of different size and shape are superimposed, we can examine the relationship between PSP and PSTH characteristics for a number of simulated synaptic potentials applied under identical conditions in the same motoneuron (cf. Poliakov et al., 1997).

Our procedures also involve constructing an additional random noise waveform that when added to the current transient waveform results in a total signal that approximates white noise, i.e. it has a nearly flat power spectrum over the range of frequencies of interest and a Gaussian distribution of amplitudes (see Poliakov et al., 1997 for details). The use of a white noise signal allows us to develop a more general input-output model of spike encoding based on the white noise method of system identification (Marmarelis and Marmarelis, 1978).

The white noise analysis procedure that we use was originally developed by Lee and Schetzen (1965) and is schematically illustrated in the bottom set of traces in Fig. 3. The procedure involves calculating the mean motoneuron firing rate, and the first and second-order crosscorrelations between motoneuron spikes and the injected current noise. These quantities are then used to calculate the zero-, first- and second-order Wiener kernels (h_0, h_1 and h_2), using the expressions presented at the bottom of Fig. 3. The zero-order kernel (h_0) is simply the background firing rate, i.e. the number of motoneuron spikes (N) divided by the duration of the discharge period (T). The first-order kernel (h_1) is derived from the average current trajectory that precedes the motoneuron spike (ACT; Bryant and Segundo, 1976). The value of the ACT at a particular time before a motoneuron spike (τ) is simply the average of all the white noise current values (X) that occurred at τ ms before the spike, i.e. the sum of these current values divided by the number of spikes: $(1/N)\Sigma(X(\tau - t_i)$, where t_i is the time of the ith spike and the summation is carried out from $i = 1$ to N. The first-order kernel is obtained by reversing the spike-triggered average in time (i.e. $(1/N)\Sigma X(t_i - \tau)$, in nA) and multiplying the result by the ratio of the background firing rate (h_0, in imp/s) to the power of the noise stimulus (P, in nA^2-ms). The resultant quantity has units of (imp/s)/(nA-ms), and represents the best linear approximation to the change in firing rate produced by a brief pulse of current with an area of 1 nA-ms.

The second-order Wiener kernel, which represents nonlinear interactions between two inputs, is related to the average product of current values that precede the spike at times τ_1 and τ_2. The lower middle trace represents this average product for $\tau_1 = \tau_2$. The values of the second-order kernel for $\tau_1 = \tau_2$ are obtained by reversing this average

product in time, subtracting the value of the autocorrelogram (R) at $\tau_1 - \tau_2$ and multiplying the result by ($h_0/2P_2$). The resultant quantity has units of $(imp/s)/(nA\text{-}ms)^2$, and represents the difference between the change in firing rate produced by combining two unit pulses of current at times τ_1 and τ_2 and the change in firing rate expected from the linear sum of the effects of each pulse alone. In other words, if the effects of the two pulses sum linearly, then the corresponding value of the second-order kernel is zero. Supralinear and sublinear summation result in positive and negative kernel values, respectively. The entire second-order kernel is represented as a three-dimensional surface or contour diagram with τ_1 and τ_1 along the x and y axes, and the kernel value at this pair of time lags

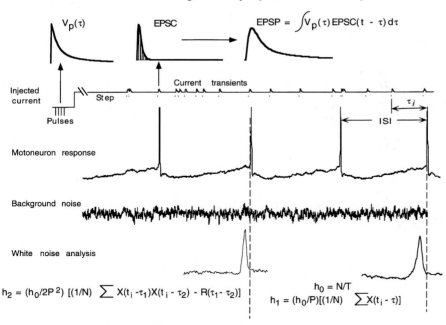

Fig. 3. Simulation of PSPs and background synaptic noise with injected current waveforms. The second trace from the top shows the injected current waveform, consisting of a set of hyperpolarizing current pulses, followed by a step of current with superimposed current transients. The upper set of traces shows the estimate of the passive impulse response ($V_p(\tau)$), based on the average response to the hyperpolarizing current pulses, a typical excitatory current transient (EPSC), and an EPSP estimated from the convolution of the current transient with the passive impulse response. The third trace from the top shows a portion of the motoneuron response to the injected current waveform, along with measurements of interspike interval (ISI) and lag from the ith current transient to a motoneuron spike (τ_i). In many cases, an additional noise waveform is added to the injected current waveform, and if the sum of the current transient waveform and the noise waveform approximates white noise, white noise analysis can be used to derive a general model of spike encoding (see text for further details).

along the z axis (see Fig. 5B). However, it turns out that for motoneurons (and perhaps many other neurons as well), the second-order kernel can be approximated from the first-order kernel (see below), so that explicit representation of this three-dimensional surface may not be necessary. In any case, if these first three Wiener kernels are sufficient to describe the input–output properties of the neuron, then the response of the neuron to any current waveform can be predicted by convolving that waveform with the kernels.

Effects of background synaptic noise on the PSP-to-PSTH transform

The first issue that we addressed with these techniques was the effect of the amplitude of background synaptic noise on the spike-triggering efficacy of a simulated PSP (Poliakov et al., 1996). We used a single train of depolarizing current transients, each of which produced simulated EPSPs with peak amplitudes of slightly less than 1 mV. We compared the changes in firing probability produced when these EPSPs were applied alone and in combination with different levels of background noise. The effects of background noise on the PSP-to-PSTH transform are shown in Fig. 4 (adapted from Fig. 3 of Poliakov et al., 1996). The top thin trace in the upper left panel shows the PSTH obtained under noiseless conditions and the thick trace shows the PSTH obtained in the same motoneuron in the presence of background noise. In both cases, the PSTH is characterized by a

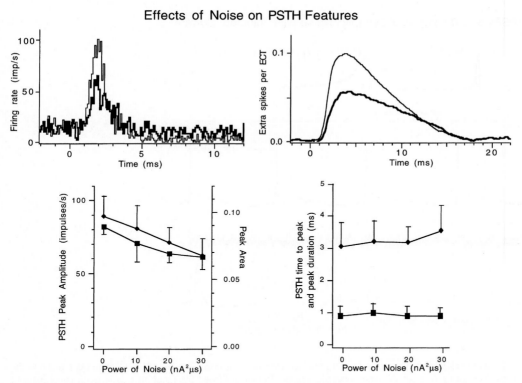

Fig. 4. Effect of background noise on the features of the post-stimulus time histogram (PSTH) compiled between a set of excitatory current transients and motoneuron spikes (adapted from Figure 3 of Poliakov et al., 1996). The upper left panel shows PSTHs illustrating the effects of an excitatory current transient on the firing probability of a rat hypoglossal motoneuron in the presence (thick trace) and absence (thin trace) of noise. The upper right panel shows the associated cumulative summations (CUSUMS) obtained by subtracting the baseline firing rate and integrating the remainder (cf. Ellaway, 1978). The lower panels show the means and standard deviations for PSTH peak amplitude, area, duration and time to peak as a function of the power of the noise stimulus for 6 rat hypoglossal motoneurons. See text for further details.

transient increase in firing rate that begins about 1 ms after the onset of the current transient (reflecting the time taken for spike initiation and detection) and returns to baseline about 3 ms later. Both the amplitude and the area of the PSTH peak were reduced by noise.

The average results for six rat hypoglossal motoneurons are shown in the bottom panels. As the power of the noise was increased, both the peak amplitude and the area of the PSTH peak were reduced, but neither the location of the PSTH peak nor the duration of the increase in firing probability changed. The decrease in PSTH peak amplitude with increasing noise is in qualitative agreement with previous theoretical predictions (H. Bostock's model as cited in Kirkwood and Sears, 1991). However, our finding that the time course of the PSTH peak is unchanged by noise is contrary to previous predictions based on threshold-crossing

neuron models (Midroni and Ashby, 1989; Polyakov, 1991).

Functional identification of a second-order model of synaptic transduction in motoneurons

Our use of white-noise analysis on both cat and rat motoneurons revealed that spike encoding in these cells can be predicted by a second-order model based on the zero-, first- and second-order Wiener kernels (Poliakov et al., 1997). Figure 5 (adapted from Fig. 6 of Poliakov et al., 1997) shows the first- (A) and second-order (B) kernels obtained from a cat lumbar motoneuron firing at a mean background rate of 17 imp/s. As discussed above, the first-order kernel represents the change in firing probability produced by a current pulse with an area of 1 nA ms, and for both cat and rat

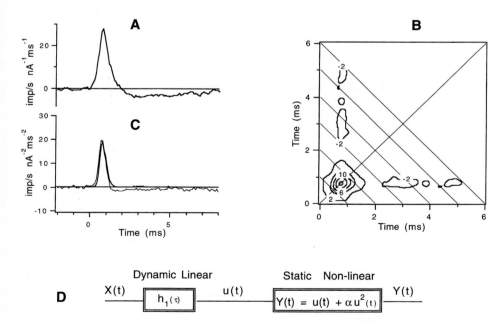

Fig. 5. Second-order model of synaptic transduction in motoneurons (adapted from Figure 6 of Poliakov et al., 1997). A. First-order Wiener kernel calculated for a cat spinal motoneuron. B. Contour diagram of the second-order Wiener kernel. C. Main diagonal of the second-order Wiener kernel (thin line) along with an approximation based on the square of the first-order kernel. D. The entire transduction can be represented as a cascade of a dynamic linear filter followed by a static nonlinearity.

92

motoneurons exhibits a characteristic shape, consisting of an increase in firing probability followed by a prolonged decrease. This biphasic shape is characteristic of a high-pass filter, and the duration of the kernel for this motoneuron indicates that firing probability can be affected by the values of the injected current over about a 10 ms period.

Figure 5B is a contour map of the second-order Wiener kernel, which exhibits two salient characteristics: (1) a short-latency peak near the origin (i.e. at short time lags) and two symmetric troughs that occur when one time lag is slightly under 1 ms, and the other ranges from 3–6 ms. Figure 5C shows a diagonal slice along the second-order kernel to illustrate what happens when two inputs are applied simultaneously (i.e. $\tau_1 = \tau_2$). The short-latency peak in the diagonal indicates that the increase in firing probability produced by an excitatory input grows in a greater-than-linear fashion with input amplitude, whereas the decrease in firing probability

produced by an inhibitory input grows in a less-than-linear fashion with increasing input amplitude.

In both this example and in the other motoneurons studied, the main features of the second-order kernel can be approximated by a scaled version of the square of the first-order kernel (i.e. $h_2 (\tau_1, \tau_2) = \alpha h_1 (\tau_1) h1 (\tau_2)$). For the results presented in Fig. 5, if both τ_1 and τ_2 are between about 1 and 2 ms, the value of h_1 is large and positive so that the product of $h_1 (\tau_1)$ and $h_1 (\tau_2)$ will also be large and positive, leading to the peak in the second-order kernel. In contrast, if one time lag occurs during the peak of h_1 and the other during the subsequent trough, the product of $h_1 (\tau_1)$ and $h_1 (\tau_2)$ will be negative, leading to the troughs in the second-order kernel. As shown in Fig. 5D, the adequacy of this approximation indicates that the entire input-output transformation can be represented as the sum of the output of a dynamic linear filter, represented by the

Linear and Nonlinear Predictions of PSTHs Produced by Current Transients

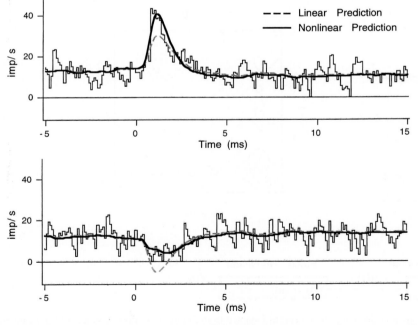

Fig. 6. Linear and nonlinear predictions of the PSTHs produced by depolarizing (upper panel) and hyperpolarizing (lower panel) current transients. The thin lines in each panel are the calculated PSTHs, thick solid lines the predictions based on the second-order (nonlinear) model and dashed lines the predictions of a first-order (linear) model.

first-order kernel, and a second term representing a static nonlinearity.

Our method of testing the accuracy of this second-order model of spike encoding differs from previous approaches to the problem of predicting a discontinuous output (i.e. a series of spikes) from a continuous input. One approach that has been used is to derive a continuous output from a model and then convert this output into spike train by assuming that a spike will occur whenever the output value exceeds a fixed threshold (e.g. Korenberg et al., 1988). The alternative method we used, which was originally employed by Moore and Auriemma (1985), is to obtain a continuous output by compiling PSTHs in response to the repetitive application of the transient waveforms embedded in the white noise input. Figure 6 shows the observed and predicted PSTHs associated with one set of symmetric depolarizing and hyperpolarizing current transients. A linear prediction (dashed line) based only on the zero- and first-order kernels, tends to underestimate the effects of an excitatory input and overestimate the effects of an inhibitory input. However, the second-order model (solid line) accurately predicts the PSTHs associated with this particular set of transients and also predicts the effects of a range of simulated PSPs on firing probability.

Limitations of the second-order model

Although the second-order model presented above represents an improvement over previously developed models, it is not truly general. The results presented thus far indicate that the relation between the characteristics of a synaptic potential and its effects on firing probability are complex: spike-triggering efficacy is reduced by increasing background synaptic noise and is also related in a nonlinear fashion to the amplitude of the input. In addition, the input-output properties of motoneurons change as function of their mean discharge rate. Figure 7 shows the effects of mean discharge rate on the shapes of the Wiener kernels. The lower left panel shows the relationship between background firing rate and the peak amplitude of the first-order kernel for a cat spinal motoneuron. In this case and in all other cells, the amplitude of the first-order kernel increases with increasing background discharge rate. The duration of the kernel decreases with increasing discharge rate. Thus, when the kernels are normalized by dividing their amplitude by the background discharge rate and expressing their duration as a fraction of the mean interspike interval, these normalized kernels superimpose (upper panel in Fig. 7).

The second-order model of spike encoding continues to hold as background discharge rate is changed, so that the second-order kernel is always well approximated by a scaled version of the square of the first-order kernel. The lower right panel in Fig. 7 shows the relationship between the amplitude of the scaling coefficient, α, and background firing rate for our entire sample of motoneurons. The scaling coefficient is inversely related to the background firing rate. Since the amplitude of u(t) is linearly related to firing rate, the contribution of the second term ($\alpha u_2(t)$) also increases linearly with firing rate. In other words, the relative contributions of the linear and nonlinear terms are independent of firing rate over the range of firing rates that we studied.

Extension of the white-noise approach to other experimental conditions

The predictions based on our white-noise analysis cover relatively small inputs corresponding to unitary or small compound PSPs. In contrast, the stimuli used in most human experiments probably produce somewhat larger PSPs, since the PSTH peaks obtained in these experiments are typically larger than those obtained in our experiments (e.g. Ashby and Zilm, 1982a; Miles et al., 1989; Miles, 1997). It is possible that higher-order nonlinear terms would be required to describe the effects of larger PSPs on firing probability. In addition, as mentioned above, the interspike interval (ISI) distributions obtained at the lowest firing rates in human experiments suggest that the net depolarization produced by the synaptic input may be subthreshold for repetitive discharge, so that many of the interspike intervals are longer than the AHP duration. If there were no AHP, and the average difference between the membrane potential and threshold were constant regardless of the amount of time since the previous spike, then the ISI distribution should follow a Poisson distribution, i.e. the percentage of intervals observed will decline exponentially with interval length as illustrated by the dotted curve in the upper left panel of Fig. 8. At low discharge rates, ISI distributions of human motoneurons (solid curve) do in fact show an exponential tail, which may indicate that at this point the AHP is over and the membrane potential is a constant distance from threshold.

Matthews (1996) has proposed that an estimate of the difference between the membrane potential and spike threshold (i.e. 'distance to threshold') can be obtained by calculating the 'death rate' from the interspike interval histogram. The death rate provides a measure of the instantaneous probability of an interval being terminated (i.e. dying) as a

function of time from the preceding spike (see Matthews, 1996 for details). The upper right panel of Fig. 8 illustrates the ISI histogram and death rate obtained for a rat hypoglossal motoneuron in response to a subthreshold current step combined with superimposed noise. If the membrane potential fluctuations produced by the current noise are known, then the death rate can be transformed into an estimate of the distance to firing threshold as a function of time since the last spike. In our experiments, we can estimate the noise-driven membrane potential fluctuations by convolving the noise stimulus with the passive membrane response (cf. Fig. 3).

The lower left panel of Fig. 8 shows our estimates of the distance to threshold for a rat hypoglossal motoneuron firing at a number of

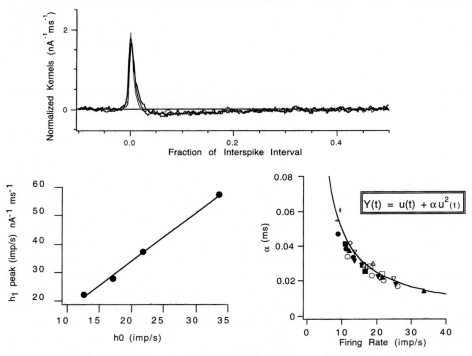

Changes in Motoneuron Responsiveness with Background Firing Rate

$$Y(t) = u(t) + \alpha u^2(t)$$

Fig. 7. Changes in motoneuron responsiveness with background firing rate (adapted from Figure 7 of Poliakov et al., 1997). Upper panel: first-order kernels obtained at three different background firing rates in a cat spinal motoneuron, normalized in amplitude by dividing by the background firing rate and in duration by expressing time as a fraction of the interspike interval at each mean rate. Lower left panel: relation between peak amplitude of the first-order kernel and the background firing rate (h_0). Lower right panel: Relation between the scaling factor (α) relating the first and second order kernels and background firing rate. Data for all of the motoneurons in our sample is superimposed on the graph.

different rates. As the firing rate increases, the distance to threshold decreases. A simulated synaptic potential is superimposed on one of these 'distance to threshold' trajectories. At the highest discharge rate, the PSP exceeds threshold for a little less than 50% of the mean interspike interval. The lower right panel shows the spike-triggering efficacy (calculated by dividing the number of extra spike counts in the PSTH peak by the number of stimuli) of this current transient as a function of discharge rate. The spike-triggering efficacy exhibits a complex dependence on firing rate, first increasing and then decreasing. Moreover, there is

a considerable amount of variance in the estimates of efficacy at a given rate. These results may help explain why some human studies have reported that the spike-triggering efficacy of a synaptic input increases with increasing motoneuron firing rate (cf. Jones and Bawa, 1997), whereas others have reported that the efficacy is independent of firing rate (Ashby and Zilm, 1982a; Miles et al., 1989). The right hand axis and the asterisks show the percentage of the mean ISI during which the EPSP exceeds threshold. It appears that over this range of firing rates, the decrease in efficacy may reflect the fact that as firing rate goes up the EPSP exceeds

Interval Statistics, Distance from Threshold and Spike-Triggering Efficacy

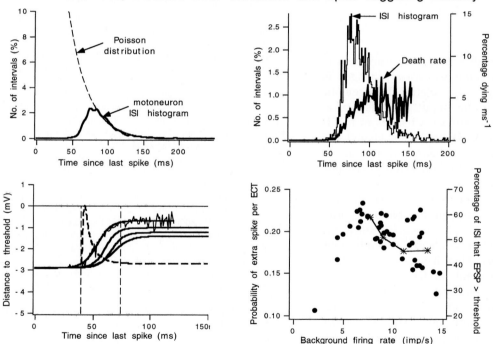

Fig. 8. Interval statistics, distance from threshold and spike-triggering efficacy. Upper left panel: a typical interspike interval (ISI) histogram from a motoneuron is compared to that expected for a Poisson process (dotted line). Upper right panel: ISI histogram and death rate calculated from the discharge of a rat hypoglossal motoneuron in response to an injected current waveform consisting of a subthreshold current step with superimposed noise. Lower left panel: Estimates of distance to threshold derived from the death rate. Solid noisy trace is based on the death rate curve illustrated in the upper right panel. The smooth solid lines are sigmoidal fits to estimates from this death rate curve and those calculated at other mean rates. The dashed curved line is an estimate of the PSP produced by current transients embedded in the injected current noise. The left vertical dashed line shows the first point in the interspike interval (for the highest firing rate) when the PSP can cross threshold and the right vertical dashed line represents the mean duration of the interspike interval at the highest firing rate. Lower right panel: Left axis and solid circles show the relation between background firing rate and the spike-triggering efficacy of the current transient for 48 trials. Right axis and asterisks illustrate estimates at four different mean rates of the proportion of the interspike interval in which the EPSP exceeds the distance to threshold.

96

threshold for a smaller percentage of the interspike interval. At a background rate of about 8 imp/s, the EPSP exceeds threshold for almost 60% of the interspike interval, and yet at this background rate, slightly less than 25% of the current transients triggered extra motoneuron spikes. This discrepancy may reflect the fact that the arrival rate of the current transients was higher than the motoneuron discharge rate, so that more than one current transient could occur during an interspike interval. As a result, the apparent spike-triggering efficacy of a given current transient may have been obscured by the closely spaced arrival of another transient. Thus, the PSP arrival rate must be another factor that can influence the PSP-to-PSTH transform.

Conclusions

In summary, considerable caution is warranted in the interpretation of stimulus-evoked changes in motoneuron discharge. The relation between the amplitude of a synaptic input and its spike-triggering efficacy is nonlinear. Changes in PSTH features can occur that depend upon changes in background noise and motoneuron firing rate in addition to changes in the underlying synaptic potential. The second-order model of spike encoding derived from our white noise analysis predicts discharge behavior solely on the basis of prior values of the input signal. However, since the distance to spike threshold clearly depends upon the time since the last spike, it may be possible to formulate a more general model of the PSP-to-PSTH transform that is independent of background rate by incorporating a term which reflects prior activity of the cell (Berry and Meister, 1998). Finally, as mentioned in the Introduction, our experiments do not address the role of factors that affect the transfer of current from the synapse to the soma (cf. Rose and Cushing, Chapter 8, this volume).

Acknowledgements

We would like to acknowledge our colleagues A. Sawczuk, C. Madore, and A.V. Poliakov for their contributions to the work presented here. We would also like to thank Douglas G. Stuart for his unwavering support of our research efforts, regardless of how idiosyncratic they may have become. This work was supported by Grants NS–01650, NS–26840 and NS–31925 from the National Institute of Neurological Disorders and Stroke, and a Human Frontier Science Program (LT 144/94) grant to A.V. Poliakov.

References

Ashby, P. and Zilm, D. (1982a) Characteristics of postsynaptic potentials produced in single human motoneurons by homonymous group 1 volleys. *Exp. Brain Res.*, 47: 41–48.
Ashby, P. and Zilm, D. (1982b) Relationship between EPSP shape and cross-correlation profile explored by computer simulation for studies on human motoneurons. *Exp. Brain Res.*, 47: 33–40.
Baldissera, F. and Gustafsson, B. (1974) Afterhyperpolarization time course in lumbar motoneurones of the cat. *Acta Physiol. Scand.*, 91: 512–527.
Bennett, D.J., Hultborn, H., Fedirchuk, B. and Gorassini, M. (1998) Synaptic activation of plateaus in hindlimb motoneurons of decerebrate cats. *J. Neurophysiol.*, 80: 2023–2037.
Bernander, O., Koch, C. and Douglas, R.J. (1994) Amplification and linearization of distal synaptic input to cortical pyramidal cells. *J. Neurophysiol.*, 72: 2743–2753.
Berry, M.J. and Meister, M. (1998) Refractoriness and neural precision. *J. Neurosci.*, 18: 2200–2211.
Binder, M.D., Heckman, C.J. and Powers, R.K. The physiological control of motoneuron activity. In: L.B. Rowell and J.T. Shepherd (Eds). *Handbook of Physiology. Section 12. Exercise: Regulation and Integration of Multiple Systems.* New York: Oxford University Press, pp. 3–53, 1996.
Bras, H., Gogan, P. and Tyc, D.S. (1987) The dendrites of single brain-stem motoneurons intracellularly labelled with horseradish peroxidase in the cat. Morphological and electrical differences. *Neuroscience*, 22: 947–970.
Bryant, H.L. and Segundo, J.P. (1976) Spike initiation by transmembrane current: a white-noise analysis. *J. Physiol. (Lond.)*, 260: 279–314.
Calvin, W.H. (1974) Three modes of repetitive firing and the role of threshold time course between spikes. *Brain Res.*, 69: 341–346.
Calvin, W.H. and Stevens, C.F. (1968) Synaptic noise and other sources of randomness in motoneuron interspike intervals. *J. Neurophysiol.*, 31: 574–587.
Coombs, J.S., Curtis, D.R. and Eccles, J.C. (1957) The generation of impulses in motoneurones. *J. Physiol. (Lond.)*, 139: 232–249.
Cope, T.C., Fetz, E.E. and Matsumura, M. (1987) Cross-correlation assessment of synaptic strength of single Ia fibre connections with triceps surae motoneurones in cats. *J. Physiol. (Lond.)*, 390: 161–188.
Cullheim, S., Fleshman, J.W., Glenn, L.L. and Burke, R.E. (1987) Membrane area and dendritic structure in type-

identified triceps surae alpha motoneurons. *J. Comp. Neurol.*, 255: 68–81.

Ellaway, P.H. (1978) Cumulative sum technique and its application to the analysis of peristimulus time histograms. *Electroenceph. Clin. Neurophys.*, 45: 302–304.

Fetz, E.E. and Gustafsson, B. (1983) Relation between shapes of post-synaptic potentials and changes in firing probability of cat motoneurones. *J. Physiol. (Lond.)*, 341: 387–410.

Gustafsson, B. and McCrea, D. (1984) Influence of stretch-evoked synaptic potentials on firing probability of cat spinal motoneurones. *J. Physiol. (Lond.)*, 347: 431–451.

Hodgkin, A.L. and Huxley, A.F. (1952) A quantitative description of membrane current and its application to conduction and excitation in nerve. *J. Physiol. (Lond.)*, 116: 500–544.

Jack, J.J.B., Noble, D. and Tsien, R.W. *Electric Current Flow in Excitable Cells.* Oxford: Clarendon Press, 1975.

Jones, K.E. and Bawa, P. (1997) Computer simulation of the responses of human motoneurons to composite 1A EPSPS: Effects of background firing rate. *J. Neurophysiol.*, 77: 405–420.

Kernell, D. (1965) The limits of firing frequency in cat lumbosacral motoneurones possessing different time course of afterhyperpolarization. *Acta Physiol. Scand.*, 65: 87–100.

Kernell, D. (1979) Rhythmic properties of motoneurones innervating muscle fibres of different speed in m. gastrocnemius medialis of the cat. *Brain Res.*, 160: 159–162.

Kirkwood, P.A. (1979) On the use and interpretation of cross-correlations measurements in the mammalian central nervous system. *J. Neurosci. Methods*, 1: 107–132.

Kirkwood, P.A. and Sears, T.A. (1978) The synaptic connexions to intercostal motoneurones as revealed by the average common excitation potential. *J. Physiol. (Lond.)*, 275: 103–134.

Kirkwood, P.A. and Sears, T.A. (1991) Cross-correlation analyses of motoneuron inputs in a coordinated motor act. In: J. Kruger (Ed.). *Neuronal Cooperativity.* Heidelberg: Springer-Verlag, 225–248.

Knox, C.K. (1974) Cross-correlation functions for a neuronal model. *Biophys. J.*, 14: 567–582.

Korenberg, M.J., French, A.S. and Voo, S.K. (1988) White-noise analysis of nonlinear behavior in an insect sensory neuron: kernel and cascade approaches. *Biol. Cybern.*, 58: 313–320.

Lee, R.H. and Heckman, C.J. (1996) Influence of voltage-sensitive dendritic conductances on bistable firing and effective synaptic current in cat spinal motoneurons in vivo. *J. Neurophysiol.*, 76: 2107–2110.

Lee, Y.W. and Schetzen, M. (1965) Measurement of the Wiener kernels of a non-linear system by cross-correlation. *Int. J. Control*, 2: 237–254.

Marmarelis, P.Z. and Marmarelis, V.Z. *Analysis of Physiological Systems. The White Noise Approach.* New York: Plenum Press, 1978.

Matthews, P.B.C. (1996) Relationship of firing intervals of human motor units to the trajectory of post-spike after-hyperpolarization and synaptic noise. *J. Physiol. (Lond.)*, 492: 597–628.

Mauritz, K.H., Schlue, W.R., Richter, D.W. and Nacimiento, A.C. (1974) Membrane conductance course during spike intervals and repetitive firing in cat spinal motoneurons. *Brain Res.*, 76: 223–233.

Midroni, G. and Ashby, P. (1989) How synaptic noise may affect cross-correlations. J Neurosci Methods, 27: 1–12.

Miles, T.S. (1997) Estimating post-synaptic potentials in tonically discharging human motoneurons. *J. Neurosci. Meth.*, 74: 167–174.

Miles, T.S. and Turker, K.S. (1987) Decomposition of the human electromyogramme in an inhibitory reflex. *Exp. Brain Res.*, 65: 337–342.

Miles, T.S., Turker, K.S. and Le, T.H. (1989) Ia reflexes and EPSPs in human soleus motor neurones. *Exp Brain Res.*, 77: 628–636.

Moore, G.P. and Auriemma, R.A. (1985) Prediction of muscle stretch receptor behavior using Wiener kernels. *Brain Res.*, 331: 185–189.

Moore, G.P., Segundo, J.P., Perkel, D.H. and Levitan, H. (1970) Statistical signs of synaptic interaction in neurons. *Biophys. J.*, 10: 876–900.

Nordstrom, M.A., Fuglevand, A.J. and Enoka, R.M. (1992) Estimating the strength of common input to human motoneurons from the cross-correlogram. *J. Physiol. (Lond.)*, 453: 547–574.

Pol, S., Vidailhet, M., Meunier, S., Mazavet, D., Agid, Y. and Pierrot-Deseilligny, E. (1998) Overactivity of cervical premotor neurons in Parkinson's disease. *J. Neurol. Neurosurg. Psychiat.*, 64: 166–171.

Poliakov, A.V., Powers, R.K. and Binder, M.D. (1997) Functional identification of the input-output transforms of motoneurones in the rat and cat. *J. Physiol. (Lond.)*, 504: 401–424.

Poliakov, A.V., Powers, R.K., Sawczuk, A. and Binder, M.D. (1996) Effects of background noise on the response of rat and cat motoneurones to excitatory current transients. *J. Physiol. (Lond.)*, 495: 143–157.

Polyakov, A.V. (1991) Synaptic noise and the cross-correlation between motoneuron discharges and stimuli. *NeuroReport*, 2: 489–92.

Powers, R.K.D.B. and Binder, M.D. (1996) Experimental evaluation of input-output models of motoneuron discharge. *J. Neurophysiol.*, 75: 367–379.

Rall, W. (1967) Distinguishing theoretical synaptic potentials computed for different soma-dendritic distributions of synaptic input. *J. Neurophysiol.*, 30: 1138–1168.

Rall, W., Burke, R.E., Holmes, W.R., Jack, J.J., Redman, S.J. and Segev, I. (1992) Matching dendritic neuron models to experimental data. *Physiol. Rev.*, 86: S159–S185.

Reyes, A.D. and Fetz, E.E. (1993) Effects of transient depolarizing potentials on the firing rate of cat neocortical neurons. *J. Neurophysiol.*, 69: 1673–1683.

Rose, P.K., Keirstead, S.A. and Vanner, S.J. (1985) A quantitative analysis of the geometry of cat motoneurons

98

innervating neck and shoulder muscles. *J. Comp. Neurol.*, 239: 89–107.

Schwindt, P.C. and Calvin, W.H. (1972) Membrane-potential trajectories between spikes underlying motoneuron rhythmic firing. *J. Neurophysiol.*, 35: 311–325.

Schwindt, P.C. and Calvin, W.H. (1973) Nature of conductances underlying rhythmic firing in cat spinal motoneurons. *J. Neurophysiol.*, 36: 955–973.

Schwindt, P.C. and Crill, W.E. (1982) Factors influencing motoneuron rhythmic firing: results from a voltage-clamp study. *J. Neurophysiol.*, 48: 875–890.

Schwindt, P.C. and Crill, W.E. (1995) Amplification of synaptic current by persistent sodium conductance in apical dendrite of neocortical neurons. *J. Neurophysiol.*, 74: 2220–2224.

Stein, R.B. and Capaday, C. (1988) The modulation of human reflexes during functional motor tasks. *Trends Neurosci.*, 11: 328–332.

Traub, R.D. (1977) Motoneurons of different geometry and the size principle. *Biol. Cybern.*, 25: 163–176.

Traub, R.D. and Llinas, R. (1977) The spatial distribution of ionic conductances in normal and axotomized motorneurons. *Neuroscience*, 2: 829–849.

M.D. Binder (Ed.)
Progress in Brain Research, Vol 123

CHAPTER 8

Non-linear summation of synaptic currents on spinal motoneurons: lessons from simulations of the behaviour of anatomically realistic models

P.K. Rose* and S. Cushing

MRC Group in Sensory-Motor Neuroscience, Department of Physiology, Queen's University, Kingston, ON K7L 3N6, Canada

Introduction

The input/output properties of spinal motoneurons are deceptively simple. As described thirty years ago by Granit, Kernell and co-workers, the steady-state frequency of action potentials generated by motoneurons, the output, is related to the current reaching the soma due to presynaptic activity, the input, in a close to linear manner (Granit et al., 1963, 1966). This straightforward relationship, however, conceals a large number of non-linear factors that play critical roles in transforming presynaptic activity into trains of action potentials. Some of these factors become more apparent if the input/output function is expanded to include the relationship between the current arriving at the soma due to presynaptic activity and the magnitude of presynaptic activity. This function depends on several factors, such as the frequency of action potentials arriving at synapses on the surface of the motoneuron and the number of active synapses. These factors have the potential to introduce large non-linearities into the relationship between the level of presynaptic activity and the frequency of action potentials generated by motoneurons.

Most synapses on motoneurons are located on the dendritic tree (Rose et at., 1985; Cullheim et al.,

1987; Ulfhake and Cullheim, 1988). The current that these synapses transmit to the soma depends on the location of the synapse and the electrotonic structure of the dendritic tree (Rall, 1977). Thus, the total current reaching the soma from different synapses will not be a simple function of the frequency of action potentials in the presynaptic terminals or the number of active synapses. At the site of each synapse, the magnitude of the synaptic current is determined by another non-linear property. In a highly branched dendritic tree, cable theory predicts that the input resistance at distal sites is much larger than at proximal sites (Rall and Rinzel, 1973). Thus, post-synaptic potentials generated at the sites of distal synapses will be much larger than post-synaptic potentials generated at proximal sites. This will differentially reduce the current delivered by distal synapses, since the current delivered by each synapse is determined by the product of the conductance change caused by the opening of ligand-dependent channels and the driving potential. Activation of additional synapses in the same region will deliver even less current due to further reductions in the driving potential. Hence, summation of the current generated by multiple synapses, especially if they are located on distal dendrites, will be less than linear.

The importance of non-linear summation of synaptic currents in determining the input/output properties of motoneurons is poorly understood.

---
*Corresponding author. Tel.: (613) 545-2804;
e-mail: ken@biomed.queensu.ca

This problem can be partially attributed to the difficulty of measuring the magnitude of the non-linearity in experimental situations where the precise number and location of active synapses are known. To address this problem, we have built compartmental models of motoneurons, based on detailed measurement of the geometry of their dendritic trees. Simulated synapses on the dendritic trees of these models were activated and the resulting current that reached the cell body was measured. The results of these simulations indicate that a substantial fraction of the current generated by individual synapses is 'lost' due to non-linear summation.

The model

Three compartmental models were constructed. Their characteristics were based on the dendritic geometry of three motoneurons innervating the dorsal neck muscles, biventer cervicis and complexus of the cat. These motoneurons were antidromically identified and intracellularly stained with horseradish peroxidase. The dendritic trees of these motoneurons were reconstructed by using a Wild–Leitz microscope equipped with a X63 oil immersion objective (N.A. 1.40) and a Eutectic neuron tracing system. This system converts tracings of each dendrite into a series of data points describing the XYZ coordinates and diameters of points along the dendritic tree. To maximize the accuracy of these reconstructions, each change in direction or change in diameter (greater than 0.2 μm) was entered as a new data point during the tracing procedure. The number of data points describing the structure of the three dendritic trees ranged from 7500 to 13 500. The surface area of the soma was calculated using the formula for the surface area of a prolate spheroid where the maximum and minimum diameters of the soma equalled the maximum and minimum diameters of the largest ellipse that could be fitted within the contour of the cell body drawn at a magnification of X500.

Successive pairs of data points were used to construct a series of cylindrical compartments whose lengths were determined by the difference between the XYZ coordinates of adjacent data points. The diameter of each compartment was determined by the average diameter of the proximal and distal data points. If adjoining compartments had the same diameter, they were merged, unless the total length of the compartment exceeded 30 μm. The number of compartments after this merging process ranged from 4000 to 5000. The electrical properties of each compartment were represented by two equal resistances that linked the compartment to adjoining proximal and distal compartments. A parallel resistor-capacitor circuit was used to represent the electrical properties of the membrane of each compartment. The values assigned to these resistors and capacitors were determined by the geometry of each compartment and the specific membrane properties using formulae previously described by Rall (1977). For the present simulations, the specific internal resistivity was set at 70 Ωcm. Specific membrane capacitance was 1 μF cm^{-1} and specific membrane resistivity was varied from 6000 to 60 000 Ω cm^2.

The conductance change caused by each synapse was modelled by means of the following equation (cf. Bernander et al., 1991):

$$g(t) = g_{peak} \exp(1)\ t/t_{peak} \exp(-\ t/t_{peak}) \qquad (1)$$

For excitatory synapses, t_{peak} was set at 0.2 msec and g_{peak} was assigned a value of 5.0 nS based on the experimental data reported by Finkel and Redman (1983). For inhibitory synapses, t_{peak} and g_{peak} were increased to 0.65 msec and 9.0 nS, respectively. These values correspond to the time course and magnitude of the conductance caused by activation of single axons of Ia inhibitory interneurons (Stuart and Redman, 1990). Since simulations using multiple time-variant conductance changes of the type described in equation 1 are time-consuming, these time-dependant synaptic conductances were often replaced by a constant, equivalent time-averaged conductance change, as described by Bernander et al., (1991). The synaptic conductance in each compartment was defined by the following equation:

$$\bar{g} = g_{peak} \exp(1)\ t_{peak} nfP \qquad (2)$$

where n is the number of synapses, f is the activation frequency and P is the probability of neurotransmitter release (cf Walmsley et al., 1988).

For some simulations, synapses were distributed uniformly, i.e. same number of synapses per unit area, over the entire dendritic tree. The maximum synaptic density was set at $1/14.3$ μm^2 based on the electron microscopic observations of Rose and Neuber-Hess (1991). The position of the synapses were assigned using the following protocol. Beginning at the cell body, the cumulative area of successive compartments was determined. If addition of the next distal compartment resulted in a cumulative area exceeding a pre-defined value (eg. for a density of 1 in 50 synapses, one synapse was located every 715 μm^2), a synapse was placed on that compartment. n was adjusted to include a factor that took into account the 'excess area' of that compartment if the cumulative area exceeded the pre-specified value. The number of synapses on the last compartment of each segment was determined by the ratio of the 'leftover area' to the pre-defined area interval. The current generated by each synapse i_{sy} was defined by:

$$i_{sy} = \bar{g}(E_{rev} - V_m) \qquad (3)$$

where V_m is the membrane potential and E_{rev} is the equilibrium potential. E_{rev} was set at 0 and -80 mv, respectively, for excitatory synapses and inhibitory synapses. The difference between E_{rev} and V_m is the driving potential.

Simulations were performed using Saber Simulator (Analogy Inc.) running in the Windows NT environment on a Pentium based computer (Carnevale et al., 1990). In order to calculate the total current reaching the cell body due to synaptic activity, the membrane potential of the cell body was voltage-clamped to the resting membrane potential. This procedure is equivalent to the experimental technique developed by Heckman and Binder (1988) and widely used by Binder and his colleagues (for a review, see Binder et al., 1996) to determine the effective synaptic current produced by tonic activation of a wide variety of segmental and descending connections to lumbosacral motoneurons. Thus, the values of the simulated currents can be compared directly to those obtained experimentally.

Results

Figure 1 shows the responses of one of the compartmental models following activation of either a proximal or distal synapse. Despite the fact that the time-course and magnitude of the conductance change caused by each of these synapses are identical, the EPSP at the site of the proximal synapse is less than 1 mV, while the EPSP at the site of the distal synapse is approximately 15 mV. This difference is due to the higher input impedance of the distal dendritic site and has important consequences for the summation of post-synaptic currents. The small proximal EPSP has little effect on the driving potential for the current generated by nearby synapses. In contrast, the 15 mV EPSP at the site of the distal synapse, reduces the driving potential by more than 20%.

The charge reaching the cell body from the proximal and distal synapses was calculated by using two different models for synaptic current injection. In one model, the driving potential was kept constant. In the other model, the driving potential varied with the membrane potential, i.e. a physiological synapse. The differences between the charge reaching the soma using these models provide a means of quantifying the effects of changes in driving potential. If the driving potential remains constant, activation of one synapse produces a charge injection of 190 fC. At the proximal synapse, most of this charge, 171.7 fC, travels towards the cell body and, due to the proximal location of this synapse, 99% of this charge, 169.1 fC, reaches the cell body (Fig. 2). Using the constant driving potential model for the synapse, simultaneous activation of a second synapse will deliver the identical charge to the cell body. As shown in Fig. 2B, the use of the more physiological representation of the synapse where the charge injection is determined by the driving potential, causes a small decrease in the charge reaching the cell body. The charge injected by the first synapse is reduced by 2.6 fC and the charge injected by a second simultaneously active synapse is decreased further, but it is still almost 95% of the charge injected using the synapse model where the driving potential is constant. These results suggest that changes in driving potential has little effect on the

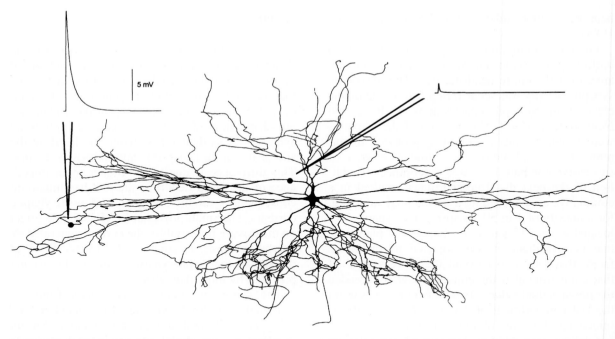

Fig. 1. Relationshp between synaptic current reaching the soma and the number of active synapses. A: total current. B: current per synapse. See text for further details.

charge reaching the cell body and hence, non-linear summation of synaptic potentials play a small role

A Constant driving potential

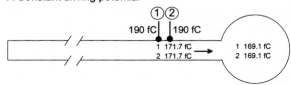

B 'Physiological' synapse

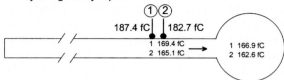

Fig. 2. Responses of a compartmental model of a biventer cervicis/complexus motoneuron following activation of an excitatory synapse located either proximally or distally. The sites of the synaptic contacts are indicated by the filled circles. The EPSPs 'recorded' at these sites are shown above or beside the pseudo electrodes. The resting membrane potential for these simulations was + 70 mV.

in determining the input/output properties of motoneurons.

The results shown in Fig. 3 lead to a different conclusion. Once again, both synapses deliver 190 fC at the site of synaptic contact. Due to the distal location of these synapses, almost 75% of this charge is lost en route to the cell body. The charge reaching the cell body is reduced even further using the more physiological representation of the synapse model where the charge injected at each synapse is determined by the driving potential. Using this model, the first synapse delivers 40.7 fC to the soma, a reduction of almost 20%. A second synapse, simultaneously activated with the first synapse, delivers 27.8 fC, a reduction of over 40%. Thus, the total charge arriving at the soma is 68.5 fC. The same synapses, but in the absence of changes in driving potential, deliver 99 fC to the soma.

The effect of changes in the driving potential can be described by calculating a ratio where the charge reaching the soma from the physiological model of the synapse is divided by the charge delivered by

A Constant driving potential

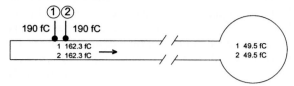

B 'Physiological' synapse

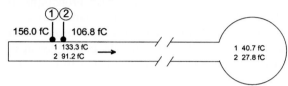

Fig. 3. Charge transfer to the soma from the position of the proximal synapse shown in Figure 1. The charge was calculated by integrating the currents flowing into the compartment contacted by the synapse, the current leaving this compartment en route to the soma, and the current that reached the soma. A and B compare the charge transfer for two models of synaptic current. The charge delivered by activation of one synapse is shown by the charges associated with synapse ①. The charge transfer by a second, simultaneously active, synapse is shown by the charges associated with synapse ②.

the constant driving potential model. For the two proximal synapses, the total charge reaching the soma is: $166.9/169.1 + 162.6/169.1 = 1.95$, very close to a linear summation. For the distal synapses, summation is markedly sublinear: $40.7/49.5 + 27.8/49.5 = 1.38$.

The results of the simulation shown in Figs 2 and 3 indicate that the non-linear summation of post-synaptic potentials is highly dependent on the location of the synapses. Thus, simulations of the current or charge reaching the soma from distal or proximal synapses both provide a biased perspective of the importance or lack of importance of non-linear summation. To provide a more representative assessment of the significance of non-linear summation, other compartmental models were constructed in which many synapses were placed on the dendritic and somatic membrane. In these models, the density innervation was uniform, i.e. same number of synapses per unit area. Thus, the distribution of synapses was determined by the relative availability of membrane at different distances from the cell body. For these simulations,

the synapses were activated tonically, i.e. Equation 3 was used to determine the current injected by each synapse, and the membrane potential was voltage-clamped to a resting membrane potential of -64 mV. The current required to maintain the membrane potential at this value is equivalent to the effective synaptic current measured by Binder and colleagues (Binder et al., 1996).

Figure 4A summarizes the results of a simulation in which 4 to 100% of all of the excitatory synapses on one of the motoneurons were activated. Each synapse was activated at 100 Hz and the probability of release was set at 0.5. The dotted line indicates the total current that was injected by all synapses as measured at the site of each synapse and keeping the driving potential constant. This simulation is

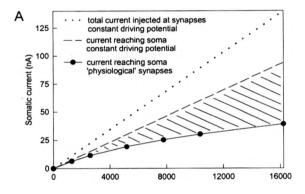

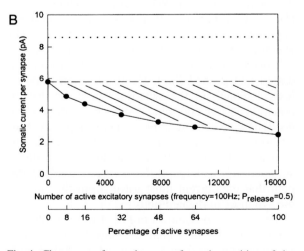

Fig. 4. Charge transfer to the soma from the position of the distal synapse shown in Figure 1. Same format as Fig. 2.

equivalent to placing all of the synapses on the cell body. As expected, there is a linear relationship between the number of active synapses and the total somatic current. The maximum current generated exceeds 100 nA. The effect of redistributing these synapses on the dendritic tree with a uniform density is shown by the dashed line. As before, the driving potential at each synapse was held constant and, as a consequence, there is a linear relationship between the total current reaching the cell body and the number of active synapses. The difference between the dotted and dashed line provides a measure of the average current from all synapses that is lost en route to the cell body. Removing the constraint of a constant driving potential causes a further reduction in the total current reaching the cell body. In this simulation, the relationship between somatic current and total number of active synapses is highly non-linear. The difference between the current measured using a constant driving potential model versus the current using the more physiological model grows progressively as the number of active synapses increases. This difference reflects the magnitude of non-linear summation and is illustrated by the diagonal lines.

The non-linearity introduced by changes in driving potential can also be seen by examining the relationship between the number of active synapses and the current delivered per synapse (Fig. 4B). Assuming that there is no change in driving potential, synaptic activation at a frequency of 100 Hz with probability of release of 0.5 delivers approximately 8 pA to the site of each synapse. On average, 2.8 pA of this current is lost on route to the cell body (indicated by the difference between the dotted and dashed line). Using the more physiological model for the synapse, where the driving potential is not constant, results in a progressive decline in the current delivered per synapse as more synapses are activated. If 50% of the synapses are activated, the 'loss' of current due to non-linear summation is as large as the average loss along the path that the current must travel from the sites of the synapses to the cell body.

The simulations shown in Fig. 4 were conducted using a model in which the specific membrane resistivity was assigned a value of 15 000 Ω cm^2. Further simulations using values of specific mem-

brane resistivity between 6000 and 60 000 Ω cm^2 had little effect on the total current reaching the cell body. Superimposing a low level of background activity in a small number of excitatory (16% of the total activated at 50 Hz) and inhibitory synapses (20% of the total activated at 55 Hz) reduced the total current reaching the cell body further. Activation of 50% of the excitatory synapses in this model (frequency of activation, 100 Hz; probability of release, 0.5) resulted in a total somatic current of 10.4 to 17.9 nA for the three motoneurons examined. With 100% of all excitatory synapses activated, the somatic current ranged from 19.6 to 33.9 nA.

Discussion

Previous attempts to measure the magnitude of non-linear summation in motoneurons, either experimentally or by means of simulations, have usually examined the effects of transient changes in membrane conductance. The results of the experimental studies concluded that non-linear summation was negligible (Kuno and Miyahara, 1969, Clements et al., 1986) or, at the most, caused a 20% reduction in the peak height of the EPSP (Burke, 1967; Burke et al., 1971). In contrast, Barrett and Crill (1974) and more recently, Ulrich et al. (1994), calculated that the current delivered by a *single* synapse on a distal dendrite of compartmental models of a motoneurons was reduced by approximately 20% due to a reduction in driving potential. This result was confirmed in the present study. The charge delivered by a second, simultaneously active, synapse on a distal dendrite was reduced by more than 40%.

These are several possible explanations for the discrepancy between the experimental observations and the predictions generated by the modelling studies. An obvious concern is the similarity of the geometry of the compartmental model and the morphology of the dendritic tree of 'real' motoneurons. However, one of the strengths of the compartmental modelling strategy is the ability to incorporate very detailed measures of dendritic tree geometry into the model. This strategy ensures that the geometry of the model is a faithful representation of the morphology of each motoneuron, although it leaves open questions related to the effects of histological processing and the accuracy of measurements obtained at the light microscope level. The errors introduced by these factors likely lead to an overestimate of dendritic diameter (Ornung and Ulfhake, 1990; Kincaid et al., 1998). This would result in an underestimate of the magnitude non-linear summation, since the input impedance of the distal dendrites would be under-estimated. Hence, these factors cannot explain the discrepancy between the degree of non-linear summation predicted from the simulations and observations obtained experimentally.

One important feature that is not incorporated in the simulations is the presence of voltage-dependent channels on the dendritic tree. Could these alter the degree of non-linear summation? The addition of voltage-dependent sodium or calcium channels would be expected to cause supra-linear, not sub-linear, summation. In contrast, as shown by Bernander et al. (1994), activation of voltage-dependent potassium channels can almost eliminate non-linear summation. Thus, 'real' motoneurons may solve the problem of non-linear summation through other non-linear elements. This solution, however, causes a second problem. The total current reaching the soma will be reduced due to the voltage-dependent potassium channels. In the present study, the total somatic current only exceeded the average rheobase for type FF motoneurons (cf. Zengel et al., 1985), if more than 50% of all excitatory synapses were activated. Thus, a further reduction in the total somatic current could make many motoneurons inexcitable.

The relatively modest non-linear summation seen experimentally is most likely due to the fact that only a small number of synapses are excited in most experiments. Doubling the number of active synapses from 1298 to 2596 in the simulation shown in Fig. 5, increased the total current reaching the soma by a factor of 1.8. This magnitude of non-linear summation is close to that seen experimentally and in simulations of composite EPSPs generated by synapses of group Ia afferents on triceps surea motoneurons (Segev et al., 1990). The latter connection involves approximately 300 synapses. Moreover, if the active synapses were preferentially distributed on the proximal dendrites,

the magnitude of the non-linearity would be expected to be even smaller. This may explain the close to linear summation of excitatory synaptic currents described by Binder et al., (1996) following stimulation of the red nucleus and group Ia afferents.

The results of the simulations reported in this study indicate that non-linear summation of synaptic currents can significantly reduce the magnitude of the current reaching the cell body following activation of dendritic synapses. This effect, in combination with the loss of current due to the remote electrical position of many of the synapses, causes a large reduction in the total current reaching the cell body. As a consequence, activation of more than 50% of all excitatory synapses appears to be necessary just to reach threshold, assuming that at least some of the motoneurons examined in this study were type FF and that the rheobase of neck and hindlimb motoneurons are similar. Although the precise number of synapses that must be activated to generate sustained activity in neck motoneurons is not known, the logistics of tonically activating more than 5000 synapses would seem to preclude the possibility that motoneurons would rely on this massive synaptic bombardment as a routine mechanism for achieving sustained activity. Increasing the specific resistivity of the membrane does not solve this problem. Although this will reduce the current lost en route to the soma, the magnitude of the non-linear summation will increase due to the resulting increase in input resistance.

The dilemma of an apparently ineffectual synaptic current may be solved by other properties that are intrinsic to motoneurons. Synaptic current can be augmented by persistent inward currents generated by voltage-dependent channels on the dendritic tree of motoneurons (eg. Hounsgaard and Kiehn, 1993; Lee and Heckman, 1998; Bennett et al., 1998). In addition, a 'noisy' resting membrane potential or a modest synchronization of the presynaptic activity can increase the frequency of motoneuron discharge (Bernander et al., 1991; Poliakov et al., 1996). Regardless of which of these mechanisms are used, the results of the present simulations suggest that tonic synaptic activity, by itself, is insufficient to drive most motoneurons to physiologically meaningful (ie. in terms of muscle tension) levels of activity.

Acknowledgements

This research was supported by the Medical Research Council of Canada. The authors thank A. Pollett and S. Woods for writing the software that converted the Eutectic NTS data to a file structure suitable for building morphologically-based compartmental models in the Saber software environment.

References

Barrett, J.N. and Crill, W.E. (1974) Influence of dendritic location and membrane properties on the effectiveness of synapses on cat motoneurones. *J. Physiol.*, 239: 325–345.

Bennett, D.J., Hultborn, H., Fedirchuk, B. and Gorassini, M. (1998) Synaptic activation of plateaus in hindlimb motoneurons of decerebrate cats. *J. Neurophysiol.*, 80: 2023–2037.

Bernander, O., Douglas, R.J., Martin, K.A. and Koch, C. (1991) Synaptic background activity influences spatiotemporal integration in single pyramidal cells. *Proc. Natl. Acad. Sci.*, 88: 11569–11573.

Bernander, O., Koch, C. and Douglas, R.J. (1994) Amplification and linearization of distal synaptic input to cortical pyramidal cells. *J. Neurophysiol.*, 72: 2743–2753.

Binder, M.D., Heckman, C.J. and Powers, R.K. (1996) The physiological control of motoneuron activity. In: L.B. Rowell and J.T. Shepherd (Eds), *Handbook of Physiology, Exercise: Regulation and Integration of Multiple Systems*, section 12, chapter 1, Oxford University Press, New York, Oxford, pp. 3–53.

Burke, R.E. (1967) Composite nature of the monosynaptic excitatory postsynaptic potential. *J. Neurophysiol.*, 30: 1114–1137.

Burke, R.E., Fedina, L. and Lundberg, A. (1971) Spatial synaptic distribution of recurrent and group Ia inhibitory systems in cat spinal motoneurones. *J. Physiol.*, 214: 305–326.

Carnevale, N.T., Woolf, T.B. and Shepherd, G.M. (1990) Neuron stimulations with SABER. *J. Neurosci. Meth.*, 33: 135–148.

Clements, J.D., Nelson, P.G. and Redman, S.J. (1986) Intracellular tetraethylammonium ions enhance group Ia excitatory post-synaptic potentials evoked in cat motoneurones. *J. Physiol.*, 377: 267–282.

Cullheim, S., Fleshman, J.W., Glenn, L.L. and Burke, R.E. (1987) Membrane area and dendritic structure in type-identified triceps surae alpha motoneurons. *J. Comp. Neurol.*, 255: 68–81.

Finkel, A.S. and Redman, S.J. (1983) The synaptic current evoked in cat spinal motneurones by impulses in single group Ia axons. *J. Physiol.*, 342: 615–632.

Granit, R., Kernell, D. and Shortess, G.K. (1963) Quantitative aspects of repetitive firing of mammalian motoneurones, caused by injected currents. *J. Physiol.*, 168: 911–931.

Granit, R., Kernell, D. and Lamarre, Y. (1966) Algebraical summation in synaptic activation of motoneurones firing within the 'primary range' to injected currents. *J. Physiol.*, 187: 379–399.

Heckman, C.J. and Binder, M.D. (1988) Analysis of effective synaptic currents generated by homonymous Ia afferent fibers in motoneurons of the cat. *J. Neurophysiol.*, 60: 1946–1966.

Hounsgaard, J. and Kiehn, O. (1993) Calcium spikes and calcium plateaux evoked by differential polarization in dendrites in turtle motoneurones in vitro. *J. Physiol.*, 468: 245–259.

Kincaid, A.E., Zheng, T. and Wilson, C.J. (1998) Connectivity and convergence of single corticostriatal axons. *J. Neurosci.*, 18: 4722–4731.

Kuno, M. and Miyahara, J.T. (1969) Non-linear summation of unit synaptic potentials in spinal motoneurones of the cat. *J. Physiol.*, 201: 465–477.

Lee, R.H. and Heckman, C.J. (1998) Bistability in spinal motoneurons in vivo: systematic variations in persistent inward currents. *J. Neurophysiol.*, 80: 583–593.

Ornung, G. and Ulfhake, B. (1990) Changes in size and shape during histochemical preparation for light and electron microscopy of neurons intracellularly labelled with horseradish peroxidase. *Acta Physiol. Scand.*, 140: 501–506.

Poliakov, A.V., Powers, R.K., Sawczuk, A. and Binder, M.D. (1996) Effects of background noise on the response of rat and cat motoneurones to excitatory current transients. *J. Physiol.*, 495: 143–157.

Rall, W. (1977) Core conductor theory and cable properties of neurons. In: J.M. Brookhard and V.B. Mountcastle (Eds), *Handbook of Physiology, The Nervous System*, Vol. 1, American Physiological Society, Bethesda, Maryland, pp. 39–97.

Rall, W. and Rinzel, J. (1973) Branch input resistance and steady attenuation for input to one branch of a dendritic neuron model. *Biophys. J.*, 13: 648–687.

Rose, P.K., Keirstead, S.A. and Vanner, S.J. (1985) A quantitative analysis of the geometry of cat motoneurons innervating neck and shoulder muscles. *J. Comp. Neurol.*, 239: 89–107.

Rose, P.K. and Neuber-Hess, M. (1991) Morphology and frequency of axon terminals on the somata, proximal dendrites and distal dendrites of dorsal neck motoneurons in the cat. *J. Comp. Neurol.*, 307: 259–280.

Segev, I., Fleshman, J.W. Jr. and Burke, R.E. (1990) Computer simulation of group Ia EPSPs using morphologically realistic models of cat α-motoneurons. *J. Neurophysiol.*, 64: 648–660.

Stuart, G.J. and Redman, S.J. (1990) Voltage dependance of Ia reciprocal inhibitory currents in cat spinal motoneurones. *J. Physiol.*, 429: 111–125.

Ulfhake, B. and Cullheim, S. (1988) Postnatal development of cat hind limb motoneurons. III: Changes in size of motoneurons supplying the triceps surae muscle. *J. Comp. Neurol.*, 278: 103–120.

Ulrich, D., Quadroni, R. and Luscher, H.R. (1994) Electronic structure of motoneurons in spinal cord slice cultures: a comparison of compartmental and equivalent cylinder models. *J. Neurophysiol.*, 72: 861–871.

Walmsley, B., Edwards, F.R. and Tracey, D.J. (1988) Nonuniform release probabilities underlie quantal synaptic transmission at a mammalian excitatory central synapse. *J. Neurophysiol.*, 60: 889–908.

Zengel, J.E., Reid, S.A., Sypert, G.W. and Munson, J.B. (1985) Membrane electrical properties and prediction of motor-unit type of medial gastrocnemius motoneurons in the cat. *J. Neurophysiol.*, 53: 1323–1344.

M.D. Binder (Ed.)
Progress in Brain Research, Vol 123
© 1999 Elsevier Science BV. All rights reserved.

CHAPTER 9

Selectivity of presynaptic inhibition: a mechanism for independent control of information flow through individual collaterals of single muscle spindle afferents

P. Rudomin

Department of Physiology and Biophysics, Centro de Investigación y de Estudios Avanzados del Instituto Politécnico Nacional, Ap. 14740, México D.F., Mexico

Mechanisms of presynaptic inhibition

In the early sixties, Eccles and collaborators related primary afferent depolarization (PAD) to presynaptic inhibition (Eccles et al., 1961, 1962a, b). They proposed that PAD results from the activation of GABAergic interneurons synapsing with the intraspinal terminals of the afferent fibers. Pharmacological studies have subsequently shown that presynaptic inhibition and PAD are both reduced by the $GABA_A$ antagonists, picrotoxin and bicuculline (Eccles et al., 1963; Curtis et al., 1971). On the basis of these results, it has been suggested that the effects of GABA are mediated through $GABA_A$-type receptors, i.e. GABA receptors coupled to chloride channels (for review see Alvarez-Leefmans et al., 1998). The existence of GABAergic axo-axonic synapses on the intraspinal terminals of group I and II muscle and cutaneous afferents has been amply confirmed by means of immunohistochemical methods (Fyffe and Light, 1984; Maxwell et al., 1990, 1997; Nicol and Walmsley, 1991; Alvarez, 1998; Lamotte d'Incamps et al., 1998).

The prevailing hypothesis about the cellular mechanisms involved in presynaptic inhibition is that GABA inhibits the release of neurotransmitter from primary afferent axons, either by preventing action potential invasion into their terminals, or by reducing the amplitude of propagated action potentials, thereby blocking or reducing Ca^{2+} influx. Actually, the blocking of action potential invasion or the reduction in its amplitude is thought to result mainly from the depolarization of the terminals and to a lesser extent from the change in conductance produced by GABA (Graham and Redman, 1994; Walmsley et al., 1995).

Patterns of PAD

Studies made in the eighties by measuring the intraspinal threshold of single muscle afferents (Rudomin et al., 1983, 1986), or by intrafiber recording of PAD from functionally identified afferent fibers (Jiménez et al., 1988), have expanded the initial observations of Eccles et al. (1962b), and of Lundberg and collaborators (1964, 1982). These studies indicate that stimulation of group I afferents and of the vestibular nuclei, produces PAD in many muscle spindle (Ia) afferents, while stimulation of cutaneous nerves, the bulbar reticular formation, the red nucleus and the pyramidal tract produce no PAD. These inputs are instead able to inhibit the PAD produced by group I and by vestibulospinal fibers (type A PAD pattern). In contrast, many of the intraspinal

*Corresponding author. Tel.: (525) 747 7099; Fax: (525) 747 7105; e-mail: rudomin@fisio.cinvestav.mx

terminals of the tendon organs are depolarized by stimulation of group I muscle afferents and also by stimulation of rubrospinal, reticulospinal and corticospinal fibers. Quite interestingly, stimulation of cutaneous nerves appears to have a dual action on Ib afferents: it produces PAD in some fibers (type B PAD pattern), and inhibits the PAD in other fibers (type C PAD pattern; see Rudomin et al., 1986, for a more detailed description of the PAD patterns).

Based on these findings, it was thought that type A PAD patterns were almost an exclusive feature of muscle spindle afferents, while type B and type C PAD patterns were shared by tendon organ afferents (for example see Rudomin et al., 1986; Harrison and Jankowska, 1989). However, in a recent and more detailed study made by intrafiber recording of PAD in functionally identified afferents, Enríquez et al. (1996a) found that only 52% of muscle spindle afferents in the cat medial gastrocnemius had a type A PAD pattern. In addition, 26% of these fibers had a type B PAD pattern and the 13% had a type C PAD pattern. In contrast, only 11% of the tendon organ afferents had a type A PAD pattern, 35% a type B and 54% a type C PAD pattern.

Quite interestingly, two to twelve weeks after crushing the cat medial gastrocnemius nerve, the number of fibers reconnected to muscle spindles, in which stimulation of the bulbar reticular formation produced PAD, was significantly increased. There was also a decrease in the number of fibers that were depolarized by cutaneous volleys (Enríquez et al., 1996b). This reduced the proportion of fibers with a type A PAD pattern to 35%, while the proportion of afferent fibers with a type C PAD pattern was increased to 65%. On the other hand, all afferents that reconnected with tendon organs appeared to be depolarized by stimulation of cutaneous nerves and also by stimulation of the bulbar reticular formation. That is, all tendon organs acquired a type C PAD pattern. The changes in the PAD patterns produced by the peripheral nerve crush were partly recovered six months after the nerve lesion.

The alterations in the PAD patterns of muscle afferents after a peripheral nerve crush have been explained by assuming that there are independent changes in the effectiveness of the spinal pathways leading to PAD of muscle spindles and of tendon organs. These changes could form part of a compensatory reaction aimed at limiting 'inadequate' information generated in damaged afferents (Enríquez et al., 1996b). These observations indicate very clearly that the PAD patterns of muscle afferents are not invariant features of the afferent fibers. They can be changed by a peripheral nerve lesion, or, as it will be shown below, by suppressing the descending influences acting on the spinal circuitry that mediates PAD (Lomelí et al., 1998).

Local control of PAD

In 1987, Hultborn et al. devised a non-invasive method that allowed measurement of changes in presynaptic inhibition of muscle spindles synapsing with motoneurons. These investigators found that at the onset of a voluntary contraction in humans, there is a *reduction* of the tonic presynaptic inhibition of the muscle spindle afferents arising from the muscle to be activated, and *increased* presynaptic inhibition of group Ia fibers innervating the synergistic, non-contracting muscles. They proposed that during voluntary contractions this differential control would be exerted on different collaterals of the same muscle spindle afferent. According to Meunier and Pierrot-Deseilligny (1989), the decreased presynaptic inhibition of the Ia input to motoneurons of the contracting muscle would increase the gain of the monosynaptic stretch reflex, which could be functionally important in compensating rapidly for the actual load at the beginning of the movement.

Based on the observations of Hultborn et al. (1987), we have investigated the spinal circuitry that underlies the selective modulation of PAD of muscle spindle afferents in the anesthetized cat. To this end, we measured the effects of sensory and descending stimuli on the electrical thresholds of pairs of collaterals of the same Ia afferent. In some experiments both collaterals ended in the intermediate nucleus within the L6 spinal segment (Eguibar et al., 1994, 1997; Quevedo et al., 1997), while in other experiments one collateral ended in the intermediate nucleus at L6, and the other in Clarke's column at L3 (Lomelí et al., 1998). Our main finding was that although stimulation of the posterior biceps and semitendinosus (PBSt) nerve often produced PAD of about the same magnitude in both collaterals, conditioning stimulation of cutaneous afferents, and of supraspinal structures, could almost completely inhibit the PAD elicited in one collateral leaving the PAD in the other collateral practically unaffected.

Figure 1 illustrates this situation. Stimulation of the sural (SU), superficial peroneus (SP) and posterior articular nerves (PAN) completely inhibited the PBSt-induced PAD in the L3 collateral of a Ia afferent fiber, while the PAD in the L6 collateral of the same fiber was slightly reduced. A similar differential inhibition of the PAD was produced by stimulation of the reticular formation (RF) and of the nucleus raphe magnus (NRM). To the extent that PAD is related to presynaptic inhibition, this implies that the presynaptic inhibition exerted by PBSt stimulation on the L3 collateral would be decreased, or removed by cutaneous and descend-

ing inputs, while keeping the L6 collateral presynaptically inhibited. As a consequence, the afferent input would be directed towards L3 to activate spinocerebellar neurons in Clarke's column that relay information from muscle afferents to the cerebellum (Osborn and Poppele, 1993), of relevance for sensory acquisition and discrimination (Gao et al., 1996) and motor learning (Raymond et al., 1996). Such a local control of information transmission appears possible because separate sets of interneurons mediate PAD of segmental and ascending branches of individual muscle spindle afferents (Jankowska and Padel, 1984; Harrison and Jankowska, 1984).

We also found that in some muscle spindle afferents the inhibition of PAD was stronger in the L6 than in the L3 collateral. The relative rostral or caudal dominance of the inhibition of the evoked PAD was not a fixed feature of individual afferents. It could be modified in many fibers by changing the

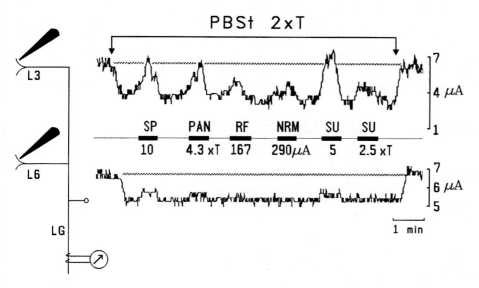

Fig. 1. Selective inhibition of PAD in segmental and ascending collaterals of a single muscle spindle afferent. Two separate stimulating micropipettes were placed at the L3 and L6 segmental levels within Clarke's column and intermediate nucleus, respectively. Antidromic action potentials produced by stimulation through each micropipette were recorded from a fine gastrocnemius nerve filament. Interaction between the antidromic potentials, because of refractoriness, was taken as evidence for activation of two collaterals of the same afferent fiber (as in Fig. 3A). Conditioning stimulation of sensory nerves (superficial peroneus, SP; sural, SU and posterior articular nerve, PAN) and of supraspinal structures (bulbar reticular formation, RF and nucleus raphe magnus, NRM) inhibits the PAD produced in both collaterals by stimulation of the posterior biceps and semitendinosus (PBSt) nerve. However, the inhibition of PAD is stronger in the L3 than in the L6 collateral. The PBSt stimulus was a train of 4 pulses, 400 Hz, 1.6 xT, applied 25 ms before the threshold testing pulse. SU and SP nerves were stimulated with one pulse applied 50 ms before the threshold testing pulse. PAN, NRM and RF, with a train of 8 pulses at 700 Hz preceding the threshold testing pulse by 75 ms. Stimulus strengths are indicated (Lomelí, Linares and Rudomin, unpublished observations).

intensity of stimulation of the PBSt nerve and of the pathways used to inhibit the PAD. It also depended on the location of the supraspinal stimuli, as well as on descending influences, as could be inferred from the effects produced by cold-block of impulse conduction in the mid-thoracic spinal cord (Lomelí et al., 1998).

The experiment of Fig. 2 illustrates the effects of spinalization on the PAD patterns of a pair of collaterals of a single muscle spindle afferent. One collateral of this afferent ended within the L6 segment and the other ascended to L3 within Clarke's column. Before the spinal cold block, conditioning stimulation of the PBSt nerve with trains of pulses 1.3 xT, reduced the intraspinal threshold of the L3 and L6 collaterals to 88.4 and 79.5% of control, respectively. Conditioning stimulation of the posterior articular nerve inhibited the PBSt-induced PAD to about the same extent in both collaterals. In contrast, stimulation of the SU and SP nerves almost completely suppressed the PAD in the L6 collateral and had only a minor effect on the PAD in the L3 collateral (Fig. 2A). During spinalization, the magnitude of the PBSt-induced PAD in the L3 collateral was about the same as before the spinal block, and was slightly reduced in

the L6 collateral (86.5 and 88.5% of control, respectively). Nevertheless, the inhibitory effects of sural and superficial peroneus were *largely reversed*. They now produced a strong inhibition of the PBSt-PAD elicited in the L3 collateral, and had a rather small effect on the PAD elicited in the L6 collateral (Fig. 2B).

These observations indicate that the *direction* of information flow within the intraspinal arborizations of single afferents is subject to central control, and depends on the balance of the sensory and descending inputs received by the spinal circuitry mediating the PAD of individual collaterals, or small groups of collaterals. In this context, one important question is why cutaneous afferents inhibit the PAD of muscle spindle afferents as strongly as do descending inputs. By studying changes in soleus H reflexes of healthy subjects, Iles (1996) found that electrical stimulation of cutaneous nerves, as well as mechanical stimulation of skin afferents (light brushing) reduced the presynaptic inhibition of monosynaptic reflexes produced by stimulation of the common peroneal nerve. The most effective inhibitory regions in the skin that reduced presynaptic inhibition of monosynaptic reflexes were those located in the distal

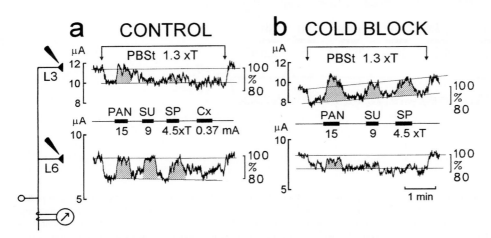

Fig. 2. Spinalization reverses the differential inhibition of PAD in segmental and ascending collaterals of a single muscle spindle afferent. A and B, inhibition of the PBSt-induced PAD by conditioning stimulation of SU, SP and PAN nerves, before and during spinal block, as indicated. Before the spinal block, conditioning stimulation of the SU and SP nerves produced a stronger inhibition of PAD in the L6 collateral ending within the intermediate nucleus, than in the L3 collateral ending in Clarke's columns. During spinal block, the inhibition of PAD produced by these same stimuli was stronger in the L3 collateral than in the L6 collateral. Peripheral threshold of the afferent fiber 1.14 xT; mean conduction velocity 84.3 ms^{-1}. Separation between microelectrode tips 2.5 cm. Reproduced with permission from Lomelí et al. (1998).

dorsal and plantar surfaces of the ipsilateral foot. These regions are precisely those that would be activated during the termination of a programmed movement, or when the limb encounters an unexpected obstacle. Mechanical stimulation of these skin areas would then remove the presynaptic inhibition of muscle spindle afferents and allow the information on the state of the muscles to reach the spinal cord to be utilized in the processing of the compensatory movement.

Conduction of action potentials in L3 and L6 collaterals

The mechanisms leading to the differential control of presynaptic inhibition in individual collaterals of muscle spindle afferents have not been completely elucidated. Analysis of the PAD produced by intraspinal microstimulation in pairs of collaterals of single afferents has disclosed the existence of local mechanisms that modulate transmitter release (Quevedo et al., 1997). They appear to involve activation of axo-axonic synapses made by the GABAergic interneurons with the intraspinal terminals of the afferent fibers (see also Rudomin, 1990, and Rudomin et al., 1998). However, it is possible that during PAD impulses also fail to invade some of the terminal arborizations of the muscle spindle afferents (Henneman et al., 1984; Luscher, 1990, 1998), and that this failure is relieved during the inhibition of PAD. In this context, the observations of Wall and colleagues (see Wall, 1994; Wall and McMahon, 1994) are of particular interest. They have shown that in the rat spinal cord, a substantial number of cutaneous afferents extend their arborizations beyond the spinal area within which cells respond to their activation, and that impulses fail to propagate in the long-range reach of myelinated fibers caudally in the dorsal columns. Application of $GABA_A$ receptor antagonists relieves impulse blockade, probably because of the suppression of a tonic GABA-operated Cl^- conductance operating in the terminals.

We have examined the contribution of conduction block in the control of information flowing through specific sets of segmental and ascending collaterals of single muscle spindle afferents. To this end we measured the changes in the activation threshold produced in a given L3 or L6 collateral, by an action potential initiated in the other collateral in the anesthetized cat (Castillo et al., 1998). It was assumed that the collaterals invaded by the action potential became relatively refractory and increase their threshold for a short period of time (1–2 ms) after their activation (Curtis et al., 1995, 1997). If PAD were to block conduction of action potentials somewhere between the stimulated and tested collateral, no refractoriness should be produced in the tested collateral by conditioning with action potentials generated in the other collateral.

Figure 3 shows the results obtained in one experiment in which we were able to place one stimulating micropipette within the gastrocnemius motor (LG) nucleus at the L6 segmental level, and another micropipette within Clarke's column region at the L3 level (Castillo et al., 1998). A single conditioning pulse was applied through the L6 micropipette at various times before the L3 threshold testing pulse. When the L6 stimulus preceded the L3 stimulus at a short time interval, the antidromic response produced by the L3 stimulus was no longer evoked (Fig. 3A). This was taken as evidence that both antidromic spikes were produced by activation of two different collaterals of the same afferent fiber (Quevedo et al., 1997; Eguibar et al., 1997; Lomelí et al., 1998).

After this test, the stimulus applied to the L3 collateral was preceded by an action potential initiated at the L6 collateral, while the intensity of the stimulus applied to the L3 collateral was changed, by means of a computer controlled circuit (Madrid et al., 1979), until it produced an antidromic action potential in the nerve filament with a constant firing probability (set to 0.5). As shown in Fig 3B, when the CT stimulus time interval was longer than 1.6 ms, the intraspinal threshold of the L3 collateral was slightly reduced. With shorter time intervals the threshold increased steadily, until it was not possible to produce an antidromic potential, despite the increase in stimulus strength (17 μA when the CT stimulus interval was of 1.0 ms). This threshold increase was taken as evidence that in resting conditions, impulses generated in the L6 collateral in the motor nucleus invaded the L3

114

collaterals, at least up to the testing site in Clarke's column region.

Conditioning stimulation of the PBSt nerve was used to produce PAD in this fiber. As shown in Fig. 3C, this conditioning stimulus reduced the intraspinal threshold of the L3 collateral to 67.7% of

resting threshold. Even so, L6 stimulation increased the threshold of the L3 collateral at the shortest CT time stimulus intervals. This suggests that during PAD, impulses generated in the L6 collateral still invaded the L3 collateral, where they produced a relative refractoriness.

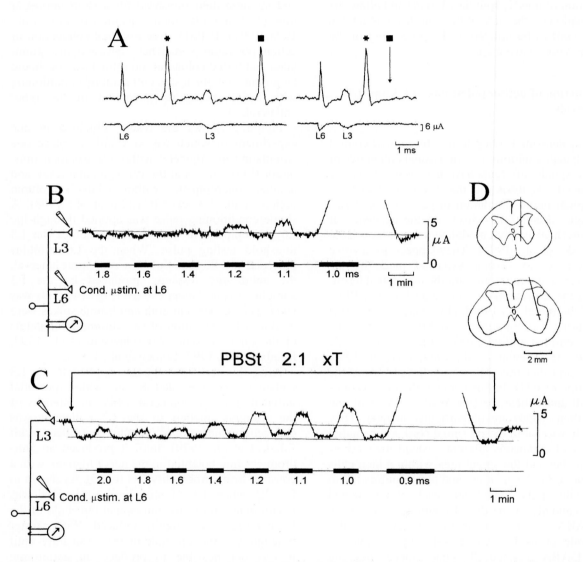

Fig. 3. Effects of PAD on conduction of action potentials between the L6 and L3 collaterals of a single muscle spindle afferent. A, interaction between the antidromic action potentials produced by L6 and L3 stimulation. B, changes in current necessary to produce an antidromic potential in the L3 collateral when preceded, at various time intervals, by an action potential generated in the L6 collateral. C, the same but during the PAD produced by stimulation of the PBSt nerve with a train of 3 pulses 2.1 xT strength applied 35 ms before the threshold testing pulse applied at L3. D, histological reconstruction of electrode tracks at L3 and L6, as indicated *(Castillo, Lomelí, Linares and Rudomin, unpublished observations)*.

At the present time we have analyzed impulse conduction and its modification during PAD in eight pairs of L3 and L6 collaterals of single Ia fibers with a mean peripheral threshold of 1.25 ± 0.24 xT. Invasion by action potentials initiated in the L3 collateral was tested in three collaterals ending within the motor nucleus region at the L6 level. We also examined invasion in five collaterals ending at L3 within Clarke's column by action potentials generated caudally at L6. The resting thresholds of the tested collaterals varied between 1.2 and 13 μA. We have assumed, in agreement with available evidence (Curtis et al., 1995), that tests made on fibers with the lowest resting thresholds (1.2–2 μA) reflect more closely changes in the terminals of the afferent fibers.

We have found that in all the examined fibers, action potentials generated in one collateral increased the intraspinal threshold of the other collateral at short CT time stimulus intervals (< 1.2 ms). In no case did PAD prevent the threshold increase during the relative refractoriness produced by a preceding action potential. It thus seems that in the spinal cord of the anesthetized cat, action potentials initiated in the L6 collaterals continue to invade the L3 collaterals of single muscle spindle afferents, even during a relatively strong PAD. The same phenomenon has been observed with action potentials initiated in the L3 collaterals invading the L6 collaterals.

It could be argued that threshold measurements were circumscribed to the coarser portions of the intraspinal arborizations and that conduction block still occurred within the finest collaterals. That is, in those collaterals with thresholds below 1–1.5 μA, which are more sensitive to anodal block and perhaps also to depolarization (Curtis et al., 1995). Although this possibility cannot be completely excluded, our data suggest that PAD produces no significant conduction block along the intraspinal segments of muscle spindle afferents coursing from L6 in the LG motor nucleus, up to the L3 collaterals ending within the Clarke's column. It then follows that relief of an already established conduction block may not play a significant role in the differential inhibition of the PBSt-induced PAD in the tested pairs of collaterals of single muscle spindle afferents. Most likely the differential inhibition results from changes in impulse transmission within the neuronal networks mediating the PAD in each collateral or in small groups of collaterals, as illustrated in the diagram of Fig. 4. The question on whether or not there is conduction block during PAD in the more caudal branches of

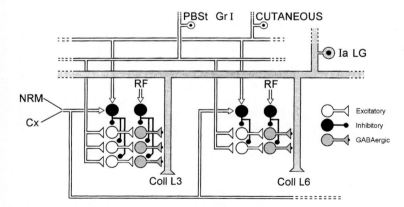

Fig. 4. Neuronal connections explaining the local character of inhibition of PAD in the L3 and L6 collaterals of individual muscle spindle afferents. The PAD produced by stimulation of group I PBSt afferents is mediated by at least two interposed interneurons. Separate groups of GABAergic interneurons produce PAD of L3 and L6 collaterals. Stimulation of cutaneous afferents and of NRM and corticospinal (Cx) fibers inhibits PAD by acting on the first order interneurons mediating PAD of muscle spindles, through separate sets of inhibitory interneurons. RF fibers reduce PAD by inhibiting the last-order GABAergic interneurons. Reproduced with permission from Lomelí et al (1998).

116

muscle spindle afferents, as in the long-range cutaneous fibers of the rat (Wall, 1994; Wall and McMahon, 1994), remains open.

Concluding remarks

The observations presented here emphasize the concept that the intraspinal arborizations of afferent fibers are not obligatory routes for the conduction of action potentials, but are instead dynamic systems that can be modified by central mechanisms to restrict information to selected neuronal targets. The differential inhibition of PAD is envisaged as a means by which different spinal postsynaptic targets coupled by sensory input from a common source could be decoupled by central control mechanisms (Rudomin et al., 1998; Lomelí et al., 1998). This could be of relevance for motor performance and sensory discrimination. The extent to which these changes are reflected at the population level, will depend on the degree of synchronization of the PAD-mediating interneurons, a feature that can be also centrally controlled (Rudomin et al., 1975). A more functional approach to the understanding of the central mechanisms involved in the presynaptic control of information flow in sensory fibers will require the use of non-invasive methods in behaving animals performing specific motor tasks.

Acknowledgements

I would like to thank J. Lomelí, J. L Castillo, J. Quevedo and P. Linares for allowing presentation of unpublished material. This work was partly supported by grants NS 09196 from NIH and grant 26402-N from CONACyT, México.

References

Alvarez-Leefmans, F.J., Nani, A. and Márquez, S. (1998) Chloride transport, osmotic balance, and presynaptic inhibition. In: Rudomin P, Romo R, Mendell L (Eds), *Presynaptic Inhibition and Neural Control*, Oxford University Press, New York, pp. 50–79.

Alvarez, F.J. (1998) Anatomical basis for presynaptic inhibition of primary sensory fibers. In: Rudomin P, Romo R, and Mendell L (Eds), *Presynaptic Inhibition and Neural Control*, Oxford University Press, New York, pp. 13–49.

Castillo, L., Lomelí, J., Linares, P. and Rudomin, P. (1998) Does PAD block spike invasion to axonal branches of individual group I afferents? *Abst. Soc. Neurosci.*, 24:1152.

Curtis, D.R., Duggan, A.W., Felix, D. and Johnston, G.A.R. (1971) Bicuculline, an antagonist of GABA and synaptic inhibition in the spinal cord of the cat. *Brain Res.*, 32: 69–96.

Curtis, D.R., Gynther, B.D., Beattie, D.T. and Lacey, G. (1995) An electrophysiological investigation of group Ia afferent fibres and terminations in the cat spinal. *Exp. Brain Res.*, 106: 403–417.

Curtis, D.R., Gynther, B.D., Lacey, G. and Beattie, D.T. (1997) Baclofen: reduction of presynaptic calcium influx in the cat spinal cord in vivo. *Exp. Brain Res.*, 113: 520–523.

Eccles, J.C., Eccles, R.M. and Magni, F. (1961) Central inhibitory action attributable to presynaptic depolarization produced by muscle afferent volleys. *J. Physiol. (Lond.)*, 159: 147–166.

Eccles, J.C., Kostyuk, P.G. and Schmidt, R.F. (1962a) Central pathways responsible for depolarization of primary afferent fibres. *J. Physiol.(Lond.)*, 161: 237–257.

Eccles, J.C., Magni, F. and Willis, W.D. (1962b) Depolarization of central terminals of group I afferent fibres from muscle. *J. Physiol. (Lond.)*, 160: 62–93.

Eccles, J.C., Schmidt, R.F. and Willis, W.D. (1963) Pharmacological studies on presynaptic inhibition. *J. Physiol. (Lond.)*, 168: 500–530.

Eguibar, J.R., Quevedo, J., Jiménez, I. and Rudomin, P. (1994) Selective cortical control of information flow through different intraspinal collaterals of the same muscle afferent fiber. *Brain Res.*, 643: 328–333.

Eguibar, J.R., Quevedo, J. and Rudomin, P. (1997) Selective cortical and segmental control of primary afferent depolarization of single muscle afferents in the cat spinal cord. *Exp. Brain Res.*, 113: 411–430.

Enríquez, M., Jiménez, I. and Rudomin, P. (1996a) Segmental and supraspinal control of synaptic effectiveness of functionally identified muscle afferents in the cat. *Exp. Brain Res.*, 107: 391–404.

Enríquez, M., Jiménez, F. and Rudomin, P. (1996b) Changes in PAD patterns of group I muscle afferents after peripheral nerve crush. *Exp. Brain Res.*, 107: 405–421.

Fyffe, R.E.W. and Light, A.R. (1984) The ultrastructure of group Ia afferent fiber synapses in the lumbosacral spinal cord of the cat. *Brain Res.*, 300: 201–209.

Gao, J.H., Parsons, L.M., Bower, J.M., Xiong, J., Li, J. and Fox, P.T. (1996) Cerebellum implicated in sensory acquisition and discrimination rather than motor control. *Science*, 272: 545–547.

Graham, B. and Redman, S.J. (1994) A simulation of action potentials in synaptic boutons during presynaptic inhibition. *J. Neurophysiol.*, 71: 538–549.

Harrison, P.J. and Jankowska, E. (1984) Do interneurones in lower lumbar segments contribute to the presynaptic depolarization of group I muscle afferents in Clarke's column. *Brain Res.*, 295: 203–210.

Harrison, P.J. and Jankowska, E. (1989) Primary afferent depolarization of central terminals of group II muscle afferents in the cat spinal cord. *J. Physiol. (Lond.)*, 411: 71–83.

Henneman, E., Lüscher, H.-R. and Mathis, J. (1984) Simultaneously active and inactive synapses of single Ia fibres on cat spinal motoneurones. *J. Physiol (Lond.)*, 352: 147–161.

Hultborn, H., Meunier, S., Pierrot-Deseilligny, E. and Shindo, M. (1987) Changes in presynaptic inhibition of Ia fibres at the onset of voluntary contraction in man. *J. Physiol.(Lond.)*, 389: 757–772.

Iles, J.F. (1996) Evidence for cutaneous and corticospinal modulation of presynaptic inhibition of Ia afferents from the human lower limb. *J. Physiol.(Lond.)*, 491: 197–207.

Jankowska, E. and Padel, Y. (1984) On the origin of presynaptic depolarization of group I muscle afferents in Clarke's column in the cat. *Brain Res.*, 295: 195–201.

Jiménez, F., Rudomin, P. and Solodkin, M. (1988) PAD patterns of physiologically identified afferent fibres from the medial gastrocnemius muscle. *Exp. Brain Res.*, 71: 643–657.

Lamotte d'Incamps, B., Destombes, J., Thiesson, D., Hellio, R., Lasserre, X., Kouchtir-Devanne, N., Jami, L. and Zytnicki, D. (1998) Indications for GABA-immunoreactive axoaxonic contacts on the intraspinal arborization of a Ib fiber in the cat: a confocal microscope study. *J. Neurosci.*, 18: 10030–10036.

Lomelí, J., Quevedo, J., Linares, P. and Rudomin, P. (1998) Local control of information flow in segmental and ascending collaterals of single afferents. *Nature*, 365: 600–604.

Lundberg, A. (1964) Supraspinal control of transmission in reflex paths to motoneurons and primary afferents. In: Eccles J, Schadé JP (Eds), *Physiology of the spinal neurons*, Elsevier, Amsterdam, pp. 197–221.

Lundberg, A. (1982) Inhibitory control from the brain stem of transmission from primary afferents to motoneurons, primary afferent terminals and ascending pathways. In: Sjölund B, Björklund A (Eds), *Brain stem control of spinal mechanisms*, Elsevier Biomed. Press, pp. 179–224.

Lüscher, H.-R. (1990) Transmission failure and its relief in the spinal monosynaptic reflex arc. In: Binder MD, Mendell LM (Eds), *The segmental motor system*, Oxford University Press, Oxford, pp. 328–348.

Lüscher, H.-R. (1998) Control of action potential invasion into terminal arborizations. In: Rudomin P, Romo R, Mendell L (Eds), *Presynaptic Inhibition and Neural Control*, Oxford University Press, New York, pp. 126–137.

Madrid, J., Alvarado, J., Dutton, H. and Rudomin, P. (1979) A method for the dynamic continuous estimation of excitability changes of single fiber terminals in the central nervous system. *Neurosci. Lett.*, 11: 253–258.

Maxwell, D.J., Christie, W.M., Short, A.D. and Brown, A.G. (1990) Direct observations of synapses between GABA-immunoreactive boutons and muscle afferent terminals in lamina VI of the cat's spinal cord. *Brain Res.*, 53: 215–222.

Maxwell, D.J., Kerr, R., Jankowska, E. and Riddell, J.S. (1997) Synaptic connections of dorsal horn group II spinal interneurons: synapses formed with the interneurons and by their axon collaterals. *J. Comp. Neurol.*, 380: 51–69.

Meunier, S. and Pierrot-Deseilligny, E. (1989) Gating of the afferent volley of the monosynaptic stretch reflex during movement in man. *J. Physiol. (Lond.)*, 419: 753–763.

Nicol, M.J. and Walmsley, B. (1991) A serial section electron microscope study of an identified Ia afferent collateral in the cat spinal cord. *J. Comp. Neurol.*, 314: 257–277.

Osborn, C.E. and Poppele, R.E. (1993) Sensory integration by the dorsal spinocerebellar tract circuitry. *Neuroscience*, 54: 945–956.

Quevedo, J., Eguibar, J.R., Lomelí, J. and Rudomin, P. (1997) Patterns of connectivity of spinal interneurons with single muscle afferents. *Exp. Brain Res.*, 115: 387–402.

Raymond, J.L., Lisberger, S.G. and Mauk, M.D. (1996) The cerebellum: a neuronal learning machine? *Science*, 272, 1126–1131.

Rudomin, P. (1990) Presynaptic inhibition of muscle spindle and tendon organ afferents in mammalian spinal cord. *Trends Neurosci.*, 13: 499–505.

Rudomin, P., Burke, R.E., Núñez, R., Madrid, J. and Dutton, H. (1975) Control by presynaptic correlation: a mechanism affecting information transmission from Ia fibers to motoneurons. *J. Neurophysiol.*, 38: 267–284.

Rudomin, P., Jiménez, F. and Quevedo, J. (1998) Selectivity of the presynaptic control of synaptic effectiveness of group I afferents in the mammalian spinal cord. In: P. Rudomin, R. Romo, L. Mendell (Eds), *Presynaptic Inhibition and Neural Control*, Oxford University Press, New York, pp. 282–302.

Rudomin, P., Jiménez, I., Solodkin, M. and Dueñas, S. (1983) Sites of action of segmental and descending control of transmission on pathways mediating PAD of Ia- and Ib-afferent fibers in cat spinal cord. *J. Neurophysiol.*, 50: 743–769.

Rudomin, P., Solodkin, M. and Jiménez, I. (1986) PAD and PAH response patterns of group Ia- and Ib-fibers to cutaneous and descending inputs in the cat spinal cord. *J. Neurophysiol.*, 56: 987–1006.

Wall, P.D. (1994) Control of impulse conduction in long range afferents. *Eur. J. Neurosci.*, 6: 1136–1142.

Wall, P.D. and McMahon, S.B. (1994) Long range afferents in rat spinal cord. III. Failure of impulse transmission in axons and relief of the failure after rhizotomy of dorsal roots. *Philos. Trans. R. Soc. Lond. (Biol.)*, 343: 211–223.

Walmsley, B., Graham, B. and Nicol, M.J. (1995) Serial E-M and simulation study of presynaptic inhibition along a group of Ia collateral in the spinal cord. *J. Neurophysiol.*, 74: 616–623.

SECTION IV

Properties and central actions of muscle receptors

M.D. Binder (Ed.)
Progress in Brain Research, Vol 123

CHAPTER 10

Why are there three types of intrafusal muscle fibers?

A. Taylor,* P.H. Ellaway and R. Durbaba

Department of Sensorimotor Control, Division of Neuroscience and Psychiatry, Imperial College School of Medicine, Charing Cross Hospital, London W6 8RF, UK

Introduction

The complexities of the mammalian muscle spindle provide a challenge for scientists interested in relating structure to function. This is particularly the case with regard to the intrafusal muscle fibers, which are well-known to consist of three quite distinct types, most simply named bag_1, bag_2 and chain. When the actions of the gamma motor system were first analysed (Matthews, 1962; Crowe and Matthews, 1964), histological studies had identified only two types of intrafusal muscle fibers: chain and bag. It is understandable, therefore, that division of gamma axons into two sub-populations designated static and dynamic (γ_s and γ_d) seemed both reasonable and satisfying. It was readily accepted that dynamic effects were expressed through bag fibers and static effects through chain fibers. The subsequent recognition of the existence of a second type of bag fiber (Banks et al., 1977) caused confusion at first, but it soon became evident that one type of bag fiber (bag_1) was responsible for dynamic effects, whilst the other (bag_2) and the chain fibers were both involved in static effects (see Boyd, 1981). Thus, one problem was solved, but another was created, namely: why are two fiber types apparently needed for the static fusimotor action?

To appreciate the difficulty we must look at the properties of the three different intrafusal muscle fiber types (Barker et al., 1978). The bag_1 fiber is very similar to the tonic extrafusal type, best seen in amphibia. It requires repetitive stimulation to be activated, it contracts slowly and weakly and does not support propagated action potentials. The chain fibers, by contrast, are very rapidly contracting twitch type, with tetanic fusion frequency in excess of 100 Hz. Bag_2 fibers are somewhat intermediate in their properties. They shorten considerably and more rapidly than bag_1 fibers and sometimes show propagated action potentials, but their tetanic fusion frequency is about 30 Hz – much lower than that for chain fibers.

The significance of the fusimotor system is usually thought of in terms of modifying spindle responses to stretch (see Fig. 1 and Boyd, 1985). In the case of the dynamic gamma action, the propensity of the bag_1 fiber for stiffening rather than shortening suits it well for increasing the stretch sensitivity of the primary afferent, without causing much biassing. The static gamma action is usually described as an increase in bias and a reduction in stretch sensitivity, but this is actually a complex effect due to the combined contraction of bag_2 and chain fibers. The capacity of bag_2 fibers for shortening appears to suit them for adding a bias to primary afferents and to those secondary afferents with bag_2 contacts. They seem not to have much influence on the stretch sensitivity (at least to ongoing movements: Boyd et al., 1985b; Taylor et al., 1997a) and their contraction does not occlude dynamic effects (Dickson et al., 1993). The function of chain fibers is more difficult to rationalise,

---

*Corresponding author. Tel.: +44 181 846 7593; Fax: +44 181 846 7338; e-mail t.taylor@ic.ac.uk

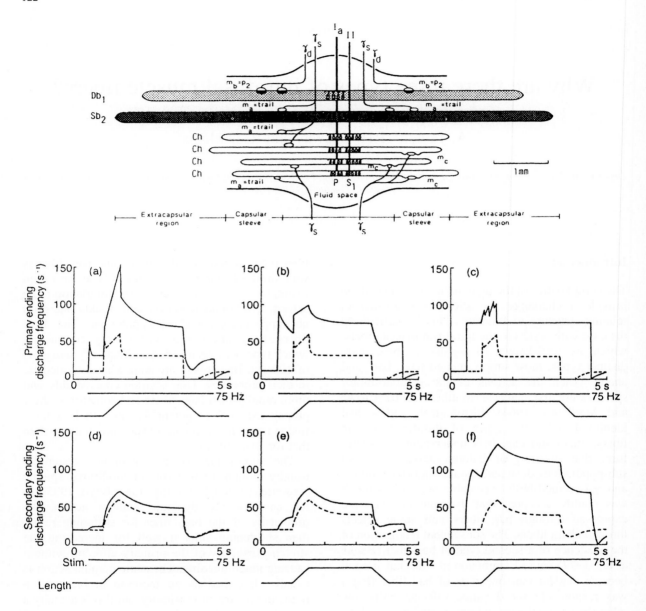

Fig. 1. Standard scheme of the structure of the mammalian muscle spindle and the effects of the contraction of the three intrafusal muscle fiber types. The top diagram shows the three intrafusal fibre types: bag$_1$ (Db$_1$), bag$_2$ (Sb$_2$) and chain (Ch). Primary endings (Ia) are shown to terminate on all three, whilst secondary endings (II) contact chain fibers. Not shown here are the frequent contacts of secondaries on bag$_2$ fibers and the lack of contacts of some primary afferents on bag$_1$ fibers (see text). Gamma dynamic (γ_d) axons, shown here restricted to bag$_1$ fibers, sometimes also contact bag$_2$ and/or chain. Static gamma (γ_s) axons contact bag$_2$, chain or bag$_2$ and chain fibers. Long chain fibers and beta innervation are not shown here. The schematic records below show the effects on primary afferents (upper row) and secondary afferents (lower row), during ramp stretches, of exciting bag$_1$ fibers (left), bag$_2$ fibers (middle) or chain fibers (right). Dashed lines are controls, continuous lines are responses during gamma stimulation at 75 Hz. Figure modified from Boyd (1980) and Boyd and Gladden (1985), with permission.

because during muscle stretch their unfused tetanic contraction may cause primary afferent driving at 1 to 1, or some subharmonic, leading to a very irregular and unpredictable afferent response to stretch (Boyd, et al., 1985a).

Variations in sensory innervation

Attempts in the past to clarify the functions of the three fiber types have been hampered because of the complexity of the innervation patterns within spindles. In the first place, there is much more variability in the distribution of sensory terminals than predicted from classical studies on the basis of separation of primary and secondary afferents by conduction velocity. Happily, this can be dealt with by quantitative tests with succinylcholine (Price and Dutia, 1989; Taylor et al., 1992a, b). Succinylcholine (SCh) causes strong contracture of bag_1 and bag_2 fibers, but has little effect on chain fibers. The wide range of sensory properties of spindles which can be attributed to the different degrees of influence of bag_1 and bag_2 fibers can be seen from Fig. 2 in which the responses of 10 medial gastrocnemius afferents are recorded simultaneously with ramp and hold stretches repeating regularly every 6 s. The control period shows that in the absence of any intrafusal activation (de-efferented), there are no very remarkable differences between units. However, shortly after an injection of SCh, some afferents show greatly increased dynamic sensitivity, whilst in others the effect is principally to raise the background firing rate or bias. The influence of the bag_1 and bag_2 fibers can be estimated by the increases caused in certain measures of dynamic sensitivity and of bias, respectively. Consequently, each afferent can be assessed according to its apparent contacts with the two bag fibers as b_1c, b_1b_2c, b_2c or c. One interesting outcome of these studies is the finding of a substantial number of primary afferents (25–30%) with conduction velocities throughout the Group I range, which have no contacts on bag_1 fibers. Another is the demonstration that most secondary afferents have functionally important contacts on bag_2 fibers (Taylor et al., 1992b).

The ability to test spindle afferents for these characteristics has put the interpretation of spindle records in terms of the underlying gamma motor activity on a much firmer basis than previously. For example, Fig. 3 shows results from a study in which a systematic search was made within the midbrain for regions from which dynamic fusimotor effects could be elicited by electrical stimulation. Stimulation in the vicinity of the red nucleus produced signs of strong dynamic fusimotor output, but this affected only 4 out of 5 primary afferents from medial gastrocnemius recorded simultaneously. The reason for this became clear when the testing with SCh showed that the unit failing to show dynamic effects was a b_2c type primary. If recordings had been restricted by chance to this afferent, it would have been concluded that no dynamic output could be elicited from this part of the midbrain. The other advantage of SCh testing is that the functional strength of the afferent contacts on bag_1 and bag_2 fibers can be estimated separately and correlated with other spindle properties. This has provided evidence that the stretch response of primary afferents in the absence of intrafusal contraction depends principally on the bag_2 contacts. It has also been possible to show that the strength of the bag_2 contacts is better than that of bag_1 contacts as a predictor of the strength of the monosynaptic central excitatory projection on alpha motoneurones and on certain interneurones (Taylor et al., 1993). This may well have developmental significance since the bag_2 fibers differentiate first. It is something which should be kept in mind when looking at the outcome of denervation and re-innervation experiments and the effects of neurotrophic factors.

Variations in motor innervation

The connections of γ axons, also, cannot be expected to conform regularly to the standard description. Even the γ_d axons, generally taken to be specific for bag_1 fibers, sometimes make bag_2 or chain contacts (Emonet-Dénand et al., 1977; Taylor, et al., 1996). Static γ axons can make contact with bag_2 or chain fibers separately or together. The earlier descriptions of intrafusal motor innervation depended heavily upon histology and upon direct visualisation of intrafusal contractions in isolated spindles (Boyd, 1981; Banks et al.,

124

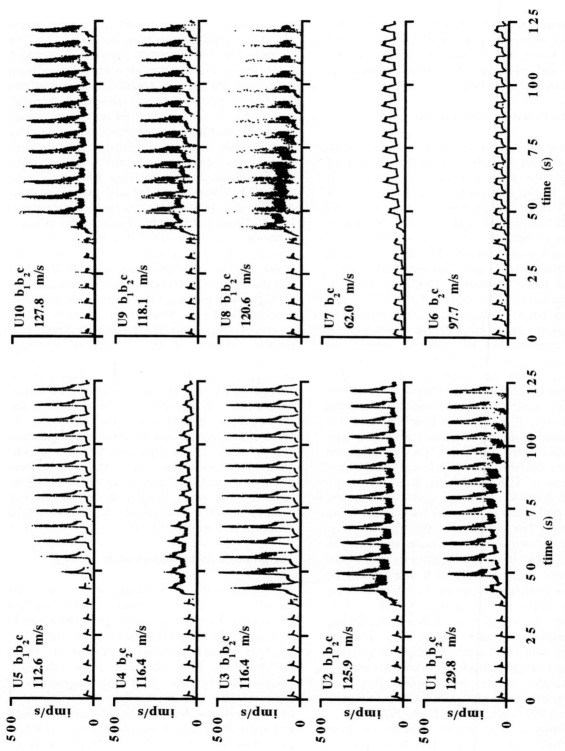

Fig. 2. To show the range of variation of spindle afferent responses to activation of bag_1 and bag_2 intrafusal fibers by succinylcholine (SCh). Ten single spindle afferents from cat medial gastrocnemius were recorded from dorsal rootlets with ventral roots cut. Ramp stretches (not shown) were applied continuously (5 mm rising and falling in 1.0 s, maintained for 1.5 s and repeated every 6 s). SCh (200 µg/kg i.v.) injected 30 s after start of record. In each panel is shown as instantaneous frequency. Afferent firing is shown as instantaneous frequency. In each panel is shown the pattern of intrafusal fiber afferent contacts as deduced from the SCh effects and the conduction velocity. Note that the primary afferents U4 and U6 show no significant increase in dynamic stretch response, but only an increase in bias. Also the secondary afferent (U7) shows signs of a bag_2 effect through increased bias.

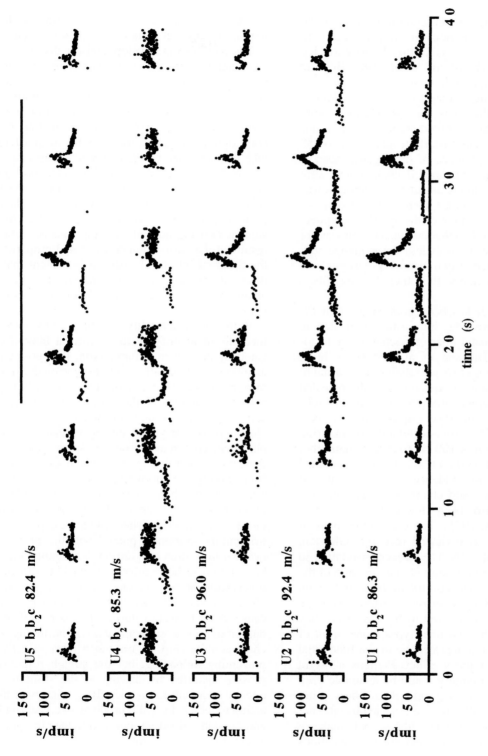

Fig. 3. Demonstration that some spindle primary afferents cannot respond to dynamic fusimotor output. Five primary afferents from medial gastrocnemius were recorded simultaneously during ramp stretches (5 mm rising and falling in 1 s and maintained for 1.5 s) repeated every 6 s. Conduction velocities and the pattern of intrafusal fiber contacts revealed by SCh testing are shown above each record. Cat under chloralose anaesthesia. Stimulation in midbrain, at the base of the red nucleus (200 Hz, 0.2 ms, 100 μA) signalled by horizontal bar. Note the strong dynamic effect on units 1, 2, 3 and 5, which are b_1b_2c type and the lack of this effect on unit 4, which is b_2c type.

1985). To examine γ_s innervation more widely and in more natural conditions it was necessary to develop physiological tests. In this the way was led by Boyd's group (Boyd and Ward, 1982; Boyd et al., 1983). It was possible to use the driving of Ia afferents, depending on the fast twitch behaviour of chain fibers, as the basis for the so-called ramp frequency test. This involved stimulating γ_s axons with a frequency rising linearly from zero up to 150 Hz in 2.5 s. The presence of driving was seen at some point during the ramp if chain fibers were being activated. With the use of this method, it was found that most γ_s axons were either driving or non-driving in all or most of the spindles supplied. Though it was admitted that the innervation was not always so specific, nevertheless the evidence suggested the existence of two distinct γ_s systems, one innervating chain fibers, the other the bag_2 fibers (Boyd, 1986).

More recently it has been pointed out that the prevalence of pure bag_2 innervation indicated in this way was greater than expected from histological studies (Dickson et al., 1993). A more sensitive test, using cross-correlation of Ia afferent firing with the ramp frequency stimuli, revealed that some of the apparently pure bag_2 innervations were actually mixed. A subsequent study in peroneus tertius, using cross-correlation of Ia firing with regular stimuli at 100 Hz to detect chain fiber activation (Celichowski et al., 1994), concluded that there was no evidence for specificity of innervation of bag_2 and chain fibers. Histological evidence has also been found to be against specificity (Banks, 1991). These and other lines of evidence have been reviewed recently (Gladden, 1995; Taylor et al., 1995). However, in relation to these studies it could be argued that rejection of the possibility of separate control of bag_2 and chain fibers was based on over-rigid criteria. Gamma axons were only considered to be specific if they supplied one of the two fiber types alone in *all* of the spindles affected, irrespective of the functional strength of the minority effect. Perhaps a useful degree of separate control could be available even though innervation of bag_2 and chain fibers is not completely separate. After all, γ_d axons are not entirely restricted to bag_1 fibers, but make a significant number of bag_2 and chain connections

and this is accepted as quite compatible with the notion of a distinct dynamic fusimotor system.

The most recent development for distinguishing chain and bag_2 fiber innervation has been the use of random stimulus trains applied to single γ axons, combined with cross-correlation of the stimuli with the afferent spikes (Taylor et al., 1995; Taylor et al., 1996; Taylor et al., 1998). As seen in Fig. 4, the correlograms observed for γ_s axons to Ia afferents take one or other of three forms. There can be a single, large, brief deflection, a weak, prolonged deflection or a combination of the two. The first two types can be fitted very well by single log-normal curves, whilst the third type is fitted by the sum of two log-normals. Taking into account the results of the ramp frequency test and properties of the different intrafusal fibers, it is evident that the different correlograms represent evidence for pure chain, pure bag_2 and mixed innervation, respectively.

With the availability of these physiological methods of identifying the intrafusal fibers innervated by any given gamma axon, it is possible to examine the effects of each fiber type on the spindle response to stretch in any muscle of interest. Figure 5 shows examples of the actions of each type on spindle primary endings in medial gastrocnemius. Notice particularly that during repeated stretches pure bag_1 contraction produces a large increase in dynamic response (Fig. 5A), but does not sustain firing during the shortening phases. The increased bias, caused when contraction of bag_1 fibres is initiated at resting length, disappears when cyclic movements are established. In fact, the presence of firing in the shortening phases, with this protocol of cyclic ramp stretches during γ_d stimulation, has been found to be regularly associated with mixed innervation of bag_2 or chain fibers (Taylor et al., 1996). In Fig. 5B pure bag_2 activation is seen to cause firing to restart during the shortened phase, but not to prevent silencing *during* shortening. Pure chain activity (Fig. 5C) is much more effective in preventing unloading, but the stretch response is grossly distorted by driving at the stimulus frequency or at sub-harmonics. Bag_2 and chain fibers acting together (Fig. 5D) produce a very strong bias and prevent unloading, but also reduce the primary afferent response to stretch.

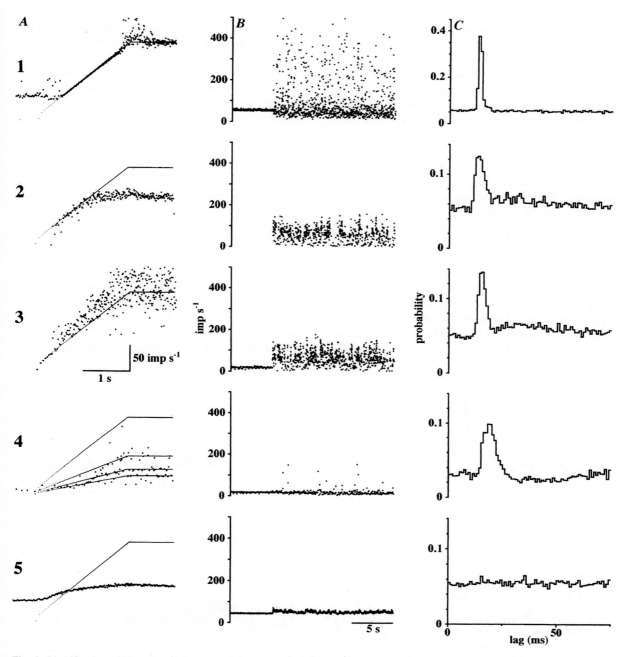

Fig. 4. Identification of intrafusal fiber types activated by γ_s motor stimulation. Left hand column (A) shows instantaneous frequency responses of Ia afferents to ramp frequency stimulation of five different static gamma axons (0–150 Hz in 2.5 s). (1): afferent driving at 1 to 1. (2) and (3): driving over a limited range together with biassing. (4): driving fluctuating between 1 to 2 and 1 to 4. (5): no trace of driving, smoothly increasing bias only. Stimulus frequency is shown by fine dotted lines. Additionally in 4, the stimulus record is shown divided by 2, 3 and 4. Middle column: instantaneous frequency plots of afferent responses to random stimuli with mean frequency of 50 Hz. Stimulation starts 5 s after the start of the record. Right hand column: correlograms formed between random stimuli and Ia afferent firing. Bin widths 1 ms. Data taken from the experiments of Taylor et al. (1998).

The new methods of detecting contraction of the different intrafusal fibers have also allowed a further examination of the question of the specificity of innervation of the bag$_2$ and chain fibers (Taylor et al., 1998). Classification of the effects of γ_s axons to medial gastrocnemius muscle in the cat showed a significant excess of pure bag$_2$ and pure chain effects over that expected from chance distribution (Fig. 6). An additional useful procedure is to take the Fourier transforms of the correlograms to generate plots of 'gain' as a function of frequency. The plots from the simple correlograms are found to be well fitted by first order lag characteristics with a corner frequency of 50–100 Hz for the fast peaks and 2–8 Hz for the slow ones. The mixed effects are fitted by the sum of two such curves. The merit of this frequency domain analysis is that from the fitted curves it is possible to make estimates of the functional strength of the particular fiber connections. Using this method, the mixed effects were reclassified as pure bag$_2$ or pure chain if the dominant effect was at least five times

stronger than the weaker. The reclassification made departure from a chance distribution statistically much more significant.

The implication of these findings is that, though the innervation of chain and bag$_2$ intrafusal fibers is by no means specific, nevertheless it may be sufficiently distinct for the CNS to be able to make use of the very different properties of these fiber types. Another line of evidence which points to the potential value of a degree of separate control is the way in which γ stimulation can modulate the afferent discharge. We have studied this in medial gastrocnemius, peroneus tertius and soleus muscles by isolating single γ axons in ventral roots and observing their effects on primary and secondary afferents, of which up to 12 were recorded at one time. The γ axons were identified as static or dynamic by their effects on responses to ramp stretches and then examined for their effects on bag$_2$ and chain fibers by the random stimulation and correlation method described above. They were then stimulated by a frequency modulated stimulus

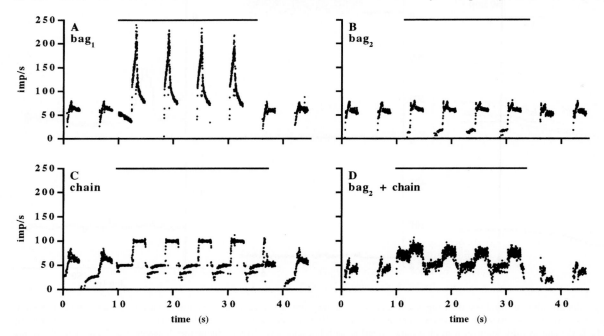

Fig. 5. The effect of contraction of the different intrafusal fibers on primary afferent responses to stretch. Each panel shows the response of a Ia afferent in MG to ramp stretches (5 mm in 1 s, every 6 s) in control conditions and during gamma stimulation at 100 Hz (solid line). A: bag$_1$ fiber active alone – note large increase in dynamic sensitivity and lack of firing between stretches. B: bag$_2$ fiber active alone – note increased bias, peak frequency unaffected. C: chain fiber active alone – note driving at 100 Hz during stretch. D: mixed bag$_2$ and chain fiber activation – note the irregular response to stretch.

source in which the mean frequency was 50 Hz and this was modulated sinusoidally at 1 Hz by various amplitudes up to 60 Hz peak to peak, while keeping muscle length constant. The results (see Fig. 7) were very clear and consistent. Neither bag_1 nor bag_2 fibers acting alone produced any appreciable modulation of the afferent discharge. Pure chain fiber activation gave modulation fluctuating between 1 to 1 or 1 to 2. Static gamma axons which acted on bag_2 and chain fibers together gave strong and linear modulation with an amplitude as much as 2.7 times the input modulation. Mixed bag_2 and chain contraction was also very effective in modulating secondary afferent discharge. It is clear that if part of the gamma motor output during rhythmic movements is to provide a lead signal or to offset the unloading of spindles during active shortening, then this would best be provided by γ_s axons activating bag_2 and chain fibers. At first sight this

conclusion seems to argue against there being any value in separate activation of bag_2 and chain fibers. However, pure bag_2 activation has the special property of providing a bias to both primary and secondary afferents, which does not conflict with the dynamic sensitivity to stretch.

Conclusions

Thus, a working scheme for the use of the three intrafusal fiber types might be as follows. The bag_1 fibers provide control of stretch sensitivity of primary afferents. Rapid changes in dynamic fusimotor output would be pointless, because of the relative slowness of response of bag_1 fibers and their inability effectively to oppose unloading. The bias levels of primary and secondary afferents could be set by bag_2 activity, but the slowness of bag_2 fiber contraction means that quick changes

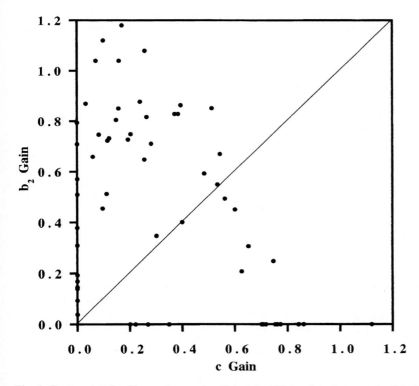

Fig. 6. Scatter plots for 60 γ_s actions on Ia afferents in MG to relate the strength of the bag_2 effect to the strength of the chain effect. Gain in each case represents the low frequency gain estimated from the Fourier transformed correlograms. The diagonal line indicates where points would lie if the bag_2 and chain effects were equal. Points lying on the vertical and horizontal axes represent pure bag_2 and chain effects, respectively. Reproduced with permission from Taylor et al. (1998).

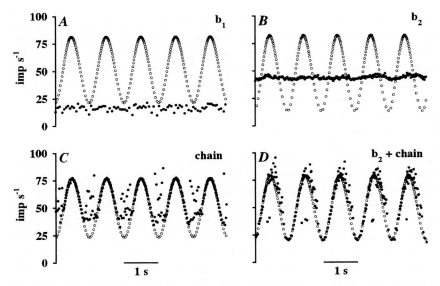

Fig. 7. Comparison of the capacity of the different intrafusal fibers to modulate Ia afferent discharge. Single γ_s axons affecting MG primary afferents were isolated in ventral roots and characterised according to their effects on intrafusal fibers. They were then stimulated with a mean frequency of 50 Hz, frequency modulated sinusoidally at 1 Hz by $\pm$ 30 Hz. The afferent frequency (filled circles) is shown superimposed on the stimulus frequency (open circles). Note the failure of bag$_1$ (A) and bag$_2$ (B) fibers acting alone to produce significant modulation of afferent firing. Pure chain activation (C) gives 1:1 driving at stimulus frequencies above resting discharge frequency (about 35 Hz) and an irregular response otherwise. Mixed bag$_2$ and chain stimulation (D) gives continuous, essentially linear modulation throughout.

could not be made in this way. Gamma axons supplying bag$_2$ fibers alone can be expected, therefore, like dynamic axons, to fire tonically rather than phasically. Finally, the γ motoneurones which would be expected to show rapid modulation during movements should be those jointly supplying bag$_2$ and chain fibers. The proposed function for the dynamic system is already well-supported by spindle recordings in natural movements (Prochazka, 1996; Taylor and Appenteng, 1981; Taylor, et al., 1997b) but the crucial test for a dual function within the static system will be to look for two distinct patterns of natural activity amongst γ_s axons. The prediction would be that one group, directed mainly to bag$_2$ fibers, will fire tonically whilst the other, directed to chain or to bag$_2$ and chain fibers will be modulated roughly in parallel with the active muscle contractions.

Acknowledgement

Supported by the UK Medical Research Council.

References

Banks, R.W. (1991) The distribution of static γ-axons in the tenuissimus muscle of the cat. *J. Physiol.*, 442: 489–512.

Banks, R.W., Harker, D.W. and Stacey, M.J. (1977) A study of mammalian intrafusal muscle fibres using a combined histochemical and ultrastructural technique. *J. Anat.*, 123: 783–796.

Banks, R.W., Barker, D. and Stacey, M.J. (1985) Form and classification of motor endings in mammlian muscle spindles. *Proc. R. Soc. (Lond.) B.*, 225: 195–212.

Barker, D., Bessou, P., Jankowska, E., Pages, B. and Stacey, M.J. (1978) Identification of intrafusal muscle fibres activated by single fusimotor axons and injected with fluorescent dye in cat tenuissimus spindles. *J. Physiol.*, 275: 149–165.

Boyd, I.A., Gladden, M.H. and Ward, J. (1983) Two types of static γ-axon having a predominantly static bag fibre action or predominantly chain fibre action in several cat muscle spindles they supply. *J. Physiol.*, 343: 110–111P.

Boyd, I.A. (1981) The action of the three types of intrafusal fibre in isolated cat muscle spindles on the dynamic length sensitivities of primary and secondary sensory endings. In: A. Taylor and A. Prochazka (Eds), *Muscle Receptors and Movement*, Macmillan, London, pp. 17–32.

Boyd, I.A. (1985) Intrafusal muscle fibres in the cat and their motor control. In: W.J.P. Barnes and M.H. Gladden (Eds), *Feedback and Motor Control in Invertebrates and Vertebrates*, Croom-Helm, London, pp. 123–144.

Boyd, I.A. (1986) Two types of static γ-axon in cat muscle spindles. *Q. J. Exp. Physiol.*, 71: 307–327.

Boyd, I.A., Murphy, P.R. and Mann, C. (1985a) The effect of chain fibre 'driving' on the length sensitivity of primary sensory endings in the tenuissimus, peroneus tertius and soleus muscles. In: I.A. Boyd and M.H. Gladden, (Eds), *The Muscle Spindle*, Macmillan, London, pp. 195–200.

Boyd, I.A., Murphy, P.R. and Moss, V.A. (1985b) Analysis of primary and secondary afferent responses to stretch during activation of the dynamic bag$_1$ fibre or the static bag$_2$ fibre separately in cat muscle spindles. In: I.A. Boyd and M.H. Gladden (Eds), *The Muscle Spindle*, Macmillan, London, pp. 153–158.

Boyd, I.A. and Ward, J. (1982) The diagnosis of nuclear chain intrafusal fibre activity from the nature of the group Ia and group II afferent discharge of isolated cat muscle spindles. *J. Physiol.*, 329: 17P–18P.

Celichowski, J., Emonet-Dénand, F., Laporte, Y. and Petit, J. (1994) Distribution of static γ-axons in cat peroneus tertius spindles determined by exclusively physiological criteria. *J. Neurophysiol.*, 71: 722–732.

Crowe, A. and Matthews, P.B.C. (1964) The effects of stimulation of static and dynamic fusimotor fibres on the response to stretching of the primary endings of muscle spindles. *J. Physiol.*, 174: 109–131.

Dickson, M., Emonet-Dénand, F., Gladden, M.H. and Petit, J. (1993) Incidence of non-driving excitation of Ia afferents during ramp frequency stimulation of static γ-axons in cat hindlimbs. *J. Physiol.*, 460: 657–673.

Emonet-Dénand, F., Laporte, Y., Matthews, P.B.C. and Petit, J. (1977) On the subdivision of static and dynamic fusimotor actions on the primary endings of the cat muscle spindle. *J. Physiol.*, 268: 827–861.

Gladden, M.H. (1995) Isolated muscle spindles, their motor innervation and central control. In: W.R. Ferrell and U. Proske (Eds), *Neural Control of Movement*, Plenum Press, New York and London, pp. 3–10.

Matthews, P.B.C. (1962) The differentiation of two types of fusimotor fibres by their effects on the dynamic response of muscle spindle primary endings. *Q. J. Exp. Physiol.*, 47: 324–333.

Price, R.F. and Dutia, M.B. (1989) Physiological properties of tandem muscle spindles in neck and hind-limb muscles. *Prog. Brain Res.*, 80: 47–56.

Prochazka, A. (1996) Proprioceptive feedback and movement regulation. In: L.B. Rowell and J.T. Sheperd (Eds), *Handbook of Physiology: Section 12. Exercise: Regulation and Integration of Multiple Systems*, American Physiological Society, New York, pp. 89–127.

Taylor, A. and Appenteng, K. (1981) Distinctive modes of static and dynamic fusimotor drive in jaw muscles. In: A. Taylor and A. Prochazka (Eds), *Muscle Receptors and Movement*, Macmillan, London, pp. 172–192.

Taylor, A., Durbaba, R. and Rodgers, J.F. (1992a) The classification of afferents from muscle spindles of the jaw-closing muscles of the cat. *J. Physiol.*, 456: 609–628.

Taylor, A., Durbaba, R. and Rodgers, J.F. (1993) Projection of cat jaw muscle spindle afferents related to intrafusal fibre influence. *J. Physiol.*, 465: 647–660.

Taylor, A., Durbaba, R. and Rodgers, J.F. (1995) Correlation methods in identifying intrafusal activity. In: A. Taylor, M.H. Gladden and R. Durbaba (Eds), *Alpha and Gamma Motor Systems*, Plenum, New York, pp. 280–283.

Taylor, A., Ellaway, P.H. and Durbaba, R. (1996) The characterisation of dynamic fusimotor action using random stimuli. In: G.N. Ganchev, V.S. Gurfinkel, D.M. Stuart, M. Wiesendanger and S. Mori (Eds), *Motor Control Symposium VIII*, Academic Publishing House, Sofia, pp. 43–46.

Taylor, A., Ellaway, P.H. and Durbaba, R. (1997a) The influence of bag$_2$ intrafusal fibre contraction on primary muscle spindle afferent behaviour in the cat. *J. Physiol.*, 505: 76P.

Taylor, A., Ellaway, P.H. and Durbaba, R. (1998) Physiological signs of the activation of bag$_2$ and chain intrafusal muscle fibers of gastrocnemius muscle spindles in the cat. *J. Neurophysiol.*, 80: 130–142.

Taylor, A., Hidaka, O., Durbaba, R. and Ellaway, P. H. (1997b) Fusimotor influence on jaw muscle spindle activity during swallowing-related movements in the cat. *J. Physiol.*, 503: 157–167.

Taylor, A., Rodgers, J.F., Fowle, A.J. and Durbaba, R. (1992b) The effect of succinylcholine on cat gastrocnemius muscle spindle afferents of different type. *J. Physiol.*, 456: 629–644.

M.D. Binder (Ed.)
Progress in Brain Research, Vol 123
© 1999 Elsevier Science BV. All rights reserved.

CHAPTER 11

Quantifying proprioception

Arthur Prochazka*

Division of Neuroscience, University of Alberta, Edmonton, AB T6G 2S2, Canada

Introduction

The papers of Douglas Stuart and his colleagues in the 1970s on the properties of neuronal ensembles controlling cat locomotion (e.g. Goslow et al., 1973b; Wetzel and Stuart, 1976; Rasmussen et al., 1978), were among the most influential of their era. They heralded a transition from studies of segmental reflexes in immobile, anesthetized animals, to those in which ensembles of sensorimotor neurons controlling complex movements in awake animals are identified and characterized. The two papers on kinematic, EMG and proprioceptive responses during locomotion (Goslow et al., 1973a, b) have become classic references for all research laboratories concerned with the neural control of locomotion.

Jasper et al. (1958) and Evarts (1964) pioneered the recording of the activity of single neurons in the brain during motor behavior in awake monkeys. This had a tremendous impact on motor control and spawned many other studies and new approaches. Within a decade, techniques were developed for recording from single sensory afferent neurons in the dorsal root ganglia of freely-moving cats (Prochazka et al., 1976; Loeb et al., 1977). In a parallel development, Hagbarth and Vallbo (1967) pioneered the technique of human miocroneurography, which for the first time revealed the firing of single sensory axons in human peripheral nerves. This technique, which also had a major impact on

the field, has the advantage that sensory activity is monitored in awake humans performing voluntary motor tasks, but it has the disadvantage that movement is greatly restricted in range and velocity because the microelectrodes are easily dislodged from the nerve.

Over the years, a consistent and puzzling difference emerged in the firing properties of human and animal muscle spindle afferents. In humans, spindle firing rates rarely exceeded 30 impulses/s, whereas in cats and monkeys performing motor tasks, the firing rate of spindle primary (Ia) afferents typically fluctuated between 25 and 200 impulses/s, transiently exceeding 500 impulses/s in demanding situations (review: Prochazka, 1996). Human neurographers have suggested that the difference in firing rates is due to a fundamental species difference. But my group has argued that it may be due merely to the large differences in muscle velocities in the human and animal experiments. The question is quite important from a control systems point of view and as we shall see, it is also relevant to another discrepancy, namely that in cats, fusimotor action appears to fluctuate dramatically with task and context (fusimotor 'set'), whereas in humans it seems to be exclusively linked to α-motoneuronal activation (Kakuda et al., 1996, 1998; Gandevia et al., 1997).

In this chapter I will argue that the data of Stuart's group on muscle velocities in gait of different speeds, when combined with a quantitative analysis of the components of spindle Ia response due to velocity, displacement and α-γ co-activation, show that the differences between the

*Corresponding author. Tel.: 1 780 492 3783; Fax 1 780 492 1617; e-mail: arthur.prochazka@ualberta.ca

firing rates of animal and human spindles may indeed be due mainly to differences in the velocities of movement studied. I arrived at this conclusion with the help of simple mathematical models of spindle response properties. These models are now very easy to realise and manipulate with graphics-based software. An important aim of this chapter is therefore to present a set of models of proprioceptive transduction in this format. The models are reasonably accurate, and yet simple enough to be incorporated into larger models of sensorimotor function. They may be downloaded via the Internet (see later).

Models of spindle and tendon organ transduction

In two recent papers, Monica Gorassini and I tested several models in the literature of the responses of cat spindle (group Ia and II) and tendon organ

(group Ib) afferents. We evaluated the accuracy of the various models in predicting the averaged firing profiles of ensembles of single afferents in the step cycle recorded with microwires implanted in the dorsal root ganglia of normal cats (Prochazka and Gorassini, 1998a, b). To our surprise, all of the Ia models, which included those of Matthews and Stein (1969), Chen and Poppele (1978), Houk et al. (1981) and Hasan (1983), fitted the chronic data well, with r^2 values ranging from 0.4 to 0.94. In retrospect, this is not too surprising, because peak muscle velocities are high in the step cycle and as all of the models have a velocity component, this dominated in a similar way in all the predictions. However, when we tested the same models, with the same gain parameters, on Ia responses to slow ramp-and-hold stretches derived from the literature, some predicted the responses better than others (Fig. 1). The most general and accurate model overall was a variant of those proposed by Houk et al. (1981) and Hasan (1983), namely:

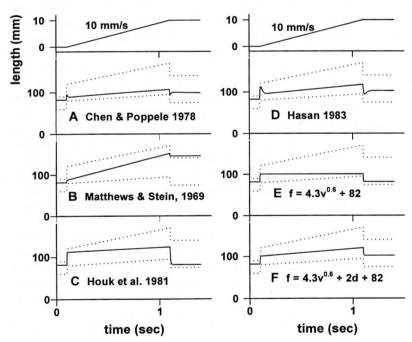

Fig. 1. Predictions of the models of spindle primary responses to ramp-and-hold stretches at a low velocity (10 mm/sec). Dotted lines show the range of spindle primary responses under moderate static fusimotor drive, estimated from the literature. Models without length-sensitive terms (e.g. C and E) did not reproduce the ramp increase in firing rate during stretch, so cannot be considered general. The responses in D and F fall in the middle of the expected range and have appropriate step and ramp components, indicating that their velocity and positional sensitivities are correctly scaled. Reproduced with permission, (Prochazka and Gorassini, 1998a).

$$\text{Ia firing rate} = 4.3 * \text{velocity}^{0.6} + 2 * \text{displacement} + K\% * \text{EMG} + \text{mean rate} \tag{1}$$

(rate: impulses/s, muscle velocity: mm/s, displacement: mm). The EMG term adds a component of Ia firing proportional to α-motoneuronal activity, representing α-linked γ_{static} action. EMG is the normalized, high-pass-filtered, averaged, rectified EMG of the receptor-bearing muscle, the high-pass transfer function being $(s+1)/(s+20)$). K% is the percentage of maximal EMG recruitment possible in the muscle. Figure 2 shows the EMG term and the overall fit achieved with Equation 1 of the mean firing rate profile of nine hamstrings Ia afferents in the cat step cycle with K% set to 50. The mean rate in the chronic data was 80 impulses/s.

I will now propose a slightly simpler and more general version of the above model, namely:

$$\text{Ia firing rate} = 65 * \text{velocity}^{0.5} + 200 * \text{displacement} + K\% * \text{EMG} + \text{mean rate} \tag{2}$$

In this case displacement and velocity are expressed in rest lengths (RL and RL/s), and velocity$^{0.5}$ replaces the velocity$^{0.6}$ term in Equation 1. Note that the Ia models as they stand in Equations 1 and 2 cannot be used for negative velocities. We dealt with this by computing the Ia response to the absolute value of velocity and then restoring the sign (see Fig. 5). Although the fits obtained with Equation 1 of the chronically recorded spindle data were slightly better than those with Equation 2, this is offset by the advantage of being able to estimate the square root of velocity easily by mental arithmetic. For example, consider the data of Fig. 2. During the swing phase of the step, hamstrings muscle length

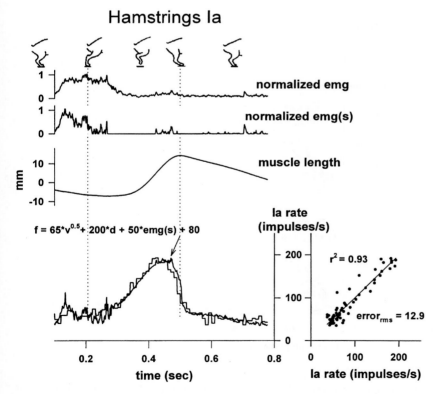

Fig. 2. Prediction of hamstrings Ia firing rate from length and EMG. 9 hamstrings Ia afferents each contributed 4 step cycles of data to the firing rate probability density function. The prediction of Ia rate was computed using Equation 2. The mean rate of the chronic data was 80 impulses/s. The plot at bottom right is of predicted Ia rates (y-axis) versus chronically recorded Ia rates (x-axis). The RMS error was 12.9 impulses/s, i.e. <8% of modulation depth.

136

increased 15 mm in about 0.05 s, i.e. velocity was 15/0.05 = 300 mm/s. The rest length of hamstrings is about 100 mm, so 300 mm/s represents 3 RL/s. Equation 2 tells us that the component of Ia firing rate due to this velocity is 65*sqrt3 = 92 impulses/s. Add to this the displacement term 200*0.15 = 30 and a mean rate of 80 from the chronic data and we have a predicted peak firing rate of 202 impulses/s, which agrees well with the peak of the firing rate profile in Fig. 2. From Fig. 3, triceps surae stretches more slowly: ~ 10 mm in 0.1s during the swing phase, i.e. 0.1 RL in 0.1 s = 1 RL/s. The mean rate

of triceps Ia's in our data was 50 impulses/s. Equation 2 thus predicts a peak firing rate of 65 + 20 + 50 = 135 impulses/s. Just before foot touchdown, muscle velocity reverses from + 1 to − 1 RL/s, leading to a predicted reduction of 2*65 = 130 impulses/s. It is here that the EMG component, representing α-linked γ_{static} action, became very significant in improving the fit of the triceps surae Ia data (compare Fig. 3A and 3B). But even with the EMG-linked term, the fit in B was not as good as that for hamstrings Ia rate profiles (Fig. 2), possibly because of muscle unloading and

Triceps Surae Ia

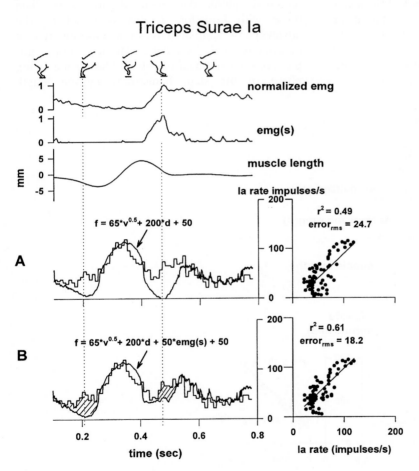

Fig. 3. Prediction of Triceps Surae Ia firing rate from length (A) and length + EMG (B). Chronic data from 9 Triceps Surae Ia afferents, each contributing 4 step cycles. Equation 2 was used to predict Ia firing rate from length and EMG. Mean rate = 50 impulses/s. In A, the EMG component of Equation 2 was set to zero. In B, adding this component (to simulate α-linked fusimotor action) improved the fit (compare B to A), but even then the fit was not as good as that in Fig. 3. This may be due to a discrepancy in origin-to-insertion muscle displacement and the internal displacement 'seen' by the spindles (see text). This Figure is based on the same chronic data as in Fig. 2 of Prochazka et al. (1998b), though with a different set of step cycles.

tendon strain effects in triceps surae, which are maximal just before and after the swing phase respectively: see the shaded portions of Fig. 3B (Hoffer et al., 1989; Elek et al., 1990; Griffiths, 1991). As we will see below, the relative sizes of the velocity and EMG terms are important in resolving some of the differences in Ia firing behavior in cats and humans.

Unfortunately, the firing of group II spindle afferents has rarely been recorded chronically in any species. Monica Gorassini and I only had access to averaged step-cycle profiles from three such afferents. Two were fitted best by a model in which muscle displacement (measured in mm) and normalized, averaged, rectified EMG (non-filtered) were the modulating terms:

$$\text{II firing rate} = 13.5*\text{displacement} + 20*\text{EMG} + \text{mean rate} \qquad (3)$$

The third profile was best fitted by filtering the displacement (again in mm) with the Poppele and Bowman group II transfer function and additional EMG_{norm} and mean rate terms:

$$\text{II firing rate} = 0.4*\text{displacement}*(s+0.4)(s+11)/ (s+0.8) + 20*\text{EMG} + \text{mean rate} \qquad (4)$$

The Poppele and Bowman transfer function is likely to be more general as it not only fitted two of the chronic profiles but was originally based on data obtained in acute experiments, so the recommendation to modellers at this stage is to use Equation 4 with a mean rate of 80 impulses/s to describe group II responses. The EMG term representing α-linked γ_{static} action, has a smaller gain constant than for Ia afferents and this is in line with the conclusion of Loeb and Duysens (1979) and Loeb and Hoffer (1985), that spindle secondaries are modulated largely by muscle length changes. The more general form of (4), in which displacement is expressed in RL is:

$$\text{II firing rate} = 40*\text{displacement}*(s+0.4)(s+11)/ (s+0.8) + 20*\text{EMG} + \text{mean rate} \qquad (5)$$

Finally, for tendon organ Ib afferents, we used the inverse of the Houk and Simon (1967) model to estimate triceps surae force from the Ib ensemble profile.

Houk and Simon model

$$\text{Ib firing rate} = K*\text{Force}*(s+0.15)(s+1.5)(s+16)/ (s+0.2)(s+2)(s+37) \qquad (6)$$

Inverse

$$\text{Force} = K^{-1}*(\text{Ib firing rate})*(s+0.2)(s+2) (s+37)/(s+0.15)(s+1.5)(s+16) \qquad (7)$$

The estimated force profile agreed well with the mean soleus force profile measured with implanted buckle transducers by Fowler et al. (1993) and Herzog et al. (1993) in freely-moving cats (Fig. 4). This indicates that if the time course of force is known (either as a measurement or as a signal computed within a biomechanical model), the ensemble Ib firing profile can be estimated with Equation 6.

The value of the gain constant K depends on whether one uses the force of a single muscle such as soleus or that of a muscle group such as the triceps surae. To simplify matters, normalized force profiles may be used and K then becomes the scale factor that produces appropriate peak Ib firing rates. The value of K^{-1} used in Equation 6 to obtain normalized force from Ib firing rate in Fig. 4 was 0.003. So the recommendation to compute Ib firing rate from normalized force is K = 333.

Typically peak soleus force in the stance phase of the cat step cycle is ~ 20 N (Herzog et al., 1993) and in the whole triceps surae it is ~ 36 N (Fowler et al., 1993). Among other things this shows that members of a synergistic group do not contribute equal forces. Furthermore, Ib firing rate may not be linearly related to whole muscle force, especially when force is large (Proske, 1981; Crago et al., 1982; Jami, 1992). For example, Walmsley et al. (1978) showed that soleus force ranges from 20 N in gait to 100 N in sudden jumps. Figure 4 shows that peak Ib rate is already over 120 impulses/sec in gait. As it is unlikely that Ib firing rates ever exceed 500–600 impulses/s (personal observations) this implies a saturation in the force-rate relationship. For these reasons and the fact that our tests of analytical models on chronic Ib data are the only ones in the literature so far, any prediction of Ib

138

responses in normal motor tasks based on Equation 6 should be viewed as approximate only.

If force is unavailable a very rough estimate of Ib firing rate may be obtained from the normalized

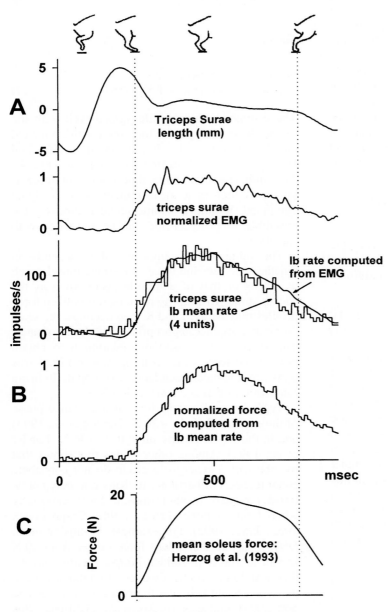

Fig. 4. Prediction of force from Ib firing rate and Ib firing rate from EMG. The chronic data were obtained from four Ib afferents each contributing 4 step cycles to the firing rate histogram (A). The inverse Houk and Simon model of Equation 7 was used to predict force from this firing rate profile (B). Compare B with C, the mean soleus force profile recorded with implanted buckle transducers. Equation 8 was used to predict Ib firing rate from the EMG profile and the result is the smooth superimposed curve in A. This is a modified version of Fig. 7 in Prochazka and Gorassini, 1998b.

EMG by adding some low-pass filtering to Equation 6 (Jacks et al., 1988) and adjusting the gain constant accordingly:

$$\text{Ib firing rate} = 4500 * \text{EMG} * (s+0.15)(s+1.5)(s+16)/(s+0.2)(s+(2)(s+37)(s+12) \quad (8)$$

Again it should be understood that EMG is only proportional to muscle force in isometric contractions. Whenever muscles lengthen or shorten appreciably the relationship starts to become non-linear and the prediction less reliable.

Object-oriented models. For the convenience of the reader, Equations 2, 5, 7 and 8 are implemented in a form suitable for use with Matlab Simulink in Fig. 5. As mentioned above, in the Ia model responses to negative velocities are dealt with by computing the response to the absolute magnitude of velocity and then restoring the sign.

Implications of the models for differences in animal and human spindle firing behavior. Equation 2 tells us that muscle spindle Ia responses are a function of muscle velocity, displacement and α-linked γ action. It is very interesting to compare the data of Douglas Stuart and his colleagues on the ranges of muscle velocity encountered in cat gait with the ranges of velocity that occur in normal human movement and in human neurography experiments. What emerges goes a long way towards explaining the puzzling differences between the animal and human spindle data over the last few years.

In the cat the changes in muscle velocity within each locomotor cycle range from 0.8 to 2.8 RL/s in walking and from 1.2 to 10.0 RL/s in running (Goslow et al., 1973). In human gait, the corresponding values are 0.4 to 0.6 RL/s for walk and 2.0 to 3.0 RL/s for run (derived from Winter, 1987, assuming the full range of motion about a joint corresponds to 0.3 RL change in muscle length). In human neurography experiments since 1967, I have estimated that muscles velocities have ranged from 0 RL/s to 0.1 RL/s (Prochazka, 1981; Prochazka and Hulliger, 1998). If we now use Equation 2 to calculate the mean modulation depth of Ia firing corresponding to the mean changes in velocity, displacement and EMG (representing α-linked γ action), we obtain:

$$\text{Ia firing rate} = 65 * \text{velocity}^{0.5} + 200 * \text{displacement} + \text{K}\% * \text{EMG(s)} \quad (9)$$

cat walk:	87	+	20	+	50
cat run:	154	+	30	+	100
human walk:	46	+	40	+	50
human run:	102	+	60	+	100
neurography:	15	+	20	+	50

In all but the human neurography situation, the estimated modulation of Ia firing due to velocity and displacement combined exceeds that due to α-linked γ action. The slowness of movement in human neurography explains why α–γ linkage has been so prominent a factor. Conversely, Ia firing recorded in freely moving animals emphasizes velocity and displacement rather than α–γ linkage except in strong, relatively isometric contractions. The figures above show that the same would probably hold true if it were possible to record from spindles in human walking and running, though α-linked γ action might be a little more prominent in humans, because muscle velocities (in RL/s) in comparable movements are lower than those in cats. The main point of all this is that the spindle models presented in this article provide a convenient means of estimating the contribution of the different modulating factors and help explain some of the differences in the human and animal data.

Conclusion

Neuromechanical modeling. The above models, along with models of load-moving behavior of muscle can be very useful in testing specific hypotheses. For example, we recently asked how it could possibly be that the reflex excitation of homonymous muscles by tendon organ input during locomotion, which represents positive force feedback, does not completely destabilize the limbs. The result, that the gain of the positive force feedback declines to stable levels as muscles shorten, was as unexpected as it was illuminating (Prochazka et al., 1997). Analytical models of spindle and tendon organ feedback similar to those above were decisive in reaching this conclusion and thanks to object-oriented software and the Internet, the models are readily available to all researchers

140

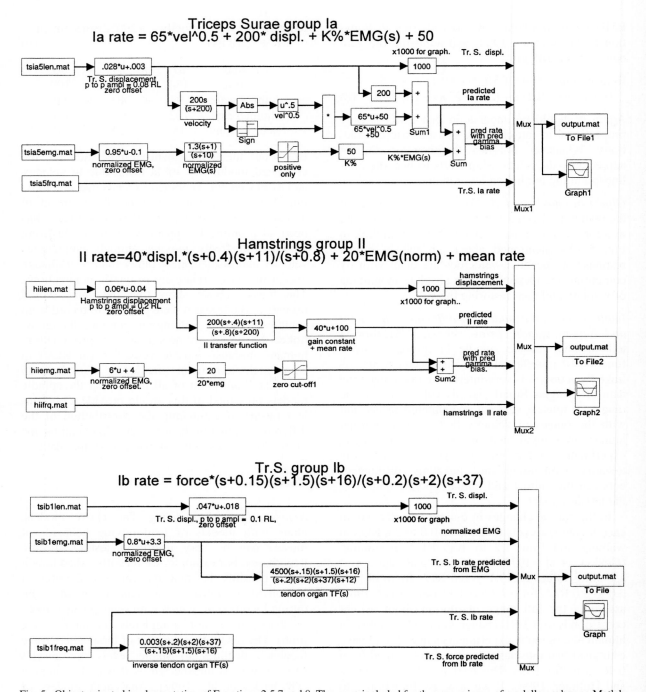

Fig. 5. Object-oriented implementation of Equations 2,5,7 and 8. These are included for the convenience of modellers who use Matlab Simulink software. The boxes at left represent the length, EMG and firing rate profiles stored as Matlab data files. The models and data files in this figure may be downloaded from the following website: http://www.ualberta.ca/ ~ aprochaz/hpage.html.

and can be used and altered with great ease (see Fig. 5 and http://www.ualberta.ca/~aprochaz/hpage.html.). Other control systems approaches to the peripheral control of movement, including finite state control, fuzzy logic and neural networks (Prochazka, 1996) will all depend on core models of sensory feedback such as those described above. Douglas Stuart's vision of moving the field forward by studying neural responses in relation to normal movement is now more relevant than ever.

Acknowledgements

This work was supported by the Canadian Medical Research Council, Neuroscience Canada Foundation, Alberta Paraplegic Foundation and Alberta Heritage Foundation for Medical Research.

References

Chen, W.J. and Poppele, R.E. (1978) Small-signal analysis of response of mammalian muscle spindles with fusimotor stimulation and a comparison with large-signal properties. *J. Neurophysiol.*, 41: 15–27.

Crago, P.E. Houk, J.C. and Rymer, W.Z. (1982) Sampling of total muscle force by tendon organs. *J. Neurophysiol.*, 47: 1069–1083.

Elek, J., Prochazka, A., Hulliger, M. and Vincent, J. (1990) In-series compliance of gastrocnemius muscle in cat step cycle: do spindles signal origin-to-insertion length? *J. Physiol.*, 429: 237–258.

Evarts, E.V. (1964) Temporal patterns of discharge of pyramidal tract neurons during sleep and waking in the monkey. *J. Neurophysiol.*, 27: 152–171.

Fowler, E.G., Gregor, R.J., Hodgson, J.A. and Roy, R.R. (1993) Relationship between ankle muscle and joint kinetics during the stance phase of locomotion in the cat, *J. Biomech.*, 26: 465–483.

Gandevia SC. Wilson LR. Inglis JT. Burke D. (1997) Mental rehearsal of motor tasks recruits α-motoneurones but fails to recruit human fusimotor neurones selectively. *J. Physiol.*, 505: 259–66.

Goslow, G.E. Reinking, R.M. and Stuart, D.G. (1973a) The cat step cycle: hind limb joint angles and muscle lengths during unrestrained locomotion. *J. Morphol.*, 141: 1–42.

Goslow, G.E. Stauffer, E.K. Nemeth, W.C. and Stuart, D.G. (1973b) The cat step cycle: responses of muscle spindles and tendon organs to passive stretch within the locomotor range. *Brain Res.*, 60: 35–54.

Griffiths, R.I. (1991) Shortening of muscle fibres during stretch of the active cat medial gastrocnemius muscle: The role of tendon compliance. *J. Physiol.*, 436: 219–236.

Hagbarth, K.-E. and Vallbo, A.B. (1967) Afferent response to mechanical stimulation of muscle receptors in man. *Acta. Soc. Med. Upsalien*, 72: 102–104.

Hasan, Z. (1983) A model of spindle afferent response to muscle stretch. *J. Neurophysiol.*, 49: 989–1006.

Herzog, W., Leonard, T.R. and Guimaraes, A.C. (1993) Forces in gastrocnemius, soleus, and plantaris tendons of the freely moving cat. *J. Biomech.*, 26: 945–953.

Hoffer, J.A. Caputi, A.A. Pose, I.E. and Griffiths, R.I. (1989) Roles of muscle activity and load on the relationship between muscle spindle length and whole muscle length in the freely walking cat. In: J.H.J. Allum and M. Hulliger (Eds), *Afferent Control of Posture and Locomotion, Progress in Brain Res.* Vol. 80, Elsevier, New York, pp. 75–85.

Houk, J.C. Rymer, W.Z. and Crago, P.E. (1981) Dependence of dynamic response of spindle receptors on muscle length and velocity. *J. Neurophysiol.*, 46: 143–166.

Houk, J.C. and Simon, W. (1967) Responses of Golgi tendon organs to forces applied to muscle tendon. *J. Neurophysiol.*, 30: 1466–1481.

Jacks, A., Prochazka, A. and Trend, P.St.J. (1988) Instability in human forearm movements studied with feedback-controlled electrical stimulation of muscles. *J. Physiol.*, 402: 443–461.

Jami, L. (1992) Golgi tendon organs in mammalian skeletal muscle: functional properties and central actions. *Physiol. Rev.*, 72: 623–666.

Jasper, H. Ricci G.F. and Doane, B. (1958) Patterns of cortical neurone discharge during conditioned responses in monkeys. In: G. Wolstenholme and C. O'Connor (Eds), *Neurological Basis of Behavior*, Boston: Little Brown.

Kakuda, N. and Nagaoka, M. (1998) Dynamic responses of human spindle afferents to stretch during voluntary contractions. *J. Physiol.*, 513: 621–628.

Kakuda, N., Vallbo A.B. and Wessberg J. (1996) Fusimotor and skeletomotor activities are increased with precision finger movement in man. *J. Physiol.*, 492: 921–929.

Loeb, G.E., Bak, M.J. and Duysens, J. (1977) Long-term unit recording from somatosensory neurons in the spinal ganglia of the freely walking cat. *Science*, 197: 1192–1194.

Loeb, G.E. and Duysens, J. (1979) Activity patterns in individual hindlimb primary and secondary muscle spindle afferents during normal movements in unrestrained cats. *J. Neurophysiol.*, 42: 420–440.

Loeb, G.E. and Hoffer, J.A. (1985) Activity of spindle afferents from cat anterior thigh muscles. II. Effects of fusimotor blockade. *J. Neurophysiol.*, 54: 565–577.

Matthews, P.B.C. and Stein, R.B. (1969) The sensitivity of muscle spindle afferents to small sinusoidal changes of length. *J. Physiol.*, 200: 723–743.

Prochazka, A. (1981) Muscle spindle function during normal movement. In: R. Porter (Ed.), *International Review Physiol.*, 25, (Neurophysiol. IV), University Park Press, Baltimore, pp. 47–90.

Prochazka, A. (1996) Proprioceptive feedback and movement regulation. In: L. Rowell and T. Sheperd (Eds), *Handbook of Physiology. Section 12. Exercise: Regulation and Integration of Multiple Systems*, American Physiological Society, New York, pp. 89–127.

Prochazka, A., Gillard, D. and Bennett, D.J. (1997) Implications of positive force feedback in the control of movement. *J. Neurophysiol.*, 77: 3237–3251.

Prochazka, A and Gorassini, M. (1998a) Ensemble firing of muscle afferents recorded during normal locomotion in cats. *J. Physiol.*, 507: 277–291.

Prochazka, A and Gorassini, M. (1998b) Models of ensemble firing of muscle afferents recorded during normal locomotion in cats. *J. Physiol.*, 507: 293–304.

Prochazka, A. and Hulliger, M. (1998) The continuing debate about CNS control of proprioception *J. Physiol.*, 513.2: 315.

Prochazka, A., Westerman, R.A. and Ziccone, S. (1976) Discharges of single hindlimb afferents in the freely moving cat. *J. Neurophysiol.*, 39: 1090–1104.

Proske, U. (1981) The Golgi tendon organ: properties of the receptor and reflex action of impulses arising from tendon organs. In: R. Porter (Ed.), *International Review Physiol.*, 25, (Neurophysiol. IV), University Park Press, Baltimore, pp. 127–171.

Rasmussen, S., Chan, A.K. and Goslow, G.E. (1978) The cat step cycle: electromyographic patterns for hindlimb muscles during posture and unrestrained locomotion. *J. Morphol.*, 155: 253–270.

Walmsley, B. Hodgson, J.A. and Burke, R.E. (1978) Forces produced by medial gastrocnemius and soleus muscles during locomotion in freely moving cats. *J. Neurophysiol.*, 41: 1203–1216.

Wetzel, M.C. and Stuart, D.G. (1976) Ensemble characteristics of cat locomotion and its neural control. *Prog. Neurobiol.*, 7: 1–98.

Winter, D.A. (1987) *The Biomechanics and Motor Control of Human Gait*. University of Waterloo Press, Waterloo Canada, p. 72.

M.D. Binder (Ed.)
Progress in Brain Research, Vol 123
© 1999 Elsevier Science BV. All rights reserved.

CHAPTER 12

Movement detection thresholds at the human elbow joint

U. Proske,* A.K. Wise and J.E. Gregory

Department of Physiology, Monash University, Clayton, Victoria 3168, Australia

Introduction

When we close our eyes, we are able to touch the tip of our nose with remarkable accuracy. The sense which we rely on to achieve such an accomplishment is the kinaesthetic sense, the sense of position and movement of our limbs. Speculations about the neural basis of the kinaesthetic sense have been ongoing since the last century (Goldscheider, 1889). Views have changed remarkably over the years as the debate has raged over the importance of one or other sensory receptor type which might provide the relevant signal. It is interesting to look back and read about the case put for joint receptors and the arguments used to discount a contribution from muscle receptors (Mountcastle and Powell, 1959). The third class of receptor considered was receptors in skin adjacent to the joint. The present-day view is that all three play a role. The evidence suggests that skin and joint receptors are especially important at distal joints while muscle receptors play a more prominent role at proximal joints (Horch et al., 1975). Presumably for a particular task the central nervous system can extract the information it requires from the responses of each kind of afferent. It emphasises a feature commonly encountered in central sensory processing, that of multiple, parallel inputs with overlapping information content providing the necessary background and 'textural' information to generate the sensation.

*Corresponding author. Tel.: 61 3 9905 2526; Fax: 61 3 9905 2531; e-mail: uwe.proske@med.monash.edu.au

The importance of muscle receptors in kinaesthesia has been demonstrated by experiments in which vibration of a muscle produces illusions of position and movement of a joint (Goodwin et al., 1972). Since in a passive muscle only the primary endings of spindles are vibration sensitive, they must be primarily responsible for the illusions. In fact we know rather little about the role of spindle secondary endings in kinaesthesia.

It might have been thought that the debate about the role of muscle receptors in kinaesthesia would have subsided following the reports by Goodwin et al. Yet the arguments continue (for a review see Gandevia, 1995). Only very recently it was reported that knowledge about a spatial location acquired by the left arm, and indicated by the right arm, was disturbed by elbow joint anaesthesia but not by vibration of forearm flexor and extensor muscles. It led the authors to conclude "that in this test, joint afferent input is more important than spindle input in target localisation" (Amassian et al., 1998).

Work in our laboratory has been concerned with a property of muscle called thixotropy, where the mechanical state of the passive muscle is dependent on what has happened to it beforehand, that is, on its recent history of contraction and length changes (Proske et al., 1993). More important for this discussion is the finding that the intrafusal fibres of muscle spindles show similar thixotropic properties (Morgan et al., 1984). We have taken advantage of intrafusal thixotropy to re-examine the question of the role of muscle receptors in the detection of movements at the human elbow joint (Wise et al.,

144

1996, 1998). We observed systematic changes in detection thresholds, dependent upon the form of muscle conditioning which preceded each measurement and have concluded that muscle spindles do play an important role in the kinaesthetic sense at that joint. Muscle history dependent changes in detection threshold are not expected for elbow skin and joint receptors.

Passive detection thresholds

The experiments which form the basis of our conclusions were carried out on young, healthy volunteers, after ethical approval had been given. The blindfolded subjects had their forearm held in a cushioned support which was attached to a hinged bar that could be moved by a servo-regulated motor. Subjects were asked to either flex or extend their arm, carry out a co-contraction of elbow muscles in that position and, after they had relaxed, the experimenter moved the passive arm into a position where the forearm subtended an angle of 90° at the elbow. Small, slow extension or flexion movements ($0.2° \text{ s}^{-1}$), presented in random order, were then applied by the servo-motor and subjects had to report the direction of the movements.

It was found that after conditioning of elbow muscles with the arm flexed, subjects correctly detected smaller movements in the direction of extension than in the direction of flexion (Fig. 1). Conversely, after conditioning with the arm extended, thresholds were lower in the direction of flexion. We have attributed these threshold changes to changes in stretch sensitivity of muscle spindles.

During a voluntary contraction there is co-activation of skeletomotor and fusimotor neurones (Vallbo, 1974). Therefore any pre-existing slack in the intrafusal fibres of spindles will be taken up by the resulting intrafusal contraction. If, for example, biceps is contracted with the arm held flexed, when the passive arm is moved to the 90° position, biceps spindles will remain taut and therefore sensitive to movements which stretch them (extension, see diagram Fig. 1). Movements in the direction of flexion will lead to interruption of biceps spindle activity as the muscle is shortened. If elbow muscles undergo conditioning contractions with the

arm extended, biceps will be shortened on return to the 90° test position and its spindles are likely to fall slack (diagram Fig. 1). Therefore test movements will not evoke a prompt response from biceps spindles. All of these arguments can also be applied to the spindles of elbow extensor muscles. These will only play an important role after extension conditioning. Here thresholds for movement detection will be low in the direction of

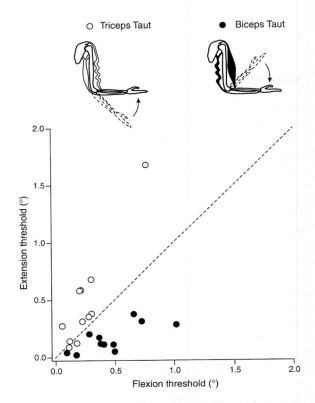

Fig. 1. A plot, for each of eleven human subjects, of movement detection thresholds at the elbow joint for movements applied in the direction of extension, versus thresholds for movements into flexion. Two forms of conditioning of elbow muscles were used, indicated by the drawings at the top of the figure. After a conditioning contraction with the arm held flexed ('biceps taut', filled symbols) when the passive arm was returned to the 90° test position detection thresholds for imposed movements at $0.2° \text{ s}^{-1}$ were lower in the direction of extension (biceps stretched). This is indicated by the fact that all filled symbols lie below the dashed line of equal thresholds. After a conditioning co-contraction with the arm held extended ('triceps taut', open symbols) thresholds were systematically lower in the direction of flexion (triceps stretched) as indicated by values lying above the line of equality.

flexion, and high in the direction of extension (Fig. 1).

In this experiment the 2 s co-contraction carried out with the arm held either flexed or extended meant that when the arm had been moved back to the test position, one of the antagonist pair would always be shortened and therefore would be expected to lie slack and not provide a kinaesthetic signal. It means that responses were coming predominantly from the taut muscle. In a second experiment we asked the question, if at the test length both antagonists are kept taut, is the central nervous system able to access, not only the increase in spindle discharge coming from the muscle undergoing stretch, but receive an additional cue from the fall in discharge in spindles of the muscle being shortened?

To put this question to the test, subjects were asked to carry out their conditioning co-contraction with the arm already in the 90° test position. It was found that under these conditions movement detection thresholds were about the same in the direction of flexion and extension, and they were not significantly lower than thresholds measured under conditions where spindles of only one of the antagonist pair was providing the kinaesthetic signal (Fig. 2). The result suggested that the muscle being lengthened provided the main signal.

Active detection thresholds

In a third experiment, movement detection thresholds were measured, not in the passive arm, but while elbow muscles were actively contracting at 15–20% of their maximum. It was found that under these conditions detection thresholds were significantly higher than for the passive arm (Fig. 2). Given that during a voluntary contraction there is co-activation of skeletomotor and fusimotor neurones, this result suggests that the fusimotor-evoked afferent discharge, produced in addition to the stretch-evoked activity, did not lead to an improvement of subjects' ability to detect small, slow movements at the elbow joint. In fact it reduced their ability to detect such movements. There are a number of possible explanations for this result. One is that there are central mechanisms operating during a voluntary contraction which lead to a

reduction of perception of muscle afferent signals (see Collins et al., 1998). A quite different explanation would be that the fusimotor activity during the contraction reduces spindle stretch sensitivity and therefore raises movement detection thresholds.

Responses of cat spindles

In a series of experiments on the soleus muscle of the anaesthetised cat we have examined the effect of fusimotor stimulation on spindle stretch

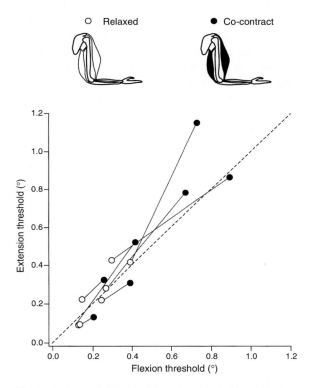

Fig. 2. A plot, as in Fig. 1 of detection thresholds at the elbow joint, for each of seven subjects, for movements in the direction of extension against thresholds in the direction of flexion. Here, however, the form of muscle conditioning was different. Subjects were asked to carry out a conditioning co-contraction of elbow muscles at the test angle (90°) and then to relax ('relaxed', open symbols) or to continue to maintain a contraction at 15–20% of maximum ('co-contract', filled symbols) while the test movements were applied to the elbow. Active and passive thresholds for each subject are joined by a line showing that active thresholds were invariably higher. All values lie scattered about the dashed line of equal thresholds indicating that there was no significant difference in thresholds measured in the directions of flexion and extension.

146

responses (Wise et al.,1999). The muscle was subjected to test stretches which had been scaled in size and speed to correspond approximately to the movements we had applied to the human forearm. After a conditioning contraction of the muscle at the test length, at fusimotor strength, responses of single primary endings of soleus muscle spindles to stretch of the passive muscle were compared with stretch responses during stimulation of single, identified fusimotor fibres. It was found that during stimulation of either kind of fusimotor fibre, static or dynamic, stretch responses were smaller than passive stretch responses (Fig. 3). This reduced stretch sensitivity therefore represents one explanation for the rise in movement detection threshold observed at the human elbow joint during a voluntary contraction.

It might be asked, why did dynamic fusimotor stimulation lower stretch responses, given that the definition of a dynamic action is to raise the response of the spindle above its passive value during the length change? The answer lies in the size and speed of the test stretches used in this study. It is known from the responses of spindles to sinusoidal movements that at low stretch frequencies responses during dynamic fusimotor stimulation are below the passive value (Goodwin et al., 1975). The explanation for the phenomenon probably resides in the high resting stiffness to small movements of passive muscle.

Conclusions

To conclude, our experiments have shown three things. First, there are systematic changes in movement detection thresholds, observable at the human elbow joint, which cannot be assigned to signals from skin or joint receptors and which must therefore be attributed to muscle spindles in elbow muscles. Only muscle spindles show changes in sensitivity dependent on contraction history. So while joint receptors at this joint may be important in the laying down of memories of spatial locations of the limb (Amassian, 1998), they do not play a major role in determining detection levels when the passive limb is moved.

Secondly, we have shown that when only one of a pair of antagonist muscles generates proprioceptive signals, movement detection thresholds are no higher than when the two antagonists are in a mechanically identical state and are therefore both potentially able to generate signals. Movements which stretched one muscle and increased its spindles' output would be accompanied by decreases in spindle output from the antagonist. It appears from our results that the additional cue available to the central nervous system of a decrease in spindle discharge, does not lead to a further lowering of movement detection thresholds.

Thirdly, we have observed significant rises in movement detection thresholds when they are measured while elbow muscles are actively contracting. One explanation for this result is that the fusimotor activity accompanying the extrafusal contraction lowers spindle stretch sensitivity. It still remains to be shown that the principal mechanism for the rise in detection threshold does not have a central origin. In any case, our findings suggest that

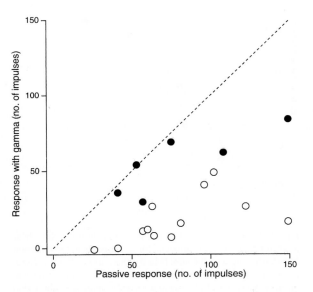

Fig. 3. Responses of muscle spindles of the soleus muscle of the anaesthetised cat to stretch of the muscle (100 μm at 20 μms^{-1}) during stimulation of single, identified static fusimotor fibres (open symbols) or dynamic fusimotor fibres (filled symbols), plotted against passive stretch responses. Each response was scored as the total impulse count during a stretch. It can be seen that all values lie on or below the dashed line of equal responsiveness, indicating that passive responses were invariably larger than during fusimotor stimulation.

there is a peripheral mechanism available which can adequately explain the result.

This finding, of a rise in detection threshold during a contraction, compared to that in a passive muscle, is contrary to some earlier observations (see Gandevia et al., 1992) and the different result can probably be explained by the way in which the muscle was conditioned before each test. When considered more broadly, our result is also unexpected. It is well known that when limbs are moved passively, position sense is poor (McCloskey, 1978). In a forearm matching task, for example, subjects are much more accurate when they place their arms voluntarily than when the passive arm is positioned by the experimenter. Perhaps here there is an additional cue, that of gravity, providing positional information. In future experiments kinaesthetic performance in actively contracting muscles should be explored further. It may help to resolve the problem of the role of muscle spindles as proprioceptors, given that during active movements they are likely to be under fusimotor control. Any scheme involving reafference does not seem, at least in its simplest form, to be able to provide a satisfactory explanation.

References

Amassian, V.E., Cracco, R.Q., Maccabee, P.J., Vergara, M. and Capaday, C. (1998) Joint afferents subserve human proprioception that is interhemispherically transferred. *J. Physiol.*, 509: 162P.

Collins, D.F., Cameron, T., Gillard, D.M. and Prochazka, A. (1998) Muscular sense is attenuated when humans move. *J. Physiol.*, 508(2): 635–643.

Gandevia, S.C., McCloskey, D.I. and Burke, D. (1992) Kinaesthetic signals and muscle contraction. *Trends Neurosci.*, 15: 62–65.

Gandevia, S.C. (1995) Kinesthesia: Roles for afferent signals and motor commands. In: L.P. Rowell and J.T. Shepherd (Eds), *Handbook on Integration of Motor, Circulatory, Respiratory and Metabolic Control During Exercise*, American Physiological Society, Oxford University Press, New York, pp. 128–172.

Goldscheider, A. (1889) Untersuchungen über den Muskelsinn. *Arch. Anat. Physiol., Leipzig*, 3: 369–502.

Goodwin, G.M., McCloskey, D.I. and Matthews, P.B.C. (1972) The contribution of muscle afferents to kinaesthesia shown by vibration induced illusions of movement and by the effects of paralysing joint afferents. *Brain*, 95: 705–748.

Goodwin, G.M., Hulliger, M. and Matthews, P.B.C. (1975) The effects of fusimotor stimulation during small amplitude stretching on the frequency-response of the primary ending of the mammalian muscle spindle. *J. Physiol.*, 253: 175–206.

Horch, K.W., Clark, F.J. and Burgess, P.R. (1975) Awareness of knee joint angle under static conditions. *J. Neurophysiol.*, 38: 1436–1447.

McCloskey, D.I. (1978) Kinaesthetic sensibility. *Physiol. Rev.*, 58, 763–820.

Morgan, D.L., Prochazka, A. and Proske, U. (1984) The after-effects of stretch and fusimotor stimulation on the responses of primary endings of cat muscle spindles. *J. Physiol.*, 356: 465–477.

Mountcastle, V.B. and Powell, T.P. (1959) Central nervous mechanisms subserving position sense and kinesthesis. *Bull. Johns Hopkins Hosp.*, 105(1): 173–200.

Proske, U., Morgan, D.L. and Gregory, J.E. (1993) Thixotropy in skeletal muscle and in muscle spindles: a review. *Prog. Neurobiol.*, 41: 705–721.

Vallbo, A.B. (1974) Human muscle spindle discharge during isometric voluntary contractions. Amplitude relations between spindle frequency and torque. *Acta Physiol. Scand.*, 90: 319–336.

Wise, A.K., Gregory, J.E. and Proske, U. (1996) The effects of muscle conditioning on movement detection thresholds at the human forearm. *Brain Res.*, 735: 125–130.

Wise, A.K., Gregory, J.E. and Proske, U. (1998) Detection of movements of the human forearm during and after co-contractions of muscles acting at the elbow joint. *J. Physiol.*, 508: 325–330.

Wise, A.K., Gregory, J.E. and Proske, U. (1999) The responses of muscle spindles to small, slow movements in passive muscle and during fusimotor activity. *Brain Res.*, 821: 87–94.

M.D. Binder (Ed.)
Progress in Brain Research, Vol 123
© 1999 Elsevier Science BV. All rights reserved.

CHAPTER 13

A positive feedback circuit involving muscle spindle secondaries and gamma motoneurons in the cat

E. Jankowska[1,*] and M.H. Gladden[2]

[1] *Department of Physiology, Göteborg University, Box 432, SE 405 30 Göteborg, Sweden*
[2] *Institute of Biomedical and Life Sciences, University of Glasgow, G12 8QQ, UK*

Introduction

Many more negative than positive feedback neuronal circuits are known in the mammalian nervous system. Negative feedback is represented for example by recurrent inhibition of motoneurons via their axon collaterals and Renshaw cells, by recurrent inhibition of several other neurons, or by autogenetic inhibition of motoneurons following contractions of the muscles that they innervate. Examples of a clear-cut positive-feedback are more difficult to find; in a recent review on proprioceptive feedback and movement regulation (Prochazka, 1996) positive feedback was mentioned only once (p. 113), and in addition only in the context of force feedback.

Results and conclusions

Coupling between group II muscle afferents and γ-motoneurons

Positive feedback involving muscle spindle afferents was proposed some time ago between these afferents and γ-motoneurons which innervate the same muscle (Ellaway and Trott, 1976; Fromm and Noth, 1976; Ellaway and Trott, 1978; Noth and

*Corresponding author. Tel.: +46 (31) 77 33 508; Fax: +46 (31) 77 33 512;
e-mail: Elzbieta.Jankowska@physiol.gu.se

Thilmann, 1980; Appelberg et al., 1982, 1983; Gladden et al., 1995). The coupling should involve primarily muscle spindle secondaries, because they provide strong input to γ-motoneurons. Selectively activated group Ia afferents have, on the other hand, not been found to excite these neurons (Eccles et al., 1960; Appelberg et al., 1983), or might excite them only negligibly (Fromm and Noth, 1976; Ellaway and Trott, 1978).

An effective positive feedback would require the connection between muscle spindle afferents and γ-motoneurons to be as direct as possible, preferably to be monosynaptic. Previous studies led to the conclusion that group II afferents excite γ-motoneurons only via di-, tri- or even polysynaptic pathways because of the rather long latencies of their actions (Appelberg et al., 1983). Latencies of EPSPs and IPSPs evoked in α-motoneurons by electrical stimulation of group II afferents in muscle nerves were similarly classified as evoked polysynaptically (Laporte and Lloyd, 1952; Eccles and Lundberg, 1959). A number of subsequent observations have, however, shown that at least some synaptic actions of group II muscle afferents on α-motoneurons might be evoked disynaptically, or even monosynaptically. Both morphological and functional studies of projections of group II afferents demonstrated that some of their collaterals terminate in motor nuclei (Fu and Schomburg, 1974; Fyffe, 1979; Lundberg et al., 1987; Hongo, 1992). Using the spike triggered averaging technique several groups have revealed weak but distinct synaptic actions of single group II afferents (identified as secondary muscle spindle afferents) on α-motoneurons (Kirkwood and Sears, 1975; Stauffer et al., 1976; Munson et al., 1982). The most direct interneuronal pathways between group II muscle afferents and α-motoneurons likewise turned out to be simpler than originally thought and to include only single interneurons (Cavallari et al., 1987; Edgley and Jankowska, 1987; Lundberg et al., 1987). The latter are represented in Fig. 3 by the interneuron labelled 'interm'.

We have recently analysed the possibility that the coupling between group II afferents and γ-motoneurons is similar to that with α-motoneurons, i.e. not only via interneuronal pathways but also monosynaptic and that group II afferents – represented by the lowest projecting group II axon collateral in Fig. 3 – synapse upon them (Gladden et al., 1998). To this aim we reinvestigated latencies of excitation of lumbar γ-motoneurons following electrical stimulation of hindlimb muscle nerves and compared them to minimal latencies of disynaptically evoked excitation of other neurons by group II afferents. Responses evoked at central latencies *shorter than the minimal latencies of disynaptic actions* of these afferents on previously investigated interneurons, α-motoneurons, and ascending tract neurons (Edgley and Jankowska, 1987; Lundberg et al., 1987; J.S. Riddell and M.R. Hadian, personal communication) were considered to be compatible with monosynaptic actions, even if they were longer than the latencies of responses which are conventionally classified as evoked monosynaptically. Longer latencies of directly evoked actions of group II than of group I muscle afferents are explained by slower conduction velocities both along the stem axons of group II afferents within peripheral nerves (see e.g. Boyd and Davey, 1968; Matthews, 1972) and along their intraspinal collaterals (Fu and Schomburg, 1974; Lundberg et al., 1987).

The border lines between latencies of responses that might be evoked disynaptically, and of those that would be too short to be evoked disynaptically, were taken to be 2.2 and 2.5 ms for intracellularly recorded EPSPs (with respect to the earliest

components of group I volleys in proximal and distal nerves, respectively). For extracellularly recorded action potentials they were 2.4 and 2.7 ms. Using these borderlines, responses of about 1/3 of the 76 investigated γ-motoneurons were found to be evoked monosynaptically, or both mono- and polysynaptically. It should be stressed that the ranges of latencies of excitation of γ-motoneurons by group II afferents found in our study were similar to those reported previously (Appelberg et al., 1983), and that there is no disagreement between our and previous experimental data. The only difference is in their interpretation. Our interpretation finds an additional support in the similar distribution of minimal latencies of responses evoked by group II afferents in γ-motoneurons and in α-motoneurons of the sample of Stauffer et al. (1976) when these latencies are related to the arrival of nerve impulses in group II afferents to the spinal cord.

Positive feedback sensu stricto would require that γ-motoneurons are excited by muscle spindle afferents of the muscle that is innervated by these γ-motoneurons. However, earlier observations indicating positive feedback were made when γ-motoneurons were excited by afferents of three or four muscles stimulated together within the hamstring or triceps surae nerves (Noth and Thilmann, 1980; Appelberg et al., 1983), or following stretches of the whole triceps surae (Fromm and Noth, 1976; Ellaway and Trott, 1978), or both posterior biceps and semitendinosus (Appelberg et al., 1982). Under these conditions it was impossible to differentiate between effects of afferents from synergists and from the muscle innervated by them. We verified that γ-motoneurons are indeed excited by group II afferents of their target muscle by recording from their axons in a muscle nerve (Gladden et al., 1995) and from their somata (Gladden et al., 1998). In the latter study we found for instance that 1/3 of extracellularly recorded and 1/2 of intracellularly recorded medial gastrocnemius γ-motoneurons with group II input (a total sample of 43 neurons) were excited by medial gastrocnemius group II afferents. However, most of these and other γ-motoneurons were excited by group II afferents of not only one, but two, three or even four other muscles, showing that

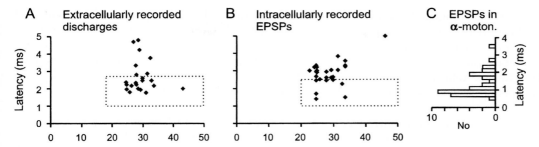

Fig. 1. The shortest latencies of responses evoked by group II afferents in γ-motoneurons of gastrocnemius, soleus, plantaris and flexor digitorum longus. A, Minimal central latencies of extracellularly recorded responses (ordinate) in neurons with different conduction velocities (abscissa). The latencies were measured from group I afferent volleys. B, As in A but for EPSPs evoked by group II afferents in intracellularly recorded γ-motoneurons. The dotted rectangles encompass latencies that were shorter than the estimated minimal latencies of disynaptically evoked responses (see text). C, For comparison, histogram of latencies of EPSPs evoked in α-motoneurons following nerve impulses in single group II afferents of triceps surae recorded close to their entry to the spinal cord, re-plotted from Fig. 1 of Stauffer et al. (1976) using 0.2 ms bins. Zero latency in C corresponds to 0.9 ms on the ordinates in A and B to account for the 0.9 ms later arrival of incoming volleys in triceps surae group II afferents relative to group I afferents. Note that the majority of latencies of EPSPs evoked in α-motoneurons overlapped with latencies of EPSPs classified as evoked monosynaptically in γ-motoneurons. Modified from Fig. 3 in Gladden et al., 1998.

positive feedback from a homonymous muscle would be considerably enhanced by group II input from other muscles. Such an enhancement does not need to be interpreted in terms of either diffuse or non-specific actions of group II afferents because marked differences have been found in the patterns of origin of group II input to γ-motoneurons belonging to different muscles, as illustrated in Fig. 2. Because of these differences, the effectiveness of positive feedback via γ motoneurons innervating various muscles may be linked to the length of other muscles in different combinations, providing a mechanism for co-ordination between these muscles.

Receptor origin of the direct group II input to γ-motoneurons

Results of experiments in which natural stimuli (muscle stretches and vibration) were used to excite γ-motoneurons indicate that secondaries are the main source of origin of muscle spindle input to these neurons, but cannot define the coupling between them. More synchronous activation of muscle afferents by electrical stimuli provides a much better opportunity for defining the latency of their synaptic actions and thereby the kind of coupling (as discussed in the preceding section). It allows however only a facultative identification of

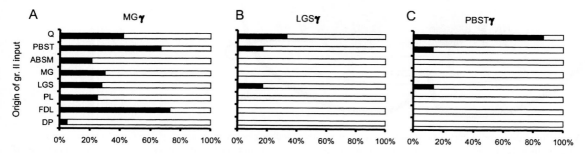

Fig. 2. Muscles of origin of group II afferents providing input to different populations of γ-motoneurons. Percentages of 43 medial gastrocnemius (MG), 6 lateral gastrocnemius – soleus (LGS) and 15 posterior biceps – semitendinosus (PBST) extracellularly recorded γ-motoneurons (abscissa) responding to stimulation of group II afferents from the nerves indicated on the ordinate are shown in A, B and C. Black and white, percentages of activated and non-activated γ-motoneurons respectively. Modified from Fig. 6 in (Gladden et al., 1998).

the receptor origin of the stimulated afferents. We will therefore indicate here three main arguments for our proposal that monosynaptically evoked excitation of γ-motoneurons by electrically stimulated group II afferents reflects direct contacts between muscle spindle secondaries and γ-motoneurons.

First, the minimal latencies of disynaptically evoked synaptic actions of electrically stimulated group II afferents were calculated for the actions of the fastest conducting group II afferents, and non-spindle group II afferents would be likely to conduct at slower conduction velocities (Boyd and Davey, 1968). Secondly, the properties of single group II afferents shown to project to motor nuclei (Fu and Schomburg, 1974; Fyffe, 1979; Lundberg et al., 1987; Hongo, 1992) and/or to have direct synaptic actions on α-motoneurons (Kirkwood and Sears, 1975; Stauffer et al., 1976; Munson et al., 1982) fulfilled criteria for muscle spindle secondaries. Thirdly, the effects of the fastest and lowest threshold electrically stimulated group II afferents were reproduced by muscle stretches on both γ-

motoneurons (Ellaway and Trott, 1976; Fromm and Noth, 1976; Ellaway and Trott, 1978; Appelberg et al., 1982; Gladden et al., 1995) and other neurons. Some of these effects were also reproduced following activation of muscle spindles via γ-motoneurons (Harrison et al., 1988).

Neuronal network in which positive feedback between muscle spindle secondaries and γ-motoneurons is utilised and in which its operation is modulated

Figure 3 summarises the main elements of this network. It shows that muscle spindle afferents may affect γ-motoneurons through 2 parallel pathways: both directly and via intermediate zone interneurons (labelled 'interm') that are activated by their other collaterals (Edgley and Jankowska, 1987). There are strong indications that of a number of interneuronal populations with input from group II muscle afferents, only those in the intermediate zone project to motor nuclei (Edgley and Jankowska, 1987; Bras et al., 1989; Jankowska

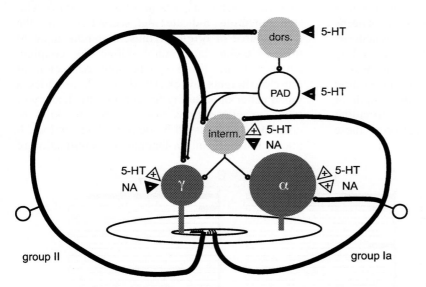

Fig. 3. A simplified diagram of connections in the circuit of positive feedback between group II afferents and γ-motoneurons. The circles represent different populations of spinal neurons (dark grey, γ- and α-motoneurons innervating muscle spindles and extrafusal muscle fibers respectively; light grey, two first order interneurons in pathways from group II afferents, in the intermediate zone (interm.) and in the dorsal horn (dors.); white, a last order interneuron mediating primary afferent depolaristion (PAD). Thick lines represent secondary and primary muscle spindle afferents and their intraspinal collaterals. Thin lines represent axons of the interneurons. Small circles indicate terminals of the afferents and excitatory interneurons. Triangles represent sites of release of 5-HT and NA; their excitatory and inhibitory actions are indicated by + and − . For further explanation see text.

et al., 1993). Interneurons mediating di- or tri-synaptic excitation of γ-motoneurons should thus be among them. The proposal that the same interneurons synapse on γ- as on α-motoneurons is more hypothetical. It is based on observations that a high proportion of intermediate zone interneurons projecting to motor nuclei had synaptic actions on α motoneurons (Cavallari et al., 1987). It is therefore more likely that the same rather than separate interneurons provide excitatory input to α- and γ-motoneurons. Another sub-population of intermediate zone interneurons (not shown in the diagram) might be considered to mediate post-synaptic inhibition of both α- and γ-motoneurons from group II afferents. Two other populations of interneurons would be involved in mediating pre-synaptic inhibition of transmission from group II afferents to their various target neurons. There are indications that both the first order excitatory interneurons (labelled 'dors.') and the last order interneurons (labelled 'PAD') of these latter populations are located in the dorsal horn (Edgley and Jankowska, 1987; Bras et al., 1989; Jankowska et al., 1993; Jankowska and Riddell, 1995).

The operation of this neuronal network will, as in the case of any other networks, depend on the excitability of its constituent neurons, in this case both γ-motoneurons and all of the involved inter-neurons. The excitability of these neurons will in turn depend on the excitatory and inhibitory input to them from a number of sources. Of these, only two modulatory neuronal systems that may play a particular role are indicated in Fig 3, those of the descending noradrenergic and serotoninergic neurons.

Noradrenaline (NA) strongly depresses synaptic actions of group II afferents on γ-motoneurons (Jankowska et al., 1998) and on the intermediate zone interneurons (Bras et al., 1990) which provide input to them. NA releasing neurons should thus effectively depress the positive feedback from group II afferents to any γ-motoneurons. Morpho-logical studies also indicate that NA releasing axons have close contacts with both γ-motoneurons (Sahal et al., 1998) and intermediate zone inter-neurons (Maxwell et al., 1997).

Serotonin turned out to have opposite effects – to enhance activity of γ-motoneurons (Ellaway and

Trott, 1975; Jankowska et al., 1998) as well as of the intermediate zone interneurons (E. Jankowska, I. Hammar Simonsberg, B. Chojnicka and Ch Heden, in preparation). This facilitatory effect might be strengthened by depression of activity of dorsal horn interneurons (Bras et al., 1990) which mediate presynaptic inhibition of transmission from group II afferents (those labelled 'dors.' and 'PAD' in Fig. 3). 5-HT releasing neurons should thus effectively enhance the positive feedback from group II afferents to γ-motoneurons. Again, mor-phological studies indicate that serotoninergic fibers have a considerable number of contacts with γ-motoneurons (Sahal et al., 1998) as well as with intermediate zone (Maxwell et al., 1997) and dorsal horn (Jankowska et al., 1997) interneurons.

Changes in the balance between the opposite effects of NA and 5-HT releasing neurons on γ-motoneurons may be used to adjust the effectiveness of positive feedback to these neurons to the needs of different movements. These mod-ulatory actions will therefore supplement effects of any other neuronal systems that select optimal fusimotor sets (Prochazka et al., 1985; Hulliger et al., 1989). Potent changes in the patterns of fusimotor drive following systemic application of precursors of NA and 5-HT indicate however, that some of these other neuronal systems are also affected by NA and 5-HT. For example, the NA precursor L-DOPA differently modifies tonic dis-charges of static and dynamic γ-motoneurons, and those innervating flexor and extensor muscles in non-anesthetised decerebrated animals (see e.g. Grillner et al., 1967).

The effectiveness of positive feedback between muscle spindle secondaries and γ-motoneurons

Positive feedback between group II muscle spindle secondaries and γ-motoneurons involves feedback from and to γ-motoneurons as well as from and to muscle spindles. Discharges of γ-motoneurons enhance muscle spindle output, which in turn should enhance their own discharges. Similarly, nerve impulses in muscle spindle afferents should enhance activity of γ-motoneurons, which in turn would increase the frequency of their responses and/or lower the threshold of these responses. On the basis of previous studies it is well established that single γ-motoneurons may modify muscle spindle output in a very potent way, while nerve impulses in single afferents have only marginal effects on any neurons. Both facets of the positive feedback between muscle spindle afferents and γ-motoneurons will therefore depend primarily on how effectively group II afferents excite γ-motoneurons.

In some movements activation of γ-motoneurons during muscle contraction is strong enough to prevent effects of unloading of muscle spindles, e.g. during voluntary movements in the man (Vallbo, 1971) or during locomotion in the cat (Bessou et al., 1989). In other cases activity of γ-motoneurons is apparently too weak to prevent a drop in the frequency of discharges of muscle spindle afferents during contraction (see Prochazka, 1996). However, even in the latter cases positive feedback may assist in adding excitatory input to γ-motoneurons by any nerve impulses in muscle spindle secondaries that *are* induced during muscle contractions, and thus counteract the effects of unloading of muscle spindles.

Under experimental conditions, the strength of group II input to γ-motoneurons may appear to be low, because effective activation of γ-motoneurons often requires near maximal activation of group II afferents by electrical stimuli. Intracellular records show also that the peak amplitudes of EPSPs evoked by these afferents are not very high (Eccles et al., 1960; Appelberg et al., 1983). However, some interneurons in the excitatory pathways from group II afferents to γ-motoneurons will be co-excited by Ia afferents (Edgley and Jankowska, 1987) so that when several muscles are stretched synchronously, the two groups of afferents will jointly induce discharges in these interneurons; this will strengthen the excitatory input to γ-motoneurons. Furthermore, effects of either direct or indirect actions of group II afferents on γ-motoneurons will always be superimposed on the effects of other sources of input to these neurons which are suppressed by anesthesia and muscle denervation. In non-anesthetised decerebrate preparations (Bessou et al., 1984) and in anesthetised preparations (Gladden et al., 1995) in which denervation was kept to a minimum, muscle stretches have indeed been found to be much more effective in activating γ-motoneurons, and in turn the spindle afferents.

Even if synaptic actions of group II afferents on γ-motoneurons are not very strong, their attenuation by noradrenergic neurons is apparently needed to prevent an excessive activation of α-motoneurons by either group Ia, or group II afferents. An excessive activation of α-motoneurons following spinal or central injuries that result in exaggerated stretch reflexes and spasticity, is effectively counteracted by the NA agonists clonidine and tizanidine, or the NA precursor L-DOPA. Since NA does not depress the synaptic actions of group Ia afferents, it has been proposed that failure in the attenuation of activation of spinal interneuronal pathways by group II muscle afferents by damage of the axons of noradrenaline releasing neurons may be one of the reasons for the exaggerated stretch reflex (Eriksson et al., 1996). Recently this proposal has been extended by the suggestion that excessive activation of γ-motoneurons by group II afferents might, secondarily, lead to a pathological enhancement of reflex actions of group Ia muscle afferents as well as those of group II afferents (Jankowska et al., 1998). Stronger actions of γ-motoneurons on muscle spindles would obviously be followed by stronger responses of both primaries and secondaries.

Acknowledgments

The study was supported by grants no 05648 from the Swedish Medical Research Council to EJ and from the Wellcome Trust to MHG.

List of abbreviations

α-motoneuron	alpha motoneuron
EPSP	excitatory postsynaptic potential
γ-motoneuron	gamma motoneuron
5-HT	serotonin
L-DOPA	L–3,4, dihydroxyphenylalanine
LGS	lateral gastrocnemius – soleus
MG	medial gastrocnemius

NA	noradrenaline
PAD	primary afferent depolarization
PBST	posterior biceps – semitendinosus

References

Appelberg, B., Hulliger, M., Johansson, H. and Sojka, P. (1982) Fusimotor reflexes in triceps surae elicited by natural stimulation of muscle afferents from the cat ipsilateral hind limb. *J. Physiol. (Lond.)*, 329: 211–229.

Appelberg, B., Hulliger, M., Johansson, H. and Sojka, P. (1983) Actions on γ-motoneurones elicited by electrical stimulation of group II muscle afferent fibres in the hind limb of the cat. *J. Physiol. (Lond.)*, 335: 255–273.

Bessou, P., Dupui, P., Cabelguen, J.M., Joffroy, M., Montoya, R. and Pages, B. (1989) Discharge patterns of γ-motoneurone populations of extensor and flexor hindlimb muscles during walking in the thalamic cat. In: J.H.J. Allum and M. Hulliger (Eds), *Afferent Control of Posture and Locomotion, Progress Brain Research*. Vol. 80, Elsevier, Amsterdam, pp. 37–45.

Bessou, P., Joffroy, M., Montoya, R. and Pages, B. (1984) Effects of triceps stretch by ankle flexion on intact afferents and efferents of gastrocnemius in the decerebrate cat. *J. Physiol. (Lond.)*, 346: 73–91.

Boyd, I. and Davey, M. (1968) *Composition of Peripheral Nerves*. Livingstone: Edinburgh and London, pp. 1–57

Bras, H., Cavallari, P., Jankowska, E. and Kubin, L. (1989) Morphology of midlumbar interneurones relaying information from group II muscle afferents in the cat spinal cord. *J. Comp. Neurol.*, 290: 1–15.

Bras, H., Jankowska, E., Noga, B. and Skoog, B. (1990) Comparison of effects of various types of NA and 5-HT agonists on transmission from group II muscle afferents in the cat. *Eur. J. Neurosci.*, 2: 1029–1039.

Cavallari, P., Edgley, S.A. and Jankowska, E. (1987) Postsynaptic actions of midlumbar interneurones on motoneurones of hind-limb muscles in the cat. *J. Physiol. (Lond.)*, 389: 675–689

Eccles, J. C., Eccles, R. M., Iggo, A. and Lundberg, A. (1960) Electrophysiological studies on γ-motoneurones. *Acta Physiol. Scand.*, 50: 32–40.

Eccles, R. and Lundberg, A. (1959) Synaptic actions in motoneurones by afferents which may evoke the flexion reflex. *Arch. Ital. Biol.*, 97: 199–221.

Edgley, S.A. and Jankowska, E. (1987) An interneuronal relay for group I and II muscle afferents in the midlumbar segments of the cat spinal cord. *J. Physiol. (Lond.)*, 389: 647–674.

Ellaway, P.H. and Trott, J.R. (1975) The mode of action of 5-hydroxytryptophan in facilitating a stretch reflex in the spinal cat. *Exp. Brain Res.*, 22: 145–162.

Ellaway, P.H. and Trott, J.R. (1976) Reflex connections from muscle stretch receptors to their own fusimotor neurones. In: S. Homma (Ed.), *Understanding the Stretch Reflex*, Progress in Brain Research, Vol. 44, Amsterdam, Elsevier, pp 113–122.

Ellaway, P.H. and Trott, J.R. (1978) Autogenetic reflex action on to γ-motoneurones by stretch of triceps surae in the decerebrated cat. *J. Physiol. (Lond.)*, 276: 49–66.

Eriksson, J., Olausson, B. and Jankowska, E. (1996) Antispastic effects of L-dopa. *Exp. Brain Res.*, 111: 296–304.

Fromm, C. and Noth, J. (1976) Reflex responses of γ-motoneurones to vibration of the muscle they innervate. *J. Physiol. (Lond.)*, 256: 117–136.

Fu, T.C. and Schomburg, E.D. (1974) Electrophysiological investigation of the projection of secondary muscle spindle afferents in the cat spinal cord. *Acta Physiol. Scand.*, 91: 314–329.

Fyffe, R. (1979) The morphology of group II muscle afferent fibre collaterals. *J. Physiol. (Lond.)*, 296: 39–40P.

Gladden, M.H., Dickson, M. and Lumsdon, T. (1995) Reflex activation of γs- and γd-motoneurones observed in isolated muscle spindles of cat hindlimb muscles. In: A. Taylor, M.H. Gladden and R. Durbaba (Eds), *Alpha and Gamma Motor System*, New York, Plenum, pp. 129–136.

Gladden, M., Jankowska, E. and Czarkowska-Bauch, J. (1998) New observations on coupling between group II muscle afferents and feline γ-motoneurones. *J. Physiol. (Lond.)*, 512.2: 507–520.

Grillner, S., Hongo, T. and Lundberg, A. (1967) The effect of DOPA on the spinal cord. 7. Reflex activation of static γ-motoneurones from the flexor reflex afferents. *Acta Physiol. Scand.*, 70: 403–411.

Harrison, P.J., Jami, L. and Jankowska, E. (1988) Further evidence for synaptic actions of muscle spindle secondaries in the middle lumbar segments of the cat spinal cord. *J. Physiol. (Lond.)*, 402: 671–686.

Hongo, T. (1992) Patterns of spinal projection of muscle spindle group II fibres. In: L. Jami, E. Pierrot-Deseilligny and D. Zytnicki (Eds), *Muscle Afferents and Spinal Control of Movement*, Oxford, Pergamon Press, pp. 389–394.

Hulliger, M., Durmuller, N., Prochazka, A. and Trend, P. (1989) Flexible fusimotor control of muscle spindle feedback during a variety of natural movements. In: J.H.J. Allum and M. Hulliger (Eds), *Afferent Control of Posture and Locomotion, Progress Brain Research*. Vol. 80, Elsevier, Amsterdam, pp. 87–101.

Jankowska, E., Gladden, M.H. and Czarkowska-Bauch, J. (1998) Modulation of responses of feline γ-motoneurones by noradrenaline, tizanidine and clonidine. *J. Physiol. (Lond.)*, 512.2: 521–531.

Jankowska, E., Maxwell, D.J., Dolk, S. and Dahlstrom, A. (1997) A confocal and electron microscopic study of contacts between 5-HT fibres and feline dorsal horn interneurons in pathways from muscle afferents. *J. Comp. Neurol.*, 387: 430–438.

Jankowska, E. and Riddell, J.S. (1995) Interneurones mediating presynaptic inhibition of group II muscle afferents in the cat spinal cord. *J. Physiol. (Lond.)*, 483: 461–471.

156

Jankowska, E., Riddell, J.S., Szabo Lackberg, Z. and Hammar, I. (1993) Morphology of interneurones in pathways from group II muscle afferents in sacral segments of the cat spinal cord. *J. Comp. Neurol.*, 337: 518–528.

Kirkwood, P.A. and Sears, T.A. (1975) Monosynaptic excitation of motoneurones from muscle spindle secondary endings of intercostal and triceps surae muscles in the cat. *J. Physiol. (Lond.)*, 245: 64p–66p.

Laporte, Y. and Lloyd, D.P.C. (1952) Nature and significance of the reflex connections established by large afferent fibres of muscles. *Am. J. Physiol.*, 169: 609–621.

Lundberg, A., Malmgren, K. and Schomburg, E.D. (1987) Reflex pathways from group II muscle afferents. 1. Distribution and linkage of reflex actions to alpha-motoneurones. *Exp. Brain Res.*, 65: 271–281.

Matthews, P. (1972) *Mammalian Muscle Spindles and Their Central Action*. Arnold, London.

Maxwell, D.J., Riddell, J.S. and Jankowska, E. (1997) A confocal microscopic analysis of contacts formed by serotoninergic and noradrenergic axons with electrophysiologically characterized spinal interneurons in the anaesthetized cat. *J. Physiol. (Lond.)*, 501P: 40–41P.

Munson, J.B., Sypert, G.W., Zengel, J.E., Lofton, S.A. and Fleshman, J.W. (1982) Monosynaptic projections of individual spindle group II afferents to type-identified medial gastrocnemius motoneurons in the cat. *J. Neurophysiol.*, 48: 1164–1174.

Noth, J. and Thilmann, A. (1980) Autogenetic excitation of extensor γ-motoneurones by group II muscle afferents in the cat. *Neurosci. Lett.*, 17: 23–26.

Prochazka, A. (1996) Proprioceptive feedback and movement regulation. In: L.B. Rowell and J.T. Shepard (Eds), *Exercise: Regulation and Integration of Multiple Systems*, American Physiological Society, New York, pp. 89–127.

Prochazka, A., Hulliger, M., Zangger, P. and Appenteng, K. (1985) 'Fusimotor set': new evidence for alpha-independent control of γ-motoneurones during movement in the awake cat. *Brain Res.*, 339: 136–140.

Sahal, A., Maxwell, D.J., Jankowska, E. and Gladden, M.H. (1998) Relationships between noradrenaline and serotonin-immunoreactive axons and γ-motoneurones. *J. Physiol. (Lond.)*, 509P: 172P.

Stauffer, E.K., Watt, D.G., Taylor, A., Reinking, R.M. and Stuart, D.G. (1976) Analysis of muscle receptor connections by spike-triggered averaging. 2. Spindle group II afferents. *J. Neurophysiol.*, 39: 1393–1402.

Vallbo, A.B. (1971) Muscle spindle response at the onset of isometric voluntary contractions in man. Time difference between fusimotor and skeletomotor effects. *J. Physiol. (Lond.)*, 218: 405–431.

M.D. Binder (Ed.)
Progress in Brain Research, Vol 123
© 1999 Elsevier Science BV. All rights reserved.

CHAPTER 14

Neurotrophin–3 and maintenance of muscle afferent function

John B. Munson[1], Richard D. Johnson[1,2] and Lorne M. Mendell[3,*]

[1] *Department of Neuroscience, University of Florida, Gainesville, FL 32610, USA*
[2] *Department of Physiological Sciences, University of Florida, Gainesville, FL 32610, USA*
[3] *Department of Neurobiology and Behavior, State University of New York at Stony Brook, Stony Brook, NY 11794, USA*

Introduction

It has long been known that axotomizing peripheral cutaneous and muscle nerves and thus depriving them of contact with their peripheral targets results in slowed conduction of their action potentials (e.g. Kiraly and Krnjevic, 1959). Furthermore, reinnervation of their peripheral targets results in recovery of conduction velocity (e.g. Collins et al., 1986). These results suggest the sufficiency of the normal peripheral target for maintenance of at least this one measure of normal physiological function (conduction velocity), and further suggest the presence of some substance(s) in the target tissue that is capable of acting in a supportive trophic manner on the innervating afferent fibers.

Groups I and II muscle afferents of cats uniformly exhibit several physiological properties: they are rapidly conducting (24–120 m/s), have mechanosensitive receptive fields in muscle, are slowly adapting in response to a maintained stimulus, and are stretch-sensitive (Collins et al., 1986), and generate monosynaptic EPSPs in homonymous and heteronymous spinal motoneurons (Eccles 1964). In the experiments summarized here we have investigated: (a) whether maintenance of these various other physiological properties of

peripheral sensory nerves also depends upon target innervation, and (b) whether the reinnervation by afferents of *foreign* as well as *native* target tissue is sufficient for maintenance of these properties.

The neurotrophin NT–3 along with its high affinity receptor trkC has been shown to be essential for aspects of normal development during the prenatal period (reviewed in Mendell, 1995, and Lindsay, 1996). In particular, group I muscle afferents and their receptors (muscle spindles and tendon organs) are absent in NT–3-deficient newborns (Ernfors et al., 1994). Interestingly, the trkC receptor and its NT–3 ligand continue to be expressed in both muscle and skin during adult life (Copray and Brouwer, 1994; McMahon et al., 1994; McMahon and Priestley, 1995). We speculated that a role for NT–3 in the adult might be to maintain the normal physiological properties of muscle stretch receptor afferent fibers. Thus we also tested (c) whether provision of exogenous NT–3 to cut peripheral muscle nerves can substitute for NT–3-containing biological tissue in this regard.

Methods

In this chapter we summarize experiments in adult female cats in which the medial gastrocnemius (MG) muscle nerve was axotomized and capped for varying periods (Johnson and Munson, 1991); or axotomized and either capped or directed into its native or a foreign tissue for 6–30 months (e.g. the

*Corresponding author. Tel: (516) 632-8616; Fax: (516) 632-5723; e-mail: lmendell@notes.cc.sunysb.edu

muscle nerve regrown into muscle or into skin, respectively: Mendell et al., 1995), or axotomized and provided with NT–3 applied chronically to the cut end of the nerve for five weeks (Munson et al., 1997a). In terminal acute experiments using pentobarbital anesthesia the sensitivity of individual afferents was then tested in response to mechanical stimulation of the periphery (details in Johnson et al., 1995), and EPSPs were generated in response to electrical stimulation of the treated afferents (Mendell et al., 1995).

Results

A. Conduction velocity (Fig. 1A)

The mean conduction velocity (CV) for tested normal groups I and II muscle afferents was 66 ± 2 m/s (SEM) ($n = 325$). After 6 d axotomy and capping with a blind Gore-Tex sleeve, mean CV dropped only to 64 ± 3 m/s ($n = 75$); it then declined progressively to 44 ± 1 m/s ($n = 251$) and 27 ± 1 m/s ($n = 208$) following axotomy of 3 mo and 7 mo respectively. Immediate reunion to the MG nerve (regeneration into muscle: CV $= 67 \pm 2$ m/s, $n = 69$) or the sural nerve (regeneration into skin: CV $= 68 \pm 2$ m/s, $n = 87$)) fully restored CV to normal values. Five weeks' treatment with NT–3 also sustained normal CV (67 ± 2 m/s, $n = 100$) which instead declined to 59 ± 2 m/s ($n = 100$) if treated with vehicle for five weeks.

B. Mechanosensitive receptive fields of muscle afferents (Fig. 1B)

'Receptive field' refers to the location in the periphery where an adequate physiological stimulus activates a particular sensory neuron. Receptive fields for normal muscle afferents are located within muscle, where they may be localized by exploration with a blunt probe (Collins et al., 1986). All or virtually all normal large MG afferents are activated by mechanical manipulation of the MG muscle (Collins et al., 1986). In experiments in which the MG nerve was axotomized for six days and capped with a blind Gore-Tex sleeve, about half the tested afferents were excited by gently probing the sleeve (Johnson

et al., 1991). This fraction declined to about one-fourth at 3 mo and one-eighth at 7 mo.

When the MG nerve was cut and self-reunited, about three-fourths of the afferents had mechanosensitive receptive fields in the muscle after 3 to 9 months (Collins et al., 1986). It is likely that most or all of those afferents not having receptive fields in the muscle had failed to regenerate through the neuroma and into the muscle, and that most that had regenerated into the muscle could be activated by probing the muscle.

Interestingly, when the MG nerve was directed into the sural nerve for up to 30 mo, essentially all of the 'muscle' afferents were excited by gently probing the area of skin normally innervated by the sural nerve (Johnson et al., 1995). Thus muscle afferents, most of which would have become insensitive to mechanical stimulation had they remained axotomized for that period, retained or recovered their mechanosensitivity by making functional contact with skin.

Lastly we have axotomized the MG nerve and provided the neurotrophin NT–3 continuously to the cut end for up to five weeks. While fewer than half of MG afferents were excitable if simply axotomized for six days, 60–70% were excitable (had receptive fields) if axotomized and NT–3-treated for five weeks. We are unable to explain why fewer afferents were excitable following six days axotomy than following five weeks axotomy with vehicle.

In summary, these experiments have shown that muscle afferents are normally activated by mechanical stimulation of the host muscle, that this property is rapidly lost over a few days to months if the afferents are deprived of their normal target by axotomy, and that regeneration into either muscle or skin retains or restores this ability. Furthermore, directly applied NT–3 is also capable of sustaining mechanosensitivity in axotomized afferents, suggesting that NT–3 obtained from skin or muscle may perform a similar role in the other normal or experimental cases.

C. Slow adaptation property of muscle afferents (Fig. 1C)

Virtually all large normal muscle afferents can be identified as innervating either muscle spindles or tendon organs (Collins et al., 1986) and are considered slowly adapting; i.e. the afferents discharge continuously in response to a maintained stimulus. Ninety percent of muscle afferents retain this property following six days' axotomy, but by 3 mo only 1 in 3 and by 7 mo only 1 in 5 axotomized mechanosensitive muscle afferents is still slowly adapting, giving rather only a brief burst of action

potentials in response to sustained steady probing of the blind Gore-Tex sleeve.

Following axotomy and immediate reunion with muscle or cutaneous nerves, virtually all mechanosensitive afferents which regenerated into muscle or skin retained their slowly adapting capability. This is particularly interesting with regard to regeneration into skin because only about 25% of

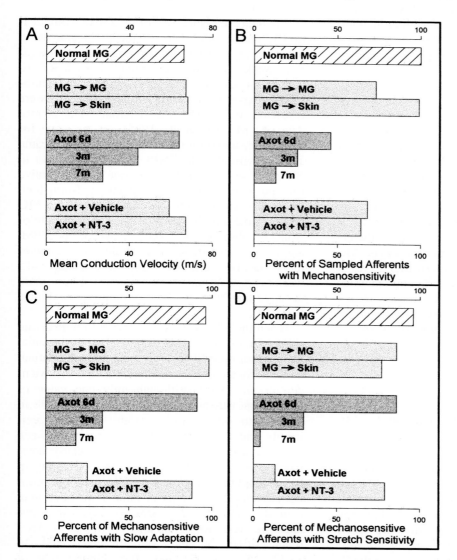

Fig. 1. Properties of large muscle afferents in cats. MG nerve was transected and coapted with the MG (MG→MG) or distal portion of axotomized caudal cutaneous sural nerve (MG→skin) for 6–30 mos. Axotomized afferents were transected and capped with a blind Gore-Tex sleeve for periods as stated. Axotomized nerves treated with either vehicle or NT–3 were transected and provided with the named substance by osmotic pump for 5 weeks.

cutaneous afferents are normally slowly adapting, the rest being rapidly adapting (Burgess et al., 1968). Thus regeneration into skin does not respecify the adaptive property of muscle afferents, suggesting that rapid or slow adaptation is an inherent property of the afferent fiber, not determined by its peripheral innervation. Provision of NT–3 (but not vehicle) to axotomized afferents also sustained the slowly-adapting ability of most muscle afferents, again consistent with an hypothesis of NT–3 being the target-derived substance critical for maintaining this property in normal animals.

D. Stretch-sensitivity (Fig. 1D)

The adequate stimulus for normal spindle and tendon organ afferents is stretch of the receptor within the muscle. Six days following axotomy of the MG nerve, 86% of the mechanosensitive afferents were activated by gentle stretch of the enclosing Gore-Tex sleeve (Johnson and Munson, 1991). This declines to 30% at 3 mo and to 4% at 7 mo. If the axotomized MG nerve is immediately redirected back into the distal portion of the MG nerve or into the sural nerve, 86% (if MG nerve) or 77% (if sural nerve) of the afferents may be activated by stretch of the MG muscle or the innervated skin territory, respectively. And as in the tests above, the stretch-sensitive property of 86% of axotomized muscle afferents was retained by NT–3 treatment.

E. Excitatory postsynaptic potentials

We have investigated EPSPs produced by MG group Ia afferents in intact LGS motoneurons after axotomy of the MG nerve, or after it was allowed to reinnervate muscle or skin, or after provision of NT–3 to the axotomized nerve in order to assess recovery of their central synaptic function. Two forms of stimulation were employed: low frequency stimulation (0.5 Hz) to measure EPSP amplitude, and high frequency stimulation (32 shocks at 167 Hz delivered every 2 s with the 32 EPSPs being averaged in register, 1, 2, 3, . . . , 32) to measure the modulation of EPSP amplitude. Modulation is defined as $100[\{(EPSP_{30} + EPSP_{31})/$

$2\}/\{EPSP_1\}-1]\%$ and is > 0 if the mean of $EPSP_{30}$ and $EPSP_{31}$ is larger than $EPSP_1$ and is < 0 if the later EPSPs in the burst are smaller in amplitude than the initial EPSP. In control preparations there are substantial data both with composite and with single fiber EPSPs that small EPSPs tend to facilitate during the burst whereas large ones tend to depress (Collins et al., 1984, 1988; Mendell et al., 1995).

The data are displayed in Fig. 2. One complication is that for the data for the peripheral nerve regeneration experiments (Fig. 2A) a period of 5–15 weeks' axotomy was used (1 cat each at 5, 10 and 15 weeks after axotomy) whereas the neurotrophin experiments displayed here (Fig. 2B) were restricted to 5 weeks after axotomy. The control data (▲: Mendell et al., 1995) are the same for both. After axotomy (■) EPSP amplitude became smaller (virtually all EPSPs < 2 mV in contrast to controls) and modulation became more negative (no positive values of modulation from high frequency stimulation of the axotomized MG nerve). Note that this correlation is the opposite of what is observed in controls where as EPSP amplitude becomes smaller, modulation becomes more positive (▲). After axotomy lasting 5–15 weeks (Fig. 2A) modulation is substantially more negative than after 5 weeks axotomy plus vehicle (Fig. 2B).

When the MG nerve was allowed to reinnervate skin (+) or muscle (○) there was substantial recovery of both EPSP amplitude and modulation, particularly after reinnervation of the muscle (Mendell et al., 1995). Although only one value of modulation was > 0, many values were $> -40\%$ in contrast to values after axotomy that were uniformly more negative. This difference between axotomy and reinnervation was particularly noteworthy for small EPSPs where the variability in EPSP amplitude modulation is normally greatest. For EPSPs < 2 mV the mean value of modulation in controls was $+7 \pm 32\%$ (SD) ($n = 24$). After axotomy it fell to $-63 \pm 14\%$ ($n = 32$). After reinnervation of the skin it recovered to $-34 \pm 16\%$ ($n = 17$) and after reinnervation of muscle, to $-16 \pm 27\%$ ($n = 19$). The negative correlation between EPSP amplitude modulation and EPSP amplitude recovered towards normal.

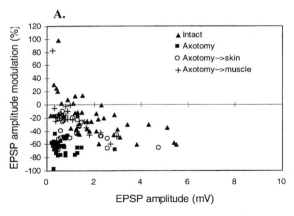
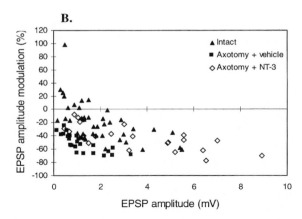

Fig. 2. Modulation of amplitude of EPSPs during high-frequency burst (167 Hz) (ordinate) as a function of EPSP amplitude at low frequency (0.5 Hz) (abscissa). EPSPs were generated in intact LGS motoneurons by intact or experimental MG afferents. Data from intact cats are same for both plots (Mendell et al., 1995). A. Many small EPSPs generated by intact group Ia afferents show positive modulation during burst. Low frequency EPSP amplitude is reduced by afferent axotomy but is partially restored by regeneration into either muscle or skin. Modulation becomes more negative following axotomy and is partially restored by regeneration into skin, and even more so by regeneration into muscle. B. Similarly, EPSP amplitude is reduced and modulation is made more negative during 5 wks treatment of axotomized group Ia afferents with vehicle. Similar treatment with NT–3 greatly enlarges EPSPs and partially restores EPSP modulation to less negative values.

Five weeks' treatment of the axotomized afferents with vehicle resulted in EPSPs of reduced size, all of which exhibited negative modulation (Figure 2B). After five weeks' NT–3 treatment ($\diamond$) EPSP amplitudes were *larger* than in normal controls (note the presence of EPSP amplitudes >6 mV and none <0.4mV, in contrast to normal controls) (Munson et al., 1997a; Mendell et al., 1999). Values of EPSP amplitude modulation for EPSPs <2 mV recovered only modestly, from $-47 \pm 12\%$ ($n=21$) after vehicle treatment, to $-29 \pm 15\%$ ($n=10$) after NT–3 treatment. All experimental EPSPs exhibited negative values of EPSP amplitude modulation, whether vehicle- or NT–3-treated.

We conclude that both reinnervation of the periphery and provision of NT–3 to axotomized Ia afferent fibers result in some recovery of central synaptic function. At a qualitative level reinnervation of the muscle led to values of EPSP amplitude and EPSP amplitude modulation that were the most similar to what was observed in controls. Reinnervation of the skin was the next most effective treatment in promoting recovery to normal values. Treatment with NT–3 led to exaggeration of EPSP amplitude well above normal values, and to

modulation values that were somewhat more negative than those observed after reinnervation of the periphery. This might have been anticipated for the very largest EPSPs (Mendell et al., 1995). However, even when the analysis was confined to small EPSPs (<2 mV), the values of EPSP amplitude modulation remained more negative than after reinnervation of the periphery, particularly the muscle.

We carried out spike-triggered-averaging experiments (Mendell and Henneman, 1971) on NT–3-treated axotomized MG afferents in order to investigate the mechanism of the increase in EPSP amplitude (Mendell et al., 1999). Part of the explanation is the increased projection frequency of the ~60 individual MG group Ia afferents: whereas in normal animals each MG afferent projects to (i.e. generates EPSPs in) about 60% of LGS motoneurons, that projection was raised to about 85% following NT–3 treatment. We believe that the 'single-fiber' EPSPs generated by each individual afferent are also larger in amplitude following NT–3 treatment; however we were unable to test this rigorously because the discharge rates of the triggering afferents were very high, thereby reducing the amplitude of the elicited EPSPs in comparison with those generated at lower rates in the normal control experiments.

Discussion

The neurotrophins are known to serve essential roles in the differentiation and survival of neurons during development. These substances and their receptors continue to be expressed postnatally, however, suggesting that they then serve some different role after these first functions are complete. Our experiments in adult cats may provide a partial answer to the question of the roles of the neurotrophins in adult animals.

We have shown that the various mechanosensitive properties of large muscle afferents as well as their ability to generate EPSPs are lost if the afferents are deprived of contact with their normal target tissue because of peripheral axotomy. These abilities are instead sustained or restored if the afferents regenerate into their native target (muscle). Interestingly, regeneration of these muscle afferents into skin is similarly effective. These facts suggest the presence of some trophic substance common to both muscle and skin that is capable of supporting these functions. We have found that provision of the neurotrophin NT–3 directly to the cut end of the axotomized MG nerve can also serve these rescue functions. NT–3 is expressed in both muscle and skin in adult animals and its associated high affinity receptor trkC is expressed on spindle afferent fibers. We suggest therefore that the dependence upon target innervation by muscle afferents is in fact a dependence upon NT–3, which has an essential role in the maintenance of the normal physiological properties of the afferents (see also Munson et al., 1997b).

We believe that the action of NT–3 comes about at least in part through the retrograde transport of the protein from the periphery to the dorsal root ganglion (DRG). Subcutaneous administration of the same dose of NT–3 was without effect, only NT–3 supplied directly to the cut end of the nerve was effective. Its role in the DRG may be multiple. The slowly-adapting stretch-specific mechanosensitivity of the terminal may be dependent upon specific stretch-activated membrane channels being transported distally from the DRG. The production and/or the transport of the channels could require NT–3. Conduction velocity of the neurons is related to nerve caliber, which in turn is related to neurofilament content and transport, all of which are reduced following axotomy (Verge et al., 1990). We suggest that in the absence of NT–3, neurofilament production and/or transport by the DRG are down-regulated and fiber caliber is thus reduced. Consistent with this, Verge et al. (1990) reported that exogenous NGF restores neurofilament mRNA in the subpopulation of DRG cells with high affinity NGF receptors.

The role of NT–3 in not only rescuing but also augmenting the amplitude of EPSPs generated by NT–3-treated afferents could be achieved at least in part by similar mechanisms, for example by DRG-initiated reversal of the changes to central processes of group Ia afferents brought about by axotomy. Also to be considered is a possible *anterograde* effect of NT–3. Recent work by von Bartheld et al. (1996) showed that NT–3 injected into the eye of chick embryos was transported anterogradely to the optic tectum where it appeared postsynaptically in dendrites and cell bodies. Precisely how the NT–3 would alter synaptic function once transported to the central terminals remains to be determined. However, the fact that trkC receptors are expressed on motoneurons (Johnson et al., 1996) suggests that NT–3 from some source is involved in normal motoneuron function.

Comparison of the recovery of synaptic function from axotomized afferent fibers after peripheral reinnervation and after provision of neurotrophins normally present in the terminal fields of these afferent fibers reveals similarities and differences. Both provision of NT–3 and reinnervation of the periphery lead to enhancement of EPSP amplitude. Both result in some recovery of EPSP amplitude modulation from the extreme negative values observed for axotomized fibers. Our data do not allow a perfect comparison because the periods of axotomy were different in these cases. However, the function of the system appears to be closer to normal after peripheral reinnervation than after NT–3 administration, particularly when one restricts the analysis to small EPSPs where modulation is most variable. This is indicative of the complexity of the signaling from the periphery: NT–3 is probably only one of a complex group of peripheral molecules responsible for functional recovery of afferents and their central synapses. Whether other neurotrophins are the only molecules that are involved or whether other classes of signaling molecules are also involved is not known. Nonetheless, the group Ia afferent/motoneuron system is a good model system to examine these important questions related to trophic interactions between periphery and center.

Acknowledgements

We thank our colleague Julian Taylor who collaborated in many of these experiments. The authors' work was supported by NIH grants NS 15913 (JBM and RDJ), NS 16996 (LMM), NS 14899 (LMM) and NS 32264 (LMM). We thank Regeneron Pharmaceuticals for providing the NT–3 used in these experiments.

References

Burgess, P.R., Petit, D. and Warren, R.M. (1968) Receptor types in cat hairy skin supplied by myelinated fibers. *J. Neurophysiol.*, 31: 833–848.

Collins. W.F., III, Davis, B.M. and Mendell, L.M. (1988) Modulation of EPSP amplitude during high frequency stimulation depends on the correlation between potentiation, depression and facilitation. *Brain Res.*, 442: 161–165.

Collins,W..F, III, Honig, M.G. and Mendell, L.M. (1984) Heterogeneity of group Ia synapses on homonymous a-motoneurons as revealed by high frequency stimulation of Ia afferent fibers. *J. Neurophysiol.*, 52: 980–993.

Collins, W.F., III, Mendell, L.M. and Munson, J.B. (1986) On the specificity of sensory reinnervation of cat skeletal muscle. *J. Physiol. (Lond.)*, 375: 587–609.

Copray, J.C. and Brouwer, N. (1994) A selective expression of neurotrophin–3 messenger RNA in muscle spindles of the rat. *Neuroscience*, 63: 1125–1135.

Eccles, J.C. *The Physiology of Synapses*, Berlin, Springer. 1964.

Ernfors, P., Lee, K–F., Kucera, J. and Jaenisch, R. (1994) Lack of neurotrophin–3 leads to deficiencies in the peripheral nervous system and loss of limb proprioceptive afferents. *Cell*, 77: 503–512.

Johnson, H., Hokfelt, T. and Ulfbake, B. (1996) Decreased expression of TrkB and TrkC mRNAs in spinal motoneurons of aged rats. *Eur. J. Neurosci.*, 8: 494–499.

Johnson R.D. and Munson J.B. (1991) Regenerating sprouts of axotomized cat muscle afferents express characteristic firing patterns to mechanical stimulation. *J. Neurophysiol.*, 66: 2155–2158.

Johnson, R.D., Taylor, J.S., Mendell, L.M. and Munson, J.B. (1995) Rescue of motoneuron and muscle afferent function in cats by regeneration into skin. I. Properties of afferents. *J. Neurophysiol.*, 73: 651–661.

Kiraly, J.K. and Krnjevic, K. (1959) Some retrograde changes in function of nerves after peripheral section. *Q. J. Exp. Physiol.*, 44: 244–257.

Lindsay, R.M. (1996) Role of neurotrophins and trk receptors in the development and maintenance of sensory neurons: an overview. *Phil. Trans. R. Soc. Lond. B. Biol. Sci.*, 351: 365–373.

McMahon, S.B., Armanini, M.P., Ling, L.H. and Phillips, H.S. (1994) Expression and co-expression of trk receptors in subpopulations of adult primary sensory neurons projecting to identified peripheral targets. *Neuron*, 12: 1161–1171.

McMahon, S.B. and Priestley, J.V. (1995) Peripheral neuropathies and neurotrophic factors: animal models and clinical perspectives. *Curr. Opin. Neurobiol.*, 5: 616–624.

Mendell L.M. (1995) Neurotrophic factors and the specification of neural function. *Neuroscientist*, 1: 26–34.

Mendell, L.M. and Henneman, E. (1971) Terminals on single Ia fibers: location, density and distribution within a pool of 300 homonymous motoneurons. *J. Neurophysiol.*, 34:171–187.

Mendell, L.M., Johnson, R.D. and Munson, J.B. (1999) Neurotrophin modulation of the monosynaptic reflex after peripheral nerve transection. *J. Neurosci.*, 19: 3162–3170.

Mendell, L.M., Taylor, J.S., Johnson, R.D. and Munson, J.B. (1995) Rescue of motoneuron and muscle afferent function in cats by regeneration into skin. II. Ia-motoneuron synapse. *J. Neurophysiol.*, 73: 662–673.

Munson, J.B., Johnson, R.D. and Mendell, L.M. (1997a) NT–3 increases amplitude of EPSPs produced by axotomized group Ia afferents. *J. Neurophysiol.*, 77: 2209–2212.

Munson, J.B., Shelton, D.L. and McMahon, S.B. (1997b) Adult mammalian sensory and motor neurones: roles of endogenous neurotrophins and rescue by exogenous neurotrophins following axotomy. *J. Neurosci.*, 1997 17: 470–476.

Verge, V.M.K., Tetzlaff, W., Bisby, M.A. and Richardson, P.M. (1990) Influence of nerve growth factor on neurofilament gene expression in mature primary sensory neurons. *J. Neurosci.*, 10: 2018–2025.

von Bartheld, S., Byers, M.R., Williams, R. and Bothwell, M. (1996) Anterograde transport of neurotrophins and axodendritic transfer in the developing visual system. *Nature*, 379: 830–833.

Motor unit properties
and recruitment

M.D. Binder (Ed.)
Progress in Brain Research, Vol 123

CHAPTER 15

Revisiting the notion of 'motor unit types'

R.E. Burke

Laboratory of Neural Control, NINDS, NIH, Bethesda, MD 20892, USA

Introduction

Sherrington introduced the term 'motor unit' to embody his recognition that all skeletal muscle action is quantized by the fact that motoneurons are the only route out of the central nervous system (CNS) for somatic movement. He hypothesized that each motoneuron controls the action of a unique group of muscle fibers (now called the 'muscle unit'), so that the combination of motoneuron and its muscle unit form the irreducable output element in motor control (Liddell and Sherrington, 1925). Sherrington's student, Derek Denny-Brown, elaborated on Sherrington's notion of 'recruitment' to demonstrate that the motor units making up an anatomical muscle are brought into action, or 'recruited', in more-or-less repeatable sequences depending on their output force (Denny-Brown, 1929a; Denny-Brown and Pennybacker, 1939). These terms and the ideas that they represent are now second nature to all neuroscientists.

Marc Binder asked me to contribute a chapter about motor unit types, despite the fact that I have not worked in this field for over a decade and therefore have no new information to impart. Nevertheless, this topic is one to which Douglas Stuart and his group in Tucson made important contributions and it seems appropriate to put those contributions into context in this tribute volume. What follows is an essay that briefly reviews the history of the idea of 'motor unit types' up to 1980, including some personal observations that may be of interest to readers of this volume.

Why classify motor units?

My friend the late Elwood Henneman told me several times in conversation that he thought classifying motor units into distinct categories was probably a bad idea because, unless used with care, classifications tend to distort reality. I agreed, and still do, that taxonomies can lead to overly rigid thinking (and sometimes even lack of thinking) but they are necessary for communication, which requires that things be named; and scientific communication demands that things be named precisely, according to their attributes (e.g. Sokal, 1974). A taxonomy for motor units is actually inevitable, given the well known fact that mammalian muscles come in two colors (and flavors), 'red' and 'white,' with differences in speed of twitch contraction and resistance to fatigue (Ranvier, 1874), as well as differences in histological appearance (see Denny-Brown, 1929b). After detailed histological work and examination of whole muscle mechanical properties, Denny-Brown (1929b) discounted Grützner's (Grützner, 1884) hypothesis that some 'white' muscle could actually contain admixtures of slow and fast twitch muscle fibers, and by inference slow and fast twitch motor units. Twenty years later, Grützner's conclusion was shown to be correct by physiological methods (Gordon and Holbourne, 1949; Gordon and Phillips, 1953).

*Corresponding author. Tel.: 301-496-4306; Fax: 301-402-4836; e-mail: reburke@helix.nih.gov

How many kinds of motor units?

The early physiological studies of individual motor units in mixed muscles or cats or rats had rather disparate outcomes. Some workers reported finding two kinds, fast and slow twitch, within nominally 'fast' muscles (Gordon and Holbourne, 1949; Gordon and Phillips, 1953; Andersen and Sears, 1964; Steg, 1964). Other studies found populations of units with relatively similar twitch contraction times but wide ranges in force output (Devanandan et al., 1965; Eccles et al., 1968). Still others demonstrated a wide spectrum of properties that did not suggest distinct groupings (Bessou et al., 1963; Appelberg and Emonet-Denand, 1967). Perhaps wisely, none of these studies suggested criteria to distinguish motor unit 'types.' The impetus for typing came from the emerging field of muscle cytochemistry.

Building on early histological studies, the development of muscle histochemistry in the early 1960s suggested that there were three basic kinds of muscle fibers, called A, B and C, on the basis of increasing density of oxidative enzyme staining (Stein and Padykula, 1962). This view was soon supported by the advent of reliable histochemical methods to distinguish three different species of myosins (e.g. Guth and Samaha, 1969; Brooke and Kaiser, 1970; Dubowitz and Brooke, 1973), which led to the type I, IIA, and IIB nomenclature that is still in common use.

The pioneering studies of motor unit populations in the cat hindlimb in Elwood Henneman's laboratory were much influenced by the view that there should be three corresponding kinds of motor units because they assumed that all muscle fibers in a given motor unit should be of the same muscle fiber type. Wuerker et al. (1965) systematically studied a large sample of single motor units in the cat medial gastrocnemius (MG). They used their data from motor units in the histochemically homogeneous and clearly slow twitch cat soleus (SOL; (McPhedran et al., 1965) to try to identify similar motor units in the mixed MG. The slow twitch units (contraction times >70 ms) in MG were called 'type-B' because the SOL fibers had type B histochemistry. More fatigable units with faster contraction times (<70 ms) and larger force

outputs were called 'type-A' but they could find no group that clearly fit expectations for the 'type-C' fiber type.

Shortly thereafter, Camille Olson and Chester Swett, working in Henneman's laboratory at Harvard, looked at motor units in the cat flexor digitorum longus (FDL; (Olson and Swett, 1966)) and proposed a tentative scheme for separating three types of units based on muscle unit mechanical properties. As in the earlier work, they did not specify criteria to distinguish their unit groups but they stated that "... small, fast-contracting units are distinguishable from small, slow-contracting units as well as from large, fast-contracting one." (Olson and Swett, 1966, p. 496) In a later study in the cat MG (Olson and Swett, 1969), these authors introduced somewhat more specific criteria to distinguish three motor unit types, mainly having to do with post-tetanic repetitive activity.

Two kinds of motor units?

My own interest in motor units arose mainly because I was excited about testing the predictions of Henneman's 'size principle' hypothesis (Henneman and Olson, 1965; Henneman et al., 1965) that was published shortly after I arrived at NIH. In early work using intracellular recording I had been struck by the wide range in composite group Ia EPSP amplitudes in different triceps surae motoneurons. Henneman's hypothesis predicted that such variations in synaptic strength should be systematically linked to variations in size-related motoneuron properties like input resistance, as well as to the kind of muscle fiber innervated by individual cells. Devanandan and coworkers (Devanandan et al., 1965) had already shown that it was feasible to study single motor units using intracellular recording and stimulation. It therefore seemed clear that the intracellular approach was the best way to examine many of the 'size principle' predictions.

In my first study of this issue, muscle units in the medial gastrocnemius (MG) of the cat appeared to fall into two groups, one with relatively long twitch contractions times (≥ 40 ms) and uniformly small force output ('type S') and another with faster contraction times (<30 ms) and a remarkably wide range in output forces ('type F'). In contrast, units in the soleus muscle (SOL) were uniformly slow twitch (i.e. all 'type S'), with force outputs that were somewhat larger than those of the S units in gastrocnemius, as already noted by McPhedran and colleagues (McPhedran et al., 1965). On the motoneuron end, despite quite a lot of scatter, the input resistances of type S motoneurons were on average higher than those of type F, and the strength of group Ia EPSPs (Burke, 1968b) and the recruitability of the motor units in the stretch reflex (Burke, 1968a) generally fit the predictions of the size principle. The recruitment study also suggested that the fast twitch units with relatively small muscle unit forces (then called type F*) might be systematically different from the large-force F units (Burke, 1968a).

Back to three kinds of motor units?

The connection between cytological/histochemical characteristics and the mechanical properties of muscle fibers within a mixed muscle was entirely a matter of speculation until the appearance in 1968 of a landmark paper by Edström and Kugelberg (1968). They demonstrated that it was possible to use activity-dependent depletion of intra-fiber glycogen to identify the muscle fibers belonging to individual motor units that had been functionally characterized. Working in the rat tibialis anterior (TA), they classified fiber types according to increasing oxidative enzyme activity (succinic dehydrogenase; the same A, B, C system discussed above) and noted a corresponding increase (types A to C) in resistance to fatigue during continuous stimulation, as well as an inverse relation with twitch tension. However, they found no corresponding differences in twitch contraction times in their rather small sample (seven type A, six type B, and two type C units).

Felix Zajac, David Levine, and I had worked out a new scheme for motor unit classification in the cat triceps surae. The classification criteria that we eventually used (fatigue index and the presence or absence of 'sag' in unfused tetani) emerged only after examining a variety of mechanical motor unit properties that could be tested conveniently (Burke et al., 1971, 1973). Like everyone else, we were biased in that we were looking for properties that

would divide motor units into three categories. We were very excited by Edström and Kugelberg's paper, as was Peter Tsairis, whom we did not know at the time. Peter had come to NIH as a neuromuscular disease fellow in W.K. Engel's group and was learning how to do muscle histochemistry. He called me one afternoon to introduce himself and to ask if we might be interested in a collaboration on motor unit histochemistry. Within milliseconds the deal was sealed. The NIH Intramural Program was, and happily still is, a place where such fortuitous conjunctions can happen without formalities.

We already had a fair sample of physiologically-characterized MG motor units and had begun using an 'FF–FR–S' rubric as shorthand for three groups or units. These acronyms respectively stood for 'fast twitch, fatigable', 'fast twitch, fatigue resistant' and simply 'slow twitch' (all were resistant to fatigue). As the sample of glycogen-depleted units grew, so did our elation, because all of the units with a given physiological type had the same histochemical profile, whereas the different unit types had different profiles. Moreover, it appeared that all fibers within a given muscle unit were histochemically uniform. We wound up with a sample of 28 functionally and histochemically-defined, one unit of which we called 'unclassified' (later referred to as 'F(int)'; Burke et al., 1976) that had a histochemical profile slightly different from any of the others. The final report of this work was published in 1973 (Burke et al., 1973) without referring to histochemical type designations because at the time these were in flux. However, the fiber type profiles that we found fit exactly with the IIB, IIA, and I terminology that soon came into wide use (Dubowitz and Brooke, 1973).

Peter sat with us through long nights of searching for stable gastrocnemius motoneurons despite his full clinical schedule, often working on our material at night and on weekends because of his other duties. Without Peter's skill and enormous energy, not to mention good humor, the study could not have been carried out. It seemed useful to recount this history in some detail because the 'FF–FR–S' nomenclature has, for better or worse, now come into wide use. These terms are sometimes even dubbed 'the conventional unit types' with no indication of where they came from or what they imply, perhaps validating Elwood Henneman's worry.

Is this classification scheme useful?

To be useful, a taxonomic system should be robust and repeatable. 'Robust' means that the system encompasses data that are not themselves part of the classification criteria and does not fall apart as new information accumulates. For example, the FF–FR–S system, based purely on muscle unit mechanical properties, successfully predicted the histochemical profiles of the muscle units in the mixed gastrocnemius muscle. Not surprisingly, the same criteria applied to the red, slow cat SOL showed that all units studied were type S by our definition, although their mechanical properties differed quantitatively from those of gastrocnemius S units. Indeed, the histochemical profiles of SOL fibers and those of type S muscle units in mixed muscles like MG are clearly not identical (Burke et al., 1974; see their Plate 2), which led to the earlier problems in guessing the links between fiber type and muscle unit mechanical properties (Wuerker et al., 1965; Olson and Swett, 1966; Burke, 1967).

On the motoneuron end, the muscle unit type seemed to make sense of the spectrum of conduction velocities (Burke et al., 1973; Zengel et al., 1985; Emonet-Denand et al., 1988), afterhyperpolarization durations (Zengel et al., 1985), and input resistance and rheobase (Fleshman et al., 1981b; Zengel et al., 1985). Furthermore, the organization of synaptic inputs was also meaningfully correlated with unit type (Burke et al., 1970; Burke et al., 1976; Dum and Kennedy, 1980; Fleshman et al., 1981a; Friedman et al., 1981). However, there were overlaps between the data from adjacent type groups in all of these data sets; the mapping between motor unit type and motoneuron properties and synaptic organization were recognizable but blurred. Nevertheless, Zengel and coworkers (1985) showed that it was possible to predict muscle unit type for about 95% of cat MG motor units from the distributions of the motoneuron input resistance and rheobase.

No motor unit types?

Early attempts to replicate the FF-FR-S classification scheme using the original criteria met varying levels of success. It worked reasonably well for Proske and Waite (Proske and Waite, 1974) in cat MG, although 7/67 units showed contradictory combinations of properties. A series of important 'beta tests' were done in Doug Stuart's laboratory in Tucson. Doug began to study the properties of motor units because of his intense interest in the function of Golgi tendon organs and their activation by individual muscle units, a field to which he made major contributions. He and his colleagues found little in their early data on cat tibialis anterior (TA) motor units that suggested distinct types (Mosher et al., 1972). When John Stephens joined Doug's group in the early 1970s, they produced a series of papers about MG motor units (Stephens and Stuart, 1975a, b in which they explored a variety of inter-relations between motoneuron conduction velocity and muscle unit properties that tested whether there were consistent clusters in these data. This work was summarized (Reinking et al., 1975) in a paper entitled "The motor units of cat medial gastrocnemius: Problem of their categorization on the basis of mechanical properties." The group found a much more continuous distribution of fatigue indicies than we had, albeit using a different way of analyzing the raw data (the cumulative fatigue index). They also noted that ". . . a fast-slow categorization based on the sag test was not without its own ambiguities . . ." (Reinking et al., 1975, p. 311).

Doug and I had a number of discussions about why so many fast twitch units in Tucson cats were more resistant to fatigue than those found in Bethesda. There was much joking about Arizona cats being consitutionally tougher than animals in the effete East, but eventually we agreed that it was probably due to the fact that NIH animals were quarantined longer than those in Tucson, leading to a difference in exercise histories (see Goslow et al., 1977; McDonagh et al., 1980). It is also important to remember that tests of fatigue resistance are critically dependent on the history of muscle activation, on time scales ranging from minutes to months. Less obvious but also relevant is the fact that the sag property is also history dependent, in that it tends to disappear with incipient muscle fiber fatigue. It seems likely that such history dependence – the exact order and timing of the sequence of stimuli delivered to individual units – could be one factor that explains some of the variable results obtained in different laboratories.

Four kinds of motor units?

The tide in Tucson (if there is such a thing) began to turn a few years later when Doug, with Ted Goslow and Bill Cameron (Goslow et al., 1977), published a study of large samples of fast twitch motor units (defined by contraction times less than 45 ms) in the cat TA and extensor digitorum longus (EDL) muscles. Using their cumulative fatigue index criterion, they found that fast units in these flexor muscles ". . . can be clearly separated into FR and FF categories, in contrast to our own MG fast twitch units which illustrate a more continuous spectrum of fatigability." (Goslow et al., 1977, p. 41). Even so, there was a relatively high proportion of units (about one third of each sample) with intermediate fatigability, which they called 'FI' units. The correlation between fatigue index and peak tetanic force output was the same as predicted from earlier MG data, and they discounted their earlier view that force output is closely related to twitch/tetanus force ratios. A sigh of relief was heard in Bethesda.

The icing on this particular cake came in 1980 with the publication of two papers which replicated the FF–FR–S classification scheme for motor unit populations in other cat hindlimb muscles, along with glycogen depletion to check the mapping between fiber histochemistry and muscle unit mechanical properties. Richard Dum and Thelma Kennedy published a survey of cat TA and EDL motor units using intracellular recording and stimulation (Dum and Kennedy, 1980a). They found that the original sag and fatigue index criteria were suitable to discrimate four motor unit groups. Only about 9% of the fast twitch units were type F(int) and the sag property seemed to work as originally advertised. They also found that the histochemical profiles of glycogen-depleted type F units matched those expected from the MG results, except for one unit which had an unusual constellation of both mechanical and histochemical characteristics. Type S units were rare in their sample, as found earlier

by Golsow et al. (1977), and no type S units were glycogen-depleted. In addition, Dum and Kennedy surveyed a variety of synaptic inputs (Dum and Kennedy, 1980b) and found distributions of synaptic strength that closely matched the ones we had observed in the cat MG (Burke et al., 1976).

The second paper (McDonagh et al., 1980) came from Doug Stuart's lab and was based on Jennifer McDonagh's careful and thorough thesis work (McDonagh, 1979) that surveyed motor units in the relatively small but functionally important tibialis posterior (TP) muscle. The TP contains only about 60 motor units, of which over 40% are type S units. The fast twitch group (mostly distinguished by the sag property) were pretty well divided into FF and FR groups, with only about 8% type FI. Eleven units did not conform completely to the expectations of the original typing scheme but ten of these were classifiable by their other properties. Twelve units were glycogen-depleted and subjected to systematic histochemical fiber type analysis. Functionally identified FF, FR and S each had a distinct histochemical profile corresponding to those we had described earlier (Burke et al., 1971, 1973). None of the depleted units were type FI but a small proportion of TP muscle fibers had histochemical profiles intermediate between those characteristic of identified FF and FR muscle units, rather similar to the profile that we found in one depleted 'unclassified' unit noted above (see also McDonagh et al., 1980). A follow-up paper from the Tucson group confirmed the physiological to histochemical type mapping in considerable detail, using quantitative single fiber biochemical analysis (Hamm et al., 1988). These studies were important validations because they came from respected research groups, at least one of which began with a high level of skepticism.

Lump or split?

The motor unit populations in certain small, distal muscles like the lumbricals in cats (Kernell et al., 1975), small muscles in the human hand (Thomas et al., 1991), and in extraocular muscles (e.g. Goldberg, 1990) are not readily classified into 'types' because the distributions of their mechanical properties do not exhibit clear clusters (cf. however, Gates et al., 1991; Ridge and Rowlerson, 1996). On the other hand, there seems little doubt that the motor units that make up larger limb muscles in cats (e.g. Botterman et al., 1985; Bodine et al., 1987), rats (e.g. Kanda and Hashizume, 1992), rhesus monkeys (Scheiber et al., 1997), and even perhaps in humans (Garnett et al., 1979), can be grouped into a small number of relatively clearly-defined categories that resemble the FF, FR, and S motor units found in the cat MG. Moreover, these physiological types are relatively robust in the face of marked alterations in motor unit usage (Walsh et al., 1978; Mayer et al., 1981; Mayer et al., 1984; Pierotti et al., 1991). Most studies have also shown that the fast twitch group can be divided into fatigable and fatigue-resistant sub-categories, although as noted above there has been some question about how bimodal the distributions are. The functional differences in fatigue resistance are directly correlated with the relative activity of oxidative enzymes (Kugelberg and Lindegren, 1979; see also Hamm et al., 1988). However, it is clear that the fibers of physiologically identified FF and FR muscle units differ not only in myosin ATPase characteristics but also in myosin isozyme immunoreactivity (Gauthier et al., 1983; Unguez et al., 1993).

Whether or not there is an advantage to recognizing a third, 'intermediate' type of fast unit (the F(int) or FI type) is not so clear. If one tends to be a 'lumper' rather than a 'splitter', it is always possible to select some dividing line that will give just two subgroups irrespective of the shape of the fatigue index distribution. In the rat, muscle fibers with the type IIB myosin profile (associated with physiological type FF units in the cat) can exhibit very wide ranges in oxidative enzyme activity (Nemeth and Pette, 1981), and presumably in corresponding relative fatigue resistance. Lumping definitely has the virtue of simplicity (Botterman et al., 1985).

On the other hand, there is some evidence that 'F(int)' units may have a distinct profile of myosin isoforms (Burke et al., 1973; McDonagh et al., 1980). The case for the splitting has been strengthened by recent work on muscle fiber types in a variety of muscles and species using quantitative biochemical and cytochemical methods. For example, there appear to be four recognizable fiber types in rat muscle (Lind and Kernell, 1991). There is an expanding catalog of myosin isoforms and correlations with metabolic enzyme activities, plus evidence for interconversions under certain conditions, which argues that the biochemically-defined muscle fiber types are both more numerous and more malleable than previously believed (e.g. Nemeth and Pette, 1981; Pette and Staron, 1990; Pette and Staron, 1993). Individual muscle fibers within glycogen-depleted muscle units in self-reinnervated cat TA can show different myosin isoforms, in contrast to the homogeneity of normal units (Unguez et al., 1993). Moreover, mixtures of myosin isoforms have been reported in single, physiologically-characterized muscle units in the rat lumbrical muscles (Gates et al., 1991; Ridge and Rowlerson, 1996) and in some glycogen-depleted fast-twitch muscle units in rat MG (De Ruiter et al., 1996). The last study also found that units of physiolgical type FR had the recently described 'IIX' histochemical profile, rather than the type IIA characteristic of cats. Perhaps most disturbing of all, Barker and coworkers (Barker et al., 1992) found evidence that histochemical myosin types may change along the length of some individual fibers. The case clearly is not closed.

Summary

Like many areas of biology, the study of motor units and their types has progressed from apparent simplicity to intimations of deep complexities as information has accumulated from different muscles, species, and methodolgical approaches. In my own (not unbiased) view, the general notion of motor units 'types' has been amply validated by over two decades of work from many laboratories. From the standpoint of function, it still seems valid to think of three basic types in mammalian limb muscles. However, it is clear that the details of how these types are best recognized, and how their mechanical properties are mapped onto muscle fiber biochemistry, are still open questions. The organization of motor units clearly remains an exciting and interesting field.

References

Andersen, P. and Sears, T.A. (1964) The mechanical properties and innervation of fast and slow motor units in the intercostal muscles of the cat. *J. Physiol. (Lond.)*, 173: 114–129.

Appelberg, B. and Emonet-Denand, F. (1967) Motor units of the first superficial lumbrical muscle of the cat. *J. Neurophysiol.*, 30: 154–160.

Barker, D., Scott, J.J.A. and Stacey, M.J. (1992) A study of glycogen depletion and the fibre-type composition of cat skeletofusimotor units. *J. Physiol. (Lond.)*, 450: 565–579.

Bessou, P., Emonet-Denand, F. and Laporte, Y. (1963) Relation entre la vitesse de conduction des fibres nerveuses motrices at la tempe de contraction de leurs unites motrices. *C.R. Acad. Sci., Ser. D (Paris)*, 256: 5625–5627.

Bodine, S., Roy, R., Eldred, E. and Edgerton, V. (1987) Maximal force as a function of anatomical features of motor units in the cat tibialis anterior. *J. Neurophysiol.*, 57: 1730–1745.

Botterman, B.R., Iwamoto, G.A. and Gonyea, J. (1985) Classification of motor units in flexor carpi radialis muscle of the cat. *J. Neurophysiol.*, 54: 656–690.

Brooke, M.H. and Kaiser, K.K. (1970) Muscle fibre types: how many and what kind? *Arch. Neurol. (Chicago)*, 23: 369–379.

Burke, R.E. (1967) Motor unit types of cat triceps surae muscle. *J. Physiol. (Lond.)*, 193: 141–160.

Burke, R.E. (1968a) Firing patterns of gastrocnemius motor units in the decerebrate cat. *J. Physiol. (Lond.)*, 196: 631–645.

Burke, R.E. (1968b) Group Ia synaptic input to fast and slow twitch motor units of cat triceps surae. *J. Physiol. (Lond.)*, 196: 605–630.

Burke, R.E., Jankowska, E. and ten Bruggencate, G. (1970) A comparison of peripheral and rubrospinal synaptic input to slow and fast twitch motor units of triceps surae. *J. Physiol. (Lond.)*, 207: 709–732.

Burke, R.E., Levine, D.N., Salcman, M. and Tsairis, P. (1974) Motor units in cat soleus muscle: Physiological, histochemical and morphological characteristics. *J. Physiol. (Lond.)*, 238: 503–514.

Burke, R.E., Levine, D.N., Tsairis, P. and Zajac, F.E. (1973) Physiological types and histochemical profiles in motor units of the cat gastrocnemius. *J. Physiol. (Lond.)*, 234: 723–748.

Burke, R.E., Levine, D.N., Zajac, F.E., Tsairis, P. and Engel, W.K. (1971) Mammalian motor units: Physiological-histochemical correlation in three types in cat gastrocnemius. *Science*, 174: 709–712.

Burke, R.E., Rymer, W.Z. and Walsh, J.V. (1976) Relative strength of synaptic input from short latency pathways to motor units of defined type in cat medial gastrocnemius. *J. Neurophysiol.*, 39: 447–458.

De Ruiter, C.J., De Hann, A. and Sargeant, A.J. (1996) Fast-twitch muscle unit properties in different rat medial gastrocnemius muscle compartments. *J. Neurophysiol.*, 75: 2243–2254.

Denny-Brown, D. (1929) On the nature of postural reflexes. *Proc. Roy. Soc., Ser. B.*, 104: 252–301.

Denny-Brown, D. and Pennybacker, J.B. (1939) Fibrillation and fasciculation in voluntary muscle. *Brain*, 61: 311–334.

Denny-Brown, D.E. (1929) The histological features of striped muscle in relation to its functional activity. *Proc. Roy. Soc., Ser. B*, 104: 371–410.

Devanandan, M.S., Eccles, R.M. and Westerman, R.A. (1965) Single motor units of mammalian muscles. *J. Physiol. (Lond.)*, 178: 359–367.

Dubowitz, V. and Brooke, M.J. (1973) Muscle biopsy: a modern approach. In: *Book Muscle Biopsy: A Modern Approach*, Saunders, Philadelphia.

Dum, R.P. and Kennedy, T.T. (1980a) Physiological and histochemical characteristics of motor units in cat tibialis anterior and extensor digitorum longus muscles. *J. Neurophysiol.*, 43: 1615–1630.

Dum, R.P. and Kennedy, T.T. (1980b) Synaptic organization of defined motor-unit types in cat tibialis anterior. *J. Neurophysiol.*, 43: 1631–1644.

Eccles, R.M., Phillips, C.G. and Wu, C.-P. (1968) Motor innervation, Motor unit organization and afferent innervation of M. extensor digitorum communis of the baboon's forearm. *J. Physiol. (Lond.)*, 198: 179–192.

Edström, L. and Kugelberg, E. (1968) Histochemical composition, distribution of fibres and fatiguability of single motor units. Anterior tibial muscle of the rat. *J. Neurol. Neurosurg. Psychiat.*, 31: 424–433.

Emonet-Denand, F., Hunt, C., Petit, J. and Pollin, B. (1988) Proportion of fatigue-resistant motor units in hindlimb muscles of cat and their relation to axonal conduction velocity. *J. Physiol. (Lond.)*, 400: 135–158.

Fleshman, J.W., Munson, J.B. and Sypert, G.W. (1981a) Homonymous projection of individual group Ia-fibers to physiologically characterized medial gastrocnemius motoneurons in the cat. *J. Neurophysiol.*, 46: 1339–1348.

Fleshman, J.W., Munson, J.B., Sypert, G.W. and Friedman, W.A. (1981b) Rheobase, input resistance, and motor-unit type in medial gastrocnemius motoneurons in the cat. *J. Neurophysiol.*, 46: 1326–1338. (a).

Friedman, W.A., Sypert, G.W., Munson, J.B. and Fleshman, J.W. (1981) Recurrent inhibition in type-identified motoneurons. *J. Neurophysiol.*, 46: 1349–1359.

Garnett, R., O'Donovan, M., Stephens, J. and Taylor, A. (1979) Motor unit organization of human medial gastrocnemius. *J. Physiol. (Lond.)*, 287: 33–43.

Gates, H.J., Ridge, R.M.A.P. and Rowlerson, A. (1991) Motor units of the fourth deep lumbrical muscle of the adult rat – isometric contractions and fibre type compositions. *J. Physiol. (Lond.)*, 443: 193–215.

Gauthier, G.F., Burke, R.E., Lowey, S. and Hobbs, A.W. (1983) Myosin isozymes in normal and cross-reinnervated cat skeletal muscle fibers. *J. Cell Biol.*, 97: 756–771.

Goldberg, S.J. (1990) Mechanical properties of extraocular motor units. In: M.D. Bindeer and L.M. Mendell (Eds), *The Segmental Motor Sytem*, Oxford University Press, New York, pp. 222–238.

Gordon, G. and Holbourne, A. (1949) The mechanical activity of single motor units in reflex contraction of skeletal muscles. *J. Physiol. (Lond.)*, 110: 26–35.

Gordon, G. and Phillips, C.G. (1953) Slow and rapid components in a flexor muscle. *Quart. J. Exp. Physiol.*, 38: 35–45.

Goslow, G.E., Cameron, W.E. and Stuart, D.G. (1977) The fast twitch motor units of cat ankle felxors: Tripartite classification on the basis of fatigability. *Brain Res.*, 134: 35–46.

Grützner, P. (1884) Zur anatomie und physiologie der quergestreiften muskeln. *Recl. Zool. Suisse*, 1: 665–684.

Guth, L. and Samaha, F.J. (1969) Qualitative differences between actomyosin ATPase of slow and fast mammalian muscle. *Exp. Neurol.*, 25: 138–152.

Hamm, T.M., Nemeth, P.M., Solanki, L., Gordon, D.A., Reinking, R.M. and Stuart, D.G. (1988) Association between biochemical and physiological properties in single motor units. *Muscle and Nerve*, 11: 245–254.

Henneman, E. and Olson, C.B. (1965) Relations between structure and function in the design of skeletal muscles. *J. Neurophysiol.*, 28: 581–598.

Henneman, E., Somjen, G.G. and Carpenter, D.O. (1965) Functional signifcance of cell size in spinal motoneurons. *J. Neurophysiol.*, 28: 560–580.

Kanda, K. and Hashizume, K. (1992) Factors causing difference in force output among motor units in the rat medial gastrocnemius muscle. *J. Physiol. (Lond.)*, 448: 677–695.

Kernell, D., Ducati, A. and Sjöholm, H. (1975) Properties of motor units in the first deep lumbrical muscle of the cat's foot. *Brain Res.*, 98: 37–55.

Kugelberg, E. and Lindegren, B. (1979) Transmission and contraction fatigue of rat motor units in relation to succinate dehydrogenase activity of motor unit fibres. *J. Physiol. (Lond.)*, 288: 285–300.

Liddell, E.G.T. and Sherrington, C.S. (1925) Recruitment and some other factors of reflex inhibition. *Proc. Roy. Soc., Ser. B*, 97: 488–518.

Lind, A. and Kernell, D. (1991) Myofibrillar ATPase histochemistry of rat skeletal muscles – a two-dimensional quantitative approach. *J. Histochem. Cytochem.*, 39: 589–597.

Mayer, R.F., Burke, R.E., Toop, J., Kanda, K. and Walmsley, B. (1981) The effect of long-term immobilization on the motor unit population of the cat medial gastrocnemius muscle. *Neuroscience*, 6: 725–739.

Mayer, R.F., Burke, R.E., Toop, J., Walmsley, B. and Hodgson, J.A. (1984) The effect of spinal cord transection on motor units in cat medial gastrocnemius muscles. *Muscle and Nerve*, 7: 23–31.

McDonagh, J.C. (1979) *The Muscle Units of Cat Tibialis Posterior: Calassification Based on Unit Neuromecahncial Properties and Whole Muscle Histochemistry*. Ph.D., University of Arizona .

McDonagh, J.C., Binder, M.D., Reinking, R.M. and Stuart, D.G. (1980) Tetrapartite classification of motor units of cat tibialis anterior. *J. Neurophysiol.*, 44: 696–712.

McPhedran, A.M., Wuerker, R.B. and Henneman, E. (1965) Properties of motor units in a homogeneous red muscle (soleus) of the cat. *J. Neurophysiol.*, 28: 71–84.

Mosher, C.G., Gerlach, R.L. and Stuart, D.G. (1972) Soleus and anterior tibial motor units of the cat. *Brain Res.*, 44: 1–11.

Nemeth, P. and Pette, D. (1981) Succinate dehydrogenase activity in fibres classified by myosin ATPase in three hind limb muscles of rat. *J. Physiol. (Lond.)*, 320: 73–80.

Olson, C.B. and Swett, C.P. (1966) A functional and histochemical characterization of motor units in a heterogeneous muscle (flexor digitorum longus) of the cat. *J. Comp. Neurol*, 128: 475–498.

Olson, C.B. and Swett, C.P. (1969) Effect of prior activity on properties of different types of motor units. *J. Neurophysiol.*, 34: 1–16.

Pette, D. and Staron, R.S. (1990) Cellular and molecular diversities of mammalian skeletal muscle fibers. *Rev. Physiol. Biochem. Pharmacol.*, 116: 2–76.

Pette, D. and Staron, R.S. (1993) The molecular diversity of mammalian muscle fibers. *News in Physiol. Sci.*, 8: 153–157.

Pierotti, D.J., Roy, R.R., Bodine-Fowler, S.C., Hodgson, J.A. and Edgerton, V.R. (1991) Mechanical and morphological properties of chronically inactive cat tibialis anterior motor units. *J. Physiol. (Lond.)*, 444: 175–192.

Proske, U. and Waite, P.M.E. (1974) Properties of types of motor units in the medial gastrocnemius muscle of the cat. *Brain Res.*, 67: 89–101.

Ranvier, L. (1874) De quelques faits relatifs à l'histologie et à la physiologie des muscles striés. *Arch. Physiol. Norm. Pathol.*, 1: 5–18.

Reinking, R.M., Stephens, J.A. and Stuart, D.G. (1975) The motor units of cat medial gastrocnemius: problem of their categorisation on the basis of mechanical properties. *Exp. Brain Res.*, 23: 301–313.

Ridge, R.M.A.P. and Rowlerson, A. (1996) Motor units of juvenile rat lumbrical muscles and fibre type compositions of the glycogen-depleted component. *J. Physiol. (Lond.)*, 497: 199–210.

Scheiber, M.H., Chua, M., Petit, J. and Hunt, C.C. (1997) Tension distribution of single motor units in multitendoned muscles: comparison of a homolgous digit muscle in cats and monkeys. *J. Neurosci.*, 17: 1734–1747.

Sokal, R.R. (1974) Classification: purposes, principles, progress, prospects. *Science*, 185: 1115–1123.

Steg, G. (1964) Efferent muscle innervation and rigidity. *Acta Physiol. Scand.*, 61, Suppl. 225: 1–53.

Stein, J.M. and Padykula, H.A. (1962) Histochemical classification of individual skeletal muscle fibers of the rat. *Am. J. Anat.*, 110: 103–124.

Stephens, J.A. and Stuart, D.G. (1975a) The motor units of cat medial gastrocnemius: speed-size relations and their significance for the recruitment order of motor units. *Brain Res.*, 91: 177–195.

Stephens, J.A. and Stuart, D.G. (1975b) The motor units of cat medial gastrocnemius: twitch potentiation and twitch-tetanus ratio. *Pflügers Arch.*, 356: 359–372.

Thomas, C.K., Johansson, R.S. and Bigland-Ritchie, B. (1991) Attempts to physiologically classify human thenar motor units. *J. Neurophysiol.*, 65: 1501–1508.

Unguez, G.A., Bodine-Fowler, S., Roy, R.R., Pierotti, D.J. and Edgerton, V.R. (1993) Evidence of incomplete neural control of motor unit properties in cat tibialis anterior after self-reinnervation. *J. Physiol. (Lond.)*, 472: 103–125.

Walsh, J.V., Burke, R.E., Rymer, W.Z. and Tsairis, P. (1978) The effect of compensatory hypertrophy studied in individual motor units in the medial gastrocnemius muscle of the cat. *J. Neurophysiol.*, 41: 496–508.

Wuerker, R.B., McPhedran, A.M. and Henneman, E. (1965) Properties of motor units in a heterogeneous pale muscle (m. gastrocnemius) of the cat. *J. Neurophysiol.*, 28: 85–99.

Zengel, J.E., Reid, S.A., Sypert, G.W. and Munson, J.B. (1985) Membrane electrical properties and prediction of motor-unit type of cat medial gastrocnemius motoneurons in the cat. *J. Neurophysiol.*, 53: 1323–1344.

M.D. Binder (Ed.)
Progress in Brain Research, Vol 123

CHAPTER 16

Orderly recruitment tested across muscle boundaries

Timothy C. Cope* and Alan J. Sokoloff

Department of Physiology, 1648 Pierce Dr., Emory University, Atlanta, GA 30322, USA

Introduction

The movements and postures of limb and body segments are achieved through partial activation of multiple muscles. For example, multiple muscles are co-active during a variety of movements in the cat, e.g. treadmill locomotion, landing, paw shake, head turning (Abraham and Loeb, 1985; Thomson et al., 1994), and in the human, e.g. hand grip and elbow flexion (Buchanan et al., 1989; Maier and Hepp-Reymond, 1995). Described in another way, there are tens to hundreds of heteronymous motor units, i.e. motor units belonging to different muscles, which are recruited together during discrete motor actions. The topic discussed in this presentation is whether recruitment is orderly among heteronymous motor units that are activated together.

Orderly recruitment of motor units: only within or also across muscles?

An orderly recruitment sequence is typically observed among motor units *within* muscles. Among the articles that review the extensive study of this topic (e.g. Burke, 1981; Desmedt,1981; Henneman and Mendell, 1981; Freund, 1983; Calancie and Bawa, 1990; Binder et al., 1996), the reader is referred to the scholarly critique written by Stuart and Enoka (1983). Motor units sampled from one or another muscle are recruited sequentially and along the continua from weak to strong

twitch and tetanic forces, from high to low resistance to fatigue, and from long to short twitch contraction time. These measures of isometric contraction are all taken from the muscle-unit portion of motor units. Recruitment order can also be assessed in relation to the motoneuron portion of the motor unit. Alpha motoneurons within a motor nucleus (the collection of motoneurons supplying a single muscle) are progressively recruited from slow to fast axonal conduction velocity. Recruitment that is rank ordered by these properties is commonly referred to as recruitment in order by the size principle. Throughout this article we describe recruitment order with respect either to a muscle and its motor units or to a motor nucleus and its motoneurons or motor axons.

Orderly recruitment by the size principle for motor units within a muscle is thought to have important functional benefits. One advantage may be the minimization of fatigue; whole-muscle fatigue would be prevented or delayed when those motor units that are the first and most frequently recruited are also those which are most resistant to fatigue (see Kernell, 1992). Minimization of fatigue by this means would pertain to any set of motor units, whether from the same or different muscles. Another potential benefit of recruitment order by the size principle among motor units belonging to a single muscle is that it assists in smoothing incremental changes in muscle force during graded contractions (Henneman and Mendell, 1981). Expanding this view to the multiple muscles that produce different directions of torque about a given joint, we have argued that the sequential

*Corresponding author. Tel.: (404) 727–8901; Fax: (404) 727–2648; e-mail: cope@physio.emory.edu

recruitment of motor units from these muscles in order by the size principle would smooth the net trajectory of joint torque (Cope and Sokoloff, 1998). Thus, order among the set of motor units recruited from different muscles, if it occurs, could have functional benefits, just as it appears to among motor units recruited from the same muscle.

The possibility of recruitment order among heteronymous motor units has not escaped attention. Bawa and Calancie (1989) hypothesized "that orderly recruitment will occur in any group of motoneurons that are activated for a particular function." They suggested the possibility that motor units from different muscles acting at the human wrist might be collectively recruited in order during wrist flexion, and furthermore, that the same scheme may even apply for muscles that, despite being anatomical antagonists, act synergistically during certain movements. While the hypothesis has not been tested across muscles, Riek and Bawa (1992) demonstrate that recruitment order holds among motor units recruited during the co-contraction of different slips of a single muscle operating independent digits in the human hand. The contrasting viewpoint is expressed by Windhorst et al. (1991) in a group report from a Dahlem Workshop. Many in this group felt that the set of motor units making up a complete recruitment sequence should be restricted to a single motor nucleus, because supersets "can get immensely large and are hardly definable at all." Certainly the potential difficulty in defining large recruitment groups is not reason enough to preclude the possibility of their existence. A more substantial argument against orderly recruitment among heteronymous motor units was mounted by Stuart and Enoka (1983), who suggest that the differential recruitment of soleus and gastrocnemius muscles "refute[s] an applicability of the size principle across motor nuclei, but not within a single nucleus." However, the recruitment behavior of motor units cannot be reliably inferred from the 'recruitment' of whole muscles (see Sokoloff and Cope, 1996). There is no consensus of opinion, therefore, and no data available, to our knowledge, to resolve the issue of whether a set of motor units (motoneurons) belonging to different muscles (motor nuclei) are recruited in order by the size principle.

Naming the group of motoneurons recruited in order by the size principle

We have used the term 'ensemble' to name the group of motor units recruited in order by the size principle. An ensemble is a collection of elements, motor units in this case, that act together to produce a particular motor effect. Specific features of a movement, e.g. joint torque and speed, will depend upon the mix of physiologically distinct motor units recruited in that movement. Our term ensemble is synonymous with the term 'task group' as used by Reik and Bawa (1992). Unfortunately, 'task group' has had multiple definitions since its introduction by Loeb (1985). It is used by Chanaud et al. (1991) to describe recruitment organization of motor units restricted to a single muscle, the scheme illustrated for our Ensemble #1 (Fig. 1B). The potential confusion caused by the multiple definitions of a task group (see also Windhorst et al., 1991) explains our use of the term 'ensemble'. We also avoid the term 'motor pool', owing again to the uncertainty in its meaning that derives from inconsistent usage (see Wyman et al., 1974; Burke, 1991). Still, we acknowledge that the term 'motor pool' in the form recommended by Burke (1991), seems equivalent to our term 'ensemble'.

Motor unit ensembles

Different kinds of ensembles are conceivable on the basis of which motor units (motoneurons) combine to yield recruitment in order by the size principle. The potential ensembles described by Wyman et al. (1974) based upon data available at the time of that report, remain feasible today. These ensembles are illustrated below with reference to motoneurons that comprise two different motor nuclei and which send motor axons through two different ventral roots (Fig. 1A).

Ensemble 1 (Fig. 1B): order by the size principle among motoneurons restricted to a single motor nucleus. Among motoneuron members of single motor nuclei and among motor units making up single muscles, recruitment order by the size principle has been demonstrated many times over (see review articles cited in Introduction). Because the group of motor axons supplying individual muscles generally traverse more than one ventral root, it is likely, although unproven, that order extends across ventral roots. The occurrence of order within nuclei and possibly across roots supports the scheme in Figure 1B, but whether order by the size principle is exclusive to motoneurons within a motor nucleus is addressed for the first time to our knowledge, by our studies presented below. The formal possibility that order might be restricted to anatomically identifiable portions of muscles, e.g. neuromuscular compartments (Windhorst et al., 1989; Calancie and Bawa, 1990), is a corollary of this scheme, but is not considered further in this article.

Ensemble #2 (Fig. 1C): order by the size principle among motoneurons from different nuclei, but restricted to those with a common ventral root exit. This grouping represents order among heteronymous motoneurons, a possibility suggested to Wyman et al. (1974) by the early studies of Henneman and colleagues (1965). Those studies revealed recruitment in order by the size of action potentials, small before large, recorded extracellularly from the central cut ends of motor axons. The motor axons compared in this way were recorded from fine filaments dissected from one ventral root, and the recruitment stimuli, e.g. electrical stimulation of cutaneous nerves, were likely to have recruited motoneurons from multiple nuclei. Thus it seems reasonable that the order observed was expressed by heteronymous motoneurons traversing a single ventral root. There is

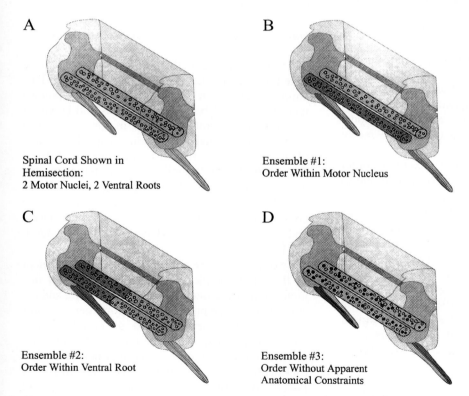

A

Spinal Cord Shown in
Hemisection:
2 Motor Nuclei, 2 Ventral Roots

B

Ensemble #1:
Order Within Motor Nucleus

C

Ensemble #2:
Order Within Ventral Root

D

Ensemble #3:
Order Without Apparent
Anatomical Constraints

Fig. 1. Three potential ensembles of motoneurons recruited in order by the size principle in relation to the model shown in (A): circles represent recruited motoneurons that are contained within one of two motor nuclei (cylinders) and that exit the spinal cord (shown in hemisection) via one of two ventral roots. For Ensembles 1, 2, 3 (B, C, D), order by the size principle occurs only among motoneurons with the same shading, either light or dark. In Ensemble #1 (B), recruitment in order by the size principle is restricted to motoneurons within a motor nucleus, but independent of motor axon ventral root exit. In Ensemble #2 (C), recruitment in order by the size principle occurs among motoneurons from different motor nuclei, but only when their axons exit the same ventral root. In Ensemble #3 (D), recruitment order by the size principle is not restricted either to a motor nucleus or ventral root.

room for doubt, however, because the identity of the motor axons was not determined, and details of the experiment permit that the orderly recruitment observed was produced predominantly by motoneurons from the same nucleus (see Cope and Sokoloff, 1998). In the absence of any other data known by us to demonstrate order among heteronymous motoneurons, this scheme receives its first definitive test in the studies described below.

Ensemble #3 (Fig. 1D): order by the size principle among motoneurons from different nuclei, irrespective of ventral root exit. This group as presented is derivative and not completely representative of the third possible recruitment grouping suggested by Wyman et al. (1974). For those authors, one recruitment group included all motoneurons activated by a particular stimulus. Our Fig. 1D is consistent with this formulation, with the explicit feature that the motoneurons in a single motor nucleus are recruited into different ensembles. While we are uncertain as to whether this depiction was intended by Wyman et al., it is supported by electrophysiological observations that synaptic sources may distribute excitation to some motoneurons and inhibition to others (see recent review by Binder et al., 1996).

Like Ensemble #2, Ensemble #3 expresses order by the size principle among heteronymous motoneurons. In distinction with Ensembles 1 and 2, order in Ensemble #3 is not bounded by any obvious anatomical limits – either nucleus or ventral root. In the absence of structural boundaries, this scheme implies a functional organization. Precedent for functionally but not anatomically distinct subsets of motor units within a muscle is reported by Hoffer et al. (1987b) for the cat sartorius muscle. Ensemble #3 suggests a similar arrangement, but across nuclei. Up to this time, there have been no data to support the existence of this group.

A prerequisite for recruitment order by the size principle

A prerequisite for Ensembles 2 and 3 (Fig. 1C, D) is that the parent muscles are at least partially recruited in the same phase of movement. In other words, there is a temporal requirement for order among heteronymous motor units, one that is met during co-contraction of different muscles. When muscles are activated out-of-phase, as they may be, for example, during alternating flexion and extension or in the sequential movement of different limb segments during reaching (e.g. Flanders et al., 1994), the motor units in these muscles cannot be recruited collectively in order by the size principle. In these cases, recruitment order by the size principle would be possible only among motor units recruited either in flexion or extension or in one phase of sequential movement. Temporal restrictions would also apply theoretically to Ensemble #1 (Fig. 1B) in cases when order by the size principle is tested among motor units from neuromuscular compartments capable of differential contraction.

Our experimental tests of motor-unit ensembles

The provisional ensembles described above were tested by us in acutely decerebrated cats. This animal preparation affords reliable and precise measurements of both the properties and behavior of individual motor units and motor axons. The relevance to normal recruitment behavior is made plain by the fact that data obtained first from decerebrate cats established the template for recruitment order by the size principle, which has since been verified in essentially all of its details in conscious humans (see Calancie and Bawa, 1990) and other animals (see Henneman and Mendell, 1981).

Two measures are needed to test for recruitment by the size principle: (1) the onset of firing of one motor unit or motoneuron relative to others, and (2) at least one of the physiological properties of motor units that is typically found to correlate with recruitment order. We obtain both measures by penetrating two α-motor axons simultaneously, one each with a single micropipette as shown in Fig. 2. Penetrations are made in ventral roots as opposed to peripheral nerves in order to prevent the damage to sensory axons that would be caused by multiple passes of the electrode tips through a muscle nerve. The identity of a penetrated axon is determined when antidromic action potentials recorded through the micropipette are initiated by electrical stimulation (bipolar electrodes in periphery not shown) of one or another of the selected muscle nerves (MG, LG, or pBF in these studies).

The recruitment sequence is determined by activating the two axons in reflexes evoked by stimulating the skin or skin afferents or by muscle stretch. Sequence is scored simply on the basis of which of the two axons begins firing first in the simultaneous records of intra-axonal voltage. Figure 2 shows a trial in which axon #1 began firing first.

Axonal conduction velocity (CV) is the motor-unit parameter compared against recruitment sequence in these studies (see below). This parameter is measured from the time and distance measured for the propagation of orthodromic action potentials initiated in the ventral root by suprathreshold current pulses injected through a micropipette and recorded extracellularly via a monopolar electrode positioned on a peripheral nerve. The evoked action potentials are discriminated in averages of 16–32 sweeps of stimulus-triggered voltage traces (see Fig. 2). The longer delay of motor axon #1 in Fig. 2 corresponds with a slower conduction velocity compared with axon #2.

In this pair-wise analysis, recruitment is judged to follow the size principle when the first axon to produce an action potential in response to a sensory stimulus (see below) also has the slower axonal conduction velocity. This pattern is illustrated in comparison of axon #1 vs. axons #2 in Fig. 2.

We have argued (Cope and Clark, 1995; Cope and Pinter, 1995) that order can be unequivocally determined only in cases in which both motor units of a pair are actually recruited in the same stimulus trial. Assessment of order when only one of the motor axons of a pair is recruited can only be made if one assumes that the inactive motor axon belongs to some fixed recruitment group; our criterion of co-activity requires no such supposition.

The relative excitability or recruitability of individual motor units can also be measured as force threshold, defined as the force of muscular contraction measured at the moment the isolated unit fires an action potential. This measure rests on the premise that the force produced by a muscle at any point in time represents the summed forces of all motor units recruited up to that moment. An isolated unit that begins to discharge when muscle force is low, therefore, has a lower threshold than a unit that begins to fire when muscle force is high. Based upon this same reasoning, we have measured force threshold, as have others (see Cope et al., 1997), in order to assess stability in the recruitment order of individual motor units over multiple recruitment trials. Wide-ranging variation in force threshold from one recruitment trial to the next might suggest, although does not prove (see Cope et al., 1997), instability in recruitment order of the isolated motor unit. Measurement of this parameter is illustrated in Fig. 3. Force threshold was measured for one MG and/or one LG motor unit in relation to the force generated by the MG and LG muscles combined. Units were recruited in reflexes generated by replicate trials of ramp-hold-release stretch of the MG and LG muscles combined. Note that we measure force threshold at the first occurrence of an action potential recorded from the motor axon in ventral roots rather than in the muscle-unit portion of a motor unit. This means the unit's force threshold is measured slightly prior to its actual contribution to muscle force, by the amount of time taken to conduct action potentials to the muscle and to initiate contraction (ca. < 10 ms). By this measure then, the isolated unit's actual force threshold is underestimated.

As mentioned above, recruitment order by the size principle can be assessed from a number of physiological properties of motor units. In our studies we find that axonal conduction velocity is at least as good a predictor of recruitment order as any of the conventional measures of motor-unit contraction (Cope and Clark, 1991). This finding corroborates a number of earlier reports that CV accurately predicted recruitment order in more than 90% of the motor-unit pairs tested (Bawa et al., 1984; Dick et al., 1987; Hoffer et al., 1987a). The use of CV to test for recruitment order by the size principle across muscles seems as valid as it was to test for order within muscles, under the conditions of our experimental paradigm. Axonal CV is easily measured (see above), and, unlike contractile properties, it can be measured with the cat paralyzed, thereby improving data yield by eliminating instability in data collection caused by the decerebrate cat's forceful movements.

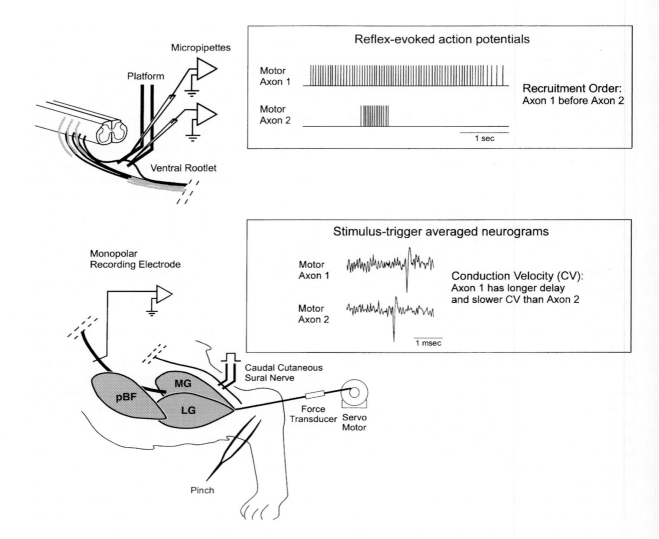

Fig. 2. Diagram of experimental setup for studying recruitment order in acutely decerebrated cats. Top: two motor axons are simultaneously penetrated, each by one of two micropipettes driven into a ventral rootlet positioned on a rigid platform. Each axon is identified by the muscle it supplies (medial gastrocnemius (MG), lateral gastrocnemius (LG), posterior biceps femoris (pBF)), when electrical stimulation of one or the other nerve (stimulating electrodes not shown) produces an antidromic action potential recorded by the micropipette. Once identified, motor axons are recruited in various reflexes. The relative onset of reflex-evoked action potentials recorded by the micropipettes establishes the recruitment sequence for the axon pair, axon #1 before #2 in this case. Vertical event markers represent the occurrence times of action potentials. Bottom: Reflexes are evoked by various stimuli presented in the hindlimb, including muscle stretch through a servomotor, cutaneous stimulation by skin pinch or electrical stimulation of the nerve, or nociceptive stimulation by penetrating the skin over the calcaneous with the tips of jeweler's forceps. When recruitment order is determined, reflex-stimulation is discontinued, and brief pulses of suprathreshold current are passed through one and then the other micropipette in order to obtain averaged records of orthodromic action potentials recorded extracellularly from a monopolar electrode positioned on a peripheral nerve. Conduction velocity for each axon is calculated from the time delay of and distance traveled by orthodromic action potentials. These data are sufficient to test for the size principle of recruitment, supported in this example by the earlier recruitment of the motor axon (#1) with the slower conduction velocity.

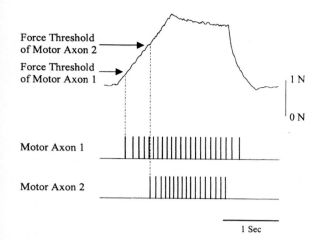

Force Threshold
of Motor Axon 2

Force Threshold
of Motor Axon 1

1 N

0 N

Motor Axon 1

Motor Axon 2

1 Sec

Fig. 3. Illustration of force threshold measurements. Top trace: force measured by force transducer during ramp-hold-release stretch of muscle applied by servo motor (see Fig. 2). Middle and bottom traces: action potentials (illustrated as vertical event markers) recruited by muscle stretch in two separate motor axons. Force threshold determined for each motor axon from the amount of force measured at the occurrence of the first reflex-evoked action potential (see dashed vertical lines).

In other studies, axonal CV is not strongly correlated with recruitment sequence under all experimental conditions or across the entire spectrum of motor units. These observations were made using electrical stimulation of muscle nerves (Zajac and Faden, 1985) or brain stem (Tansey and Botterman, 1996) at stimulation strengths and frequencies sufficiently high to recruit motor units that are typically not recruitable by the stimuli used in our studies (see Cope and Clark, 1991). Among these higher-threshold and more forceful motor units, Zajac and Faden (1985) and Tansey and Botterman (1996) report that CV is not a good predictor of recruitment order. This weakness in the relationship of recruitment sequence with CV, although apparently not pertinent to results obtained under the differing conditions of our studies, does raise the issue of the generalizability of our findings to the whole range of motor units. We cannot comment on units that are not recruited and therefore not tested. Still, our earlier study (Cope and Clark, 1991) shows that at least some of the more forceful, high-threshold motor units are recruited by muscle stretch and by skin pinch, and in order by CV. In addition, Tansey and Botterman

(1996) found that CV predicted recruitment order for all but the highest force producing motor units. These observations suggest that axonal CV is adequate for testing recruitment order over a large portion of the physiological range of motor units.

The aim of testing for the ensembles listed above required comparison of motor axons supplying different muscles. First we sought to determine whether motor units from different muscles can be recruited in order by the size principle. To answer this question we chose the medial and lateral gastrocnemius muscles (MG and LG, respectively), because these two muscles are often co-activated, as they are in natural, unrestrained locomotion (Abraham and Loeb, 1985). In decerebrate cats, these muscles are readily activated together in the stretch reflex elicited by controlled stretch, via a servomotor, of their common tendon, the Achilles tendon (Nichols, 1989). We also applied a noxious stimulation, penetration of the skin over the calcaneous with the sharp tips of fine forceps, because we found this stimulus to produce vigorous co-contractions of MG and LG muscles in decerebrate cats. Upon finding order among pairs of MG/LG motor axons (results described next), we asked whether all co-active motor units are necessarily recruited in order by the size principle. The muscle pair used in this test was identified in a separate study (Siegel et al., 1999) which demonstrated that MG muscle and the posterior biceps femoris (pBF) muscle are strongly co-activated either by pinching the dermatome of the caudal cutaneous sural nerve or by electrically stimulating the nerve.

Additional methodological detail and many of the findings described in the next section are reported by Sokoloff et al. (1999).

Can motor units from different muscles be recruited in order by the size principle?

The affirmative answer to this question is given in Fig. 4 for those pairs of motor units that exhibited no switches in order over multiple recruitment trials. The figure shows that pairs made up of heteronymous axons were recruited in order by the size principle, irrespective of whether the MG or LG axon in a pair was recruited first. This

184

recruitment pattern is essentially the same as that shown for pairs of homonymous, MG/MG, axons (unpublished data from Prather and Cope). A different depiction of these data for this sample of heteronymous axons (Fig. 1 in Sokoloff et al., 1999) shows that this recruitment pattern extended over a wide range of conduction velocity, a range having considerable overlap with that known for the whole population of MG and LG axons. From these observations we conclude that MG and LG motor axons recruited in a muscle stretch reflex comprise an ensemble, in which heteronymous axons are recruited in order by the size principle.

Because of their skeletal attachments, LG and MG muscles are commonly stretched together in the intact animal. It is possible, therefore, that in

Recruitment Order of Motor Axon Pairs During Muscle Stretch

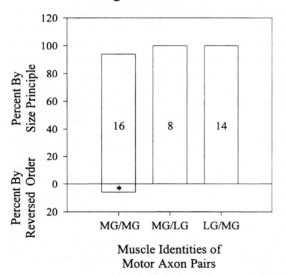

Fig. 4. Bar chart showing the percentages of motor-axon pairs recruited by muscle stretch in the order predicted by the size principle (slow before faster axonal conduction velocity) or in the reverse order. Axon pairs classified by the muscles they supply (medial or lateral gastrocnemius, MG or LG, respectively). In category labeled MG/LG, the MG axon of the pair is recruited first; in category LG/MG, the LG axon is recruited first. Numbers of pairs recruited in order or reverse order by size principle printed in bars; asterisk denotes one pair. All 22 pairs of heteronymous axons recruited in order by the size principle. Pairs exhibiting inter-trial variability in recruitment order are not included in this presentation, but are discussed in text.

intact animals and in our experiments, order depends upon coincident stretch of these two muscles. In order to assess this possibility we attempted to recruit motor units via a reflex stimulus applied outside LG and MG muscles. Success was achieved with four pairs of motor units, for which we found that, just as for muscle stretch, a noxious stimulus applied to the skin overlying the calcaneous recruited heteronymous motor axons in order by the size principle. Thus, the orderly recruitment of MG/LG motor axons does not require precise mechanical manipulation of the parent muscles. This observation parallels our finding that pairs of MG motor axons are recruited in order by the size principle whether recruited by either muscle stretch or cutaneous stimulation (Cope and Clark, 1991; Clark et al., 1993).

These findings are consistent with Ensembles 2 and 3 (Figs. 1C and D). Because motor axon pairs studied here were generally sampled from the same ventral root, our data cannot distinguish between these possible groups.

Stability in order among LG/MG axons

The combined stretch of the LG and MG muscles through their common tendon evoked reflex recruitment of each pair of motor axons in at least four and up to 60 stretch trials. Each trial was evaluated in order to assess the stability of recruitment order: were there switches in order from one trial to the next for a given pair of axons? The findings illustrated in Fig. 4 apply to the 22 pairs for which recruitment order was the same in every trial. For the 12 remaining MG/LG pairs in our sample, the sequence of recruitment switched in some trials. For 11 of these 12 pairs, a preferred order was observed, and the opposite order occurred in relatively few trials (ca. 25% or fewer). Moreover, the preferred order was according to the size principle in most of these pairs (7/11). Still, the proportion of heteronymous pairs exhibiting variability in stretch reflexes (35%) exceeds that found by us for homonymous MG/MG pairs (2/19 pairs or 11%; unpublished data, Prather and Cope).

To further explore instability in recruitment behavior of heteronymous axon pairs, we examined inter-trial variation in force threshold (see Fig. 3). The force thresholds of three different axons are plotted in Fig. 5 together with muscle force measured just before (base) and at peak contraction of MG and LG muscles combined. Measurements were taken in each of 23 consecutive trials of ramp-hold-release stretch of MG and LG muscles combined. The cases in Fig. 5 were selected to illustrate the extremes in force-threshold variation found in a sample of 9 LG and 9 MG motor axons. The MG axon shown in Fig. 5A reached action potential threshold at essentially the same level of force in repeated stretch-evoked contractions of the

MG and LG muscles combined. Force thresholds for a pair of axons are shown in Fig. 5B, with data from the LG axon exhibiting the greatest amount of variation observed in the sample of 18 axons. We have quantified inter-trial variation in terms of the coefficient of variation (force threshold standard deviation/mean). The range in coefficient of variation for the force thresholds of 9 MG and 9 LG motor axons measured against the force of MG and LG muscles combined (1.3% to 37.3%) was similar to that found by Cope et al. (1997) for 29 MG motor axons measured against the force of the MG muscle alone (2.3% to 82%). Still, the median value was somewhat greater for the heteronymous than for the homonymous pairs (19% vs. 10%).

Taken together, the tendency toward a greater proportion of axon pairs exhibiting switches in recruitment sequence and the slightly greater variation in force threshold suggest that the process of recruitment order by the size principle is somewhat less secure for heteronymous than for homonymous motor units. One source of this instability could be fluctuations in synaptic input (see Gossard et al., 1994), which may be greater across than within nuclei. Whatever the cause of instability, it does not obscure the tendency toward recruitment order by the size principle. Of relevance to this conclusion is a position which we share with other authors (e.g. Henneman and Mendell, 1981; Burke, 1991), namely that a modest amount of variation is expected in biological systems, and therefore, the variation just described seems an insufficient basis for rejecting recruitment order by the size principle.

Are motor units from different muscles necessarily recruited in order by size?

The negative answer to this question was obtained by studying pairs of MG/pBF axons recruited reflexively by electrical stimulation of the sural nerve. For these pairs of heteronymous motor axons, recruitment order by the size principle was observed no more frequently than was recruitment in the reverse order. Half of the 14 pairs that exhibited no variation in recruitment order were recruited in order by the size principle, regardless of whether the pBF or MG axon was recruited first

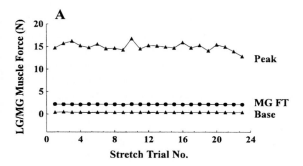
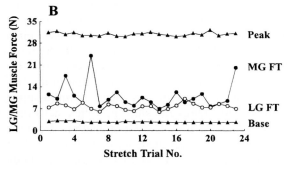

Fig. 5. Variation in motor axon force threshold. In each of two examples (A and B), peak and base force of the combined LG/MG muscles are plotted together with the force thresholds (FT) of isolated motor axons for 23 consecutive trials of LG/MG muscle stretch. Trials selected for low variation in base force and peak force. (A) Motor axon with the lowest percent coefficient of variation (1.3% = force threshold standard deviation/mean x 100). (B) Motor axon (MG) with the highest percent coefficient of variation of 37.3%. Also shown in this case is the FT of a co-active LG axon having percent coefficient of variation (13.2%) near the sample median of 19%. Despite the greater variation in FT of the MG axon, recruitment was reversed (high before low conduction velocity) in only one trial (stretch trial #17).

(Fig. 6). Ten additional pairs exhibited inter-trial variation, and six of these were recruited predominantly in order by the size principle. Over the entire sample, recruitment order by the size principle was recognizable in only 13/24 or 54% pairs of MG/pBF axons.

The apparently random recruitment order *across* muscles (motor nuclei) might have been explained by a failure of the sural cutaneous reflex to produce recruitment order by the size principle *within* either one or both of these muscles. To the contrary, our earlier studies demonstrate plainly that sural

reflexes, whether evoked by electrical stimulation (Cope and Clark, 1991) or by skin pinch (Clark et al., 1993), recruit the majority of pairs of homonymous MG/MG motor axons in order by the size principle. This finding is illustrated in Fig. 6 using previously unpublished data (Haftel, Prather, and Cope). Similarly, we have recently found (Sokoloff et al., 1999) that pairs of homonymous pBF/pBF axons also exhibit recruitment order by the size principle in the sural reflex (Fig. 6). Thus the absence of orderly recruitment across these nuclei together is not attributable to disorderly recruitment within either one separately.

Another possible explanation for disorder is that, despite obvious overlap in the reflex activation of the MG and pBF muscles, a delay in the activation of one motor nucleus relative to the other might preclude recruitment order across these nuclei. Indeed, examination of the EMG records collected by Siegel et al. (1999) revealed that sural reflex contraction begins consistently earlier (ca. 25–45 ms) in the pBF muscle than in the MG muscle. These two motor nuclei are activated by the same primary afferents, and overlap spatially in the ventral horn (Romanes, 1951). Furthermore, we estimate that only a small portion (<5 ms) of the earlier activation of pBF muscle is attributable to the shorter conduction distance from the spinal cord to the pBF muscle as compared to the more distal MG muscle. Therefore, the locus for this difference in onset of reflex contraction in the two muscles is probably to be found in intra-spinal circuits. This temporal shift in reflex activation might be sufficient to cause motoneurons from the two nuclei to be recruited out of register in their rank order by CV. However, this explanation cannot explain the observation made for three axon pairs in which the MG axon was recruited first, even though the MG's axonal CV was faster than that of the pBF axon. Thus, disorderly recruitment cannot be explained solely on the basis of the pBF muscle beginning reflex contraction before MG muscle.

The independence in recruitment order among MG and pBF motor nuclei establishes that not all co-active motoneurons are recruited in order by the size principle, even when the nuclei are recruited by the same peripheral stimulus. Although this finding is consistent with the Ensemble #1 shown

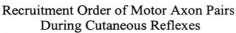

Recruitment Order of Motor Axon Pairs During Cutaneous Reflexes

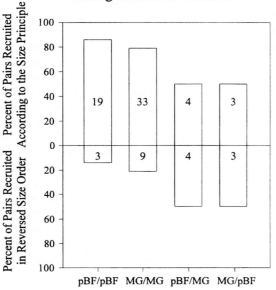

Fig. 6. Bar chart showing percentages of motor-axon pairs recruited by electrical stimulation of the caudal cutaneous sural nerve in the order predicted by the size principle (slow before faster axonal conduction velocity) or in the reverse order. Axon pairs classified by the muscles they supply (medial gastrocnemius (MG) or posterior biceps femoris (pBF)). Pairs exhibiting inter-trial variation in order (5/27 pBF pairs; 5/47 MG pairs; 10/24 heteronymous pairs) are not included. In category pBF/MG, the pBF axon of the pair is recruited first; in category MG/pBF, the MG axon is recruited first. Numbers of pairs recruited in order or reverse order by size principle printed in bars. Only half (7/14) of the pairs of heteronymous axons recruited in order by the size principle.

in Figure 1B, it does not prove that order can be restricted to single motor nuclei. The MG and pBF motor nuclei are not the only ones activated in the sural nerve reflex (e.g. Siegel et al., 1999). It remains possible, therefore, that motoneurons from the MG or the pBF nucleus are recruited in order together with motoneurons from other nuclei, peroneus longus or brevis for example. In other words, the MG and pBF motoneurons that are recruited in the sural nerve reflex might comprise portions of two different but co-active ensembles. Of particular interest to the present study would be determination of whether LG motor axons belong to an ensemble with either MG or pBF incutaneous reflexes. The former case would suggest a strong tendency toward order regardless of the synaptic input, while the latter would indicate flexibility in ensemble composition. Unfortunately, the LG muscle is not always strongly activated in the sural reflex, and therefore, has not been tested.

What establishes the limits of recruitment order?

We offer a provisional answer to this question by comparing the MG and LG muscles, for which order by the size principle was observed, against the MG and pBF muscles, for which order was not seen. One of the differences between these muscle pairs is that MG/LG share muscle-spindle feedback, while MG/pBF do not. The medial and lateral gastrocnemius muscles are each strongly excited by stretch of the other, and stimulation of group Ia afferents in the nerve supplying one muscle produces excitatory potentials in motoneurons supplying the other (see Nichols et al., 1999). By contrast, stretch of either the MG or pBF muscle does not facilitate reflex contraction of the other muscle (Nichols unpublished data), and no group I monosynaptic excitation is found across these motor nuclei (Eccles et al., 1962). The mechanism by which shared muscle-spindle feedback may form motor-unit ensembles is not established, but is suggested by the computer simulations of Heckman and Binder (1993). In these simulations supported by data collected from adult cats, the effective synaptic current injected into MG motoneurons from group Ia afferents promotes recruitment by the size principle and reduces the incidence of

disorder that can be generated by synaptic current from other sources. This same effect on MG and LG motoneurons collectively has not been tested but might apply, depending upon the distribution of effective synaptic current from MG and LG Ia afferents combined onto these motoneurons.

The importance of muscle-spindle feedback to ensemble formation requires additional tests. Further support would come from finding orderly recruitment among other muscles that share this feedback, e.g. peroneus brevis and longus or extensor digitorum longus and tibialis anterior (see Nichols et al., 1999). If recruitment order by the size principle depends exclusively upon muscle-spindle feedback, then it should not be found among any of the muscle pairs that do not share this feedback, e.g. soleus and tibialis anterior (see Nichols et al., 1999). If shared muscle-spindle feedback is critical, then we would not expect to find orderly recruitment of muscles classified as anatomical antagonists, even when they co-contract as they might to stabilize a joint. These additional tests are necessary, because MG/LG and MG/pBF muscle pairs differ in ways other than muscle-spindle feedback. For example, the pBF muscle is unique among these muscles in acting across the hip joint. Therefore, our data thus far are also consistent with the possibility that ensembles are limited to those muscles acting at the same joint. In this case, we should find orderly recruitment among co-contracting antagonists.

Our perspective on recruitment order by the size principle

The scheme illustrated in Ensemble #3 (Fig. 1D) was supported by our finding of recruitment order across the LG and MG muscles, and in its fullest exposition, describes our thinking about the functional organization of motor units. The foremost feature of Ensemble #3 is that recruitment order by the size principle can occur among motoneurons that are not confined to an anatomically defined group. This feature means that in a partially activated muscle, some motor units, even ones with the lowest intrinsic excitability, may not be selected into activity at all. Exclusion of these low-threshold units in an otherwise active muscle violates The

188

Law of Combinations (Henneman et al., 1974), which states that motor-unit thresholds are fixed and that the last motor unit recruited in a contraction must be preceded by the recruitment of all motor units in the muscle having relatively lower thresholds. This law can be discounted based on earlier findings. Kanda et al. (1977) report suppression of activity of early recruited motor units at a time when units with higher conduction velocity are recruited (but see Clark et al., 1993). Nardone et al. (1989) report that motor units in the human gastrocnemius muscle that are easily recruited during concentric contractions are not recruited in eccentric contractions. It should be noted that the latter finding has generally not been repeated in other muscles (e.g. Howell et al., 1995, and Bawa, Chapter 19, this volume) and has been challenged on the basis of technical considerations (Bawa, this volume). Finally, we have shown that some motor units in the cat soleus muscle that are recruited at low levels of force are completely inhibited during stronger reflex contraction of the whole soleus muscle (Sokoloff and Cope, 1996). All of these examples violate the Law of Combinations. However, none of these examples violates the size principle if motor units in the ensemble are not assigned a priori to fixed anatomical boundaries, e.g. a muscle. In our view, the size principle is no more violated by these examples than it is by the failure of all low-threshold motor units throughout the body to be recruited during every movement. The size principle in our formulation is simply a sequencing principle that orders the firing sequence of motor units that are selected into activity on the basis of other principles.

A scheme in which selection principles and the size principle operate in combination could yield the exclusive recruitment of, for example, type F (fast-twitch) motor units in order by the size principle. Selective recruitment of type F motor units might also be achieved by a different scheme, in which motor units are recruited in reverse order of the size principle (in Burke, 1991, see Fig. 1B, recruitment order by synaptic input from B alone). The mechanisms underlying these schemes are fundamentally different. In the former scheme, motor units are selected into activity depending upon synaptic input and are ordered predominantly

by the intrinsic excitability of their motoneurons. By contrast, activation of motor units progressively from high to low axonal conduction velocity and/or motor-unit force, i.e. recruitment in reverse order of the size principle, requires sources of synaptic drive that overcome the order that would otherwise be established by the intrinsic excitability of motoneurons. We do not favor the scheme of recruitment in reverse order of the size principle, because in contrast to the usual order for which there is abundant evidence, there is sparse evidence for functionally-relevant reversals (see Cope and Clark, 1995). Moreover, apparent cases of reversed recruitment order (e.g. Herrmann and Flanders, 1998) can be alternatively interpreted as evidence that individual motor units can be recruited into different ensembles, depending on the task (see Burke, 1991; Cope and Pinter, 1995).

A second important feature of Ensemble #3, indeed a feature of all three Ensembles shown in Fig. 1, is that co-active motor units can be broken up into multiple ensembles. This feature is verified by our finding that co-active MG and pBF motor units are independently, but not collectively recruited in order by the size principle. The basis for the formation of multiple ensembles probably reflects differential synaptic input to motoneurons. In this formulation, each ensemble shares synaptic drive that permits or promotes the recruitment order determined by intrinsic properties of motoneurons. From this viewpoint, we predict that MG and pBF motoneurons receive excitation from the sural nerve via distinct synaptic pathways. These kinds of predictions may prove useful in further study of spinal motor circuits. Another potential benefit of studying ensembles is that they might provide insight into the strategy used by the central nervous system to produce purposeful movement. It is possible, for example, that all of the motor units in a given ensemble produce similar torque trajectories, meaning that an ensemble may be selected for the torque direction it provides.

Acknowledgements

This work was supported by grants from the National Institutes of Health, R01-NS21023 and P01-HD32571. We gratefully acknowledge Mr.

Jonathan Prather for his critical review of this paper, and Dr. Sondra Siegel, Mr. Prather and Ms. Valerie Haftel for their assistance in collecting some of the data.

References

Abraham, L.D. and Loeb, G.E. (1985) The distal hindlimb musculature of the cat: Patterns of normal use. *Exp. Brain Res.*, 58: 580–593.

Bawa, P. and Calancie, B. (1989) Have studies of motor unit recruitment been too restrictive? *Behav. Brain Sci.*, 12: 647–648.

Bawa, P., Binder, M.D., Ruenzel, P. and Henneman, E. (1984) Recruitment order of motoneurons in stretch reflexes is highly correlated with their axonal conduction velocity. *J. Neurophysiol.*, 52: 410–420.

Binder, M.D., Heckman, C.J. and Powers, R.K. (1996) The physiological control of motoneuron activity. In: L.B. Rowell and J.T. Shepherd (Eds), *Handbook of Physiology Section 12: Exercise: Regulation and Integration of Multiple Systems.* American Physiological Society, Bethesda, MD, pp. 3–53.

Buchanan, T.S., Rovai, G.P. and Rymer, W.Z. (1989) Strategies for muscle activation during isometric torque generation at the human elbow. *J Neurophysiol.*, 62: 1201–1212.

Burke, R.E. (1981) Motor units: anatomy, physiology, and functional organization. In: V.B. Brooks (Ed.*), Handbook of Physiology Section 1: The Nervous System: Motor Control*, Vol. 2, part 1, American Physiological Society. Bethesda, MD , pp. 345–422.

Burke, R.E. (1991) Selective recruitment of motor units. In: D.R. Humphrey and H.-J. Freund (Eds), *Report of the Dahlem Workshop on Motor Control: Concepts and Issues*, John Wiley and Sons, Chichester, pp. 5–21.

Calancie, B. and Bawa, P. (1990) Motor unit recruitment in humans. In: M.D. Binder and L.M. Mendell (Eds), *The Segmental Motor System,* Oxford University Press, New York, pp. 75–95.

Chanaud, C.M., Pratt, C.A. and Loeb, G.E. (1991) Functionally complex muscles of the cat hindlimb: V. The roles of histochemical fiber-type regionalization and mechanical heterogeneity in different muscle activation. *Exp. Brain Res.*, 85: 300–313.

Clark, B.D., Dacko, S.M. and Cope, T.C. (1993) Cutaneous stimulation fails to alter motor unit recruitment in the decerebrate cat. *J. Neurophysiol.*, 70: 1433–1439.

Cope, T.C. and Clark, B.D. (1991) Motor unit recruitment in the decerebrate cat: several unit properties are equally good predictors of order. *J. Neurophysiol.*, 66: 1127–1138.

Cope, T.C. and Clark, B.D. (1995) Are there important exceptions to the size principle of α-motoneurone recruitment? In: A. Taylor, M.H. Gladden, and R. Durbaba (Eds), *Alpha and Gamma Motor Systems*. Plenum Press, New York, pp. 71–78.

Cope, T.C. and Pinter, M. (1995) The size principle: still working after all these years. *News in Physiol. Sci.,* 10: 280–286.

Cope, T.C. and Sokoloff, A.J. (1998) Orderly recruitment among motoneurons supplying different muscles. *J. Physiol. (Paris)*, 92: 1–5.

Cope, T.C., Sokoloff, A.J., Dacko, S.M., Huot, R. and Feingold, E. (1997) Stability of motor unit force thresholds in the decerebrate cat. *J. Neurophysiol.*, 78: 3077–3082.

Desmedt, J.E. (1981) The size principle of motoneuron recruitment in ballistic or ramp voluntary contractions in man. In: J.E. Desmedt (Ed.), *Motor Unit Types, Recruitment and Plasticity in Health and Disease. Prog. Clin. Neurphysiol.*, Vol. 9, S. Karger, Basel. pp. 97–136.

Dick, T.E., Kong, F.J. and Berger, A.J. (1987) Correlation of recruitment order with axonal conduction velocity for supraspinally driven diaphragmatic motor units. *J. Neurophysiol.*, 57: 245–259.

Eccles, J.C., Eccles, R.M., and Shealy, C.N. (1962) An investigation into the effect of degenerating primary afferent fibers on the monosynaptic innervation of motoneurons. *J. Neurophysiol.*, 25: 544–558.

Flanders, M., Pellegrini, J.J. and Soechting, J.F. (1994) Spatial/temporal characteristics of a motor pattern for reaching. *J. Neurophysiol.*, 71: 811–813.

Freund, H.J. (1983) Motor unit and muscle activity in voluntary motor control. *Physiolog. Rev.*, 63: 387–436.

Gossard, J.-P., Floeter, M.K., Kawai, Y., Burke, R.E., Chang, T. and Schiff, S.J. (1994) Fluctuations of excitability in the monosynaptic reflex pathway to lumbar motoneurons in the cat. *J. Neurophysiol.*, 72: 1227–1239.

Heckman, C.J. and Binder, M.D. (1993) Computer simulations of the effects of different synaptic input systems on motor unit recruitment. *J. Neurophysiol.*, 70: 1827–1840.

Henneman, E., Somjen, G. and Carpenter, D.O. (1965) Excitability and inhibitability of motoneurons of different sizes. *J. Neurophysiol.*, 28: 599–620.

Henneman, E. and Mendell, L. (1981) Functional organization of motoneuron pool and its inputs. In: J.M. Brookhart and V.B. Mountcastle (Eds), V.B. Brooks (Vol. Ed.), *Handbook of Physiology Section 1: The Nervous System: Motor Control*, Vol. II, pt. 1, chapt.11, American Physiological Society. Bethesda, MD, p. 423–507.

Henneman E., Clamann H.P., Gillies J.D. and Skinner, R.D. (1974) Rank order of motoneurons within a pool: law of combination. *J. Neurophysiol.*, 37: 1338–1349.

Herrmann, U. and Flanders, M. (1998) Directional tuning of single motor units. *J. Neurosci.* 18: 8402–8416.

Hoffer, J.A., Loeb, G.E., Marks, W.B., O'Donovan, M.J., Pratt, C.A. and Sugano, N. (1987a) Cat hindlimb motoneurons during locomotion. I. Destination, axonal conduction velocity and recruitment threshold. *J. Neurophysiol.*, 57: 510–529.

Hoffer, J.A., Loeb, G.E., Sugano, N., Marks, W.B., O'Donovan, M.J. and Pratt, C.A. (1987b) Cat hindlimb motoneurons during locomotion. III. Functional segregation in sartorius. *J. Neurophysiol.,* 57: 554–562.

Howell, J.N., Fuglevand, A.J., Walsh, M.L. and Bigland-Ritchie, B. (1995) Motor unit activity during isometric and concentric-eccentric contractions of the human first dorsal interosseus muscle. *J. Neurophysiol.,* 74: 901–904.

Kanda, K., Burke, R.E. and Walmsley, B. (1977) Differential control of fast and slow twitch motor units in the decerebrate cat. *Exp. Br. Res.,* 29: 57–74.

Kernell, D. (1992) Organized variability in the neuromuscular system: a survey of task-related adaptations. *Archives Italiennes de Biologie,* 130: 19–66.

Loeb, G.E. (1985) Motoneuron task groups – coping with kinematic heterogeneity. *J. Exp. Biol.,* 115: 137–146.

Maier, M.A. and Hepp-Reymond, M.-C. (1995) EMG activation patterns during force production in precision grip. I. Contribution of 15 finger muscles to isometric force. *Exp. Brain Res.,* 103: 108–122.

Nardone, A., Romano, C. and Schieppati, M. (1989) Selective recruitment of high threshold human motor units during voluntary isotonic lengthening of active muscle. *J. Physiol. (Lond.),* 410: 463–477.

Nichols, T.R., Cope, T.C. and Abelew, T.A. (1999) Rapid spinal mechanisms of motor coordination. *Exer. Sport Sci. Rev.,* 27: 255–284.

Nichols, T.R. (1989) The organization of heterogenic reflexes among muscles crossing the ankle joint in the decerebrate cat. *J. Physiol. (Lond.),* 410: 463–477.

Riek, S. and Bawa, P. (1992) Recruitment of motor units in human forearm extensors. *J. Neurophysiol.,* 68: 100–108.

Romanes, G.J. (1951) The motor cell columns of the lumbosacral spinal cord of the cat. *J. Comp. Neurol.,* 94: 313–364.

Siegel, S.G., Nichols, T.R. and Cope, T.C. (1999) Reflex activation in relation to multidirectional ankle torque in decerebrate cats. *Motor Control,* 3: 135–150.

Sokoloff, A.J. and Cope, T.C. (1996) Recruitment of triceps surae motor units in the decerebrate cat. II. Heterogeneity among soleus motor units. *J. Neurophysiol.,* 75: 2005–2016.

Sokoloff, A.J., Siegel, S.G. and Cope, T.C. (1999) Recruitment order among motoneurons from different motor nuclei. *J. Neurophysiol.,* 81: 2485–2492.

Stuart, D.G. and Enoka, R.M. (1983) Motoneurons, motor units and the size principle. In: R.N. Rosenberg (Ed.): *Clinical Neurosciences Section 5, Neurobiology* (W.D. Willis, Ed.) New York: Churchill Livingston, pp. 471–518.

Tansey, K.E. and Botterman, B.R. (1996) Activation of type-identified motor units during centrally evoked contractions in the cat medial gastrocnemius muscle. I. Motor-unit recruitment. *J. Neurophysiol.,* 75: 38–50.

Thomson, D.B., Loeb, G.E. and Richmond, F.R. (1994) Effect of neck posture on the activation of feline neck muscles during voluntary head turns *J. Neurophysiol.,* 72: 2004–2014.

Windhorst, U.R, Burke, R.E., Dieringer, N., Evinger, C., Feldman, A.G., Hasan, Z., Hultborn, H., Illert, M., Lundberg, A., Macpherson, J.M., Nichols, T.R., Schwarz, H.R.M. and Vilis, T. (1991). Group report: what are the output units of motor behavior and how are they controlled? In: D.R.Humphrey and H.-J. Freund (Eds), *Report of the Dahlem Workshop on Motor Control: Concepts and Issues,* John Wiley and Sons, Chichester, pp. 101–119.

Windhorst, U., Hamm, T.M. and Stuart, D.G. (1989) On the function of muscle and reflex partitioning. *Behav. Brain Sci.,* 12: 629–681.

Wyman, R.J., Waldron, I. and Wachtel, G.M. (1974) Lack of fixed order of recruitment in cat motoneuron pools. *Exp. Br. Res.,* 20: 101–114.

Zajac, F.E. and Faden, J.S. (1985) Relationship among recruitment order, axonal conduction velocity, and muscle-unit properties of type-identified motor units in cat plantaris muscle. *J. Neurophysiol.,* 53: 1303–1322.

M.D. Binder (Ed.)
Progress in Brain Research, Vol 123
© 1999 Elsevier Science BV. All rights reserved.

CHAPTER 17

Limited plasticity of adult motor units conserves recruitment order and rate coding

T. Gordon,[1,]* N. Tyreman,[1] V.F. Rafuse[1] and J.B. Munson[2]

[1] *Department of Pharmacology, Division of Neuroscience, University of Alberta, Edmonton, T6G 2S2, Canada*
[2] *Department of Neuroscience, University of Florida College of Medicine, Gainesville, FL 32610–0244, USA*

Introduction

Motoneuron and muscle unit properties are remarkably well matched for function. Normally, motoneurons and their muscle fibers, the motor units, are recruited according to size with the smallest and slowest motor units recruited before the larger and faster motor units (Henneman and Mendell, 1981). The duration of the afterhyperpolarization of the motoneuron's action potential limits the rate of firing and is well matched to the contraction time of the muscle units (Kernell, 1992). The slow motor units which are the most excitable and are the most readily recruited, are also the most fatigue resistant. They contract with little or no fatigue. Progressively, larger and faster motor units are recruited into activity as muscle force is increased by voluntary effort. The low force fast motor units are fatigue resistant (FR) in contrast to the large forceful fast motor units which are classified as fast fatigable (FF) units in accordance with their high susceptibility to fatigue (Burke, 1981).

The basis for the matching of motoneuron and their muscle unit properties is not fully understood. Experiments which demonstrated that contractile speed of fast and slow muscles was altered by cross-reinnervation by the slow and fast nerves, respectively, suggested that either the novel innervation of the muscles exerted different trophic effects on the muscles or that the reinnervated muscle fibers responded to the novel activation by the foreign innervation (Buller et al., 1960). Findings that chronic stimulation of fast-twitch muscles with low frequency tonic stimulation mimicked the effects of cross-reinnervation or reversed the effects of cross-reinnervation of slow muscle by fast nerves, favored the second possibility (Salmons and Vrbova, 1969; Salmons and Sreter, 1976; Ausoni et al., 1990). Kernell et al. (1987a, b) demonstrated that the contractile properties of chronically stimulated muscle varied with the total daily activity to which they were subjected, indicating that the daily amount of neuromuscular activity was an important determinant of muscle phenotype. They demonstrated that stimulation for 50% of the day at any frequency was associated with conversion of muscle properties towards the S type whilst stimulation for 5% of the day was associated with the FR phenotype and for 0.5% of each day with the FF phenotype (Eerbeek et al., 1984). One possibility is that neuromuscular activity of motor units, which is dictated by their order of recruitment according to size, determines their properties.

Methods and results

Chronic stimulation of intact motor units

To test the hypothesis that the relative activity of motor units during orderly recruitment establishes

---

*Corresponding author: Tel.: (780) 492-1668; Fax: (780) 492-1617; e-mail: tessa.gordon@ualberta.ca

the wide range of motor unit properties, we have imposed one pattern of neuromuscular activity on all motor units and examined whether that level restricts the normal wide range of motor unit properties to a very narrow range corresponding to those motor units which would be recruited at that level of excitation. In the cat, we imposed one pattern of activity on the medial gastrocnemius (MG) muscle by electrically stimulating the MG nerve at 20 Hz in a 50% duty cycle to impose activity patterns demonstrated previously to convert muscle to a slow phenotype (Eerbeek et al., 1984; Kernell et al., 1987a, b). Alternatively, we eliminated all ongoing activity by unilateral deafferentation and hemisection of the spinal cord and imposed either 20 Hz at a 50% duty cycle for direct comparison with the intact cat or at a 6.3% duty cycle which had been demonstrated previously to convert muscle to the FR phenotype (Kernell et al., 1987a, b; Gordon et al., 1997).

Bipolar stainless steel electrodes were implanted around the MG nerve in 21 cats. The wires were led through the skin on the back of the animal for attachment to a portable and locally made stimulator which was carried on a external basket which was secured and stabilized by a suture through the L5 vertebral process (Fig. 1; Gordon et al., 1997). At regular intervals of 10 to 14 days, evoked MG isometric twitch and tetanic contractions were recorded under halothane anesthesia. As shown in Fig. 2, chronic supramaximal stimulation at 20 Hz in a 50% duty cycle (2.5 s on 2.5 s off) resulted in an immediate and rapid exponential decline in muscle force with a somewhat longer and gradual increase in fatigue resistence and contraction time. The question which we addressed was, is this conversion of muscle properties accompanied by a complete conversion of motor unit properties to a very narrow range, as predicted if neuromuscular activity is directly responsible for controlling the properties of the motor units?

In final acute experiments carried out 37 to 240 days after initiation of chronic stimulation, MG muscles and their innervation were isolated and a laminectomy performed for intracellular recording of motoneuron properties and isometric force recordings of muscle unit properties prior to removal of the muscles for histochemical examination. The methods have been described in detail previously (Gordon et al., 1997; Munson et al., 1997a). All muscle fibers became uniformly slow histochemically, 75 days or more after initiation of daily chronic stimulation (Gordon et al., 1997). Yet, despite striking changes in motor unit properties towards the slow S type, which included slowing of the time to peak twitch force, lack of 'sag' during an unfused tetanic contraction, and fatigue indices greater than 0.5, there remained a wider range of motor unit properties than was predicted by the hypothesis that motor unit properties arise directly as a function of their daily level of activity, which in turn, is determined by their order of recruitment (Fig. 3). For example, the fatigue index, which is the ratio of peak 40 Hz muscle tetanic force recorded 2 min after repetition of 330 ms tetani every second to the peak force recorded at 0 min, varies widely over the range normally seen for all S and FI motor units (Fig. 3). Similarly, there is a wide range of contractile speeds in the converted S motor units after chronic stimulation. Similar results were obtained in paralysed muscles after unilateral deafferentation and spinal cord hemisection (Gordon et al., 1997) which showed that the wide range of motor unit properties could not be attributed to asynchronous levels of motor unit activity in the chronically stimulated muscles in normal cats. Rather the data indicated that synchronous activation of the muscle with a one level of neuromuscular activity failed to constrain the properties of the motor units to the very narrow range predicted if the daily neuromuscular activity was the sole determinant of motor unit properties. The same conclusions were drawn from results which were obtained for chronic stimulation of paralysed muscle with 20 Hz for 6.3% of each day, either by stimulating 6.3% of each day in a 24 h period or having a 50 Hz duty cycle in a block time of 3 h (Gordon et al., 1997). We found that this lower activity favored a range of contractile speed more typical of the fast motor units and higher endurance but the range of properties was again broader than expected if activity alone dictated the properties of the motor units.

Comparisons of histograms for motoneuron and motor unit properties in stimulated and control medial gastrocnemius motor units in Fig. 4 and 5

193

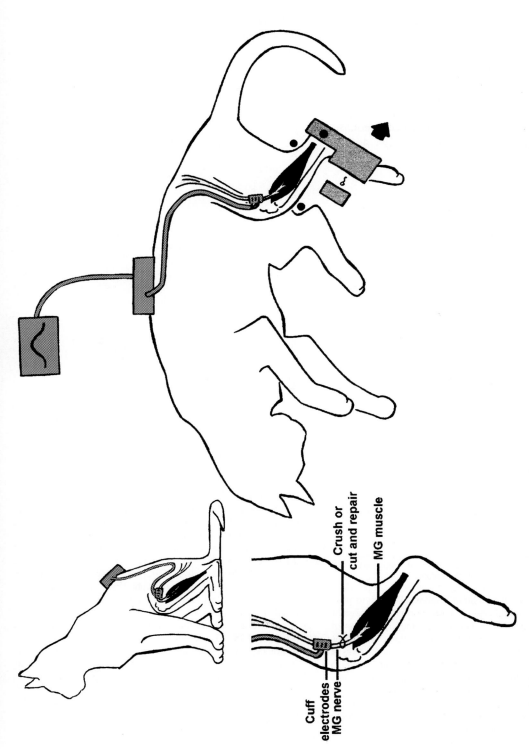

Fig. 1. Diagrammatical representation of the indwelling cuff electrodes around the nerve to the medial gastrocnemius (MG) nerve for chronic stimulation of MG motor units and monitoring of progressive changes in MG muscle isometric contractile properties. The cuff electrodes were placed on the intact MG nerve or proximal to a crush site on the MG nerve or to the site of MG nerve section and resuture of proximal and distal nerve stumps (N-N repair). The cuff electrodes were externalized via the skin overlying the lumbosacral cord and attached to an external stimulator that was mounted in a hexelite basket for 24 h stimulation in the awake cat. To monitor the changes in MG muscle properties, the cat was anesthetized with halothane and force or torque of ankle extension was recorded in response to supramaximal nerve stimulation. The knee joint was stabelized between two fixed support posts. The foot was coupled to to a strain gauge via a boot that was free to rotate about a line coaxial with the ankle joint. The ankle was rotated to a fixed point at which nerve stimulation evoked maximum twitch and tetanic isometric forces.

194

demonstrate that, although electrical stimulation narrows the range of motor unit properties towards the normal slow range, the range remains considerably larger than predicted if one pattern of stimulation was fully responsible for determining the properties of all the stimulated motor units. Perhaps the most striking reduction in the range of properties was observed for the ratio of rheobase and input resistance (Rh/Rin; compare Figs. 4c and

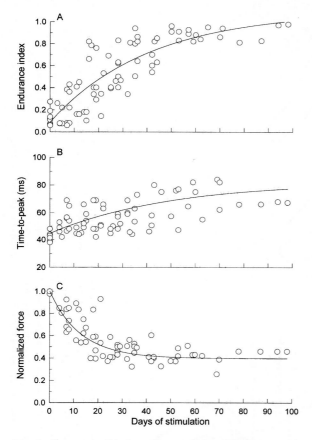

Fig. 2. Changes in (A) the endurance index, (B) time to peak twitch force and (C) muscle tetanic force, normalized to values recorded at the onset of stimulation as a function of days of chronic stimulation at 20 Hz in a 50% duty cycle of 2.5 s trains every 5 s, 24 hours per day. The endurance index is the ratio of the tetanic force at 2 minutes relative to 0 minutes after a 330 ms duration of 40 Hz tetanic contractions every second. The increase in the endurance and time to peak twitch force and the decline in tetanic force were fitted with single exponential curves. Asymptotic values were 1.1 (A), 82 ms (B) and 0.4 (C) and the time constants (time to reach 33% of asymptotic values) were 42 (A), 49 (B) and 13 (C) days.

5c). This ratio normally provides a sensitive discriminator of S type motoneurons in view of the narrow range of values for the S motor units where

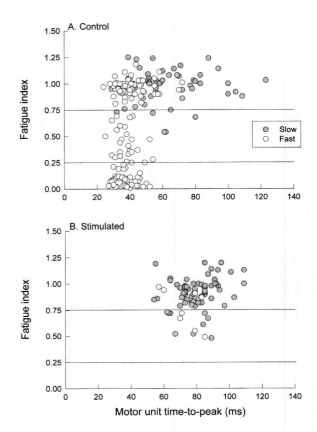

Fig. 3. The relationship between fatigue index and time to peak twitch force (TTP) in (A) normal and (B) chronically stimulated (20 Hz in a 50% duty cycle for 75–240 days) medial gastrocnemius muscles. Motor units were classified as slow (S) and fast (F) on the basis the absence and presence of 'sag' of the unfused 800 ms tetanus at $1.25 \times$ TTP as described originally by Burke et al. (1973). Fast motor units were further classified into fast fatigue resistant (FR), fast fatigue intermediate (FI) and fast fatigable (FF) motor units on the basis of whether peak force of 330 ms 40 Hz tetanic contractions repeated every second for 2 minutes declined to <0.75 (FR), >0.75 <0.25 (FI) and to <0.25 (FF) of the initial tetanic contraction. Almost all motor units, 76–240 days after chronic stimulation, were classified as S but, although the time to peak twitch tension was prolonged and the fatigue index was increased, there remained a wide range of motor units with respect to both fatigue indices and the time to peak twitch forces. The motor unit data was derived from control and chronically stimulated medial gastrocnemius muscles in seven and five cats, respectively.

Rh values are generally < 7nA and input resistance values are high (> 1 mohm) (Zengel et al., 1985). Although the change in the Rh/Rin ratio is dramatic after 20 Hz chronic stimulation for 50% of each day, the range of values is considerably larger with values up to 30 and including a value of 42 for one motor unit. The range of motor unit tetanic force is also greater than the normal slow motor unit range (Figs 4a and 5a). However, it must be remembered that, in the electrically stimulated muscles where electrical stimulation reduced muscle fiber diameters of all motor units to the same range (Gordon et al., 1997), the number of muscle fibers innervated by each motoneuron, the innervation ratio (IR) was

not changed by electrical stimulation. Since IR is an important determinant of motor unit force (Chamberlain and Lewis, 1989; Totosy de Zepetnek et al., 1992), the range of unit tetanic forces remaining after chronic stimulation reflects the normal range of IRs (Rafuse et al., 1997).

With respect to the time to peak twitch force and the half decay time of the action potential afterhyperpolarization (Figs 4 and 5; B, D), electrical stimulation moved the histograms to the right to slower values but did not reduce the range of values. The broad range of the half decay times of the afterhyperpolarization, in particular the retention of short half decay times despite slowing of the

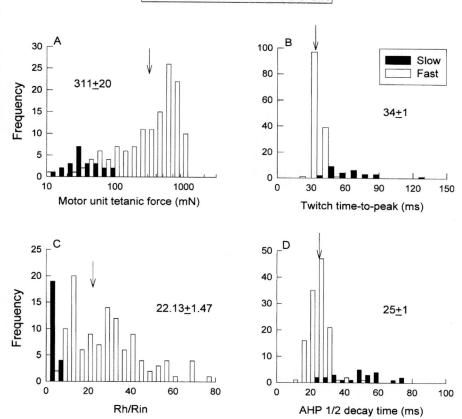

Fig. 4. Histograms of (A) motor unit tetanic force (mN), (B) twitch time to peak force (ms), (C) the ratio of rheobase to input resistence of motoneurons and (D) the 1/2 decay time for the action potential afterhyperpolarization for normal medial gastrocnemius motor units. Each plot includes data obtained from at least five animals. The number shown on each graph is the mean ± S.E. and slow and fast motor units are represented by filled and open bars, respectively.

muscle contractions, indicated an incomplete conversion of motoneuron properties. The proportion of motor units which displayed the relatively short half decay times for the afterhyperpolarization was very similar to the proportion of fast motor units in the unstimulated MG muscle, suggesting some resistance of conversion of these properties in these fast motoneurons (Munson et al., 1997a).

The Rh/Rin ratio, which provides an indicator of motoneuronal excitability relative to size, remains correlated with unit tetanic force in chronically stimulated muscles even though the range of values was reduced by the stimulation (Fig. 6A, C). In contrast, the normal relationship between the time course of the motoneuronal afterhyperpolarization and the twitch time to peak force was not observed

in chronically stimulated motor units (Fig. 6B, D). As discussed above, we had suggested that there may be incomplete conversion of F motoneurons to S on the basis of the corresponding number of motoneurons which demonstrated relative fast half-decay times of the afterhyperpolarization in chronically stimulated intact motor units. However, findings that the half-decay time of the afterhyperpolarization was significantly correlated with twitch time to peak force in reinnervated motor units after N–N suture and 20 Hz electrical stimulation in a 50% duty cycle (Fig. 7), are consistent with the view that activity modulates rather than determines neuromuscular properties.

In summary, chronic stimulation of intact motor units with the same amount of electrical activity

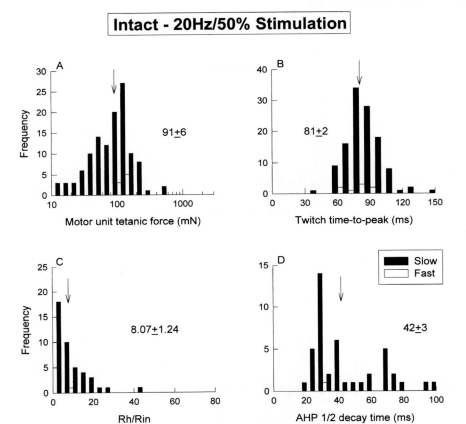

Fig. 5. Histograms of (A) motor unit tetanic force (mN), (B) twitch time to peak force (ms), (C) the ratio of rheobase to input resistence of motoneurons and (D) the 1/2 decay time for the action potential afterhyperpolarization for medial gastrocnemius motor units stimulated at 20 Hz for 50% of each day for 75–240 days. Each plot includes data obtained from 4–5 animals. The number shown on each graph is the mean ± S.E. and slow and fast motor units are represented by filled and open bars, respectively.

dramatically altered the properties of the motor units at the motoneuron and muscle unit levels. The high daily amount of activity of 50% per day converted the motor units to a S-type phenotype at both motoneuron and muscle unit levels. If, however, the daily activity experienced by each motor unit were the sole determining factor of the properties of the motoneurons and the muscle fibers that they supply, daily synchronous activation of all motor units should lead to a very narrow range of motor unit properties. Instead, the activity pattern

of 20 Hz at 50% duty cycle which converted the muscle from fast to slow with respect to muscle contraction speed and fatigability was associated with a broad range of motor unit properties which corresponded generally to the range of properties of the S-type motoneurons and their muscle units. Even then, the range of properties of the chronically stimulated motor units was generally broader than the normal range of the S-type motor units, even though, at the histochemical level and with respect to loss of the 'sag' of unfused tetani, all

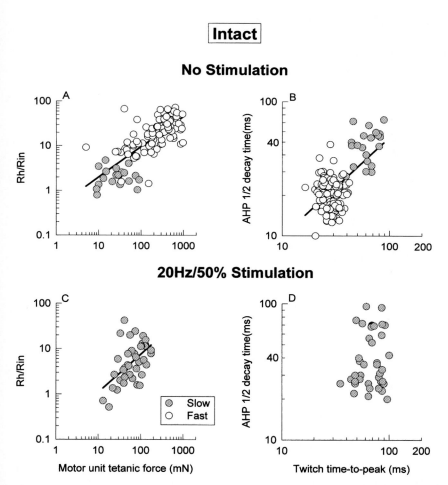

Fig. 6. Regression analysis of the relationships between motoneuronal and muscle unit properties in normal medial gastrocnemius muscles and after chronic stimulation at 20 Hz for 50% of each day. (A) and (C) Ratios of rheobase values and input resistance (Rh/Rin) of motoneurons are plotted against motor unit tetanic force and (B) and (D) half decay time of the action potential afterhyperpolarization is plotted against twitch time to peak. Regression lines are drawn only when the slope of these lines was significantly different from zero at the 0.05 confidence limit. Slow and fast motor units are shown as filled and unfilled circles, respectively. Each plot includes data obtained from at least four animals.

stimulated muscle fibers and almost all motor units were characterized as slow. Since the same findings were obtained under conditions in which all neuromuscular activity was removed by unilateral deafferentation and hemisection of the spinal cord (Gordon et al., 1997), the remaining range of motor unit properties could not simply be explained by differences in activity experienced by the motor units.

Chronic stimulation of regenerating nerve and reinnervated motor units

One possible explanation for the findings that chronic stimulation of intact motor units fails to fully transform their properties is that the differentiated adult motor units have more limited plasticity than those which have undergone dedifferentiation after axotomy and denervation.

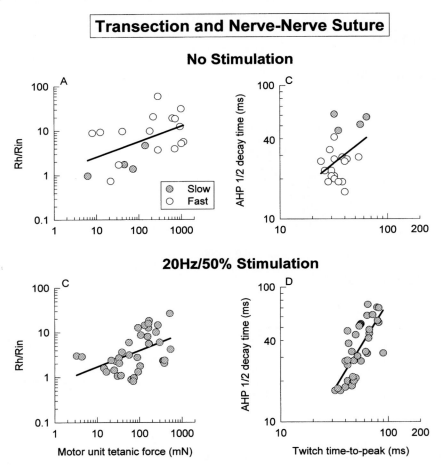

Fig. 7. Regression analysis of the relationships between motoneuron and muscle unit properties in self-reinnervated medial gastrocnemius muscles with and without chronic stimulation at 20 Hz for 50% of each day for 8–9 months. (A) and (C) Ratios of rheobase values and input resistance (Rh/Rin) of motoneurons are plotted against motor unit tetanic force and B) and D) half decay time of the action potential afterhyperpolarization is plotted against twitch time to peak. Regression lines are drawn only when the slope of these lines was significantly different from zero at the 0.05 confidence limit. Slow and fast motor units are shown as filled and unfilled circles, respectively. Data was obtained from two cats for chronically stimulated reinnervated muscles and compared with data from one cat in which reinnervation occurred after N-N suture. The latter data for the unstimulated muscles was obtained from one animal and is consistent with previous findings from larger samples (Foerhing et al., 1996).

Since axotomized motoneurons and denervated muscle fibers demonstrate dedifferentiation with respect to their properties (Gordon et al., 1988a), it could be argued that chronic stimulation may affect more dramatic changes on the dedifferentiated motoneurons and muscle fibers which would more accurately reflect the role of neuromuscular activity in determining the properties of the adult motor units. To test this possibility, we axotomized motoneurons and promoted regeneration and muscle reinnervation either by: (a) crush injury in which the axotomized motoneurons regenerate their axons in their original endoneurial pathways to reinnervate the same muscle fibers as previously, or (b) nerve section and resuture of proximal and distal nerve stumps (N–N suture) to promote the regeneration of axons to muscle fibers that they did not formerly innervate. The MG nerve was electrically stimulated central to the site of injury immediately after the surgery, as shown figuratively in Fig. 1. Nerves were chronically stimulated with 20 Hz 50% of each day, in the same manner as for the intact motor units, described above. Stimulation was continued for periods of 8 to 9 months, over which time, self-reinnervated motor units recover their normal properties and the interrelationships between motoneuronal and muscle unit properties (Gordon and Stein, 1982a, b; Foehring et al., 1986).

As shown in Fig. 7, the size relationships between motoneuron and muscle unit properties return with time after muscle reinnervation, although there is generally more overlap in properties of different motor units types (see Gordon and Stein, 1982a, b, Gordon et al., 1986, 1988b). For reinnervated motor units which were electrically stimulated throughout the period of nerve regeneration and muscle reinnervation, a wide range of properties was retained, despite chronic stimulation. Chronic stimulation affected the same conversion of fast to slow muscle fibers and slowing of all motoneuron and muscle unit parameters as demonstrated in intact motor units (Figs 4–6). In chronically stimulated reinnervated motor units, the range in properties was sufficient to demonstrate strong correlations between motoneuron and muscle unit properties, in particular the correlations between motoneuron indices of excita-bility and size, Rh/Rin ratio and axon conduction velocity, and muscle unit size in terms of tetanic force. Positive relationships between conduction velocity and motor unit tetanic forces were also statistically significant with slopes ($\pm$S.E.) of 0.37 $\pm$0.11 and 0.35 $\pm$0.14 in chronically stimulated and unstimulated reinnervated motor units, respectively. Since the relationships between electrophysiological parameters of motoneuron and muscle unit size predict the orderly recruitment of motor unit during movement, their retention in chronically stimulated muscles indicates that, even though the properties are modulated by activity, they are not determined by activity. Thus, the retention of these relationships permits control of force in the muscles by orderly recruitment according to size. In addition, the retention of the relationship between the duration of the after-hyperpolarization and twitch time to peak in chronically stimulated muscles, indicates that there remains the capacity for rate modulation of motor units for force control despite the restriction of these properties to the slow type by neuromuscular activity.

Discussion and conclusions

Chronic stimulation of intact and reinnervated motor units in the cat MG muscle led to dramatic changes in the electrical and mechanical properties of the motoneurons and the muscle fibers that they innervate, respectively. Chronic stimulation at 20 Hz for 50% of each day dramatically slowed motor unit contractions, reduced their force output and increased their resistence to fatigue. These changes were accompanied by a dramatic reduction in muscle fiber size, an increase in oxidative enzymes and conversion of myosin isoforms in the muscle fibers (Gordon et al., 1997; see also Donselaar et al., 1987). Accompanying these changes was a parallel decline in axonal conduction velocity and the Rh/Rin ratio which reflect changes in the size and excitability of the motoneurons (Munson et al., 1997a). Hence the conversion of motor units towards the S-type was accompanied by corresponding changes in the motoneuron properties toward the S-type. Nevertheless, for each motor unit parameter, there remained a wide range of physiological properties, wider than predicted if neuromuscular activity was the determining factor for the properties of the motoneurons and their muscle units. Chronic stimulation of axotomized motoneurons and reinnervating motor units did not confine the range of properties any further, as predicted if dedifferentiated motoneurons and their muscle fibers display more plasticity. Hence, the findings of this study indicate that, while neuromuscular activity has a strong modulating influence on the properties of motor units at motoneuron and muscle unit levels, the normal interrelationships between motoneuron and muscle unit properties are retained independent of neuromuscular activity. As a result, a motor nucleus containing motoneurons to one muscle retains control of muscle force by recruitment of progressively larger motor units and changes in firing rates of the recruited motor units.

Particularly striking was the finding that, chronic stimulation did not constrain motor unit forces in reinnervated muscles to a very small range despite a dramatic reduction in muscle fiber size (Gordon and Tyreman, unpublished findings). Moreover, motor unit force was directly correlated with the size of the motor nerve, as measured by conduction velocity. Under conditions in which the size of muscle fibers is no longer a determinant of motor unit force, motor unit force directly reflects the number of muscle fibers innervated by one motoneuron, the IR (Rafuse et al., 1997). Hence, the re-establishment of the relationship between Rh/Rin values and motor unit tetanic force in chronically stimulated and reinnervated motor units (Fig. 7), demonstrates that the increase in IR as a function of motoneuron size and excitability occurs independently of neuromuscular activity. In light of evidence that neuromuscular activity promotes loss of polyneuronal innervation during development and during muscle reinnervation in the adult (McArdle, 1975; O'Brien et al., 1978; Greensmith et al., 1998), these findings show that, even though neuromuscular activity may play a central role in elimination of polyneuronal innervation, the number of muscle fibers which are reinnervated by each axon is size-related and unaffected by superimposed synchronous neuromuscular activity. Since the same neuromuscular activity was imposed on all reinnervating motor units and did not eliminate the size-dependent relationship between axon conduction velocity and muscle unit force, the size ordering suggests that neuromuscular activity does not control the matching of motoneuron size and target size in the sense of the number of muscle fibers per motoneuron. In view of findings that the reduced conduction velocity of axotomized motor axons was reversed by application of neurotrophic factors, NT–3 and NT4/5, it is possible that the relationship between axons and the numbers of motoneurons is maintained by the uptake of neurotrophins from the reinnervated muscles (Munson et al., 1997b).

Clearly, neuromuscular activity strongly modulates the properties of motoneurons and their muscle units. The extensive literature on the effects of use and disuse on muscle properties strongly supports the data from this study in showing that hyperactivity strongly favors the slow muscle phenotype in contrast to hypoactivity which favors the fast fatigable muscle phenotype (reviewed by Gordon and Pattullo, 1993; Gordon and Mao, 1994; Gordon, 1995). Imposition of one activity pattern on the intact neuromuscular system or during the regeneration and reinnervation of denervated muscle, narrows the properties of the motor units toward the slow phenotype. However, the retention of a broad range of properties despite uniform neuromuscular activity (ie. same amount of daily activity), demonstrates that the activity modulates rather than determines the properties of motor units. The normal wide range of properties in individual muscles is an important determinant of the level of controls exerted by that muscle during movement. For example, in the medial gastrocnemius muscle where the slow motor units are recruited during normal standing, progressive recruitment of the fast fatigue resistant motor units is normally sufficient for limb movement (Burke, 1981). However, for rapid ballistic movements or rapid running, the brief recruitment of the larger and more fatigable motor units dramatically raises total muscle force to accomplish the required movements. Nevertheless, the plasticity of the neuromuscular system permits the specialization of the muscle according to use. Therefore, high endurance exercise can restrict muscle properties to the more fatigue resistant motor units (Gordon,

1995). However, the persistence of size relationships between motoneurons and muscle unit force retains the capacity for force control by orderly recruitment of motor units. Similarly, the relationship between duration of the afterhyperpolarization and contraction speed retains the level of control of motor unit force by rate coding.

Hence, the role of activity in controlling motor unit properties may be seen as one which modulates the range of motoneuron and muscle unit properties. Activity modulation of motoneuron excitability expands the level of motor control by expanding the range of motor units which can be recruited according to size and excitability. Modulation of the duration of the action potential afterhyperpolarization in motoneurons expands the level of control of motor unit force by rate coding. The strong relationship between duration of the afterhyperpolarization and the speed of the muscle unit expands the force control by varying the rate of firing to the maximum tetanic force levels. At the level of the muscle unit, modulation of muscle fiber size by activity expands the level of force gradation by orderly recruitment of motor units. Modulation of muscle fiber speed expands the level of control of muscle force by rate coding. Finally, the modulation of aerobic-glycolytic metabolism expands the level of force control by modulating the susceptibility to fatigue and hence the duration of muscle contraction.

The activity modulation of the range of motor control by recruitment order and rate coding can explain the range of motor unit properties normally seen in different muscles. Thus, the properties of motor units in the homogeneously slow soleus muscle in the cat, for example, lie within a relatively narrow range (McPhedran et al., 1965; Henneman and Mendell, 1981). The muscle is highly specialised for maintenance of low force levels for long periods of time for standing and has been referred to as tonic as opposed to phasic to describe the persistent low level activation during normal standing (Vrbova et al., 1995). While the range of motoneuron and muscle unit properties is constricted to the slow range, the 10 fold-range in motor unit force and contractile speed is matched by a corresponding range in motoneuronal properties which, thereby permits control by recruitment

order and rate coding. The muscle contrasts with the synergistic gastrocnemius muscles which contain a much greater breadth of properties of their motor units (Wuerker et al., 1965) which dramatically increases the range of control of force by recruitment order and rate coding. On the other hand, the antagonistic flexor muscles in the leg are more specialised toward fast motor units, in accordance with their more phasic functions during normal walking or ankle flexion. During normal walking, almost all motor units may be recruited in the tibialis anterior muscle, for example (Feiereisen et al., 1997). Motor units are recruited to flex the ankle during a relatively brief period of flexion prior to the more extended extensor phase of walking.

In summary, our experiments demonstrate that neuromuscular activity plays a strong modulatory control of motor unit properties which include both motoneuron and muscle unit properties. However, despite the restriction of properties by the amount of daily activity, a range of properties are retained which permit orderly recruitment of motor units according to size and rate coding of muscle force to a maximum of fused tetanic contractions at frequencies limited by the duration of the afterhyperpolarization. How the motoneuron-muscle unit functional matching is brought about remains to be elucidated.

Acknowledgements

Research was supported by grants from the Medical Research Council of Canada (TG) and RO1 NS–15913 (Javits Neuroscience Award) and PO1 NS–27511 (JBM). TG is an AHFMR scientist and V.F.R. was an AHFMR predoctoral fellow.

References

Ausoni, S., Gorza, L., Schiaffino,S., Gunderson, K. and. Lömo, T. (1990) Expression of myosin heavy chain isoforms in stimulated fast and slow rat muscles. *J. Neurosci.*, 10: 153–160.

Buller, A.J., Eccles, J.C. and Eccles, R.M. (1960) Interactions between motoneurones and muscles in respect of the characteristic speeds of their responses. *J. Physiol.*, 150: 417–439.

Burke, R.E. (1981) Motor units: anatomy, physiology and functional organization. In: V.B. Brooks (Ed.), *Handbook of Physiology*, Sect. 1. *The Nervous System*, Vol. II. *Motor*

202

Systems American Physiological Society: Bethesda, MD, pp. 345–422, Williams and Wilkins Co., Baltimore.

Chamberlain, S. and Lewis, D.M. (1989) Contractile characteristics and innervation ratio of rat soleus motor units. *J. Physiol.*, 412: 1–21.

Donselaar, Y., Eerbeek, O., Kernell, D. and Verhey, B.A. (1987) Fibre sizes and histochemical staining characteristics in normal and chronically stimulated fast muscle of cat. *J. Physiol.*, 382: 237–254.

Eerbeek, O., Kernell, D. and Verhey, B.A. (1984) Effects of fast and slow patterns of tonic long-term stimulation on contractile properties of fast muscle in cat. *J. Physiol.*, 352: 73–90.

Feiereisen, P., Duchateau, J. and Hainaut K. (1997) Motor unit recruitment order during voluntary and electrically induced contractions in the tibialis anterior. *Exp. Brain Res.*, 114: 117–123.

Foehring, R.C., Sypert, G.W. and Munson, J.B. (1986) Properties of self-reinnervated motor units in medial gastrocnemius of cat. I. Long-term reinnervation. *J. Neurophysiol.*, 55: 931–946.

Gordon, T. (1995) Fatigue in adapted systems. Overuse and underuse paradigms. In S.C. Gandevia, R.M. Enoka, A.L. McComas, D.G. Stuart, and C.K. Thomas (Eds.), *Fatigue: Neural and Muscular Mechanisms*, Chap. 32, pp. 429–456.

Gordon, T. and Mao, J. (1994) Muscle atrophy and procedures for training after spinal cord injury. *Phys. Ther.*, 74: 50–60.

Gordon, T. and Pattullo, M.C. (1993) Plasticity of muscle fiber and motor unit types. *Exer. Sport Sci. Rev.*, 21: 331–362.

Gordon, T. and Stein, R.B.(1982a) Time course and extent of recovery in reinnervated motor units of cat triceps surae muscles. *J. Physiol.*, 323: 307–323.

Gordon, T. and Stein, R.B. (1982b) Reorganization of motor-unit properties in reinnervated muscles of the cat. *J. Neurophysiol.*, 48: 1175–1190.

Gordon, T. Stein, R.B. and Thomas, C. (1986) Motor unit organization in extensor muscles cross-reinnervated by flexor motoneurones. *J. Physiol.*, 374: 443–456.

Gordon, T., Bambrick, L. and Orozco, R. (1988a) Comparison of injury and development in the neuromuscular system. In: D. Everad and J. Whalen, (Eds.), *Ciba Foundation Symposium on 'Plasticity of the neuromuscular System'*. John Wiley and Sons, pp. 210–226, 1988.

Gordon, T., Thomas, C.K., Stein, R.B. and Erdebil, S. (1988b) Comparison of physiological and histochemical properties of motor units after cross-reinnervation of antagonistic muscles in the cat hindlimb. *J. Neurophysiol.*, 60: 365–378.

Gordon, T., Tyreman, N., Rafuse, V.R. and Munson, J.B. (1997) Fast-to-slow conversion following chronic low-frequency activation of medial gastrocnemius muscle in cats. I. Muscle and motor unit properties. *J. Neurophysiol.*, 77: 2585–2604.

Greensmith L. Harding DI. Meyer MP. Vrbova G.(1998) Mechanical activity is necessary for the elimination of polyneuronal innervation of developing rat soleus muscles, *Dev. Brain Res.*, 110: 131–4.

Henneman, E. and Mendell, L.M. (1981) Functional organization of the motoneurone pool and its inputs. In: V.B. Brookes

(Ed.), *Handbook of Physiology*, Sect. 1. *The Nervous System*, Vol. II. *Motor Systems* American Physiological Society: Bethesda, MD, pp. 423–508, Williams and Wilkins Co., Baltimore.

Kernell, D. (1992) Organized variability in the neuromuscular system: a survey of task-related adaptations. *Arch. Ital. de Biol.*, 130: 19–66.

Kernell, D., Eerbeek, O., Verhey, B.A. and Donselaar, Y. (1987a) Effects of physiological amounts of high- and low-rate chronic stimulation on fast-twitch muscle of the cat hindlimb. I. Speed and force-related properties. *J. Neurophysiol.*, 58: 598–613.

Kernell, D., Donselaar, Y. and Eerbeek, O. (1987b) Effects of physiological amounts of high- and low-rates of chronic stimulation on the fast-twitch muscle of the cat hindlimb. II. Endurance related properties. *J. Neurophysiol.*, 58: 614–627.

McArdle, J.J. (1975) Complex endplate potentials at the regenerating neuromuscular junction of the rat. *Exp. Neurol.*, 49: 629–638.

McPhedran, A.M., Wuerker, R.B. and Henneman, E. (1965) Properties of motor units in a homogeneous red muscle (soleus) of the cat. *J. Neurophysiol.*, 28: 71–84.

Munson, J.B., Foehring, R.C., Mendell, L.M. and Gordon, T. (1997a) Fast-to-slow conversion following chronic low-frequency activation of medial gastrocnemius muscle in cats. II. Motoneuron properties. *J. Neurophysiol.*, 77: 2605–2615.

Munson JB. Shelton DL. McMahon SB. (1997b) Adult mammalian sensory and motor neurons: roles of endogenous neurotrophins and rescue by exogenous neurotrophins after axotomy. *J. Neurosci.*, 17: 470–476.

O'Brien, R.A., Ostberg, A.J. and Vrbova, G. (1978) Observations on the elimination of polyneuronal innervation in developing mammalian skeletal muscle. *J. Physiol.*, 282: 571–582.

Rafuse, V.F., Pattullo, M.C. and Gordon, T. (1997) Innervation ratio and motor unit force in large muscles: a study of chronically stimulated cat medial gastrocnemius. *J. Physiol. (Lond.)*, 499: 809–823.

Salmons, S. and Sreter, F.A. (1976) Significance of impulse activity in the transformation of skeletal muscle type. *Nature* 263: 30–34.

Salmons, S. and Vrbova, G. (1969) The influence of activity on some contractile characteristics of mammalian fast and slow muscles. *J. Physiol.*, 201: 535–549.

Totosy de Zepetnek, J.E., Zung, H.V., Erdebil, S. and Gordon, T. (1992) Innervation ratio is an important determinant of force in normal and reinnervated rat tibialis anterior muscles. *J. Neurophysiol.*, 67: 1385–1403.

Vrbova, G., Gordon, T. and Jones, R. (1995) *Nerve-Muscle Interaction*. 2nd Edn. Blackman & Hall, London.

Wuerker, R.B., McPhedran, A.M. and Henneman, E. (1965) Properties of motor units in a heterogeneous pale muscle (m.gastrocnemius) of the cat. *J. Neurophysiol.*, 29: 85–99.

Zengel, J.E., Reid, S.A., Sypert, G.W. and Munson, J.B. (1985) Membrane electrical properties and prediction of motor-unit type of medial gastrocnemius motoneurons in the cat. *J. Neurophysiol.*, 53: 1323–1344.

M.D. Binder (Ed.)
Progress in Brain Research, Vol 123
© 1999 Elsevier Science BV. All rights reserved.

CHAPTER 18

Motor cortical control of human masticatory muscles

Michael A. Nordstrom,* Timothy S. Miles, Benjamin R. Gooden, Sophie L. Butler, Michael C. Ridding and Philip D. Thompson[1]

Departments of Physiology and [1] Medicine, University of Adelaide, Adelaide SA 5005, Australia

Introduction

The trigeminally innervated masticatory muscles elevate and depress the mandible, and are involved in chewing, swallowing and speech. The motor cortex has been implicated in the initiation and subsequent control of movement of the mandible through descending corticobulbar projections to the trigeminal motor nuclei (reviewed by Luschei and Goldberg, 1981), but there are few details on the organization or operation of this pathway in humans. Anatomical evidence in humans suggests that these projections are bilateral and symmetric (Kuypers, 1958). Evidence obtained with unilateral focal transcranial magnetic stimulation (TMS) in humans suggests that corticobulbar projections are bilateral to masseter (jaw-closing) muscles (Carr et al., 1994). Corticobulbar projections to human digastric (jaw-opener) muscles have been studied with TMS in only one previous report (Cruccu et al., 1989), but the use of a circular coil in this and other studies of masticatory muscles with TMS (Benecke et al. 1988; Cruccu et al. 1989; Macaluso et al. 1990; Türk et al. 1994) means that TMS activation of both hemispheres cannot be excluded as a cause of bilateral muscle evoked potentials (MEPs). An additional complication for the anterior digastric muscle is that in rats it appears that a single muscle has motor axons arising from the

motoneuron pool on each side, as judged by horseradish peroxidase staining (Kemplay and Cavanagh, 1983). It is not known if this arrangement exists in humans; however if it does the existence of bilateral MEPs in digastric muscles following unilateral TMS would not necessarily indicate a bilateral cortical projection to the digastric motor nuclei. For this reason, analysis of single motor unit responses to TMS are needed to demonstrate a bilateral corticobulbar projection to the digastric motor nucleus.

In the present study we have used unilateral focal transcranial magnetic stimulation (TMS) to examine the nature of the projections from motor cortex to jaw-closer (masseter) and jaw-opener (anterior digastric) motoneuron pools in humans. Responses evoked by TMS in masseter and anterior digastric muscles were studied at both the whole-muscle and single motor unit level to provide information regarding: (a) the existence of bilateral projections to the motor pools from a single hemisphere; (b) the relative strength of excitatory projections from the ipsi- and contralateral hemisphere; (c) the capacity for differential control of a single motor pool via the corticobulbar projection from each hemisphere; and (d) the nature of the corticobulbar projections to trigeminal motoneurons (mono- or oligosynaptic).

Methods

Seventeen subjects (10 F, 7 M, aged from 20 to 51 years) participated in the masseter experiments, and

*Corresponding author. Tel.: + 61 8 8303 4567;
Fax: + 61 8 8303 3356;
e-mail: Michael.nordstrom@adelaide.edu.au

12 (4 F, 8 M) for digastric. Some subjects were examined on several occasions. Subjects had no history of neurological disorders and all gave informed consent. Experiments were conducted with the approval of the Human Research Ethics Committee at the University of Adelaide.

Apparatus and recording

Experiments on digastric and masseter muscles were performed in separate sessions. The surface electromyogram (EMG) of the left and right masseter muscles was recorded using self-adhesive, gel-filled bipolar Ag/AgCl electrodes in 17 subjects. For single motor unit recording in four subjects, Teflon™-insulated fine-wire electrodes (45 μm core diameter) were inserted into the muscle. For the anterior digastric muscles, surface EMG activity was recorded bilaterally with Ag/AgCl electrodes in initial experiments on five subjects. The active electrode was placed over the anterior third of the muscle belly and the reference electrode adjacent to the inferior border of the mandible. In a further seven subjects, intramuscular EMG activity was also recorded from the anterior digastric muscles bilaterally using Teflon™-insulated fine-wire electrodes (45 μm core diameter with 2 mm insulation removed from the tip). Single motor unit activity was recorded with similar electrodes bared only at the tips. The localisation of the electrodes was checked by observing the EMG when subjects performed a series of jaw opening and tongue protrusion tasks. When the electrode tips were in the anterior digastric muscle, high-amplitude EMG activity occurred during jaw opening but not during tongue protrusion. In two subjects, following recording of responses in digastric elicited by TMS applied to each hemisphere, the right mandibular nerve was blocked by the injection of 2.2 ml local anaesthetic (2% Xylocaine®) near the mandibular foramen. Paralysis of the right anterior digastric muscle was confirmed by complete absence of intramuscular EMG in the muscle during forceful isometric jaw opening. The TMS studies were then repeated.

Focal TMS was used to activate the motor cortex of one hemisphere. This was achieved using a magnetic stimulator (Magstim model 200) and a figure-of-eight stimulating coil with outer coil diameters of 9.5 cm. The stimulus artefact was suppressed by a special-purpose EMG amplifier in which the gain was reduced to unity during the period 1 ms before to 2 ms after the discharge of the stimulator. EMG signals were amplified ($1000\times$) and recorded on video tape (Data Recorder model 400 PCM, A.R. Vetter Co., Pennsylvania, USA) at sampling rates of 22 kHz per channel. For off-line analysis, the surface EMG signals were filtered (20 Hz to 1 kHz) and digitised on a personal computer. The spike trains of single motor units were discriminated with a computer-based, template matching algorithm (SPS–8701E, Signal Processing Systems, Malvern, South Australia).

Protocol

Subjects were seated comfortably in front of two oscilloscopes which provided visual feedback of the EMG of the left and right masseter or digastric muscles. In masseter surface EMG experiments, subjects bit with their teeth together in normal occlusion at 10% of maximal EMG levels. For digastric experiments, subjects were either at rest, or contracting against a resistance placed under the chin, to 10% of maximal EMG. The stimulating coil was placed over the face area of motor cortex of one hemisphere at the optimal location for producing a MEP in the active masseter or digastric muscles. Threshold TMS intensity for a MEP was determined with the muscles at rest and active.

In masseter experiments, left and right masseter muscles were co-contracted to a level of 10% maximal EMG while TMS were delivered (<0.2 s^{-1}). Fifty trials were averaged to produce the mean MEP in each masseter muscle. TMS intensity was 5–15% above active threshold. For digastric muscles the MEPs were more prominent, and MEP onset latency and peak-to-peak amplitude were measured for each trial, and averaged over 15 stimuli for both rest and active conditions.

In motor unit experiments, subjects maintained a tonic contraction of a masseter or digastric motor unit at a comfortable firing rate (in the range 8–20 Hz) with the aid of visual feedback of the smoothed discharge frequency. TMS were delivered (<0.2

s^{-1}) under computer control during periods in which the subject controlled the motor unit within acceptable limits (usually ± 2 Hz) of the target rate. Stimulus timing was incremented on successive trials in 1- or 2-ms steps with respect to the last firing time of the motor unit. The number of stimuli delivered per run (commonly 30–50) varied depending on the motor unit mean discharge rate (see Nordstrom et al., 1995 for a more detailed explanation of the stimulation protocol).

Results

Responses in digastric muscles to focal TMS

Depending on the position of the coil, TMS evoked two different responses in the anterior digastric muscles. The first occurred at short latency (2.7 ± 0.3 ms, $n = 12$) and was particularly prominent when the coil was held in more lateral scalp positions. It was observed in both the ipsilateral and contralateral surface EMG electrodes in all subjects, but only in the ipsilateral muscle with intramuscular recordings. The amplitude of the contralateral response in the surface EMG was always smaller. These responses were stable in onset latency, amplitude and waveform with repeated stimuli and were not affected by contrac-

tion of the anterior digastric muscles. Figure 1 shows an example in which the short-latency responses were recorded without the usual concurrent longer-latency response. These responses were often elicited at stimulus intensities as low as 20% of maximal stimulator output, and increased in amplitude as the stimulator intensity was increased. These responses in the ipsilateral muscle were considered to arise from stimulation of the ipsilateral trigeminal motor root, and following the terminology of Cruccu et al. (1989) these were denoted rMEPs. On the basis of other evidence (see below), responses in contralateral digastric at the same latency in the surface EMG records were considered to be cross-talk from the neighbouring ipsilateral digastric muscle.

Longer-latency responses at about 10 ms were evoked in digastric muscles of all subjects when the coil was placed more medially (Fig. 2A). The responses were always observed bilaterally in the surface EMGs, regardless of whether the muscles were relaxed or contracted. They were usually polyphasic, and varied markedly in latency, amplitude and shape from trial to trial in both the relaxed and contracting muscles. The mean onset latency of the contralateral MEPs was approximately 0.3 ms longer than that of the ipsilateral MEP in both the relaxed (10.4 ± 1.3 ms vs. 10.1 ± 1.5 ms) and

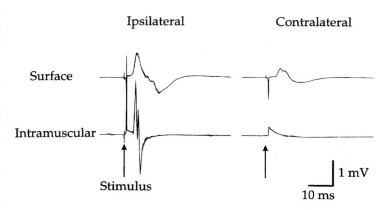

Fig. 1. Short-latency, direct motor responses evoked by TMS of the left motor cortex in left and right anterior digastric muscles in a representative subject. The responses were recorded in the surface and intramuscular EMG of relaxed anterior digastric muscles. The coil was positioned 4 cm anterior and 12 cm lateral to the vertex with the stimulator intensity at 50% of maximum output. In these and in all subsequent records, the stimulus artefact was suppressed electronically: the decay of the residual artefact can still be seen in, e.g. the lower right panel. Arrows indicate the time of stimulus onset. Four consecutive trials are superimposed. The short-latency motor potentials appeared in the surface EMG records on both sides but only in the ipsilateral intramuscular EMG record. These are direct motor responses from activation of the ipsilateral trigeminal motor nerve. (Modified from Gooden et al., 1999)

contracted states (7.7 ± 1.1 ms vs. 7.3 ± 1.0 ms); this difference between sides was significant when data from both activation states were combined (ANOVA, P < 0.05). The mean amplitude of the contralateral MEPs was larger than the ipsilateral responses in relaxed (0.13 ± 0.07 mV vs. 0.10 ± 0.04 mV) and contracted states (0.46 ± 0.31 mV vs. 0.36 ± 0.24 mV), and differences between sides were significant when data from both activation states were combined (ANOVA, P < 0.05). ANOVA revealed that muscular contraction increased the amplitude of both the ipsilateral and contralateral MEPs (P < 0.05), and significantly shortened the mean onset latency by approximately 3 ms (P < 0.05).

In six of the seven subjects in whom intramuscular recordings were made, the MEPs evoked by TMS were bilateral when the anterior digastric muscles were relaxed (Fig. 2B). In one subject responses were exclusively ipsilateral. However, with contraction of the anterior digastric muscles, responses were bilateral in all seven subjects. The short-latency (~ 3 ms) responses were seen only in the ipsilateral muscle with intramuscular recording (e.g. Fig. 2).

Cross-talk in surface EMG recordings from digastric muscle

In the surface EMG records from digastric muscles, MEPs were invariably seen on the left and right

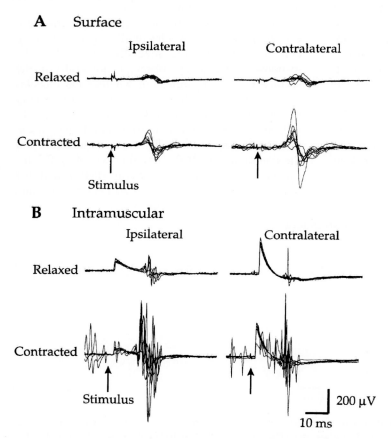

Fig. 2. Bilateral MEPs in anterior digastric muscles. A, surface EMG records from relaxed and contracted muscles, showing MEPs evoked by TMS. The coil was placed at the optimal site over the left cortex, and the stimulus intensity was 1.2 × resting threshold. Ten consecutive trials are superimposed. B. Intramuscular records for the same 10 trials. Note the appearance of the MEPs bilaterally in both the surface and the intramuscular records, and their facilitation by weak isometric contraction. (Modified from Gooden et al., 1999)

sides simultaneously. However, in intramuscular recordings, MEPs sometimes appeared in one muscle but not simultaneously in the other. To determine whether the electrical signal from one muscle was spreading to the other, in two subjects (three motor units) the action potentials of a single motor unit triggered an average of the signals recorded from surface and intramuscular electrodes of both anterior digastric muscles. This process reveals the magnitude of a given signal generated in one digastric muscle, in the surface and intra-muscular EMG of both muscles. Figure 3 shows that the motor unit action potential from one digastric muscle contributed to the surface EMG potential of both the ipsi- and contra-lateral digastric muscles: the average contribution was about 60% smaller over the contralateral muscle. However, these action potentials were not detectable in the average from the contralateral intramuscular electrode.

The appearance in the surface EMG of the contralateral digastric muscle of action potentials that clearly originated in the ipsilateral muscle is direct evidence of cross-talk in the surface EMGs: that is, the electrical activity of one muscle is recorded in the surface EMG over both muscles. On the other hand, because the electrical activity

from one digastric did not appear in the con-tralateral intramuscular recording, there was no cross-talk between the intramuscular recordings, nor did the motoneuron of the triggering motor unit innervate muscle fibres in digastric on the opposite side. To ensure that the apparently bilateral responses in digastric muscles were not the result of volume conduction, the motor nerve to the right digastric was blocked by local anaesthetic in two subjects. During complete motor block of the right digastric, MEPs could still be elicited intra-muscularly in the left digastric by focal TMS of either the left or right hemisphere, while no MEP was present in the intramuscular recording from the right digastric muscle.

Responses of digastric single motor units to focal TMS

Seventeen digastric motor units were tested with contralateral TMS and 14 with ipsilateral TMS. Figure 4 shows the most common pattern of responses to TMS applied to the ipsi- or con-tralateral motor cortex at two different stimulus intensities, while the subject maintained a tonic discharge in the motor unit. An excitatory response beginning around 10 ms is evoked by stimulation of

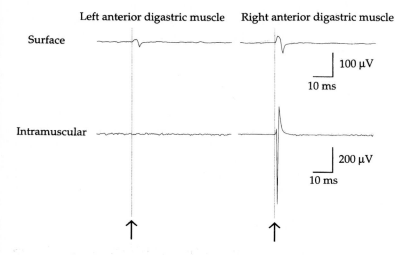

Fig. 3. Evidence for cross-talk between the two anterior digastric muscles. The records are averages of the signals recorded from left and right surface and intramuscular digastric electrodes, triggered by 250 spikes from a tonically-activated single motor unit in the right digastric muscle at the arrows. Note that the amplitude of the averaged signal in the surface EMG over the left digastric is about 40% of the amplitude over the parent muscle. However, the average of the signal recorded intramuscularly in the left muscle shows no sign of the motor unit potential. (Modified from Gooden et al., 1999)

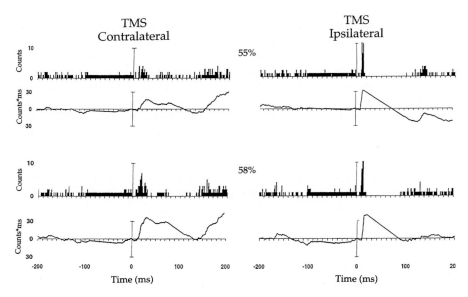

Fig. 4. Bilateral activation of a single digastric motor unit by TMS at two stimulus intensities. The PSTHs and CUSUMs show that this motor unit was activated at corticobulbar latency in a stimulus-dependent manner by stimulation of the left and right motor cortices (upper records, 55%; lower records, 58% maximal stimulator output). However, the response to ipsilateral stimulation was stronger, with less temporal dispersion than the contralateral response. (Modified from Gooden et al., 1999)

either hemisphere, and is larger at the higher stimulus intensity. The pattern of responses elicited in digastric motor units by TMS are summarised in Table 1. Contralateral TMS evoked an excitatory response in all 17 digastric motor units tested. Of these, 11 were also excited by ipsilateral stimulation (e.g. Fig. 4), one was inhibited by ipsilateral stimulation (Fig. 5), and two did not respond to ipsilateral stimulation. Three motor units were not tested with ipsilateral stimulation. The ipsilateral projection was more secure than the contralateral in

TABLE 1

Summary of responses of masseter and digastric motor units to focal TMS applied to either hemisphere

	TMS CONTRALATERAL			TMS IPSILATERAL		
	MU response (%)			MU response (%)		
	+	nil	−	+	nil	−
Digastric motor units	100	0	0	79	14	7
		(n = 17)			(n = 14)	
Masseter motor units	79	13	8	29	0	71
		(n = 24)			(n = 14)	

+, excitation; nil, no effect; −, inhibition

the 11 motor units that were excited bilaterally, as judged by a higher probability of response to ipsilateral stimulation at a given intensity, and the lower temporal dispersion. As illustrated in Fig. 4, the typical excitatory responses to contralateral stimulation were dispersed over about 10 ms, whereas the ipsilateral responses were dispersed over 5 ms or less.

It was not usually possible to obtain stimulus-response data for a motor unit over a broad range of stimulus strengths because of recruitment of other motor units at higher stimulus intensities. However, this was achieved for the digastric motor unit whose responses are shown in Fig. 5. Its threshold to contralateral TMS was between 35–40% of the maximum stimulator output. The CUSUMs reveal a progressive increase in the excitatory response of this motor unit as the contralateral stimulus intensity is increased, but even with the strongest stimulus (49%), the excitatory response was dispersed over more than 10 ms. No clear response to ipsilateral stimulation was seen until the intensity was increased to 49% where there was a suggestion of a period of reduced firing probability in the CUSUM, beginning at 9 ms. Stronger stimuli increased the duration of this silent period, which was not preceded by an excitatory response.

Responses in masseter muscles to focal TMS

TMS never produced a MEP in resting masseter muscles. Data from one subject illustrating the usual appearance of MEPs in both masseter muscles during a bilateral bite are shown in Fig. 6. In all subjects ($n = 17$), focal stimulation of the motor cortex produced a MEP in the active masseter muscle contralateral to the stimulated hemisphere. The average onset latency for this response was 7.0 ± 0.3 ms. This is consistent with a

cortical origin (Cruccu et al., 1989). In some subjects a response occurred at around 2 ms in the ipsilateral masseter, which was considered to arise from direct stimulation of the ipsilateral trigeminal motor root (rMEP). When present, the rMEP obscured responses in the ipsilateral masseter occurring at a latency consistent with cortical activation. In 12 subjects it was possible to obtain a MEP in ipsilateral masseter without contamination from an ipsilateral rMEP. The ipsilateral MEP had a mean onset latency of 6.7 ± 0.3 ms, which was not significantly different from the contralateral MEP obtained during the same bilateral biting task in

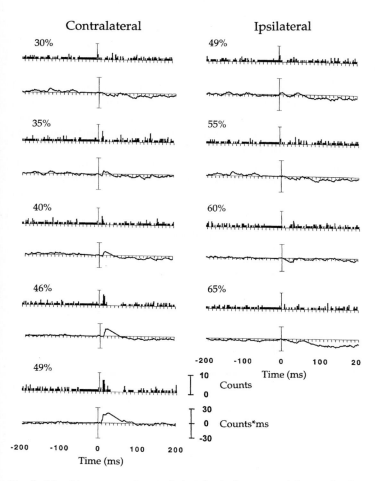

Fig. 5. Stimulus-response characteristics of a single motor unit in anterior digastric. The responses of this unit to a wide range of TMS stimulus intensities are presented as the PSTHs and CUSUMs. The motor unit was excited in a stimulus-dependent manner by contralateral TMS. Ipsilateral stimulation inhibited the same unit at a similar latency, also in a stimulus-dependent manner, but only at stronger stimulus intensities. Same calibrations for all records. (Modified from Gooden et al., 1999)

210

these subjects (6.7 ± 0.3 ms (ipsilateral) vs. 6.6 ± 0.3 ms (contralateral); paired *t*-test, $p > 0.05$, $n = 12$). These ipsilateral responses were also

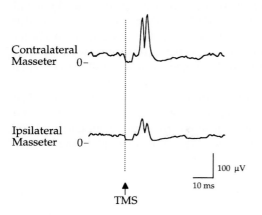

Fig. 6. Data from one subject showing averaged MEPs from surface EMG recordings of masseter following focal unilateral TMS. Traces are rectified and averaged ($n = 50$) surface EMG records with stimulus timing indicated by the arrows. An artifact suppressing amplifier gated the signal 1 ms before the stimulus, and for 2 ms afterwards. TMS intensity was 50% of maximal output. The subject activated both masseter muscles at approximately 10% of maximal contraction by performing a bilateral clench on the posterior teeth. In this example, the contralateral MEP is 80% larger than the response in the ipsilateral muscle.

considered to be cortical in origin. Contralateral and ipsilateral MEPs had a similar threshold for TMS activation during bilateral biting. TMS intensities in the trials used for analysis were 40–70% of maximum stimulator output.

With bilateral biting, the MEP was larger in the contralateral masseter in 10 of 12 subjects. When the MEP was normalised to background EMG activity the normalised MEP contralateral to the hemisphere stimulated was larger than the ipsilateral MEP in every subject. In the pooled data, the mean size of the contralateral MEP was 39% larger than the ipsilateral response during bilateral biting ($0.71 ± 0.07$ mV.ms vs. $0.51 ± 0.09$ mV.ms; paired *t*-test, $p < 0.005$, $n = 12$).

Responses of masseter single motor units to focal TMS

Figure 7 shows the most common pattern of responses in masseter single motor units to focal TMS applied to each hemisphere. With contralateral TMS there was a short-latency excitation beginning at around 6 ms, whose probability of discharge increased with increasing stimulus strength. The probability of an excitatory response in masseter motor units was generally less than that

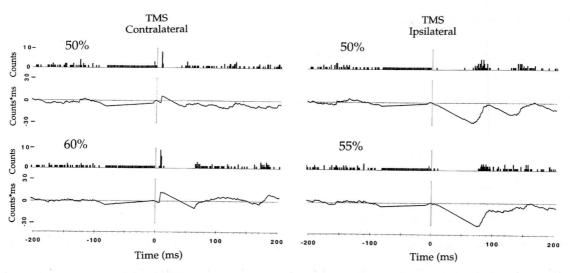

Fig. 7. Responses of a masseter single motor unit to focal TMS applied to either hemisphere. The PSTHs and CUSUMs show that this motor unit was excited at corticobulbar latency in a stimulus-dependent manner by stimulation of the contralateral motor cortex (left; 50% and 60% of maximal stimulator output), while stimulation of the ipsilateral hemisphere (right; 50% and 55% maximum output) produced a silent period lasting 70–80 ms without short-latency excitation.

seen in digastric motor units tested at comparable TMS intensities. The duration of excitatory peaks with contralateral stimulation were invariably brief (< 5 ms). In the example shown in Fig. 7, no short-latency excitatory response was evoked by ipsilateral TMS, rather a clear reduction in motor unit discharge probability (silent period) for up to 70 ms. The duration of the silent period increased with stimulus intensity.

The pattern of responses for masseter motor units is summarised in Table 1. With contralateral TMS, 19 of 24 motor units (79%) were excited, 3 of 24 (13%) did not respond at the intensities tested (which were suprathreshold for whole muscle responses), and 2 of 24 had reduced firing probabilities. With ipsilateral TMS, 4 of 14 motor units (29%) showed short-latency excitation, while firing probability was reduced in 10 of 14 (71%).

Discussion

Corticotrigeminal projections are bilateral, but not symmetrical

Several other groups have reported bilateral responses in human masticatory muscles using TMS which are consistent with activation of a fast corticobulbar pathway (Benecke et al., 1988; Cruccu et al., 1989; Macaluso et al., 1990; Carr et al., 1994; Türk et al., 1994). TMS-evoked responses in digastric have been mentioned briefly in only one report (Cruccu et al., 1989), while the others have included investigation of masseter muscles. In all but one of the previous studies (Carr et al., 1994), a circular coil was used over the vertex. This does not provide unequivocal evidence for a bilateral corticotrigeminal projection as activation of both hemispheres by TMS cannot be excluded (see for example, Fig. 6 in Cruccu et al., 1989). Carr et al. (1994) observed a bilateral response in masseter muscles using a figure–8 coil and focal TMS applied to one hemisphere. We confirm this result for masseter, and extend it to include anterior digastric muscles. In rats the anterior digastric muscle is innervated by motor axons arising from the motoneuron pool on each side, most likely from separate populations of ipsi- and contralaterally projecting motoneurons (Kemplay and Cavanagh, 1983). We found no evidence

using spike-triggered averaging that single motor neurons in humans innervate muscle fibres in the digastric muscle of both sides. If the arrangement described for rats were to exist in humans, the existence of bilateral MEPs in digastric muscles following unilateral TMS as we have observed would not necessarily indicate a bilateral cortical projection to the digastric motor nuclei. Our single motor unit data, however, provide definitive proof of a bilateral corticobulbar projection to human digastric motoneurones. The majority (11 of 14) of anterior digastric single motor units were excited at fast corticobulbar latency by stimulation of either hemisphere. These functional results are supported by anatomical evidence that corticobulbar fibres project bilaterally to the trigeminal motor nuclei (Kuypers, 1958; Iwatsubo et al., 1990). They are also consistent with the observation that bilateral responses can be elicited in jaw muscles by direct unilateral electrical stimulation of the masticatory area of human and primate motor cortex (Penfield and Boldrey, 1937; Clark and Luschei, 1974).

We found ultra-short latency responses (~ 2–3 ms) in surface EMG recordings from ipsilateral masseter and in digastric muscles on both sides following TMS when the coil was positioned laterally. Similar short-latency responses following TMS have been reported in other ipsilateral muscles supplied by the trigeminal (Benecke et al., 1988; Cruccu et al., 1989) and facial (Meyer et al., 1994) nerves. These responses were only found ipsilaterally in intramuscular recordings from digastric, and together with the demonstration of significant cross-talk in digastric surface EMG recordings (Fig. 3), led to the conclusion that responses in surface EMG recordings from contralateral digastric were due to pick-up from the ipsilateral muscle. These short-latency responses therefore occurred exclusively in the ipsilateral muscles, and are consistent with stimulation of the motor root of the ipsilateral trigeminal nerve near the foramen ovale (Cruccu, 1986). The absence of responses at 2–3 ms in the contralateral digastric following ipsilateral motor root stimulation is further evidence that single motor axons do not branch to both digastric muscles. If this were the case, the antidromic action potential would produce a response in contralateral digastric muscle.

On the basis of anatomical evidence (Kuypers, 1958), the corticobulbar projection to trigeminal motor nuclei in humans is considered to be bilateral and relatively symmetric. However recent work in normal subjects (Cruccu et al., 1989) and stroke patients (Cruccu et al., 1988) suggests that the contralateral corticobulbar projection predominates for masseter. Using focal TMS, Carr et al. (1994) reported masseter MEPs were 85% larger in the contralateral muscle, but differences between sides were not significant in their sample of seven subjects. Asymmetry of the cortical projection to digastric has not previously been studied in humans. In the present study, MEPs elicited in active muscles by focal TMS were on average 28% larger in digastric and 39% larger in masseter muscles contralateral to the hemisphere stimulated than those found in homologous ipsilateral muscles. Responses in digastric motor units were usually fairly similar with TMS applied to either hemisphere, although slightly larger with ipsilateral stimulation (Fig. 4). However, the larger amplitude of the contralateral MEPs in both the relaxed and contracted states, and the observation that all motor units tested were excited by contralateral stimulation indicates that the corticobulbar projection to the contralateral anterior digastric motoneuronal pool is stronger overall. For the masseter muscle, asymmetry of the cortical projection revealed in the surface EMG records was even more prominent in the sample of low-threshold motor units studied with TMS. The majority (79%) of masseter units tested were excited by TMS of the contralateral hemisphere, whereas with ipsilateral stimulation only 29% were excited, and 71% were inhibited.

Nature of responses elicited by TMS in masseter and anterior digastric muscles

In the present study the mean onset latency of MEPs elicited by TMS in active digastric muscles was 7.7 ± 1.1 ms in the contralateral muscles and 7.3 ± 1.0 ms ipsilaterally. Comparable values for masseter were 6.6 ± 0.3 ms vs. 6.7 ± 0.3 ms. These values are in agreement with latencies reported in other studies of trigeminal muscles using TMS (Cruccu et al., 1989; Macaluso et al., 1990; Türk et al., 1994) and are consistent with conduction via a fast corticobulbar projection (Cruccu et al., 1989). The increased latency for digastric compared with masseter is attributed to the longer path of the peripheral nerve to digastric. In rats and cats the corticobulbar projections do not terminate directly on trigeminal motor neurons in the pons, but pass to premotor interneurons in the reticular formation (Phillips and Porter, 1977). Using TMS in humans, Cruccu et al. (1989) calculated that the central delay at the trigeminal motoneuron synapse(s) was between 1.1 and 1.4 ms, leaving time for no more than two synapses. They argued that since the duration and latency variability of masseter MEPs were even shorter than for active hand muscles which are served by direct corticomotoneuronal (CM) connections, that at least some corticobulbar fibres project directly onto trigeminal motoneurons. Our motor unit data support this view. TMS produced excitatory peaks in PSTH of masseter motor units (stimulation of either hemisphere) and digastric motor units (ipsilateral hemisphere) that were brief (< 5 ms), with temporal dispersion similar to peaks in published data from motor units of intrinsic hand muscles, which are known to have strong corticomotoneuronal projections (cf. Day et al., 1989). The greater temporal dispersion (over about 10 ms) and the less secure excitatory responses of single motor units in digastric with TMS of the contralateral hemisphere suggests that the descending input may traverse at least one additional synapse en route to the contralateral digastric motor nucleus.

Masseter single motor units were frequently excited when stimulated from the contralateral hemisphere, and showed a reduction in firing probability when the ipsilateral hemisphere was stimulated with TMS. This suggests a degree of differential control of masseter motoneurons from each hemisphere. It appears that low-threshold motor units in masseter receive predominantly contralateral excitatory projections from motor cortex. The nature of the ipsilateral silent period elicited by TMS in masseter motor units is not clear. Components at various latencies could arise from inhibition of cortical neurons following TMS (Kujirai et al., 1993), an inhibitory reflex due to activation of cutaneous receptors on the scalp (Cruccu et al., 1986), or noise from the discharge of the stimulator (Meier-Ewert et al., 1974). The latter does not appear to be an important consideration, as our preliminary studies have shown that the masseter silent period following TMS is not altered by auditory masking.

Functional implications

The cortical projections to motoneurons innervating the hand and limbs are overwhelmingly contralateral, and associated with precise control of the muscles moving the limbs and digits. The present study has provided evidence of a bilateral projection from the motor cortex to anterior digastric and masseter motoneurons. However, particularly for masseter, the excitatory projection is not to all motoneurons on both sides. The excitatory bilateral projections probably account for the observation that, in contrast to the limbs, motor function is usually relatively well-preserved bilaterally in the muscles of mastication following unilateral lesions of the human and monkey primary motor cortex (Luschei and Goodwin, 1975; Willoughby and Anderson, 1984; Cruccu et al., 1988).

The anterior digastric muscles in concert with their facial nerve-innervated posterior bellies, depress the mandible during mastication and speech and raise the hyoid bone during swallowing. While the digastric muscles are clearly subject to precise control in speech and mastication, they are said to be co-activated in parallel during all basic jaw movements (Widmalm et al., 1988). The observation that an anterior digastric motoneuron may be excited by TMS activation of the contralateral hemisphere and inhibited by ipsilateral TMS (Fig. 5), suggests that the cortex has the capacity to contribute to independent activation of anterior digastric muscles on each side. Perhaps this might serve to to tilt the hyoid bone in some situations. In contrast to the digastric muscles, the masseter muscles on each side are more commonly activated independently during mastication (Luschei and Goldberg, 1981). The masseter motor nucleus receives a bilateral excitatory projection from motor cortex, which is considerably stronger from the contralateral hemisphere. Most (71%) of the low-threshold masseter motor units we studied

did not receive excitatory projections from the ipsilateral hemisphere. This organisation of cortical inputs to masseter motor nuclei provides the capacity for each hemisphere to contribute to independent activation of the masseter muscles on each side, particularly at low bite forces. This may be necessary for controlled biting on one side when food is held between the teeth.

Summary and conclusions

The corticotrigeminal projections to masseter and anterior digastric motoneuron pools that are activated by TMS are bilateral, but not symmetrical. This conclusion is supported by whole-muscle data showing larger MEPs in the contralateral muscle with unilateral focal TMS, as well as evidence that TMS stimulation of one hemisphere may produce excitation in a masseter or digastric single motor unit while stimulation of the opposite hemisphere produced inhibition of the same motor unit. The asymmetry is particularly marked for masseter, in which the low-threshold motor units were most commonly excited with contralateral TMS and inhibited with ipsilateral TMS. Spike-triggered averaging of digastric motor unit activity revealed cross-talk in surface EMG recordings from digastric muscles, and no evidence that muscle fibres in both digastric muscles were innervated by a common motor axon. Narrow excitatory peaks in the PSTH of motor unit discharge elicited by TMS in masseter (either hemisphere) and digastric motor units (ipsilateral hemisphere) suggest a direct corticomotoneuronal projection. The contralateral projection to digastric motoneurons may include additional oligosynaptic connections, as judged by the broader peaks in the PSTH with contralateral TMS. The organisation of bilateral corticotrigeminal inputs revealed with TMS suggests that: (a) the contralateral hemisphere provides relatively more of the excitatory input delivered via the fast corticotrigeminal pathway for both masseter and digastric motoneuron pools, and (b) corticotrigeminal projections from either hemisphere are capable of contributing to the voluntary command mediating activation of masseter, and (to a lesser extent) anterior digastric muscles on one side, that is independent of the homologous muscles on the other side.

214

Acknowledgments

We thank Christopher Wallace who assisted with some of the analyses. SB was supported by the Benjamin Poulton Scholarship of the Faculty of Medicine, University of Adelaide. This research was supported by a Project Grant (960485) from the NH&MRC of Australia.

References

Benecke, R., Meyer, B.-U., Schonle, P. and Conrad, B. (1988) Transcranial magnetic stimulation of the human brain: responses in muscles supplied by cranial nerves. *Exp. Brain Res.*, 71: 623–632.

Carr, L.J., Harrison, L.M. and Stephens, J.A. (1994) Evidence for bilateral innervation of certain homologous motoneurone pools in man. *J. Physiol.*, 475: 217–227.

Clark, R.W. and Luschei, E.S. (1974) Short-latency jaw movement produced by low intensity intracortical microstimulation of the precentral face area in monkeys. *Brain Res.*, 70: 144–147.

Cruccu, G. (1986) Intracranial stimulation of the trigeminal nerve in man. I. Direct motor responses. *J. Neurol. Neurosurg. Psychiat.*, 49: 411–418.

Cruccu, G., Agostino, R., Lahuerta, J. and Manfredi, M. (1986) Inhibition of jaw-closing muscles by electrical stimulation of the opthalmic division in man. *Brain Res.*, 371: 298–304.

Cruccu, G., Berardelli, A., Inghilleri, M. and Manfredi, M. (1989) Functional organisation of the trigeminal motor system in man. A neurophysiological study. *Brain*, 112: 1333–1350.

Cruccu, G., Fornarelli, M. and Manfredi, M. (1988) Impairment of masticatory function in hemiplegia. *Neurology*, 38: 301–306.

Day, B.L., Dressler, D., Maertens de Noordhout, A., Marsden, C.D., Nakashima, K., Rothwell, J.C. and Thompson, P.D. (1989) Electrical and magnetic stimulation of human motor cortex: surface EMG and single motor unit responses. *J. Physiol.*, 412: 449–473.

Gooden, B.R., Ridding, M.C., Miles, T.S., Nordstrom, M.A. and Thompson, P.D. (1999) Bilateral cortical control of the human anterior digastric muscles. *Exp. Brain Res.*, in press.

Iwatsubo, T., Kuzuhara, S., Kanemitsu, A., Shimada, H. and Toyokura, Y. (1990) Corticofugal projections to the motor nuclei of the brainstem and spinal cord in humans. *Neurology*, 40: 309–312.

Kemplay, S. and Cavanagh, J.B. (1983) Bilateral innervation of the anterior digastric muscle by trigeminal motoneurons. *J. Anat.*, 136: 417–423.

Kuypers, H.G.J.M. (1958) Cortico-bulbar connexions to the pons and lower brain-stem in man. An anatomical study. *Brain*, 81: 364–388.

Kujirai, T., Caramia, M.D., Rothwell, J.C., Day, B.L., Thompson, P.D., Frebert, A., Wroe, S., Asselman, P. and Marsden, C.D. (1993) Corticocortical inhibition in human motor cortex. *J. Physiol.*, 471: 501–519.

Luschei, E.S. and Goldberg, L.J. (1981) Neural mechanisms of mandibular control: mastication and voluntary biting. In: V.B. Brooks (Ed.), *Handbook of Physiology*, Section 1: *The Nervous System, Volume II, Motor Control, Part II.*, Williams and Wilkins, Baltimore USA, pp. 1237–1274.

Luschei, E.S. and Goodwin, G.M. (1975) Role of monkey precentral cortex in control of voluntary jaw movements. *J. Neurophysiol.*, 38: 146–157.

Macaluso, G.M., Pavesi, G., Bonanini, M., Mancia, D. and Gennari, P.U. (1990) Motor-evoked potentials in masseter muscle by electrical and magnetic stimulation in intact alert man. *Arch. Oral Biol.*, 35: 623–628.

Meier-Ewert, K., Gleitsmann, K. and Reiter, F. (1974) Acoustic jaw reflex in man: its relationship to other brain-stem and microreflexes. *Electroenceph. clin. Neurophysiol.*, 36: 629–637.

Meyer, B.-U., Werhahn, K., Rothwell, J.C., Roericht, S. and Fauth, C. (1994) Functional organisation of corticonuclear pathways to motoneurones of lower facial muscles in man. *Exp. Brain Res.*, 101: 465–472.

Nordstrom, M.A., Mapletoft, E.A. and Miles, T.S. (1995) Spike-train acquisition, analysis and real-time experimental control using a graphical programming language (LabView®). *J. Neurosci. Meth.*, 62: 93–102.

Penfield, W. and Boldrey, E. (1937) Somatic motor and sensory representation in the cerebral cortex of man as studied by electrical stimulation. *Brain*, 60: 389–443.

Phillips, C.G. and Porter, R. (1977). *Corticospinal Neurones: Their Role in Movement.* Academic Press, New York.

Türk, Ü., Rösler, K.M., Mathis, J., Müllbacher, W. and Hess, C.W. (1994) Assessment of motor pathways to masticatory muscles: an examination technique using electrical and magnetic stimulation. *Muscle Nerve*, 17: 1271–1277.

Widmalm, S.-E., Lillie, J. H. and Ash Jr., M. M. (1988) Anatomical and electromyographic studies of the digastric muscle. *J. Oral Rehab.*, 15: 3–21.

Willoughby, E. W. and Anderson, N. E. (1984) Lower cranial nerve motor function in unilateral vascular lesions of the cerebral hemisphere. *BMJ*, 289: 791–794.

M.D. Binder (Ed.)
Progress in Brain Research, Vol 123
© 1999 Elsevier Science BV. All rights reserved.

CHAPTER 19

Do lengthening contractions represent a case of reversal in recruitment order?

Parveen Bawa[1] and Kelvin E. Jones*

Department of Physiology, University of Manitoba, Winnipeg, MB, R3E 3J7, Canada
[1]*School of Kinesiology, Simon Fraser University, Burnaby, BC, Canada*

Introduction

The central nervous system recruits spinal motoneurones in an orderly fashion under most of the experimental paradigms which have been tested (Stuart and Enoka, 1983; Cope and Clark, 1995). Experimental observations suggesting selective excitation/recruitment of larger motor units during electrical stimulation of cutaneous nerves (Kanda et al., 1977; Stephens et al., 1978), electrical stimulation of rubrospinal tract (Powers et al., 1993) and during lengthening contractions (Nardone et al., 1989; Howell et al., 1995) have been reported. One could argue that the results utilizing synchronous electrical stimulation of cutaneous nerves or the red nucleus, be interpreted as non-physiological. Instead, under physiological activation of these pathways, the preferential inhibition of small motoneurons by these pathways would change the slope of the recruitment curve (Kernell and Hultborn, 1990) instead of causing selective recruitment of large motoneurons. One still needs to think about the implications and mechanisms for the selective recruitment reported during lengthening contractions.

In the following paper we present data obtained with two different experimental paradigms both of which result in lengthening of active muscles. Our observations do not support selective recruitment of fast twitch motor units during lengthening contractions. Two main papers (Nardone et al., 1989; Howell et al., 1995) where single motor unit data have been produced and interpreted to suggest selective recruitment of large motor units will be central to the discussion.

Methods

Experiments were done on three adult subjects with no known neuromuscular disease and the Ethics Committee on Human Experiments at Simon Fraser University approved the experimental procedures.

The experimental set up was identical to that described in Calancie and Bawa (1985a). Briefly, the subject's forearm was supported on a horizontal platform in a semi prone position such that their wrist joint was coaxial with the shaft of a torque motor. The subject could voluntarily contract their wrist flexors against a load to produce isometric or shortening contractions, or allow his wrist joint to be extended such that the load produced a lengthening contraction of the actively contracting wrist flexors. Single motor unit (SMU) activity of flexor carpi radialis (FCR) muscle, surface EMG of wrist flexors, angular position of the wrist joint and torque produced at the level of the metacarpophalageal joint were recorded during each experiment.

Procedure: The subject was asked to recruit at least one clearly discernible motor unit, using

---
*Corresponding author: Tel.: 204–789–3305; Fax: 204–789–3930; e-mail: kelvin@scrc.umanitoba.ca

audio-visual feed back of the SMU signal, against a constant flexor load. Once a clear stable unit(s) was obtained one of the following two paradigms were carried out.

(a) *Constant load lengthening contractions*: A constant flexor load was applied by the torque motor against which the subject contracted the wrist flexors to recruit and repetitively fire at least one clear SMU. The subject then voluntarily relaxed against the flexor load allowing the load to extend their wrist thus producing a lengthening contraction of their wrist flexors.

(b) *Ramp load lengthening contractions*: The subject contracted their wrist isometrically against a flexor load firing at least one clear SMU. An additional ramp load was applied to the torque motor resulting in extension of the wrist thus producing a lengthening contraction of wrist flexors.

For paradigms (a) and (b), a wide range of velocities of wrist extension were produced. In (a) the velocity of lengthening contraction depended on the load, the inertia of the wrist and the subject's voluntary relaxation that allowed the wrist to be extended. In (b), the subject was asked not to recruit too many units by reacting strongly to the increased load, but to maintain effort at the initial level prior to the increase in load. Again the velocity of wrist extension was determined by the velocity and amplitude of ramp load, the inertia of the wrist and the subject's reaction.

All units firing in the background were relatively low threshold during isometric contractions (< 10 % of maximum voluntary contraction).

Results

For each of the two paradigms, a variety of firing patterns of motor units were obtained. Each pattern depended on the speed of wrist extension, the load extending the wrist and the voluntary reaction of the subject. None of these patterns included selective recruitment of high threshold units. (The term 'high threshold units' implies recruitment threshold of units under isometric conditions.)

(a) *Constant load lengthening contractions*: When the lengthening was relatively fast (approx

20°/200 ms), the motor units became silent (Fig. 1A, B) or there was a burst of activity during the later part of lengthening (Fig. 1C). The torque record in all cases showed a bell shaped curve. Initially there was a decrease in tension that was followed by an increase to 'brake' the movement at the end point of extension. Motor units were recruited during this braking and these units were not different from the background units. Depending on the speed of braking, extra higher threshold units were sometimes recruited in addition to the background units, however, these were the units that were next in rank to be recruited during isometric contraction. When lengthening was relatively slow we either saw a complete silencing of the motor units, or bursts of SMUs with bursts of EMG as reported by Nardone et al. (1989). During these bursts, SMUs firing in the background were recruited. When additional units were recruited these were the next units that would be recruited during isometric contractions. Whenever additional units were recruited, derecruitment of background units was never observed.

(b) *Ramp load lengthening contractions*: Motor unit firing patterns during lengthening depended on the speed and amplitude of the ramp load, and the voluntary reaction of the subject. Motor unit activity could be silenced (Fig. 2A), remain the same (Fig. 2B), or there was recruitment of additional units (Fig. 2C). We never observed derecruitment of background units in favor of additional units being recruited. The additional units recruited were the same ones that were next to be recruited during isometric contractions.

Discussion

In our study of lengthening contractions of wrist flexors, a range of motor unit firing patterns were observed during the lengthening phase. None of these patterns consisted of selective recruitment of large units that would generally be recruited at very high thresholds during isometric contractions.

During lengthening, a subject may allow the load to smoothly extend the contracting muscle in which case there is no need to recruit additional units, slow or fast. Slowing of motor unit firing and eventually, cessation of existing activity, generally accompany such lengthening contractions. If, however, the lengthening contraction is fast and of limited amplitude, there is a cessation of ongoing activity at the beginning of lengthening followed by

bursts of motor unit firing to brake the ongoing extension at the end point of the movement. Bursts of activity consist of the units that were firing in the background, with possible addition of higher thresholds units if the amplitude was large and

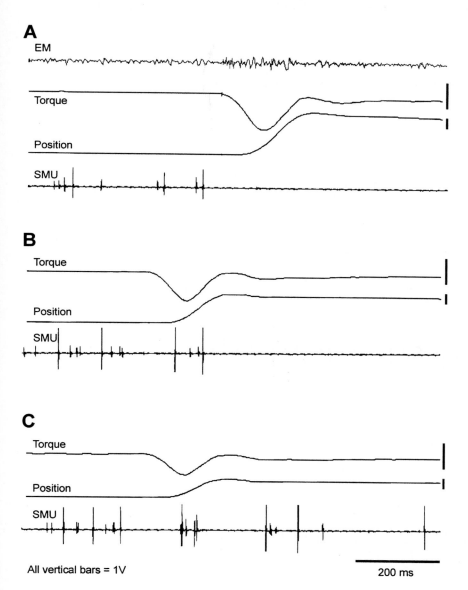

Fig. 1. The subject isometrically contracted wrist flexors against a constant flexor load. When asked by the experimenter, the subject relaxed to let the load extend their wrist thus producing a lengthening contraction of wrist flexors. Three different patterns of single motor units responses are shown during the lengthening phase: silence or silence followed by recruitment for braking the movement (C). During this re-recruitment phase, additional higher threshold units could be recruited (not shown), but not without the background units. 1 Volt = 8 deg for position trace.

218

speed of the extension fast. These higher threshold units are those that are next recruited during an isometric contraction.

If the lengthening is relatively slow, a smooth voluntary lengthening contraction is difficult. The position record may show smooth movement, but tension records show small, sharp 'braking' actions. That is, the lengthening contraction is full of 'hesitations' in the form of small, abrupt shortening contractions. As a consequence oscillatory activity is observed in tension and surface EMG. This oscillatory pattern recruits motor units

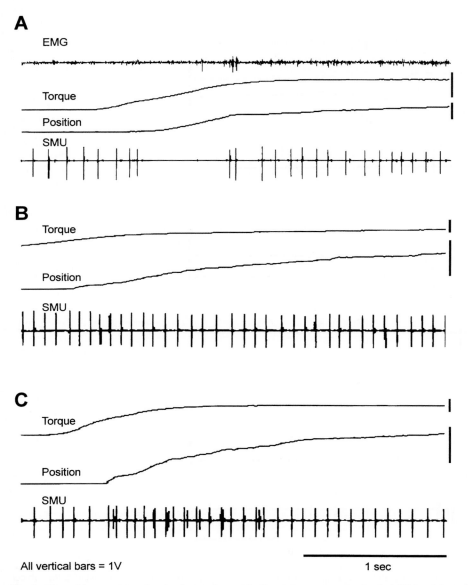

All vertical bars = 1V   1 sec

Fig. 2. The subject contracted wrist flexors isometrically against a constant load. Additional ramp load was superimposed to cause lengthening contractions. Three different patterns of motor unit firing are shown during the lengthening contractions phase. Recruitment of additional unit is seen during the lengthening phase, but no selective recruitment was seen which was accompanied by derecruitment of lower threshold background units.

219

in bursts, with both low and next higher threshold units. It has been argued that the lengthening contractions produced by torque motors are not equivalent to those produced by gravitational loads which were used by Nardone et al. (1989) and Howell et al. (1995). Considering the limits under which preferential recruitment occurs, this would imply that the central nervous system picks 'only gravitational loads' within a narrow range of velocities of extension to excite a preferred population of units.

There are two observations reported by Nardone et al. (1989). The first one is that during lengthening contractions there is a shift in activity from slow soleus to fast gastrocnemius, but only in those subjects who have a higher percentage of slow motor units in soleus. We will not dispute this observation as during postural changes, different sets of muscles may be used. It may not be a question of slow soleus versus fast gastrocnemius, but a shift from a single joint muscle to a two joint muscle.

Their second observation that lengthening contractions selectively recruit large fast twitch units in order to facilitate fast relaxation, is not justifiable either from their teleological arguments nor from a critical reinterpretation of their data. First, they argue that soleus motor units are too slow to allow relatively fast lengthening. Soleus motor units have relaxation times in the range 300–400 ms (Bawa and Stein, 1976; Nardone and Schieppati, 1988). An examination of their figures shows lengthening contractions lasting 1–2 seconds, which provide ample time for soleus motor units to relax. We are at no point compelled to believe that recruitment of fast and large units are required to provide fast relaxation as these authors have suggested. The bursts of small units we observed were sufficient during the 'braking' phase of the movement. However, bursts of large, fast twitch units may have led to oscillatory instability. Secondly, the data in Nardone et al. (1989 Fig. 1) does not necessarily support selective recruitment. The electrode during slow shortening contraction recorded no motor unit in lateral gastrocnemius (LG). But during fast shortening contraction, units were recorded which were the same units that were recorded during lengthening contractions. Obviously it is not the

case that no motor units were recruited in LG during slow shortening contractions but simply that those that were recruited were not in the vicinity of the electrode. Since it is known that there is orderly recruitment of motor units during fast/ ballistic movements (Desmedt and Godaux, 1979), we suggest that the phasic recruitment of high threshold units is the result of ballistic contractions during both the fast shortening and lengthening contractions. The recruitment during the lengthening contractions would occur as a result of interruptions by small, fast shortening contractions which are visible in the position traces, but are more evident in high sensitivity tension traces. Such oscillations can clearly be seen in the data presented by Howell et al. (1995) if one were to look at their position traces (Figure 3, for example).

One may argue that Nardone et al. (1989) have shown a wide range units recruited during lengthening contractions, not just the 'next' higher threshold units. However, the range of thresholds of units recorded by a fixed intramuscular electrode tends to be restricted to a subset of units recruited at similar force levels. If the units firing repetitively in the background are low threshold, then the next unit recorded by the electrode will, in general, be at the lower end of the threshold continuum. This seems a reasonable explanation for the results of Howell et al. (1995) where all the units recruited during lengthening contractions (3 out of 21) were low threshold. On the other hand in Nardone et al. (1989) the background load, and hence presumably the threshold of the units, were relatively high. Ballistic contractions against such loads would certainly bring in next high threshold units, which are expected to be very high threshold.

When a tonically active muscle is stretched, which may be considered a lengthening contraction, a reflex response is elicited. When the load or the velocity of stretch is small, the reflex response may be imperceptible not only because it is small, but also because neurons in the reflex arc are not discharging synchronously. With a high velocity of stretch, synchronised response of motoneurones results in a well defined reflex responses which may include spinal and transcortical reflex loops (Marsden et al., 1976). These reflexes recruit motor units according to size (Calancie and Bawa, 1985b).

We do not want to leave the impression that reversals never occur, as we ourselves have reported them (Jones et al., 1993, 1994). However we would like to suggest that these types of reversals which are limited in frequency and occur between units with a relatively small difference in recruitment threshold, arise due to noise in the biological systems rather than as special recruitment strategies and therefore do not represent an interesting phenomenon.

References

Bawa, P. and Stein, R.B. (1976) Frequency response of human soleus muscle. *J. Neurophysiol.*, 39: 788–793.

Calancie, B.M. and Bawa, P. (1985a) Firing patterns of human flexor carpi radialis motor units during the stretch reflex. *J Neurophysiol.*, 53: 1170–1193.

Calancie, B.M. and Bawa, P. (1985b) Voluntary and reflexive recruitment of flexor carpi radialis motor units in man. *J. Neurophysiol.*, 53: 1194–1200.

Cope, T.C. and Clark, B.D. (1995) Are there important exceptions to the size principle of alpha-motoneurone recruitment? In: A. Taylor, M.H. Gladden and R. Durbaba (Eds), *Alpha and Gamma Motor Systems*, Plenum Press, New York, 71–78.

Desmedt, J.E. and Godaux, E. (1979) Voluntary motor commands in human ballistic movements. *Ann. Neurol.*, 5: 415–421.

Howell, J.N., Fuglevand, A.J., Walsh, M.L. and Bigland-Ritchie, B. (1995) Motor unit activity during isometric and concentric-eccentric contractions of human first dorsal interosseous muscle. *J. Neurophysiol.*, 74: 901–904.

Jones, K.E., Bawa, P. and McMillan, A.S. (1993) Recruitment of motor units in human flexor carpi ulnaris. *Brain Res.*, 602: 354–356.

Jones, K.E., Lyons, M., Bawa, P. and Lemon, R.N. (1994) Recruitment order of motoneurons during functional tasks. *Exp. Brain Res.*, 100: 503–508.

Kanda, K., Burke, R.E. and Walmsley, B. (1977) Differential control of fast and slow twitch motor units in the decerebrate cat. *Exper. Brain Res.* 29: 57–74.

Kernell, D. and Hultborn, H. (1990) Synaptic effects on recruitment gain: a mechanism of importance for the input-output relations of motoneurone pools? *Brain Res.*, 507: 176–179.

Marsden, C.D., Merton, P.A. and Morton, H.B. (1976) Stretch reflex and servo action in a variety of human muscles. *J. Physiol.*, 259: 531–560.

Nardone, A. and Schieppati, M. (1988) Shift of activity from slow to fast muscle during voluntary lengthening contractions of the triceps surae muscles in humans. *J. Physiol. (Lond.)*, 395: 363–381.

Nardone, A, Romano, C. and Schieppati, M. (1989) Selective recruitment of high-threshold human motor units during voluntary isotonic lengthening of active muscles. *J. Physiology.*, 409: 451–471.

Powers, R.K., Robinson, F.R., Konodi, M.A. and Binder, M.D. (1993) Distribution of Rubrospinal synaptic input to cat triceps surae motoneurons. *J. Neurophysiol.*, 70: 1460–1468.

Stephens, J.A., Garnett, R. and Buller, N.P. (1978) Reversal of recruitment order of single motor units produced by cutaneous stimulation during voluntary muscle contraction in man. *Nature*, 272: 363–364.

Stuart, D.G. and Enoka, R.M. (1983) Motoneurons, motor units, and the size principles. In: R.N. Rosenberg and R.G. Grossman (Eds), *The Clinical Neurosciences*, Vol. 5 Neurobiology, Churchill Livingstone, 471–517.

M.D. Binder (Ed.)
Progress in Brain Research, Vol 123

CHAPTER 20

Motor units of extraocular muscles: recent findings

Stephen J. Goldberg[1],* and Mary S. Shall[2]

[1]*Department of Anatomy, Visual/Motor Neurosciences Division, Virginia Commonwealth University, Medical College of Virginia Campus, Richmond, VA 23298–0709, USA*
[2]*Department of Physical Therapy, Virginia Commonwealth University, Medical College of Virginia Campus, Richmond, VA 23298–0224, USA*

Introduction

The eye movement motor control system is characterized by exquisite precision and coordinated synchrony as the eyes acquire, pursue and fixate visual targets. It is logical to think that the brain stem motoneurons and the muscle fibers that they innervate exhibit comparable precision and predictability (Robinson, 1970). Consequently, the manner in which the final common path extraocular motor units are activated and how their contractile forces assemble to produce these quick, stable and repetitive movements is a significant research and clinical problem.

The aim of this chapter, then, is to summarize some of the progress made toward understanding mammalian extraocular motor units since our last review (Goldberg, 1990). The principal goals of our studies over the past ten years have been to: (a) compare and contrast extraocular motor unit types to spinal cord innervated units; (b) examine how single motor units are distributed within a particular muscle; (c) describe the motor unit forces when driven by stimulation paradigms that attempt to mimic motoneuron firing patterns observed during eye movements in alert, behaving animals; and (d) determine how single motor unit forces summate as they contract in unison. Most of the

findings over this period have been collected from deeply anesthetized, in vivo preparations involving the lateral rectus muscle in adult cats and monkeys.

There are usually six extraocular muscle subserving eye movements (Baker, 1986; Spencer and Porter, 1988). The inferior oblique muscle, plus the medial, superior and inferior recti are innervated by the oculomotor nucleus and nerve (Sasaki, 1963; Tarlov and Tarlov, 1971; Gacek, 1974). The superior oblique muscle is primarily innervated by the contralateral trochlear nucleus (Wilkinson, 1930; Miyazaki, 1985) while the lateral rectus muscle and retractor bulbi muscle (when present) are innervated by the ipsilateral principal and accessory abducens nuclei respectively (Hutson et al., 1979; Spencer et al., 1980; Crandall et al., 1981).

The morphology of the extraocular muscles has been the subject of numerous studies (Spencer and Porter, 1988). The muscles have been divided into separate global and orbital layers with at least three types of singly innervated fibers in the global layer (making up $\approx 70\%$ of the muscle fibers). The smallest-diameter of the singly innervated types can also be found in the orbital layer. In addition, there are two types of multiply innervated fibers (i.e. having more than one neural end plate per muscle fiber): one is in the global and one in the orbital muscle layer. There have also been recent investigations establishing the wide variety of

*Corresponding author. Tel.: (804) 828-9529; Fax: (804) 828-9477; e-mail: sgoldber@hsc.ucu.edu

222

myosin heavy chain isoforms that are expressed in these structurally diverse extraocular muscles (Wieczorek et al., 1985; Lucas et al., 1991; Rushbrook et al., 1994; Brueckner and Porter, 1998).

Motor unit types in extraocular muscle

The structural and histochemical diversity clearly evident in extraocular muscle (Spencer and Porter, 1988; Jacoby et al., 1989b; Davidowitz et al., 1996a, 1996b) did not seem to be matched by the contractile properties observed in earlier motor unit studies (Lennerstrand, 1974; Goldberg et al., 1976, 1981; Meredith and Goldberg, 1986; Nelson et al., 1986). Lennerstrand (1974) had distinguished two possible types of multiply innervated fibers and a singly innervated type in the cat inferior oblique muscle. One multiply innervated type displayed twitch contractions (multiply innervated twitch contracting = MIC) and one type that contracted in response to trains of stimuli, but no twitch contractions (multiply innervated non-twitch contracting = MINC). Nelson et al. (1986) systematically tested over 100 cat superior oblique muscle motor units for fatigue, twitch contraction time, fusion frequency and sag (Burke, 1981). Except for distinguishing a twitch population from a non-twitch population (comprising 5% of the units studied) the units appeared as a continuum and were not broken down into fatigue resistant and fatigable groups while sag was not apparent in any of the units (Nelson et al., 1986).

It was then decided to study one of the muscles used in horizontal eye movements, the cat lateral rectus, with a more discerning look at fusion frequency, twitch contraction time and fatigue (Shall and Goldberg, 1992). We continued with the use of one of the fatigue tests developed earlier (Nelson et al., 1986) that employed 500 msec train durations, delivered once per second, with a stimulus frequency of 150 Hz for a period of two minutes (Burke et al., 1973). This fatigue paradigm was based on the observations (Goldberg et al., 1976, 1981; Meredith and Goldberg, 1986) that lateral rectus motor units rarely exhibited fusion before 150 Hz, so they would not be unduly stressed at that frequency, and that fixations in alert

animals often lasted for over a half second (Delgado-Garcia et al., 1986; Fuchs et al., 1988). We were also able, using new equipment, to quickly and easily increment stimulation frequencies to the intracellularly identified lateral rectus motoneurons with improved precision. Rather than using stimulation frequency increments of 25 to 50 Hz until reaching 300 Hz (Nelson et al., 1986), we used frequency increments of 10 Hz (Shall and Goldberg, 1992).

While cat lateral rectus muscle motor units did show a possible bimodal distribution in contraction time, fusion frequency was unimodal as it was for superior oblique motor units (Nelson et al., 1986). However, there were clearly two groups of lateral rectus motor units based on fatigue resistance and 10% of the units were classified as non-twitch (Shall and Goldberg, 1992). So, the non-twitch units could again be considered one motor unit type and the two groups of twitch units based on fatigue could be counted as two types. We further suggested that if the continuum of fusion frequencies was divided at the mean (169.5 Hz) then units with a fusion frequency equal to or greater than 170 Hz could be considered fast and those with fusion frequencies less than 170 Hz could be considered slow (Shall and Goldberg, 1992). These distinctions indicated that there were potentially five physiological motor unit types that could be distinguished and we classified them in a manner similar to that used by Burke (1981). We found 20 FF (fast fatigable), 8 FR (fast fatigue resistant), 15 SF (slow fatigable, a 'new' classification), 10 SR (slow fatigue resistant) and 6 NT (non-twitch, not often found in other skeletal muscle). The 'attraction' of this physiological classification scheme was that it coincided with the structural and histochemical findings of five to six muscle fiber types in extraocular muscle (Spencer and Porter, 1988).

The implementation of motoneuron kt values (the slope of the motoneuron stimulation rate vs. the resultant single motor unit forces) was also introduced in this paper (Shall and Goldberg, 1992) since we now had better control over motoneuron stimulation rate. We found that muscle unit force increased linearly as stimulation frequency increased until a tension plateau was reached near a particular unit's fusion frequency. Previous studies in alert animals (Keller, 1981; Delgado-Garcia et al., 1986; Fuchs et al., 1988) have indicated a direct relationship between motoneuron activation threshold and motoneuron K value (a linear relationship between the slope of motoneuron firing frequency vs. fixated eye position (measured in degree of eccentricity from primary (straight ahead) position)). That is, the lower the K value the lower the threshold for activation and these low K value motoneurons might then innervate weaker muscle

units (Delgado-Garcia et al., 1986) recruited early in an eye movement. In contrast, we observed that the lower the motoneuron kt value the stronger the motor unit (Fig. 1). In addition, we could find no relationship between any motor unit contractile measure and lateral rectus motoneuron activation threshold in response to stimulation of the contralateral medial rectus subdivision of the oculomotor nucleus (Shall and Goldberg, 1992) which is known to have neurons that project monosynaptically to the abducens nucleus

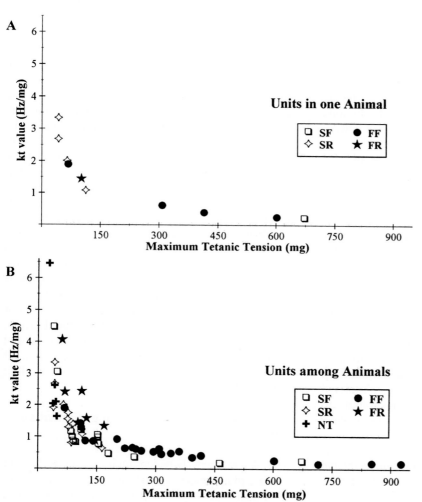

Fig. 1. kt value plotted against maximum tetanic tension of single lateral rectus muscle motor units. (A) All the units were found in one animal. (B) Units found among 13 experimental animals. Note the similarity in the graphed results between 'A' and 'B'. Motor Unit Symbols: FF = fast fatigable; FR = fast fatigue resistant; SF = slow fatigable; SR = slow fatigue resistant; NT = non-twitch. (Modified from Shall and Goldberg, 1992).

(Maciewicz et al., 1975). The possible relationship between motoneuron K and kt values as well as the sequence of extraocular motor unit recruitment needs to be pursued in future studies.

Distribution of motor unit types within a single muscle

While the contractile information discussed above helped to define extraocular motor unit types, it did not add to our knowledge regarding motoneuron distribution within the brain stem nuclei or how muscle fiber types distributed within a muscle. As mentioned at the beginning of this chapter, the anatomical division of extraocular muscles into orbital and global layers has long been recognized. The orbital layer, based both on anatomical and pharmacological data, is generally thought to be the site of slower contracting and weaker muscle units which might be used in sustained muscle contractions (Kern, 1965; Bach-y-Rita et al., 1977).

We used a preparation involving the cat inferior oblique muscle and nerve because the nerve has a relatively long and surgically accessible course through the orbit as well as clear medial and lateral divisions (Sas and Schab, 1952). We found that the lateral division of the nerve innervated slower contracting muscle units and that smaller motoneurons contributed their axons to that lateral nerve division (Shall et al., 1995). However, motoneurons were not organized by cell body size within the inferior oblique subdivision of the oculomotor nucleus (Shall et al., 1995). Furthermore, the orbital and global layers of the muscle did not appear to be differentially innervated by either of the two nerve branches. This was determined by simultaneously recording the individual orbital and global electromyographic (EMG) responses to either lateral or medial inferior oblique muscle nerve stimulation.

We also turned our attention to determining the intramuscular location of motor units within the cat lateral rectus muscle (Shall and Goldberg, 1995). We again used separate EMG recordings of the global and orbital layers and found that of 41 motor units, eight were confined to the orbital layer, 22 to the global layer (including three non-twitch units) and 11 appeared to be split between the global and orbital muscle layers ('bilayer' motor units). The bilayer units demonstrated the strongest tetanic tensions, had the lowest kt values and were classified as FF units when subjected to the fatigue test. It was noted in another study that two out of 10 bilayer units subjected to the fatigue test showed a more pronounced decline in the recorded EMG potential in the global rather than the orbital muscle layer (Shall et al., 1996). This might indicate that a single lateral rectus muscle motor unit could contain different types of muscle fibers (Edgerton et al., 1980; Gurahian and Goldberg, 1987).

In terms of how different extraocular muscle 'compartments' (English and Weeks, 1984; Windhorst et al., 1989) might be used during eye movements, it has been reported that the small diameter orbital muscle fibers in man apparently have a lower position threshold during fixation and could be recruited first (Collins, 1975; Robinson, 1978). However, a size ordered recruitment in the extraocular system has been questioned (Fuchs et al., 1988; Goldberg, 1990; Shall and Goldberg, 1992) and there did appear to be an initial coactivation of orbital and global fibers in saccades (Collins, 1975). Indeed, other investigators (Lennerstrand and Bach-y-Rita, 1974; Shall and Goldberg, 1992; Dean, 1996) have suggested that powerful motor units might be recruited early in some eye movements. The bilayer units we have found may be candidates for that initial recruitment. It is clear, however, that the force contributions and activation thresholds of motor units confined to either the global or orbital layers, as well as the bilayer unit force contributions, will need to be further clarified during various types of eye movements in order to settle the question (Shall and Goldberg, 1995).

Motor unit forces during varying stimulation patterns

The discrepancy between motoneuron K and kt values, plus concerns about finding a comprehensible sequence of motor unit recruitment (Binder et al., 1996), bothered us enough so that we wanted to try and resolve the discrepancy. It occurred to us that kt values were determined using 200 msec trains of stimuli delivered at a constant frequency

(Shall and Goldberg, 1992) while K values were determined using the observed motoneuron firing frequency during a long lasting (as much as 2 s) fixation that followed a saccade to the point of fixation; the 'pulse/step' (Fuchs et al., 1985, 1988). Although both motoneuron firing patterns, constant frequency and pulse/step, are seen in behaving animals (Delgado-Garcia et al., 1986; Fuchs et al., 1988), they are used differently. When an animal makes a saccade in a motoneuron's 'off' direction, but eye position remains within the neuron's 'on' field, the reestablishment of neuronal firing (often after a silent period during the off saccade) at the new fixation point is at a constant frequency. No pulse/step is observed as it is in a neuron's 'on' direction.

Although the kt value we observed during the step phase following the pulse (defined as the kt_{ps} value) was almost always lower (in absolute value) than the constant frequency kt value, no unit changed its relative position in the kt-kt_{ps} hierarchy. And powerful units still had the lowest values (Shall et al., 1996). So, the discrepancy between kt and K value was not resolved by using a pulse/step stimulation paradigm with a long duration step (Fig. 2).

We did, however, make some interesting observations regarding motor unit tension when comparing the constant frequency and pulse/step stimulation paradigms. It has long been known that skeletal muscle units do not always display the same force output in response to identical frequencies of motoneuronal activation, depending on their activation history (Burke et al., 1976; Binder-Macleod and Clamann, 1989; Binder-Macleod and Barrish, 1992; Binder-Macleod, 1995; Kernell, 1995). This has been termed a motor unit force 'hysteresis' (Binder-Macleod and Clamann, 1989). Other investigations have also established a hysteresis in extraocular motoneuron firing rate as the eyes attain an identical position of fixation from different directions (Eckmiller, 1974; Delgado-Garcia et al., 1986; Goldstein and Robinson, 1986; Stahl and Simpson, 1995).

Similar to the above referenced skeletal motor unit and extraocular motoneuron hysteresis, there was also a force hysteresis in single motor units of the cat lateral rectus muscle that was dependent on

activation history (Shall et al., 1996). Seventy per cent of the units studied exhibited different tensions (usually greater than a 30% difference), at the moderate stimulation rate of 100 Hz, depending on whether the 100Hz was delivered from start to finish at a constant frequency or whether it was preceded by a high frequency pulse (Fig. 2). The manner in which both the motor unit force and motoneuron firing frequency hysteresis are factored into precise eye movement control remains open to question (Goldstein and Robinson, 1986; Shall et al., 1996).

Motor units acting together

The following series of studies was embarked upon in an effort to examine the forces in simultaneously active units, but they may have also shed some light on how the observed hysteresis in single motor unit forces might be leveled out during eye movements.

Some anatomical investigations of extraocular muscles have shown the internal structure to be composed of serially arranged and branched muscle fibers: myotendinous and myomyous junctions were noted frequently (Mayr, 1975; Alvarado-Mallart and Pinçon-Raymond, 1976). Such arrangements could effect how unit forces summate (Street, 1983; Roy and Edgerton, 1992; Trotter et al., 1995). It is known that there are ≈ 1100 lateral rectus motoneurons in the cat abducens nucleus (Steiger and Büttner-Ennever, 1978; Spencer et al., 1980) and about 1000 of those innervate twitch units if some 10% of the motoneurons innervate non-twitch units (Shall and Goldberg, 1992). The cat lateral rectus muscle has been reported to contain about 15 000 muscle fibers (Peachey, 1971) resulting in an average innervation ratio of about 1 : 15 (Guéritaud et al., 1985). Stimulation of the whole muscle nerve should sum the twitch motor unit forces such that they would yield a twitch tension of ≈ 29.0 grams if the average unit twitch tension (≈ 29.0 mg) is multiplied by the 1000 of lateral rectus twitch motoneurons (Goldberg et al., 1997). However, we and others (Barmack et al., 1971) usually observe whole muscle twitch tensions of ≈ 15.0 grams in the cat. This loss of force is also evident when examining whole muscle

226

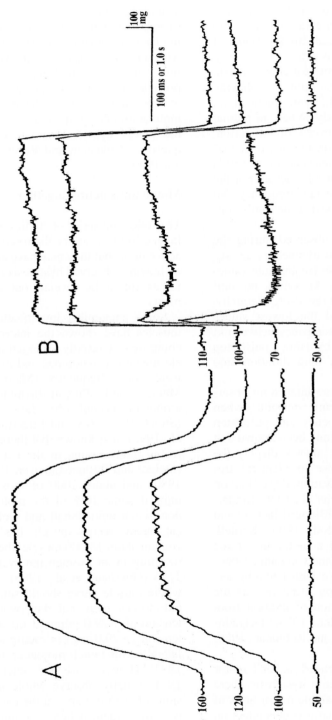

Fig. 2. Lateral rectus muscle motor unit tetanic responses showing a force hysteresis. (A) Constant frequency stimulation with 200 msec duration trains at 50, 100, 120 and 160 Hz from bottom to top. 500 mg tension at 100 Hz. (B) Pulse/step stimulation of the same motor unit as in 'A' using 2 s duration trains at 50, 70, 100 and 110 Hz step frequencies. (The total 'pulse' duration was 25 ms – 350 Hz for 10 ms and 200 Hz for 15 ms). 640 mg tension at 100 Hz step frequency measured 200 ms after the start of stimulation. (Modified from Shall et al., 1996).

tetanic tension (Goldberg and Shall, 1997). In studying lateral rectus motor units it was found that 25% of the single units lost an average of 48% of their twitch force when that unit was stimulated at the same time as an additional four or five units were activated (Goldberg et al., 1997). While the other 75% of the units did add their total force to that of the other units, we suggested that with many units active, as in normal eye movements, there might be an additional loss of force (Goldberg et al., 1997). Indeed, it has been suggested that adjacent muscle fibers, when contracting simultaneously, could in part be responsible for nonlinear additions of force (Clamann and Schelhorn, 1988). We were using a very small percentage ($\approx 0.5\%$) of the total muscle fibers in our experimental design (Goldberg et al., 1997) which would clearly lower the chances for muscle fiber interaction. Accordingly, we were somewhat surprised that a full 25% of the units studied did show a reduction of force with such a limited proportion (≈ 75 of 15 000 muscle fibers) of the muscle fibers active.

Another factor that could play a significant role in reducing 'expected' force output is the notion of polyinnervation of single muscle fibers. It is well established that many extraocular muscle fibers have multiple end plates (Spencer and Porter, 1988) but it has generally been assumed that the end plates on a particular fiber were all from the same neuron (Lennerstrand, 1974). However, recent studies have made the case that a single muscle fiber could be innervated by more than one motoneuron (Jacoby et al., 1989a; Porter and Baker, 1996) and there also appear to be different myosin isoforms along the length of a single muscle fiber (Jacoby et al., 1989b). A muscle fiber population that incorporates polyinnervation would clearly have the potential to exhibit lower than expected forces when a large proportion of the motoneuron pool was firing. That is, once a particular muscle fiber was producing force it might not be able to further increase its force when its other innervating motoneuron(s) became active. Conversely, such a muscle might also be able to sustain its force output if it somehow lost some of its innervating motoneurons.

Regardless of the mechanisms, the finding that single motor unit forces do not appear to fully

summate when contracting in unison might serve to help level out the force hysteresis observed in motor units when the are activated in isolation. Extraocular motor control, therefore, does not appear to be a straightforward linear system, even at the level of the final common path motoneurons and their muscle units.

In addition, serial arrangement, branching and polyinnervation of the muscle fibers might also serve to protect the muscle from injury if force could be transmitted through the interfiber matrix and/or against other muscle fibers with which they are in contact (Goldberg et al., 1997). In fact, there was little reduction in whole muscle force output even after excising ≈ 6.0 mm^2 from the body of the muscle (Goldberg et al., 1997).

Lateral rectus muscle motor units in the primate

After acquiring a significant amount of information about cat extraocular muscle motor unit contractile characteristics, we began to apply similar experimental procedures in order to begin studies of motor units in a primate, the squirrel monkey. For the most part, primate research has provided information for the current experimental models of man's oculomotor system although there was no data on the contractile characteristics of primate extraocular motor units (Goldberg et al., 1998).

We found a number of qualitative similarities between cat and squirrel monkey lateral rectus muscle motor units (Goldberg et al., 1998). As in the cat: (a) motor units could be categorized based on fusion frequency and fatigue; (b) kt value correlated with motor unit maximum tetanic tension; and (c) 95% of the motor units demonstrated a force hysteresis at 100 Hz. In addition, an average whole muscle force change of 0.32 gm/° and an average frequency change of 4.7 Hz/° of lateral eye displacement were seen in response to supramaximal stimulation of the abducens nerve in the brain stem (Fig. 4). A whole muscle force change of about 0.4 gm/° has been reported in man (Robinson et al., 1969).

While we do not yet know if simultaneously active primate motor units will exhibit less than the total sum of their forces as we have seen in the cat, the average maximum tetanic force observed in squirrel monkey lateral rectus muscle motor units (186.2 mg) would appear to indicate that, surprisingly, as few as two motor units might be enough to displace the eye by one degree (Fig. 4A) if the two units summed maximally (Goldberg et al., 1998).

Since little is known about innervation ratios in primates, further studies are clearly needed to

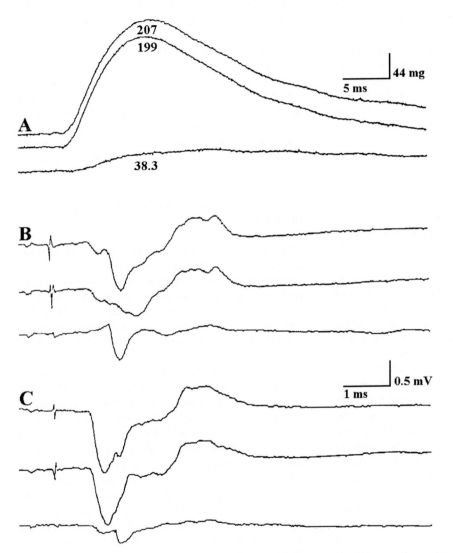

Fig. 3. Lateral rectus motor unit twitch and EMG responses showing lack of total force summation. (A) Bottom trace is single unit with a twitch tension of 38.3 mg in response to stimulation of one motoneuron. Middle trace shows several muscle units activated with low intensity nerve stimulation with a twitch tension of 199 mg. Top trace shows simultaneous activation of units in the bottom and middle traces. The combined twitch tension is 207 mg. 79% of the unit force in the bottom trace is 'lost'. (B) EMG responses from the lateral rectus muscle global layer only. Bottom trace is from the single muscle unit, middle trace from nerve activated units, and top trace from simultaneous activation. (C) EMG responses from the orbital layer only. Trace alignment is the same as in B. Note incorporation of the single unit's negative peak (bottom trace) into the simultaneous activation trace (top trace) in both 'B' and 'C'. These incorporated peaks can be seen beginning ≈1.3 msec after the stimulus artifact in the top trace of 'B' and 'C'. This shows there is no loss of EMG while the force does not sum. (Modified from Goldberg et al., 1997a.

examine the number and size of squirrel monkey lateral rectus muscle motoneurons as well as the number, possible branching patterns and possible serial arrangement of squirrel monkey lateral rectus muscle fibers. However, there have been estimates of about 5000 lateral rectus motoneurons in adult humans (Harley, 1942; Tomasch, 1973; Vijaya-shankar and Brody, 1977) with about 10,000 lateral

rectus muscle fibers in the monkey and possibly 35,000 fibers in man (Peachey, 1971).

Conclusions

The cat and monkey extraocular motor control system at the level of the final common path motor units seems to achieve its impressive precision

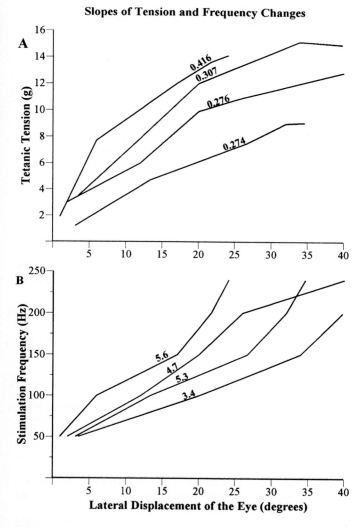

Fig. 4. (A) Slopes of whole lateral rectus muscle tetanic tension changes vs. lateral displacement of the eye in four squirrel monkeys. Note slope of tension change (gms) per degree for each animal with an average of 0.32 gm/°. (B) Constant frequency stimulation delivered to the whole sixth nerve vs. lateral displacement of the eye in four squirrel monkeys. Note slope of frequency change per degree for each animal with an average of 4.7 Hz/°. (Modified from Goldberg et al., 1998).

with, perhaps, unexpected intricacy. There do appear to be reasonably well defined physiological types of motor units to match the structural and histochemical differentiation of muscle fibers, even though some single units can have muscle fibers in both the global and orbital muscle layers. But the sequence in which the unit types are brought into play during the various types of eye movements plus the amount of tension a unit might actually contribute due to force hysteresis and/or the possible serial arrangement and branching of muscle fibers within the muscle remain to be resolved. In addition, while suggestions of poly-neuronal innervation of single muscle fibers may also help explain some of the results that have been obtained, such a complex innervation pattern reflects back on how the timing and specificity of motoneuron activation in the brain stem nuclei is achieved. That is, if a single muscle fiber could be part of more than one motor unit then a degree of obfuscation may be added to recruitment sequenc-ing. However, these proposed anatomical arrangements do tend to temper the importance of (and our ability to predict) force contributions from individual muscle fibers and motoneurons. There-fore, such 'complexity' could play a pertinent role in the maintenance of visuomotor function in the face of aging, disease or injury.

Acknowledgements

We feel privileged to be able to contribute this chapter to a volume honoring Douglas G. Stuart. He has been a wonderful and encouraging mentor (although not on the tennis court) over the years, even though neither of us formally studied with him. His intellect, energy and sustained interest in our work have helped to drive our research efforts and we are indebted to him for that, at the very least.

There have also been a number of other people who have played notable roles in shaping our research inquiries. They have done this through personal and electronic conversations and helping to review our work. While we are solely responsi-ble for any mistakes, we must share the credit for the more reliable scientific contributions. They are: Paul Bach-y-Rita, Brenda Bigland-Ritchie, Marc D. Binder, Barry R. Botterman, Nathanial A. Buchwald, Robert E. Burke, H. Peter Clamann, William F. Crandall, Paul Dean, V. Reggie Edge-rton, Albert F. Fuchs, Herschel P. Goldstein, Stephen M. Highstein, Chester D. Hull, Chris R. S. Kaneko, Edward L. Keller, Gunnar Lennerstrand, Gerald E. Loeb, J. Ross McClung, M. Alex Meredith, Jon S. Nelson, Martin J. Pinter, Charles L. Rice, David L. Sparks, Barry E. Stein, Sharyn Vanden Noven, Felix E. Zajac and especially Louis J. Goldberg.

This work was supported by National Institutes of Health-National Eye Institute Grant EY11249.

References

Alvarado-Mallart, R.M. and Pinçon-Raymond, M. (1976) Nerve endings on the intramuscular tendons of cat extra-ocular muscles. *Neurosci. Lett.*, 2: 121–125.

Bach-y-Rita, P., Lennerstrand, G., Alvarado, J., Nichols, K. and McHolm, G. (1977) Extraocular muscle fibers: ultrastructural identification of iontophoretically labeled fibers contracting in response to succinylcholine. *Invest. Ophthalmol.*, 16: 561–565.

Baker, R. (1986) Brainstem neurons are peculiar for oculomo-tor organization. *Prog. Brain Res.*, 64: 257–271.

Barmack, N.H., Bell, C.C. and Rence, B.G. (1971) Tension and rate of tension development during isometric responses of extraocular muscle. *J. Neurophysiol.*, 34: 1072–1079.

Binder, M.D., Heckman, C.J. and Powers, R.K. (1996) The physiological control of motoneuron activity. In: L.B. Rowell and J.T. Shepherd (Eds), *Handbook of Physiology. Section 12, Exercise: Regulation and Integration of Multiple Systems*, American Physiological Society, New York: Oxford, pp. 3–53.

Binder-Macleod, S.A. (1995) Variable-frequency stimulation patterns for the optimization of force during muscle fatigue. In: S.C. Gandevia, R.M. Enoka, A.J. McComas, D.G. Stuart and C.K. Thomas (Eds), *Fatigue*, Plenum Press, New York, pp. 227–240.

Binder-Macleod, S.A. and Barrish, W.J. (1992) Force response of rat soleus muscle to variable-frequency train stimulation. *J. Neurophysiol.*, 68: 1068–1078.

Binder-Macleod, S.A. and Clamann, H.P. (1989) Force output of cat motor units stimulated with trains of linearly varying frequency. *J. Neurophysiol.*, 61: 208–217.

Brueckner, J.K. and Porter, J.D. (1998) Visual system maldeve-lopment disrupts extraocular muscle-specific myosin expression. *J. Appl. Physiol.*, 85: 584–592.

Burke, R.E. (1981) Motor units: anatomy, physiology, and functional organization. In: V.B. Brooks (Ed.), *Handbook of Physiology*, Sec. 1, Vol. II, Pt. 1, *The Nervous System: Motor Control*, American Physiology Society, Bethesda, MD, pp. 345–422.

Burke, R.E., Levine, D.N., Tsairis, P. and Zajac, F.E. (1973) Physiological types and histochemical profiles in motor units of the cat gastrocnemius. *J. Physiol.*, 234: 723–748.

Burke, R.E., Rudomin, P. and Zajac, F.E. (1976) The effect of activation history on tension production by individual muscle units. *Brain Res.*, 109: 515–529.

Clamann, H.P. and Schelhorn, T.B. (1988) Nonlinear force addition of newly recruited motor units in the cat hindlimb. *Muscle Nerve*, 11: 1079–1089.

Collins, C.C. (1975) The human oculomotor control system. In: G. Lennerstrand and P. Bach-y-Rita (Eds), *Basic Mechanisms of Ocular Motility and Their Clinical Implications*, Pergamon Press, Oxford, pp. 145–180.

Crandall, W.F., Goldberg, S.J., Wilson, J.S. and McClung, J.R. (1981) Muscle units divided among retractor bulbi muscle slips and between the lateral rectus and retractor bulbi muscles in the cat. *Exp. Neurol.*, 71: 251–260.

Davidowitz, J., Rubinson, K., Jacoby, J. and Onejeme, A. (1996a) Myofibril size variation along the length of extraocular muscle in rabbit and rat. 2. Global layer. *Tissue Cell*, 28: 77–87.

Davidowitz, J., Rubinson, K., Jacoby, J. and Philips, G. (1996b) Myofibril size variation along the length of extraocular muscle in rabbit and rat. 1. Orbital layer. *Tissue Cell*, 28: 63–76.

Dean, P. (1996) Motor unit recruitment in a distributed model of extraocular muscle. *J. Neurophysiol.*, 76: 727–742.

Delgado-Garcia, J.M., del Pozo, F. and Baker, R. (1986) Behavior of neurons in the abducens nucleus of the alert cat. I. Motoneurons. *Neuroscience*, 17: 929–952.

Eckmiller, R. (1974) Hysteresis in the static characteristics of eye position coded in the alert monkey. *Pflugers Arch.*, 350: 249–258.

Edgerton, V.R., Goslow, G.E., Rasmussen, S.A. and Spector, S.A. (1980) Is resistance of a muscle to fatigue controlled by its motoneurones? *Nature*, 285: 589–590.

English, A.W. and Weeks, O.I. (1984) Compartmentalization of single muscle units in cat lateral gastrocnemius. *Exp. Brain Res.*, 56: 361–368.

Fuchs, A.F., Kaneko, C.R.S. and Scudder, C.A. (1985) Brainstem control of saccadic eye movements. *Ann. Rev. Neurosci.*, 8: 307–337.

Fuchs, A.F., Scudder, C.A. and Kaneko, C.R.S. (1988) Discharge patterns and recruitment order of identified motoneurons and internuclear neurons in the monkey abducens nucleus. *J. Neurophysiol.*, 60: 1874–1895.

Gacek, R.R. (1974) Localization of neurons supplying the extraocular muscles in kitten using horseradish peroxidase. *Exp. Neurol.*, 44: 381–403.

Goldberg, S.J. (1990) Mechanical properties of extraocular motor units. In: M.D. Binder and L.M. Mendell (Eds), *The Segmental Motor System*, Oxford University Press, Oxford: New York, pp. 222–238.

Goldberg, S.J., Clamann, H.P. and McClung, J.R. (1981) Relation between motoneuron position and lateral rectus motor unit contraction speed: and intracellular study in the cat abducens nucleus. *Neurosci. Lett.*, 23: 49–54.

Goldberg, S.J., Lennerstrand, G. and Hull, C.D. (1976) Motor unit responses in the lateral rectus muscle of the cat: intracellular current injection of abducens nucleus neurons. *Acta Physiol. Scand.*, 96: 58–63.

Goldberg, S.J., Meredith, M.A. and Shall, M.S. (1998) Extraocular motor unit and whole-muscle responses in the lateral rectus muscle of the squirrel monkey. *J. Neurosci.*, 18: 10629–10639.

Goldberg, S.J. and Shall, M.S. (1997) Lateral rectus whole muscle and motor unit contractile measures with the extraocular muscles intact. *J. Neurosci. Meth.*, 78: 47–50.

Goldberg, S.J., Wilson, K.E. and Shall, M.S. (1997) Summation of extraocular motor unit tensions in the lateral rectus muscle of the cat. *Muscle Nerve*, 20: 1229–1235.

Goldstein, H.P. and Robinson, D.A. (1986) Hysteresis and slow drift in abducens unit activity. *J. Neurophysiol.*, 55: 1044–1056.

Guéritaud, J.P., Horcholle-Bossavit, G., Jami, L., Thiesson, D. and Tyc-Dumont, S. (1985) Resistance of glycogen depletion of motor units in the cat rectus lateralis muscle. *Exp. Brain Res.*, 60: 542–550.

Gurahian, S.M. and Goldberg, S.J. (1987) Fatigue of lateral rectus and retractor bulbi motor units in cat. *Brain Res.*, 415: 281–292.

Harley, R.D. (1942) A quantitative study of the cells and fibers in the nucleus: nerve complexes of the fourth and sixth cranial nerves. *Am. J. Ophthalmol.*, 25: 1029–1042.

Hutson, K.A., Glendenning, K.K. and Masterton, R.B. (1979) Accessory abducens nucleus and its relationship to the accessory facial and posterior trigeminal nuclei in cat. *J. Comp. Neurol.*, 188: 1–16.

Jacoby, J., Chiarandini, D.J. and Stefani, E. (1989a) Electrical properties and innervation of fibers in the orbital layer of rat extraocular muscles. *J. Neurophysiol.*, 61: 116–125.

Jacoby, J., Ko, K., Weiss, C. and Rushbrook, J.I. (1989b) Systemic variation in myosin expression along extraocular muscle fibres of the adult rat. *J. Musc. Res. Cell Motil.*, 11: 25–40.

Keller, E.L. (1981) Oculomotor neuron behavior. In: B.L. Zuber (Ed.), *Models of Oculomotor Behavior and Control*, CRC Press, Boca Raton, pp. 1–19.

Kern, R. (1965) A comparative pharmacologic-histologic study of slow and twitch fibers in the superior rectus muscle of the rabbit. *Invest. Ophthalmol.*, 4: 901–910.

Kernell, D. (1995) Neuromuscular frequency-coding and fatigue. In: S.C. Gandevia, R.M. Enoka, A.J. McComas, D.G. Stuart and C.K. Thomas (Eds), *Fatigue*, Plenum Press, New York, pp. 135–145.

Lennerstrand, G. (1974) Electrical activity and isometric tension in motor units of the cat's inferior oblique muscle. *Acta Physiol. Scand.*, 91: 458–474.

Lennerstrand, G. and Bach-y-Rita, P. (1974) Activation of slow motor units by threshold stimulation of cat eye muscle nerves. *Invest. Ophthalmol.*, 13: 879–882.

Lucas, C.A., Rughani, A., Kang, L.H.D. and Hoh, J.F.Y. (1991) Immunocytochemical analysis of developmental changes in myosin isoforms in cat extraocular muscle fibres. *Proc. Aust. Physiol. Pharmacol. Soc.*, 22: 66.

Maciewicz, R.J., Kaneko, C.R.S., Highstein, S.M. and Baker, R. (1975) Morphophysiological identification of interneurons in the oculomotor nucleus that project to the abducens nucleus in the cat. *Brain Res.*, 96: 60–65.

Mayr, R., Gottschall, J., Gruber, H. and Neuhuber, W. (1975) Internal structure of cat extraocular muscle. *Anat. Embryol.*, 148: 25–34.

Meredith, M.A. and Goldberg, S.J. (1986) Contractile differences between muscle units in the medial rectus and lateral rectus muscles in the cat. *J. Neurophysiol.*, 56: 50–62.

Miyazaki, S. (1985) Bilateral innervation of the superior oblique muscle by the trochlear nucleus. *Brain Res.*, 348: 52–56.

Nelson, J.S., Goldberg, S.J. and McClung, J.R. (1986) Motoneuron electrophysiological and muscle contractile properties of superior oblique motor units in the cat. *J. Neurophysiol.*, 55: 715–726.

Peachey, L. (1971) The structure of the extraocular muscle fibers of mammals. In: P. Bach-y-Rita, C.C. Collins and J.E. Hyde (Eds), *The Control of Eye Movements*, Academic Press, New York., 47–65.

Porter, J.D. and Baker, R.S. (1996) Muscles of a different 'color': The unusual properties of the extraocular muscles may predispose or protect them in neurogenic and myogenic disease. *Neurology*, 46: 30–37.

Robinson, D.A. (1970) Oculomotor unit behavior in the monkey. *J. Neurophysiol.*, 33: 393–404.

Robinson, D.A. (1978) The functional behavior of the peripheral oculomotor apparatus: a review. In: G. Kommerell (Ed.), *Disorders of Ocular Motility*, Bergman, Munich, pp. 43–61.

Robinson, D.A., O'Meara, D.M., Scott, A.B. and Collins, C.C. (1969) Mechanical components of human eye movements. *J. Appl. Physiol.*, 26: 548–553.

Roy, R.R. and Edgerton, V.R. (1992) Skeletal muscle architecture and performance. In: P.V. Komi (Ed.), *Strength and Power in Sport*, Blackwell Press, Oxford, pp. 115–129.

Rushbrook, J.I., Weiss, C., Ko, K., Feuerman, M.H., Carleton, S., Ing, A. and Jacoby, J. (1994) Identification of alpha-cardiac myosin heavy chain mRNA and protein in extraocular muscle of the adult rabbit. *J. Muscle Res. Cell Motil.*, 15: 505–515.

Sas, J. and Schab, R. (1952) Die sogennanten 'Palisaden-Endigungen' der Augenmuskeln. *Acat Morph. Acad. Sci. Hung.*, 2: 259–266.

Sasaki, K. (1963) Electrophysiological studies on oculomotor neurons of the cat. *Jap. J. Physiol.*, 13: 287–302.

Shall, M.S. and Goldberg, S.J. (1992) Extraocular motor units: type classification and motoneuron stimulation frequency-muscle unit force relationships. *Brain Res.*, 587: 291–300.

Shall, M.S. and Goldberg, S.J. (1995) Lateral rectus EMG and contractile responses elicited by cat abducens motoneurons. *Muscle Nerve*, 18: 948–955.

Shall, M.S., Sorg, P.J., McClung, J.R., Gilliam, E.E. and Goldberg, S.J. (1995) The relationship of the mechanical properties of the cat inferior oblique muscle to the anatomy of its motoneurons and nerve branches. *Acta Anat.*, 153: 151–160.

Shall, M.S., Wilson, K.E. and Goldberg, S.J. (1996) Extraocular motoneuron stimulation frequency effects on motor unit tension in cat. *Acta Anat.*, 157: 217–225.

Spencer, R.F., Baker, R., McCrea and R.A. (1980) Localization and morphology of cat retractor bulbi motoneurons. *J. Neurophysiol.*, 43: 754–770.

Spencer, R.F. and Porter, J.D. (1988) Structural organization of the extraocular muscle. In: J.A. Büttner-Ennever (Ed), *Neuroanatomy of the Oculomotor System*, Elsevier, Amsterdam. pp. 33–79.

Stahl, J.S. and Simpson, J.I. (1995) Dynamics of abducens nucleus neurons in the awake rabbit. *J. Neurophysiol.*, 73: 1383–1395.

Steiger, H.J. and Büttner-Ennever, J.A. (1978) Relationship between motoneurons and internuclear neurons in the abducens nucleus: a double retrograde tracer study in the cat. *Brain Res.*, 148: 181–188.

Street, S.F. (1983) Lateral transmission of tension in frog myofibers: a myofibrillar network and transverse cytoskeletal connections are possible transmitters. *J. Cell. Physiol.*, 114: 346–364.

Tarlov, E. and Tarlov, S.R. (1971) The representation of extraocular muscles in the oculomotor nuclei: experimental studies in the cat. *Brain Res.*, 34: 37–52.

Tomasch, J. (1973) Cell frequencies in the abducens nucleus of man. *Confin. Neurol.*, 35: 257–262.

Trotter, J.A., Richmond, F.J.R. and Purslow, P.P. (1995) Functional morphology and motor control of series-fibered muscles. In: J. Hollizy (Ed.), *Exercise and Sports Sciences Reviews*, Vol. 23, William and Wilkins, Baltimore, pp. 167–213.

Vijayashankar, N. and Brody, H.J. (1977) A study of aging in the human abducens nucleus. *J. Comp. Neurol.*, 173: 433–438.

Wieczorek, D.F., Periasamy, M., Butler-Browne, G.S., Whalen, R.G. and Nadal-Ginard, B. (1985) Co-expression of multiple myosin heavy chain genes, in addition to a tissue-specific one, in extraocular musculature. *J. Cell Biol.*, 101: 618–629.

Wilkinson, H.J. (1930) Experimental studies on the innervation of striated muscle. *J. Comp. Neurol.*, 51: 129–151.

Windhorst, U., Hamm, T.M. and Stuart, D.G. (1989) On the functioning of muscle and reflex partitioning. *Behav. Brain Sci.*, 12: 629–681.

M.D. Binder (Ed.)
Progress in Brain Research, Vol 123

CHAPTER 21

Neuromuscular strategies underlying ballistic movements

Robert J. Callister,[1,*] Ellengene H. Peterson[2] and Alan M. Brichta[1]

[1] *The Neuroscience Group and Discipline of Anatomy, School of Biomedical Sciences, Faculty of Medicine and Health Sciences, The University of Newcastle, Callaghan, NSW 2308, Australia*
[2] *Neurobiology Program and Department of Biological Sciences, Ohio University, Athens, OH 45701, USA*

Introduction

One major goal of motor control research is to advance understanding about the central nervous system (CNS) mechanisms that bring about movement diversity. Such diversity results from two sources of variation: (a) the design of musculoskeletal elements that participate in movement, and (b) the way these elements are activated by the CNS. Conceptually, but not necessarily technically, the simplest approach to understanding how a neuromuscular system might generate a specific type of movement is to begin by studying the individual properties of its various components: e.g. the muscle fiber (MF), the motor unit (MU), and the motoneuron's (MNs). Eventually, a picture begins to emerge showing how the distinctive components might function during movement. For example, skeletal muscles are composed of MFs which have different morphological (e.g. lengths, diameters, tapering profiles) and physiological/biochemical (e.g. contraction speed, fatigability) properties. Each of these properties, and their various combinations, confer certain capabilities on the muscle. One may begin by asking how individual MFs with different properties are assembled to form whole MUs and whole muscles. One may then examine how the CNS, at both segmental and suprasegmental levels, might activate this assembly of

usually heterogeneous MFs and MUs. This approach has been applied with great success to groups of muscles that are involved in cyclical patterns of muscle activation that are driven by central pattern-generating circuits (e.g. chewing, scratching, locomotion). In contrast, much less is known about muscle systems that are involved in ballistic movements. In this article, we focus on the design of the various musculoskeletal and neural elements that participate in ballistic head retraction, the chief escape response in turtles.

Ballistic head movements in turtles

Turtles are often thought of as slow and sluggish, but they can execute movements with surprising speed and agility when threatened or acquiring prey. These rapid movements include leaping into water from a basking position (Cagle, 1946), fast swimming away from perceived danger (Silber, 1977), rapid head strikes during prey capture (Lauder and Pendergast, 1992), and, if threatened, explosive retraction of all extremities including the head/neck complex (Silber, 1977).

The fossil record shows that a retractable head and neck has been a feature of turtle anatomy for at least 150 million years (Romer, 1956; Carrol, 1969; Rougier et al., 1995). The successful performance of this movement has undoubtedly contributed to the continued survival of the species described in this report, *Pseudemys (Trachemys) scripta elegans*, and the order, Testudines, in general. We have recently analyzed turtle head movements by

---

*Corresponding author. Tel.: +61 2 4921 5608; Fax: +61 2 4921 8667; e-mail: bcrjc@mail.newcastle.edu.au

combining video monitoring and magnetic search coil (essentially accelerometer) techniques under a variety of conditions, including ballistic movements such as head strike and retraction (Brannigan et al., 1999). The feeding strike (Fig. 1) illustrates

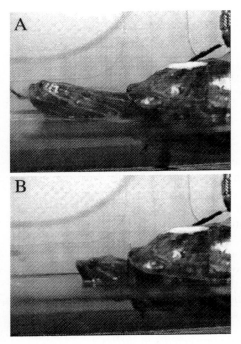

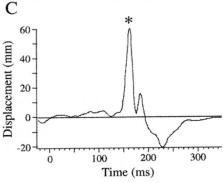

Fig. 1. Ballistic head movement in *Pseudemys*. The turtle is partially submerged, and its shell is clamped in a rigid frame. A and B show two successive frames from a video recording of the animal striking at a food reward and withdrawing its head. During this behavior, head velocity was monitored continuously by a magnetic search coil (MSC). The integrated output of the MSC is shown in C as a record of displacement vs. time. The head retraction phase of the food strike began at the asterisk and lasted ~ 40 ms.

such a ballistic movement. The animal's shell is fixed, and the turtle is lured to strike at a food target. The strike is followed by a rapid head withdrawal. A peak velocity of $1.25 \, \text{ms}^{-1}$ is generated by the animal during head retraction. This post-strike head retraction appears kinematically similar to the animal's stereotypical escape response, although comparative data on the two types of head retraction are unavailable. Our data show further that the head is withdrawn directly into the shell, regardless of its starting position. For example, if the animal is lured to strike to the left, the head is withdrawn by the shortest route from that starting position into the shell. The CNS machinery required for this fast and reproducible behavior is unknown, but a variety of indirect evidence (see below) suggests it must involve coordinated bilateral contraction of the large head retractor muscle (*retrahens capitus collique* [RCCQ]).

Figure 2 illustrates the attachments and general morphology of RCCQ in *Pseudemys*. This extensive muscle complex is composed of four successively longer bellies (R1–4) which arise from the caudal carapace and insert onto the head/neck complex. While no kinematic or electromyographic data are available to directly support this muscle's role in ballistic head retraction, its attachments, morphology and sheer size (8% of the animals muscle mass; Callister, unpublished observations) support the muscle's role in explosive retraction of the head/neck complex (Callister and Peterson, 1992). In addition, RCCQ is ideally placed to participate in movements such as positioning the head/neck complex during feeding and exploration. Thus, RCCQ can be regarded as a multifunctional muscle that participates in a variety of biologically important behaviors requiring widely different forces, velocities, displacements, and neural activation patterns.

Physical characteristics (muscle architecture) of single MFs in RCCQ

The morphology of single MFs and their arrangement within muscles (muscle architecture), albeit often ignored, plays an important role in determining muscle performance (e.g. Loeb et al., 1987).

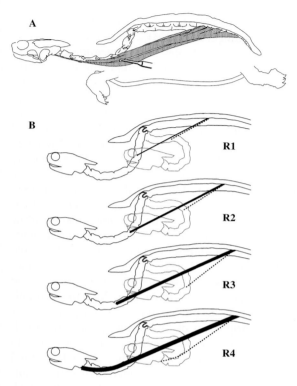

Fig. 2. Gross morphology, attachments, and action of the *retrahens capitis collique* (RCCQ) neck muscle. A: RCCQ in situ. The muscle has four bellies: the long anterior R4 attaches to the skull and the three successively shorter R3, R2, and R1, insert on vertebrae C4, 5, and 6, respectively. B: Head retraction in the mid-sagittal plane showing the approximate line of action of each belly at full protraction (solid line) and retraction (dashed line). Note that the cervical attachments of each belly undergo large excursions during head retraction. The thickness of the solid lines in B indicates the relative cross-sectional area at the mid-belly region.

MFs can be oriented in a variety of geometric patterns between a muscle's bony attachments. The consequences of arranging MFs end-to-end (in series), side-by-side (in parallel), or at an angle to the muscle's line of action, have substantial effects on muscle function (Josephson, 1975; Gans, 1982; McMahon, 1984; Trotter, 1993). The consequences of differing muscle architecture on muscle performance have also been explored theoretically (Woittiez et al., 1984; Otten, 1987; Gans and Gaunt, 1991). These theoretical approaches consider the sarcomere as the basic contractile element or building block of skeletal muscle. When equiva-

lent sarcomeres are linked together in series and shorten simultaneously, the displacements of sarcomeres are additive. For example, linking sarcomeres in series leads to greater displacements per unit time and, therefore, greater shortening velocities. In contrast, arranging equivalent sarcomeres in parallel increases the number of cross bridges that can form and so increases force production. If we ignore intrinsic properties, MF length (the number of sarcomeres in series) determines a MF's shortening velocity, while MF diameter (the number of sarcomeres in parallel) determines the force it can generate.

Using techniques that allow whole muscles to be digested into their component MFs, we removed single MFs from RCCQ and measured several of their functionally significant physical characteristics (see above). Only a brief account of these data are presented here (for a full description see Callister et al., 1992).

Single RCCQ MFs are arranged in a near-parallel fashion, and they exhibit a 10-fold variation in length, with almost 50% spanning the full muscle length. Most of the remaining MFs arise from either a bone or tendon attachment at the rostral or caudal end of the muscle and terminate intramuscularly. In RCCQ, it is rare to find MFs that have both ends terminating within the muscle's belly. MFs that terminate intramuscularly do so by tapering over several mm, and they end in fine-tapered tips (see, Loeb et al., 1987). The diameters of single MFs in RCCQ vary from 13 to 85 μm and they form two diameter classes, above and below ~ 50 μm (Fig. 3A). There is a significant positive correlation between MF diameter and length, with most MFs that span the full muscle length having large diameters (Fig. 3A).

We also assessed the morphology of the tapering regions of MFs. Those of a large-diameter tended to taper over a small percentage of their length, thereby maintaining near-maximal diameters over most of their length. In contrast, small-diameter MFs taper over a larger proportion of their total length.

In summary, the physical features of MFs in RCCQ suggest that this muscle is designed to generate a variety of movements (Table 1). Several of this muscle's features make it well suited to the

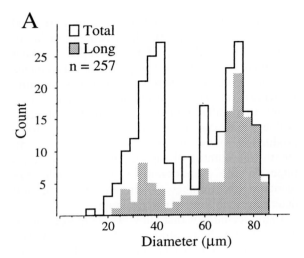

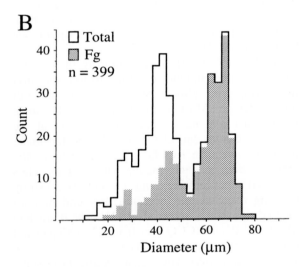

Fig. 3. Bimodal distribution of MF diameters in R4, the longest belly of RCCQ. A: The diameter distribution for MFs that span the muscle length is shown as a shaded histogram against the total sample. Note that the diameter distribution for the total MF sample is bimodal. Most MFs that span the muscle length belong to the large-diameter class. B: Distribution of MF diameters measured in histochemical material on R4. Because a significant proportion of MFs in RCCQ taper to fine tips intramuscularly, we made multiple diameter measurements of individual, histochemically-identified MFs over a distance of at least 5 mm and we accepted measurements from only those MFs having near-constant diameters over this distance (Callister et al., 1992). The diameter distribution for Fg MFs is shown as a shaded histogram vs. the total MF sample. Note that the total MF distribution has the *same* bimodal shape as in A and that the large-diameter peak in the distribution was comprised *near-exclusively* of Fg MFs.

production of ballistic movements. First, the near-parallel arrangement of MFs in all four bellies (Fig. 2) ensures that forces are transmitted to their insertions with no wasted component due to MF-angulation. Such parallel arrangements are normally found in muscles specialized for large excursions and high shortening velocities (Gans, 1982; Gans and Gaunt, 1991). Second, RCCQ contains a population of large-diameter MFs that span the full length of the muscle. These generate high forces (i.e. force $\propto$ cross sectional area). Furthermore, their long length suggests that they are capable of developing high shortening velocities, while their bone/tendon attachments allow forces to be transferred directly to the muscle ends without intervening series-elastic effects. Thus, the large-diameter MF class is well suited for producing the explosive movement needed for the turtle startle response. In contrast, most MFs in the small-diameter class terminate intramuscularly, taper over a large proportion of their length, and have small cross-sectional areas. Such MFs are not suited to explosive movement. Rather, they are better suited to assist in other head movements such as maintaining postures, and steering the head and neck complex during feeding or exploration of the environment.

Intrinsic properties of single MFs in RCCQ

A wealth of information exists on the intrinsic (metabolic and mechanical) properties of MFs in a wide range of vertebrates (for review: Van De Graaff et al., 1977; Burke, 1981; Goldspink, 1981; Rome et al., 1996; Bigland-Ritchie et al., 1998; Lutz et al., 1998; Goldberg and Shall, Chapter 20 and Richmond et al., Chapter 37 in this volume). Histochemical methods are routinely used to assess such intrinsic properties (Peter et al., 1972; McDonagh et al., 1980; Armstrong et al., 1982; Richmond and Armstrong, 1988; Selbie et al., 1993; Smits et al., 1994) because they provide insight into the functional characteristics of individual MFs: e.g. their contraction speed, force potential, and fatigue resistance. Thus, by determining a muscle's histochemical profile (i.e. by quantifying its complement of different MF types) one can obtain insight into the functional capabil-

TABLE 1

Architectural and intrinsic properties of single MFs in RCCQ

Diameter Class	Major Architectural Properties	Major Intrinsic Properties	Major Functional Implications
Large	• Large cross sectional area • Tend to be long and span muscle length • Taper over a small proportion of their length	• Dominated by Fg MFs • Fg MFs have fast myosins and low fatigue resistance	• Architecturally and histochemically specialized for brief movements requiring high forces and velocities
Small	• Small cross sectional area • Tend to be short and end intramuscularly • Taper over a large proportion of their length	• Include SO, FOG and some Fg MFs • SO and FOG MFs are resistant to fatigue	• Architecturally and histochemically suited for ongoing moments requiring low forces and velocities

ities of the whole muscle. (For the additional value of single-fiber microchemistry, see: Nemeth et al., 1986, 1991; Rosser et al., 1992).

MFs in turtle neck and hindlimb muscles can be divided into three classes on the basis of their histochemical properties: (a) slow oxidative (SO; including some non-twitch, tonic MFs; see below); (b) FOG, which have high oxidative and glycolytic capacities; and (c) Fg, which have low oxidative and low/intermediate glycolytic capacities (Callister et al., 1989; Callister et al.,1995; Laidlaw et al., 1995; for a different classification of turtle MF types, see Hermanson et al., 1986). MFs with fast myosins (i.e. Fg + FOG) predominate in all four bellies of RCCQ, accounting for 73–90% of the total MFs (Callister et al., 1992). Fg MFs account for 60% of the total in R2–R4, but are less numerous in R1. FOG MFs account for a nearly constant proportion of the total in all bellies (26–31%). Thus, the MF composition of the four bellies is very similar, with the exception that SO MFs are more numerous in R1 (the smallest belly) at the expense of Fg MFs.

The diameters of all histochemically identified MFs from one belly of RCCQ are shown in Fig. 3B. The large-diameter MFs are almost exclusively Fg, with virtually no SO and FOG MFs. Small-diameter MFs are mostly SO + FOG, but with a few Fg (Callister et al., 1992). Fig. 3B shows the same bimodal pattern is observed in the distribution of architectural features (Fig. 3A), thereby suggesting that we can reliably predict the architectural features of each histochemical MF type. For

example, large-diameter Fg MFs will tend to be long, taper over a small fraction of their total length, and many will span the full muscle belly.

In summary, the predominance of Fg MFs in RCCQ supports this muscle's primary role in developing the high forces and velocities required for rapid head retraction. The large-diameter and likely architectural features of Fg MFs make them well suited for producing ballistic movements. Nevertheless, there are a number of small-diameter, oxidative MFs (SO and FOG MFs) in all bellies of RCCQ, suggesting that this muscle may also mediate more graded movements of the head/neck complex. For example, it has been shown recently that >85% of the SO MFs in the longest belly of RCCQ (R4) are of the non-twitch type (Stuart et al., 1998). These are particularly well suited to postural functions (Morgan and Proske, 1984).

Innervation of single MFs in RCCQ

The innervation of individual MFs in RCCQ is complex (Callister and Peterson, 1992). Three of the four bellies (R2–R4) are supplied by at least two segmental nerves, and there is a well-defined boundary between the intramuscular territories of different segmental nerves supplying the same muscle belly (cf. Levine, 1966). Therefore, MFs that span the full length of RCCQ must pass through the innervation territories of more than one segmental nerve. All single MFs bear multiple terminals along their entire length. The number per MF ranges from two to 14, depending on MF

238

length. Thus, terminals are not sequestered at one end of the MF as would be expected if it was supplied by one or the other segmental nerve innervating the muscle belly. Rather, long MFs are usually innervated from two (or more) segments: i.e. they have polyneuronal innervation (for its implications, see Callister et al., 1995).

We used R4 to examine the organization of the spinal motor nucleus supplying RCCQ because it does not generally share its segmental innervation with another belly (Callister and Peterson, 1992). In addition, the nerve branches to this belly (C3–4) are readily accessible. Following application of horseradish peroxidase (HRP) to the C4 nerve, HRP-positive MNs are labeled in two spatially distinct regions of the ventral horn. One group occupies the ventral tip of the ventral horn, whereas the other lies at the dorsomedial grey/white border (Fig. 4). These two populations have been termed 'ventral' and 'medial' MNs (Yeow and Peterson, 1986; Peterson, 1989; Callister and Peterson, 1992). The two populations also differ markedly in their morphology. Ventral MNs have radiating dendrites, which project preferentially into the ipsilateral lateral funiculus and, in many respects, they resemble MNs in the turtle lumbar SC (Ruigrok et al., 1984; McDonagh et al., 1998a). In contrast, medial MNs have two distinctive dendritic systems: one projects contralaterally (Fig. 4A), and the other runs longitudinally along the medial grey/white margin of the spinal cord (SC).

In summary, each segmental nerve innervates a well-defined region of its target muscle belly, thereby forming discrete nerve-muscle compartments arranged in series. Individual MFs in RCCQ bear multiple motor terminals, and our data support an earlier suggestion by Levine (1966) that MFs spanning the entire length of the largest belly of RCCQ are polyneuronally innervated by MNs located in adjacent spinal segments. Finally, RCCQ is innervated by two populations of MNs that have distinctive dendritic morphologies and spatial distributions.

Conclusions

In conclusion, we first consider some broad implications of the architecture and innervation of

RCCQ in *Pseudemys*, and suggest how future work should advance our understanding of peripheral and segmental mechanisms subserving ballistic movements. We then consider the differing head retraction mechanisms found in the two chelonian suborders, and we propose that comparative studies of these two mechanisms may provide a useful test of the hypothesis that neuromuscular systems are conserved during the evolution of motor behaviors (cf., Pearson, 1993; Stuart and Callister, 1993).

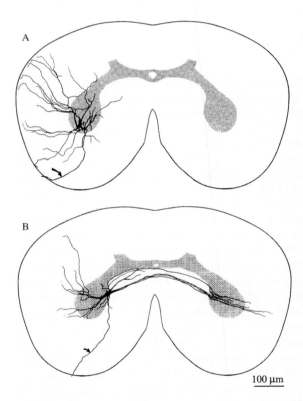

Fig. 4. Innervation of the RCCQ muscle by two spatially and morphologically distinct populations of MNs. Camera lucida drawings illustrate ventral (A) and medial (B) MNs previously labeled by applying HRP to the C4 nerve supplying R4. Each MN type has its own distinct soma position and dendritic architecture. Ventral MNs are located in the most-ventral tip of the ventral horn and they possess radial dendritic arbors, confined to the ipsilateral grey and white matter. Medial cells were at the medial grey/white border and they possess two unique dendritic systems: (1) contralateral dendrites that crossed the ventral funiculus into the opposite side of the SC; and (2) rostrocaudally-oriented longitudinal dendrites (not shown; see Callister and Peterson, 1992). Curved arrows in A–B show the cell's axon exiting the cord via a ventral root.

An hypothesis on the control of ballistic head movement in Pseudemys

Our hypothesis is that head retraction in *Pseudemys* is mediated by two peripheral effector systems, which generate distinctive movement profiles (Fig. 5). One effector system consists of large-diameter MFs that are almost exclusively of the Fg type. These MFs account for most of the muscle's cross-sectional area, tend to be long, often span the complete muscle length, and exhibit several architectural specializations for producing high forces and velocities (e.g. large cross-sectional areas, bone-to-bone attachments, minimal taper). They bear large motor terminals and receive multiple innervation, often from more than one spinal segment, and most likely from more than one MN (Levine, 1966; Callister and Peterson, 1992). *We propose that these MFs mediate the explosive head*

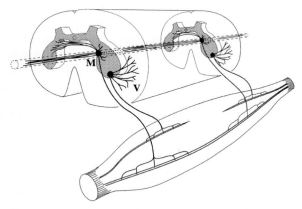

Fig. 5. Neural control of head movement in *Pseudemys*. This schematic summarizes our hypothesis on the innervation of two parallel effector channels in RCCQ. In the periphery, there exist two populations of MFs: (1) small-diameter MFs, mostly type SO and FOG, are relatively short and innervated by MNs in a *single* SC segment; and (2) large-diameter Fg MFs are long and innervated by multiple motor terminals arising from MNs in adjacent SC segments. Centrally, RCCQ is innervated by two populations of MNs, which differ in their location and dendritic morphology. Ventral MNs (V) have dendrites confined to the ipsilateral side of the cord; and medial MNs (M) have two distinctive dendritic systems, one which crosses the midline and another which runs longitudinally (indicated by dashed tube). We propose that ventral MNs innervate the small-diameter MFs, and that medial MNs innervate the large-diameter Fg MFs. The two specialized dendritic systems of medial MNs provide a substrate for the synchronous activation of ipsilateral and contralateral MNs that drive ballistic head retraction.

retraction associated with the turtle startle response.

The second effector system consists of smaller-diameter MFs. These are primarily SO and FOG MFs. They account for a small proportion of the muscle's cross-sectional area, taper over a large proportion of their lengths, and receive input from multiple, small motor terminals. Because these MFs tend to be short, they are probably innervated from a single spinal segment. We suggest that these small-diameter MFs are important for postural maintenance and more graded movements of the head during feeding, exploration, and positioning of the cranial sense organs.

The innervation of large- vs. small-diameter RCCQ MFs is unknown, but at least two lines of evidence suggest that they are innervated by medial vs. ventral MNs, respectively. First, medial MNs are uniformly large whereas ventral MNs exhibit a wider range in soma size (Callister and Peterson, 1986). In cats (Burke, 1981) and fish (Fetcho, 1986; Westerfield et al., 1986) large MNs typically innervate large-diameter MFs. Second, medial MNs possess two dendritic systems that are absent in ventral MNs. They appear well suited to subserve the kinds of synchronous activation of large-diameter (Fg) MFs that ballistic head retraction demands. The longitudinally oriented dendrites of the medial MNs could provide a substrate for synchronous activation of many Fg MFs, and of the two ends of single MFs which are innervated from adjacent spinal segments (Fig. 5). The contralaterally projecting dendrites could provide a substrate for synchronous activation of Fg MFs on both sides of the body axis, so that rapid head retraction is not compromised by lateral motion.

How might the CNS recruit these two effector channels? Much of what we know about MU recruitment is based on data from reduced preparations performing relatively simple movements and requiring low levels of force production (Enoka and Stuart, 1984; Loeb, 1987; Stuart and Enoka, 1990; Cope and Sokoloff, Chapter 16, in this volume). Until recently, it was believed that the order of MU recruitment is invariant and based on the unit's mechanical properties: slow contracting MUs, which produce low forces and are fatigue resistant, were thought to be recruited first, followed by successively faster, stronger, and more fatigue-sensitive units (Henneman and Mendell, 1981). With the advent of improved techniques, MU recruitment has now been investigated during a wider range of behaviors, and in freely moving animals. These experiments have shown that MU recruitment is not based simply on the intrinsic neuromechanical properties of the MUs but may also depend on behavioral demands. For example, MUs in the sartorius of freely moving cats can be divided into three functionally segregated groups which are preferentially recruited for different specific tasks (Hoffer et al., 1987). Distinct MU populations are active during a specific phase of locomotion and perform knee extension, knee and hip flexion, or knee extension and hip flexion, respectively. Similarly, classical recruitment order may be abandoned during certain phases of fish locomotion (Liu and Westerfield, 1988; Jayne and Lauder, 1994) and during eccentric contractions in mammals (Enoka, 1996; Bawa and Jones, Chapter 19, in this volume). Thus, activation of different MU types in a muscle's motor pool may depend on the mechanical requirements of the task being performed.

We now propose that the recruitment of MUs in RCCQ follow similar rules to those described above: i.e. specific MUs are recruited according to behavioral demands. The spatial segregation of medial and ventral MNs in the SC may simplify the task of recruiting functionally different MN populations. Such segregation of functional subpopulations within a spinal motor nucleus appears to exist in other axial muscle systems as well (Liu and Westerfield, 1988; Peterson, 1989).

Thus, our hypothesis is that RCCQ is organized into two parallel neuromuscular systems that mediate different patterns of head retraction (Fig. 5). Medial MNs drive the large-diameter Fg MFs that mediate explosive head retraction whereas ventral cells supply the small-diameter MFs that mediate graded movements of the head and neck during behaviors such as posture, feeding and exploration. This hypothesis can be tested with presently available techniques. Conventional microelectrode recording could be used to study the physiological properties (Burke, 1981) of medial and ventral MUs in an in vivo, SC-muscle preparation. MFs

belonging to MUs from each MN population could be identified via a combination of glycogen depletion and histochemical techniques (Burke, 1981). Together these experiments would allow the identification of MU territories supplied by each MN population and provide the necessary data to confirm or refute our hypothesis about the innervation of different MF types in RCCQ. If such experiments were to substantiate our hypothesis, then RCCQ will become a valuable model for the study of task-related recruitment in a multi-functional muscle.

Head retraction in cryptodyran and pleurodyran turtles

The first true chelonians appear in the fossil record from the late Triassic (over 200 million years ago). They shared several morphological features with modern species, including a highly specialized shell (Lee, 1993; Rougier et al., 1995). A retractable head/neck complex appeared considerably later in the fossil record. Subsequent musculoskeletal modifications resulted in the division of all living turtles into two suborders based in part on the mode of head/neck retraction (Fig. 6). The widespread cryptodires, such as *Pseudemys*, retract their heads into their shells in the vertical/sagittal plane (Fig. 6A). The less diverse pleurodiran ('side-neck') turtles, which are confined largely to Australia and parts of South America, retract their necks in the horizontal plane (Fig. 6B). Thus, the same important defensive behavior (ballistic head retraction) is achieved by two different mechanisms, and these require substantial differences in the joints and musculature of the neck.

What does the evolution of these two different mechanisms suggest about the segmental circuitry of the CNS that drives ballistic head retraction in cryptodiran and pleurodiran turtles? One important hypothesis about the evolution of behavioral diversity suggests that peripheral elements (e.g. muscles, muscle insertions, joint design) may undergo extensive modification, while central neural mechanisms, as assessed by muscle activation patterns and kinematics, remain relatively unchanged (Smith, 1994). Several examples support this hypothesis, including the evolution of the shoulder

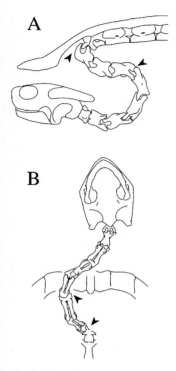

A

B

Fig. 6. The planes of retraction of the head and neck in cryptodiran vs. pleurodiran turtles. A: Cryptodiran turtles, such as *Pseudemys*, retract their necks in a sigmoid curve which lies in a vertical/sagittal plane. The arrowheads mark intervertebral articulations C5–6 and C8–D1, which allow the greatest flexion of the vertebral column. To understand neck movements in cryptodiran turtles, several workers have noted that the cervical vertebrae can be divided into two regions (Yeow and Peterson, 1986). Most articulations in the rostral half of the neck (skull to C5) are modified ball-and-socket joints which allow movement in the horizontal and vertical planes. Articulations between caudal cervical vertebrae, C5–8, occur via bicondylar joints that restrict movement to the vertical plane. These two regions are linked to the shell via a broad ellipsoidal joint (C8-D1) which serves as the main pivot point during large excursions in both the horizontal and vertical planes (Callister; unpublished observations on X-rays of freshly sacrificed preparations). Therefore, the whole cervical column is free to swing in both the vertical and horizontal planes about the highly mobile C8–D1 articulation. Note that all four bellies of RCCQ cross this joint. B: Pleurodiran turtles retract their heads in the horizontal plane. As in A, arrows point to the intervertebral articulations (C5/C6 and C8/D1), that allow the greatest flexion in the neck. According to Romer (1956), the neck flexes laterally to either side because the intervertebral articulations are simpler than those described for cryptodiran turtles.

in amniotes and feeding behavior in vertebrates but ". . . few studies have discussed how these hypoth-

eses of neuromotor conservatism may be corroborated or refuted . . ." (Smith, 1994; p. 294). We believe a careful comparison of the CNS strategies underlying head retraction in the two surviving suborders of turtles might contribute to this debate by testing whether the obvious peripheral differences in head retraction are driven by a conserved motor pattern. This would require, at a minimum, a detailed knowledge of neck structure, the neural control of head retraction, and the phylogenetic relations between a number of cryptodiran and pleurodiran species. The data obtained from such comparisons would contribute to the ever-expanding interest in the conservation vs. species specialization of motor-control systems, and it would provide valuable information about the neural control of ballistic movements.

Acknowledgements

We thank Douglas G. Stuart and Suzanne J. Farley for their helpful comments on earlier versions of this manuscript.

References

Armstrong, R.B., Saubert, C.W., Seeherman, H.J. and Taylor, C.R. (1982) Distribution of muscle fiber types in the locomotory muscles of dogs. *Am. J. Anat.*, 163: 87–98.

Bigland-Ritchie, B., Fugelvand, A.J. and Thomas, CK. (1998) Contractile properties of human motor units: is man a cat? *The Neuroscientist*, 4: 240–249.

Brannigan, J.T., Brichta, A.M. and McCrea, R.A. (1999) Context dependent changes in the vestibulo-collic reflex of the turtle. *Soc. Neurosci. Abstr.*, 25: 661.

Burke, R.E. (1981) MUs: anatomy, physiology, and functional organization. In: J.M. Brookhart and V.B. Mountcastle (Eds), *Handbook of Physiology, The Nervous System*, Vol. 2, Williams and Wilkins, Baltimore, pp. 345–422.

Cagle, F.R. (1946) The growth of the slider turtle, *Pseudemys scripta elegans. Am. Midl. Nat.*, 36: 685–729.

Callister, R.J., Callister, R. and Peterson, E.H. (1989) Histochemical classification of neck and limb muscle fibers in a turtle, *Pseudemys scripta*: a study using microphotometry and cluster analysis techniques. *J. Morphol.*, 199: 269–286.

Callister, R.J., Callister, R. and Peterson, E.H. (1992) Design and control of the head retractor muscle in a turtle, *Pseudemys (Trachemys) scripta*: I. Architecture and histochemistry of single muscles fibers. *J. Comp. Neurol.*, 325: 405–421.

Callister, R.J., Laidlaw, D.H. and Stuart, D.G. (1995) A commentary on the segmental motor system of the turtle, *Pseudemys (Trachemys) scripta elegans*: Implications for the study of muscle fatigue. *J. Morphol.*, 225: 213–227.

Callister, R.J. and Peterson, E.H. (1986) Dendritic architecture of two MN populations, supplying neck muscles in a cryptodiran turtle, *Pseudemys scripta. Soc. Neurosci.* Abstr., 12: 1420.

Callister, R.J. and Peterson, E.H. (1992) Design and control of the head retractor muscle in a turtle, *Pseudemys (Trachemys) scripta*: II. Efferent innervation. *J. Comp. Neurol.*, 325: 422–434.

Carrol, R.L. (1969) Origin of reptiles. In: C. Gans, A. Bellairs and T.S. Parsons (Eds), *Biology of the Reptilia*, Vol. 1, Academic Press, London and New York, pp. 1–44.

Enoka, R.M. (1996) Eccentric contractions require unique activation strategies by the nervous system. *J. Appl. Physiol.*, 81: 2339–2346.

Enoka, R.M. and Stuart, D.G. (1984) Henneman's 'size principle': Current issues. *Trends Neurosci.*, 7: 266–228.

Fetcho, J.R. (1986) The organization of MNs innervating the axial musculature of vertebrates. I. Goldfish *(Carassinus auratus)* and mudpuppies *(Necturus maculosus). J. Comp. Neurol.*, 249: 521–550.

Gans, C. (1982) Muscle fiber architecture and muscle function. *Exerc. Sport Sci. Rev.*, 10: 160–207.

Gans, C. and Gaunt, A.S. (1991) Muscle architecture in relation to function. *J. Biomechanics*, 24: 53–65.

Goldspink, G. (1981) Design of muscle for locomotion and maintenance of posture. *Trends Neurosci.*, 9: 218–221.

Henneman, E. and Mendell, L.M. (1981) Functional organization of the MN pool and its inputs. In: J.M. Brookhart and V.B. Mountcastle (Eds), *Handbook of Physiology, The Nervous System*, Vol. 2, Williams and Wilkins, Baltimore, pp. 423–507.

Hermanson, J.W., Lennard, P.R. and Takamoto, R.L. (1986) Morphology and histochemistry of the ambiens muscle in the red-eared turtle *(Pseudemys scripta). J. Morphol.*, 187: 39–50.

Hoffer, JA, Loeb, GE, Marks, W.B., O'Donovan, M.J., Pratt, C.A. and Sugano, N. (1987) Cat hindlimb MNs during locomotion. I. Destination, axonal conduction velocity, and recruitment threshold. *J. Neurophysiol.*, 57: 510–529.

Jayne, B.C. and Lauder, G.V. (1994) How swimming fish use slow and fast muscle fibers: implications for models of vertebrate muscle recruitment. *J. Comp. Physiol. A.*, 175: 123–131.

Josephson, R.K. (1975) Extensive and intensive factors determining the performance of striated muscle. *J. Exp. Zool.*, 194: 143–170.

Laidlaw, D.H., Callister, R.J. and Stuart, D.G. (1995) Muscle fiber-type composition of hindlimb muscles in the turtle, *Pseudemys (Trachemys) scripta elegans. J. Morphol.*, 225: 193–211.

Lauder, G.V. and Pendergast, T. (1992) Kinematics of aquatic prey capture in the snapping turtle *Chelyra serpentina. J. Exp. Biol.*, 164: 55–78.

Lee, M.S.Y. (1993) The origin of the turtle body plan: bridging a famous morphological gap. *Science*, 261: 1716–1720.

Levine, L. (1966) An electrophysiological study of chelonian skeletal muscle. *J. Physiol., (Lond.)* 183: 683–713.

Liu, D. and Westerfield, M. (1988) Function of identified MNs and co-ordination of primary and secondary motor systems during zebra fish swimming. *J. Physiol., (Lond.)*, 403: 73–89.

Loeb, G.E. (1987) Hard lessons in motor control from the mammalian SC. *Trends Neurosci.*, 10: 108–113.

Loeb, G.E., Pratt, C.A., Chanaud, C.M. and Richmond, F.J.R. (1987) Distribution and innervation of short, interdigitated muscle fibers in parallel fibered muscles of the cat hindlimb. *J. Morphol.*, 191: 1–15.

Lutz, G. J., Bremmer, S., Lajevardi, N., Lieber, R.L. and Rome, L.C. (1998) Quantitative analysis of muscle fiber type and myosin heavy chain distribution in the frog hindlimb: implications for locomotory design. *J. Muscle Res. Cell Motil.*, 19: 717–731.

McDonagh, J.C., Binder, M.D., Reinking, R.M. and Stuart, D.G. (1980) A commentary on muscle unit properties in cat hindlimb muscles. *J. Morphol.*, 166: 217–230.

McDonagh, J.C., Gorman, R.B., Gilliam, E.E., Hornby, T.G., Reinking, R.M. and Stuart, D.G. (1998a) Properties of spinal MNs and interneurons in the adult turtle: provisional classification by cluster analysis. *J. Comp. Neurol.*, 400: 544–570.

McMahon, T.A. (1984) *Muscle, Reflexes, and Locomotion*, Princeton University Press, Princeton, New Jersey.

Morgan, D.L. and Proske, U. (1984) Vertebrate slow muscle: its structure, pattern of innervation, and mechanical properties. *Physiol. Rev.*, 64: 103–169.

Nemeth P.M., Solanki, L., Gordon, D.A., Hamm, T.M., Reinking, R.M. and Stuart, D.G. (1986) Uniformity of metabolic enzymes within individual motor units. *J. Neurosci.*, 6: 892–898.

Nemeth, P.M., Rosser, B.W., and Wilkinson, R.S. (1991) Metabolic and contractile uniformity of isolated motor unit fibres of snake muscle. *J. Physiol., (Lond.)* 434: 41–55.

Otten, E. (1987) Optimal design of vertebrate and insect sarcomeres. *J. Morphol.*, 191: 49–62.

Pearson, K.B. (1993) Common principles of motor control in vertebrates and invertebrates. *Annu. Rev. Neurosci.*, 16: 265–297.

Peter, J.B., Barnard, R.J., Edgerton, V.R., Gillespie, C.A. and Stempel, K.E. (1972) Metabolic profiles of three muscle fiber types of skeletal muscle in guinea pigs and rabbits. *Biochemistry*, 11: 2627–2633.

Peterson, E.H. (1989) Motor pool organization of vertebrate axial muscles. *Am. Zool.*, 29: 123–137.

Richmond, F.J.R. and Armstrong, J.B. (1988) Muscle fiber architecture and histochemistry in the cat neck muscle, biventer cervicis. *J. Neurophysiol*, 60: 46–59.

Rome L.C., Funke, R.P., Alexander, R.M., Lutz, G., Aldridge, H., Scott F. and Freadman, M. (1988) Why animals have different muscle fibre types. *Nature*, 335: 824–827.

Rome, L., Swank, D. and Corda, D. (1993) How fish power swimming. *Science*, 261: 340–343.

Romer, A.S. (1956) *Osteology of Reptiles*, The University of Chicago Press, Chicago.

Rosser, B.W., Norris, B.J. and Nemeth, P.M. (1992) Metabolic capacity of individual muscle fibres from different anatomic locations. *J. Histochem. Cytochem.*, 40: 819–825.

Rougier, G.W., de la Fuente, M.S. and Arcucci, A.B. (1995) Late triassic turtles from South America. *Science*, 268: 855–858.

Ruigrok, T.J.H., Crowe, A. and Ten Donkelaar, H.J. (1984) Morphology of lumbar MNs innervating hindlimb muscles in the turtle, *Pseudemys scripta elegans*: an intracellular horseradish peroxidase study. *J. Comp. Neurol.*, 230: 413–425.

Selbie, W.S., Thomson, D.B. and Richmond, F.J.R. (1993) Suboccipital muscles in the cat neck: morphometry and histochemistry of the rectus capitis muscle complex. *J. Morphol.*, 216: 47–64.

Silber, G. (1977) A behavioral study of backflipping and backstroking in the turtle. Senior Honors Thesis. St Louis, Washington University.

Smith, K.K. (1994) Are neuromotor systems conserved in evolution? *Brain Behav. Evol.*, 43: 293–305.

Smits, E., Rose, P.K., Gordon, T. and Richmond, F.J.R (1994) Organization of single MUs in feline sartorius. *J. Neurophysiol.*, 72: 1885–1896.

Stuart, D.G., McDonagh, J.C., Pierce, P.A., Dalponte, D., and Abraham, K.A. (1998) Turtle non-twitch muscle fibers and their potential innervation. *Soc. Neurosci. Abstr.*, 24: 914.

Stuart, D.G. and Callister, R.J. (1993) Afferent and spinal reflex aspects of muscle fatigue: issues and speculations. In: A.J. Sargeant and D. Kernell (Ed.), *Neuromuscular Fatigue*, Amsterdam: Royal Netherlands Academy of Arts and Sciences, North-Holland, pp. 169–180.

Stuart, D.G. and Enoka, R.M. (1990) Hennerman's contributions in historical perspective. In: M.D. Binder and L.M. Mendell (Eds), *The Segmental Motor System*, New York, Oxford University Press, pp. 3–19.

Van De Graaff, K.M., Frederick, E.C., Williamson, R.G. and Goslow, G.E. Jr, (1977) Motor unit types of primary ankle extensors of the skunk (*Mephitus mephitis*). *J. Neurophysiol.*, 40: 1424–1431.

Trotter, J.A. (1993) Functional morphology of force transmission in skeletal muscle. *Acta Anat.*, 146: 205–222.

Westerfield, M., McMurray, J.V. and Eisen, J.S. (1986) Identified MNs and their innervation of axial muscles in the zebra fish. *J. Neurosci.*, 6: 2267–2277.

Woittiez, R.D., Huijing, P.A., Boom, H.B.K. and Rozendal, R.H. (1984) A three dimensional muscle model: a quantified relation between form and function in skeletal muscle. *J. Morphol.*, 182: 95–113.

Yeow, M.B.L. and Peterson, E.H. (1986) Organization of motor pools supplying the cervical musculature of a cryptodiran turtle, *Pseudemys scripta elegans*. II. Medial motor nucleus and muscles supplied by two motor nuclei. *J. Comp. Neurol.*, 243: 166–181.

Comparative physiology of pattern generators

M.D. Binder (Ed.)
Progress in Brain Research, Vol 123
© 1999 Elsevier Science BV. All rights reserved.

CHAPTER 22

General principles of rhythmic motor pattern generation derived from invertebrate CPGs

Allen Selverston*

Institute of Neurobiology, University of Peurto Rico, 201 Blvd del Valle, San Juan, Puerto Rico

Introduction

Rhythmic movements play a crucial role in the survival of all species. All animals have some form of rhythmic activity from locomotion to chewing. Understanding the neural mechanisms that underlie these rhythmic movements is an important question from the standpoint of neurophysiology, i.e. what are the mechanisms involved? But from a wider viewpoint, oscillatory activity in nerve cells, is a ubiquitous form of neural activity, and may be involved in many other functions such as sensory perception or even consciousness (Crick and Koch, 1998). While understanding oscillatory neural activity can be approached from many different levels, perhaps the most fundamental is – how do individual neurons in the central nervous system interact with one another to generate rhythmic spatio-temporal patterns? Since rhythmic behaviors are produced by appropriately timed bursts of impulses to the correct muscles, this question can be reduced to the form: how are spatio-temporal patterns produced by the nervous system? Since patterned activity forms the basis of all neuronal signalling, both sensory and motor, understanding how this one type of pattern is generated and controlled is likely to tell us much about pattern formation in general.

Invertebrate nervous systems have particular advantages in elucidating the mechanisms underlying the formation of rhythmic patterns because the circuits that generate these patterns, the central pattern generators (CPGs), are made up of fewer and larger nerve cells than are the CPGs of vertebrates. Especially useful experimentally is the fact that each of the neurons in invertebrate circuits are uniquely identifiable and thus can be studied repeatedly from animal to animal. The concept of identifiability is different from the vertebrate concept of identity. Identifiable neurons can be characterized on the basis of their anatomical location and shape, their biochemical makeup, their physiological responses to synaptic and hormonal input, even what genes they express. Vertebrate neurons can be identified and studied as a group (e.g. Purkinje cells), but the fact that it is impossible to study the same neuron in different animals means that it is impossible to know how different these neurons really are when they are actively engaged in information processing. If vertebrate neurons turn out to be as heterogeneous as invertebrate neurons, then the complexity of interactions between them would be enormous. A more parsimonious view is that the underlying circuitry is similar to that found in the invertebrates, with each unique invertebrate neuron being represented in vertebrates by multiples of the same type. If this were to be the case, it would mean that the study of

---

*Corresponding author. Tel.: (787) 721-1237; Fax: (787) 725-3804; e-mail: al@neurobio.upr.clu.edu

small invertebrate circuits can serve as models with which to investigate the fundamental properties of brain and spinal cord circuits.

From work on a simple rhythmic central pattern generator, the stomatogastric ganglion (STG) of the lobster, by many research groups, some general principles have emerged that might be useful in thinking about the CPGs of more complex systems (Harris-Warrick et al., 1992) By studying this small, well-defined neural circuit, we have learned a great deal about how single neurons and groups of interconnected neurons participate in the production of spatio-temporal patterns. Their usefulness in helping to unravel and understand more complex vertebrate circuits has become generally accepted (Stein et al., 1997).

Oscillatory circuits

Repetetive ryhthmic behaviors are a good place to begin to unravel neural circuits because by the very nature of their repetition they are easier to study than behaviors that do not repeat themselves. More recently however, the oscillatory activity of brain cell ensembles has been suggested to play important cognitive roles as well (Singer, 1990). Invertebrate CPGs are a favorable target for studying oscillatory circuits because they offers the possibility of explaining rhythmic behavior in terms of all the neurons involved. The CPGs responsible for swimming, flying, chewing, etc. in invertebrates make good experimental preparations because their basic rhythmicity occurs without sensory feedback, in fact in total isolation from the animal itself. Isolated ganglia containing one or more CPGs, can be removed from the animal, put into a dish of saline and remain viable for many hours, a self-contained neural machine. The motor rhythms, recorded from the nerves or cell bodies, continue for many hours as so-called 'fictive' patterns.

Although rhythmic patterns can be shown over and over again not to require rhythmic cycle-by-cycle feedback from sensory receptors (Delcomyn, 1980), it is clear that for most CPGs, particularly those that operate intermittently and with different stable patterns, some form of nonrhythmic excitatory drive has to be present, i.e. the neurons

comprising CPGs cannot produce rhythmic patterns unless properly activated (Nagy and Miller, 1987). Until such activation occurs, either by sensory stimulation or by exposure to an excitatory pharmacological agent, the neurons are either silent or fire continuously. The anatomical framework for the CPG is present but not in a functional state.

One fundamental question regarding oscillatory behavior is whether rhythmicity arises from one or more bursting neurons or from the synaptic interactions of non-bursty neurons. In the STG system, it is clear that all of the neurons can oscillate when properly modulated so that both the gastric and pyloric rhythms are in actuality, systems of synaptically coupled neuronal oscillators. When neurons are isolated from their synaptic inputs or put into culture and then exposed to neuromodulators, oscillatory membrane potentials can be elicited (Panchin et al., 1993). On the other hand, pairs of neurons connected with reciprocal inhibition and isolated from other cells and from modulatory inputs, can be shown to synchronize in antiphase when depolarized with injected current (Miller and Selverston, 1982). So for the STG system, while it might be parsimonious to consider cellular bursting as the basis for the rhythmicity and synaptic interactions as the basis for patterning, the latter may also play some, as yet undefined role, in the rhythmicity as well.

Oscillatory activity in single neurons arises from cyclic conductances known as bursting pacemaker potentials that are generated in the presence of certain neuromodulators. The pacemakers start with a slow inward sodium and calcium conductance and a decrease in potassium conductance that slowly ramps the voltage up to transition point where the inward current suddenly increases and gives rise to a plateau potential (Gola and Selverston, 1981). Attenuated spikes are seen on the plateau phase that can be correlated with action potentials in the peripheral nerves. Activation of a voltage sensitive potassium current combined with a calcium activated potassium current return the voltage to the 'resting' level although it does not remain there. Similar cyclic conductance patterns are found in other invertebrate neurons which burst spontaneously such as R15 in Aplysia or the small cells of the lobster cardiac ganglion.

Oscillatory activity due to reciprocal inhibitory connections can easily be demonstrated in cell pairs by computer simulation if there is a source of common excitation to both cells and a time-dependent source of fatigue for the inhibitory synapses. It has been possible to isolate pairs of biological neurons from the pyloric system that become passive and silent when modulatory inputs are removed. If these neurons are depolarized to just the right level, they will oscillate and synchronize in antiphase (Miller and Selverston, 1982).

Critical cell and synaptic properties

To study the mechanisms underlying oscillatory behavior at the cellular level we can first identify each neuron that participates in generating a rhythmic pattern and then characterize it's electrophysiological properties. Since there are so few neurons in invertebrate pattern generators, this task is an experimentally tractable one. In the lobster stomatogastric ganglion (STG), there are about thirty neurons, eleven of which make up the gastric mill CPG and fourteen of which make up the pyloric CPG. Individual stomatogastric neurons have a unique pallette of electrophysiological properties that are under the control of neuromodulators. Thus one cannot speak of a neuron's electrophysiological properties as if they were in a fixed permanent state. Under unmodulated conditions, the neurons behave passively, with almost ohmic I/V curves although some neurons can fire tonically. Synapses can still operate in this state by releasing transmitter in a graded fashion when the presynaptic terminal is depolarized. Most of the synapses are very weak; they can generate postsynaptic potentials when the terminals are invaded by action potentials but these are also weak. The application of neuromodulators to CPG neurons causes an enhanced synaptic functioning in a modulator-specific way and the expression of other phenomena that are supressed in the unmodulated ganglion. These include:

1. Bursting pacemaker potentials – oscillations of membrane potential that set the frequency of the rhythm by eliciting bursts whenever the potential crosses threshold. The frequency is cell specific and can be altered with neuromodulators.
2. Delayed excitation – a pause following excitation that delays firing of the next burst; important in determining phase relationships.
3. Plateau potentials – the rapid transition to a depolarized state which can last for many seconds and plays an important role in determining burst length.
4. Action potentials – contribute (along with graded synaptic potentials) to intraganglionic signaling and since in the stomatogastric ganglion most of the CPG neurons are also motor neurons, to signaling effectors as well.
5. Postinhibitory rebound – the rebound of membrane potential past the resting level and often past firing threshold. The kinetics of this response effects the timing of bursts following inhibition.

The changes in the electrophysiological properties are due to changes in membrane properties, in particular to the type of receptors and ionic channels present. Metabotropic receptors, specific to many kinds of peptides and amines have been found in the membranes of STG neurons. Ligands binding to these receptors lead in most cases to the initiation of second messenger cascades and the phosphorylation of membrane channels (Harris-Warrick et al., 1992). In a few cases the ligands may act directly on the channels themselves. An increased concentration of second messengers generates the electrophysiological phenomena that in turn leads to the production of specific spatio-temporal patterns (Fig. 1). The ganglion uses two neurotransmitters, Ach and Glutamate and there are Ach and Glutamate ionotropic receptors in the membranes most which produce inhibitory postsynaptic potentials. These two types of receptor channels appear to function for both fast and slow signaling between pattern-generating neurons.

The pattern and type of channel present in each neuron helps determine its identity as well as the functional role it plays in generating a pattern. Of the many voltage-gated channels present in the membrane, five play a particularly important function in pattern generation. These five are also common to vertebrate neurons where they have been studied extensively and in many cases cloned.

1. I_A is a transient potassium current that is activated by depolarization and acts to slow further depolarization. Its main effect is to delay the firing of action potentials.
2. $I_{K(Ca)}$ is a second potassium current activated by the entry of Ca into the cell and has the effect of repolarizing neurons after they burst.
3. I_{Na} is the voltaged-gated channel responsible for producing action potentials but may also contribute to slow bursting and plateau potentials.
4. I_{Ca} involved in the depolarizing phase of the bursting pacemaker potential and the generation of plateau potentials.
5. I_h is a hyperpolarization-activated potassium current very prominent in some STG pacemaker neurons. Its activation produces the depolarizing

sag seen in the membrane voltage following strong hyperpolarization and tends to limit the time a neuron spends in the hyperpolarized phase.

Intracellular properties

The proteins in the neuronal membrane transduce extracellular messengers into signals the neuron uses to control its ionic conductances. The cell for the most part relies on intracellular mechanisms to link these two events. Three of the most important intracellular properties for the pattern generating process are: (a) the activation of second messenger systems (b) an increased concentration of kinases; and (c) the movement of Ca into and out of intracellular stores. There is direct evidence that cAMP concentrations can be raised intracellularly following their binding with modulatory

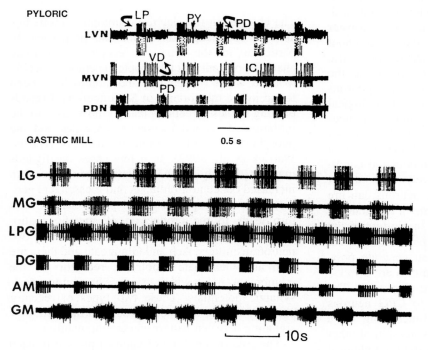

Fig. 1. Extracellular recordings of pyloric rhythm taken from a combined preparation; the three nerves contain all of the pyloric units. Note the PD unit appears in both the LVN and PDN trace and that this three phase rhythm occurs at a frequency of about 1 Hz. Extracellular recordings of the gastric mill motor pattern taken from a combined preparation. This complex five phase rhythm drives muscles responsible for moving the three teeth in the stomach in a 'chewing' rhythm. When LG and MG fire the lateral teeth close on the food particle and when LPG fires the teeth are pulled open. When DG and AM fire, the medial tooth is reset (return stroke) and when the four GMs fire the medial tooth is pulled over the food held by the lateral teeth (power stroke). Note this rhythm is much slower than the pyloric rhythm.

substances. Using the cAMP indicator FlCRhR the effect of octopamine, dopamine, acetylcholine, serotonin and proctolin were studied on identified stomatogastric neurons (Hempel et al., 1996). When bath-applied, each of these substances produced a transient increase in cAMP concentration. Each identified neuron responds differently in terms of the amplitude and time course of the response. There is some evidence that STG neurons also use IP_3 and Ca as second messengers but their effects have not been directly demonstrated. Increased concentrations of PKA and PKC appear to cause the phosphorylation of channels and receptors in STG neurons that produce a reconfiguration of the cell and synaptic properties one observes after modulator binding. Finally, the interplay between Ca entering the neuron, the metabolically driven pumping of Ca out of the cell, and Ca movements into and out of the endoplasmic reticulum, may play a role in the the chaotic oscillations in the membrane voltage time courses of isolated neurons that have been observed experimentally and analyzed using techniques of nonlinear analysis (Rabinovich et al., 1997).

Behavioral circuits are formed by synaptic interactions between individually identified neurons

The kind of analysis discussed thus far has been performed on neurons from both vertebrate and invertebrate preparations. These results have revealed that at the cellular, synaptic and molecular level, neurons operate in remarkably the same way whether they come from the cerebral cortex or from a lobster ganglion. However where a rigourous analysis of neuronal functioning begins to diverge is at the microcircuit level. Detailed circuits that consist of identified neurons linked together with invariable patterns of synaptic connectivity can really only be studied in invertebrates. This is so because in order to determine precise connectivity, neurons must be both identifiable and exist in small enough groupings that dual or triple intracellular recording and stimulating paradigms can be routinely made. Dual intracellular recordings from pre- and postsynaptic neurons in the vertebrate CNS cannot be made routinely at this time . So if we assume for the moment that the physiological

differences between vertebrate and invertebrate neurons is not large, then it is only at the circuit level that we may learn some fundamental lessons about neural circuits.

Work on the stomatogastric system, has revealed that there is a richly interconnected matrix of synaptic connections between the thirty neurons in the stomatogastric ganglion (Fig. 2). Out of this tangle of interconnections, various motor circuits are formed by specifing the biophysical properties of individual neurons and the strengths of particular synapses. How does this remarkable sculpting of defined functional circuits occur? In a normal combined preparation, the stomatogastric ganglion receives neuromodulatory inputs from higher ganglia (the commissurals and esophageal) and a very stereotyped gastric mill and pyloric motor pattern is produced (Fig. 1). This pattern is quite similar to that recorded from animals in situ. (Rezer and Moulins, 1983). However many other patterns are observed under both natural conditions and when modulatory substances are introduced into the animals bloodstream (Turrigiano and Selverston, 1989) The direct visualization of the teeth in the gastric mill by videoendoscopy has shown that the parameters of the chewing behavior can be significantly altered by modulatory substances such as proctolin or cholecystokinin (Heinzel and Selverston, 1988; Turrigiano and Selverston, 1990). As postulated previously (Harris-Warrick, 1988), the stomatogastric network is a multifunctional system capable of controlling a variety of different behaviors that are stable and useful. To some extent they parallel studies of different locomotory gaits in mammals that show that the different patterns that account for each gait are also stable but modifiable by sensory input on a cycle-by-cycle basis. The different patterns probably arise from multifunctional CPGs as well, and the mechanisms operating in each case are likely to be similar. The elegance of small systems like the stomatogastric in the study of such phenomena, is that the cellular mechanisms responsible for producing such multifunctionality can be rigorously investigated down to the cellular and molecular level. The changes that occur in the individual neurons of a defined circuit can in most cases be directly linked to the changes that occur in the motor pattern as a whole.

How are the neurons, each having sets of unique chacteristics, actually assembled into useful functional circuits? Indeed it is interesting to ask where these unique individual characteristics came from (in evolutionary terms) in the first place. Did the properties of each neuron arise primitively or were they 'tuned' as circuits of neurons were formed in response to behavioral needs or environmental constraints. It would seem that there could be many solutions to the problem of assembling circuits for particular functions and indeed many of the circuits that are found in nature, that do very similar jobs, turn out to be remarkably different in terms of their connectivity patterns. Are the circuits that have been formed the optimal ones for the task they perform? It is surprising that despite the amazing progress made at the cellular and molecular level, so little is known about how circuits are constructed, optomized and put together. Again these are questions that can be answered in defined circuits where the connectivity between neurons is known. Where it is not known, as in the extremely complicated circuitry of the mammalian CNS, the CPG is still a 'black box' in terms of it's precise connectivity. The circuits in the spinal cord that give rise to locomotion are still unknown and it is entirely possible that they will never be known in terms of interneuronal connectivity. The big question is will it matter? The lack of precise circuitry in the spinal cord has not stopped speculation about

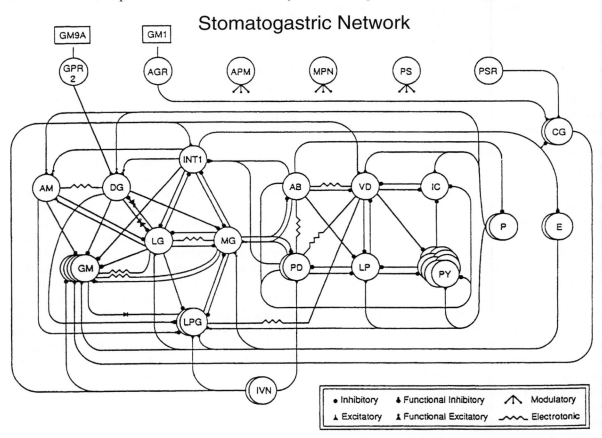

Fig. 2. The stomatogastric network consists of gastric and pyloric CPG neurons found in the stomatogastric ganglion. AB and Int 1 rhythmically inhibit the P and E cells which are located in the commissural ganglion. The P cells return rhythmic excitation to neurons in the pyloric system and the E cells return excitation to neurons in the gastric mill CPG. GPR, AGR and PSR are sensory neurons, APM, MPN and PS are all identified modulatory neurons. CG is usually found in European lobsters and is found in the commissurals. The IVNs are histaminergic fibers from the brain.

how locomotory CPGs might operate (Kiehn et al., 1997); but only if new techniques are developed, can the actual intercellular synaptic wiring of the vertebrate CNS be understood precisely.

Of course it is possible, and even likely that we will never know the microcircuitry of the brain and spinal cord with the same degree of precision that we know the circuitry of invertebrate CPGs. It may also be that even if we were to know it, the computations used when there are millions of cells and synapses involved may be totally different from when there are only a few dozen cells. But in my opinion it would be prudent to assume that the same cellular and synaptic building blocks that operate small systems are organized the same way in vertebrate circuits. That is, massive vertebrate circuits are just invertebrate circuits writ large. Each vertebrate neuron or set of neurons will probably also turn out to have different properties and the extent of connectivity will be enormous and possibly redundant but I know of no credible evidence that contradicts this possibility.

Neural circuits underlying a large number of invertebrate behaviors have now been described (Selverston et al., 1997). Their synaptic connectivity appears to be predominantly inhibitory which may be related to their ability to reduce firing irregularities (Abarbanel et al., 1996). Both excitatory synapses and electrotonic connections are found in great numbers. Overall the neural circuits that have been studied in invertebrates show as much complexity in terms of the number and types of synapses they contain, as they do in the types of cellular properties they have. Therefore the total possible number of interactions that can exist between such neurons is enormous and allows for a wide range of spatio-temporal patterns. To complicate matters further, we know that modulatory substances acting on invertebrate CPGs can alter both the cellular and synaptic properties significantly so that not even the basic cellular properties of the system are stable.

How can we begin to separate the roles of the synaptic connections from the roles of the cellular properties in producing spatio-temporal patterns? The synaptic interactions appear to be responsible for the temporal sequencing of bursts rather than in the production of the rhythmicity. Only a few CPGs

have been shown not to have endogenous or conditional bursting neurons (Getting, 1989) and these are usually associated with short-lived escape reactions. The kinetics and strengths of the synapses will be the primary organizer of the pattern. The cellular properties will generate the bursting pattern, its frequency, the length of bursts and the frequency of spike firing within a burst. So in generating a spatio-temporal motor pattern, the whole range of cellular and synaptic properties must be integrated. Patterns must be robust while at the same time flexible enough to be modified by sensory inputs and higher level commands.

Neuromodulators make circuits multifunctional

We have seen that neuromodulators play a key role in the functioning of neurons, converting them from a passive to an active state or modifying some particular biophysical property. The neurons that comprise the stomatogastric CPGs are so physiologically flexible that they are able to participate in a large number of different circuits (Dickinson and Moulins, 1992). The synaptic connectivity within the ganglion is something like a multiply interconnected central processing unit that needs to be programmed in order to produce functional circuits. The progamming consists of modifying channel properties so that the amplitude and time course of the currents they carry are altered. Individual neurons change their voltage-sensitive properties as well as their intrinsic properties. Thus a neuron that may be silent without modulation may start to generate bursting pacemaker potentials at a particular frequency. Chemical and electrical synapses that are weak and ineffective can become strong and influential.

The programing mechanism turns out to be an extremely complex one. Neuromodulatory substances released by specific neurons or by specialized neurohemal organs bind to receptors on individual neurons producing a variety of effects on their ionic channels via G proteins in the membrane. For the neurons in the STG to form *any* pattern, one or more modulatory substances must be present. Single neurons that do not receive such modulatory input do not show any form of rhythmic activity. Neurons that have the capability of bursting, but do so only when modulated are called 'conditional' bursters. There are only a few examples of neurons that have been discovered in invertebrates that are true endogenous bursters. Only when chemically activated, will conditional bursters produce the rhythmic bursts characteristic of oscillatory circuits. Not only do the neurons respond to modulators by changing their physiological properties-bursting pacemaker potentials, plateauing, postinhibitory rebound, etc., but, as mentioned, the synaptic and electrical connections between neurons are also modified. The effect of any one specific modulator on a CPG therefore is to specify a functional neural circuit that can generate a particular rhythmic motor pattern. We are only begining to get an idea about what sorts of patterns can be obtained when there are mixtures of different modulators present, as occurs in nature. But it appears that there are a finite number of stable patterns possible for any one circuit because of limitations put on them by instability and chaos.

The combined effect of all the cellular and synaptic interactions, most of which are nonlinear, should, in principle, be able to account for all of the parametric values of a rhythmic motor pattern – frequency, burst duration, burst frequency, phase relations between bursts, etc. One of the principal achievements of the invertebrate work has been the ability to incorporate cellular and synaptic phenomena into explanations of why CPGs behave the way they do. It is now possible to describe the ionic channels present in each identified cell and study how the conductance of each channel is effected by a particular modulator. We can measure the changes in strength or dynamics of a synapse between two identified neurons that result from modulatory action. There is a large and still growing data set for the properties of all of the neurons and synapses in the STG. The complexity of the thirty-celled STG is extrordinary because each neuron utilizes a different combination of ionic channels, receptors and second messenger systems. Each single neuromodulator can produce both convirgent and divergent effects and of course in the intact animal there is likely to be more than one modulator present at any one time or at any single concentration. Computer models are absolutely necessary for the synthesis of such a massive

amount of reductionistic data. Good models are able to predict the effect of experimentally altering any single cellular or synaptic property on the entire output pattern. But more fundamentally, computer models incorporating the nonlinear interactions between elements of the STG may begin to approach the theoretical question of why CPGs work at all. Why are they stable despite noise and sensory perturbations? How can they transition from one location in state space to another? To begin to answer such questions it is first necessary to be able to determine experimentally the major electrophysiological properties of the component cells and then have known circuits to plug them into.

Although the combinatorial possibilities for producing spatio-temporal patterning are huge, in fact the invertebrate CPG circuits which have been studied normally perform only a limited repertoire under natural conditions. There are probably constraints on a CPG in an intact system (sensory feedback, descending control) that are missing when the preparation is in a dish. Two such constraints are present in the stomatogastric system. One is a feedback loop between elements of both the pyloric and gastric mill CPG that provides rhythmically patterned excitation to most of the CPG neurons, even antagonists, at the same time. The precise role of these feedback loops is not known but similar loops also exist even in mammalian CPG systems.

Other types of inputs have been described by Nusbaum et al. consist of modulatory fibers with cell bodies in the commissural ganglia. Some of these neurons in addition to being modulatory have both excitatory and electrical synapses in STG. One modulatory projection neuron termed MCN_1 receives inhibitory input from a gastric mill neuron presynaptically that can switch its effect from excitation onto three neurons to electrical coupling with just one of them (Nusbaum et al., 1992). When the CPG circuits in the STG are deprived of modulatory inputs from higher ganglia or from modulators present in the blood stream, there are no interactions between neurons because the cells are for the most part silent. The particular modulator to which a ganglion is then exposed determines the functional circuit formed; the CPG circuits are therefore multifunctional and produce a pattern that is programmed by each modulator. Most studies to date on the effects of modulators use one single modulator at a time. However, in actuality, the circuitry is probably exposed to many modulators at any one time so the output states could be much more complex than we realize.

The functional rewiring of CPG circuits

Neuromodulatory substances that in some instances may be conventional neurotransmitters, can functionally rewire neural circuits to generate new patterns. If the modulators reach the ganglion from external sources such as other ganglia or as hormones they are termed extrinsic; if the substances are released by neurons that are components of a CPG, they are called intrinsic (Katz and Frost, 1995). In the lobster STG system, there is ample evidence that extrinsic modulation occurs and could play an important role in turning on and off both the gastric mill and pyloric rhythms. There is long standing evidence that Ach, a transmitter that activates relatively fast ionotropic inhibitory receptors has been released into the ganglion by identifiable neurons to produce modulatory effects as well (Nagy and Dickinson, 1983). There is also evidence for the possibility of intrinsic modulation. Recently, by using agonists for mGluR receptors, glutamate, the other fast neurotransmitter in the ganglion has been shown to have modulatory effects. While it is clear that extrinsic modulation by Ach or glutamate could occur in the STG system, it has yet to be demonstrated how it is used physiologically. If it is used intrinsically, reaching muscarinic receptors as a result of normal release by the cholinergic synapses in the ganglion, is still an open question. Similarly, although the activation of mGluRs has strong effects on the pyloric and gastric rhythms, there is as yet no evidence for how they are actually utilized by the circuit in vivo.

As already described, modulators will affect the two STG circuits by altering cellular and synaptic properties. Each known modulator changes a particular constellation of channels in each neuron by G-protein driven second messenger cascades. *The result of these changes is to produce many different motor patterns from the same circuitry by 'sculpting' out functional circuits from a single set of anatomical connections.* If the spinal circuitry underlying locomotion operated in the same way, one could conceive of a complex set of premotor interneurons and motor neurons being turned on by descending modulatory inputs and a particular gait determined by the mix of modulators selected.

For a mechanism like this to operate, the modulatory substances must activate metabotropic receptors. These receptors are specific for particular substances and their distribution on different neurons appears to vary, once again pointing out the uniqueness of individual cells and the difficulty in assuming that all neurons is any particular CNS system are the same.

In addition to the intrinsic and extrinsic modulatory sources that have been mentioned, modulators can also be released by sensory fibers entering the ganglion. The GPR receptors in the lobster are an example of how activation of a particular receptor not only affects cycle-by-cycle pattern formation but can also produce long term effects on the CPG (Simmers and Moulins, 1988).

Some general principles

The study of invertebrate central pattern generators has contributed in many ways to our understanding of rhythm generation in all animals and will, I believe, play an increasingly important role in linking today's solid advances in molecular neurobiology with more traditional systems neurophysiology. Many of the ideas that originated with invertebrate CPGs have already found their way into the vertebrate locomotion field as can be seen in this volume and in recent reviews of locomotor physiology (Kiehn et al., 1998). Perhaps the most important idea is that complex rhythmic motor patterns in simple systems can be fully explained on the basis of their circuitry and cellular properties and that these explanations can be confirmed by computer simulations. Predictions made by computer modeling have been tested experimentally and found to be valid. To this extent then it is possible to claim that we 'understand' at least some CPGs as well as we understand the ionic basis of the action potential. The most important lessons seem to be:

- The generation of rhythmicity in most networks depends on the ability of neurons to generate plateau potentials or burst endogenously. The bursting properties are usually conditional, i.e. they depend on the presence of some modulatory substance. Only a few invertebrate systems (e.g. Tritonia) still hold on to the idea that the *rhythmicity* arises from the synaptic interactions and not from bursting neurons.
- The formation of specific spatio-temporal patterns depends on the arrangement of synaptic connections as well as on the temporal properties of the cell and synaptic conductances. There appears to be little conservation of circuit arrangements between species. Many different circuit topographies of cell and synaptic building blocks are possible and indeed observed in nature.
- The function of some but not all ionic channels depends on the presence of intrinisc or extrinsic modulatory substances. Action potential currents are restricted to channels that function with or without modulation although the modulation of these channels can alter the properties of the action potentials. However channels that are heavily involved in the generation of spatio-temporal motor patterns are powerfully influenced by neuromodulators; the modification of these channels by phosphorylation can have major effects on all parameters of rhythmic patterns.
- Many neural circuits are multifunctional as a result of their exposure to different neuromodulators. Descending modulatory inputs and neuromodulators that have been released into the bloodstream can initiate and sustain distinctly different motor patterns or can elicit variations of the same pattern.

The study of invertebrate nervous systems, CPGs especially, have shown that certain principles exist between species and are likely to extend to higher nervous systems as well. Their usefulness in providing an interface between molecular biology and systems biology may make these small systems increasingly more useful.

References

Abarbanel, H.D.I., Huerta, R. et al. (1996) Synchronized action of synaptically coupled chaotic neurons: I. Simulations using model neurons. *Neural Comput.*, 8: 1567–1602.

Crick, F. and Koch, C. (1998) Consciousness and neuroscience. *Cereb. Cort.*, 8: 97–107.

Delcomyn, F. (1980) Neural basis of rhythmic behavior in animals. *Science*, 210: 492–498.

Dickinson, P.S. and Moulins, M. (Ed.) (1992) *Dynamic Biological Networks*, Cambridge, MA, The MIT Press.

Getting, P.A. (1989) Emerging principles governing the operation of neural networks. *Ann. Rev. Neurosci.*, 12: 185–204.

Harris-Warrick, R.M. (1988) Chemical modulation of central pattern generators. In: A.H. Cohen, S. Rossignol and S. Grillner (Eds), *Neural Control of Rhythmic Movements*, New York, John Wiley, pp. 285–331.

Gola, M. and Selverston, A.I. (1981) Ionic requirements for bursting activity in lobster stomatogastric neurons. *J. Comp. Physiol.*, 145: 191–207.

Harris-Warrick, R.M., Marder, E. et al. (Ed.) (1992) *Dynamic Biological Networks: The Stomatogastric Nervous System*, Cambridge, MIT Press.

Heinzel, H.G. and Selverston, A.I. (1988) Gastric mill activity in the lobster. III. Effects of proctolin on the isolated central pattern generator. *J. Neurophysiol.*, 59: 566–585.

Hempel, C.M., Vincent, P. et al. (1996) Spatio-temporal dynamics of cAMP signals in an intact neural circuit. *Nature*, 384: 166–169.

Katz, P.S. and Frost, W.N. (1995) Intrinsic neuromodulation in the Tritonia swim CPG: the serotonic dorsal swim interneurons act presynaptically to enhance transmitter release from interneuron C2. *J. Neurosci.*, 15: 6035–6045.

Kiehn, O., Hounsgaard, J. et al. (1997) Basic building blocks of vertebrate spinal central pattern generators. *Neurons, Networks and Motor Behavior*, Cambridge, MA, The MIT Press.

Kiehn, O., Harris-Warrick, R.M. et al. (Ed.) (1998) *Neuronal Mechanisms for Generating Locomotor Activity*, Annals of the New York Academy of Sciences. New York, New York Academy of Sciences.

King, D.G. (1976) Organization of crustacean neuropil. I. Patterns of synaptic connections in lobster stomatogastric ganglion. *J. Neurocytol.*, 5: 207–237.

Miller, J.P. and Selverston, A.I. (1982) Mechanisms underlying pattern generation in lobster stomatogastric ganglion as determined by selective inactivation of identified neurons. IV. Network properties of pyloric system. *J. Neurophysiol.*, 48: 1416–1432.

Nagy, F. and Dickinson, P.S. (1983) Control of a central pattern generator by an identified modulatory interneurone in crustacea. I. Modulation of the pyloric motor output. *J. Exp. Biol.*, 105: 33–58.

Nagy, F. and Miller, J.P. (1987) Appendix A: pyloric pattern generation in *Panulirus interruptus* is terminated by blockade of activity through the stomatogastric nerve. *The Crustacean Stomatogastric System*, Berlin, Springer-Verlag. 136–139.

Nusbaum, M.P., Weimann, J.M. et al. (1992) Presynaptic control of modulatory fibers by their neural network targets. *J. Neurosci.*, 12: 2706–2714.

Panchin, Y.V., Arshavsky, Y.I. et al. (1993) Lobster stomatogastric neurons in primary culture. I. Basic characteristics. *J. Neurophysiol.*, 69: 1976–1992.

Rabinovich, M.I., Abarbanel, H.D.I. et al. (1997) Self-regularization of chaos in neural systems: experimental and theoretical results. *IEEE Trans Circ. Syst.*, 44: 997–1005.

Rezer, E. and Moulins, M. (1983) Expression of the crustacean pyloric pattern generator in the intact animal. 153: 17–28.

Selverston, A.I., Panchin, Y.V. et al. (1997) Shared features of invertebrate central pattern generators. *Neurons, Networks and Motor Behavior*. Cambridge, MA, The MIT Press.

Simmers, A.J. and Moulins, M. (1988) A disynaptic sensor-imotor pathway in the lobster stomatogastric system. *J. Neurophysiol.*, 59: 740–756.

Singer, W. (1990) Search for Coherence. *Conc. Neurosci.*, 1: 1–26.

Stein, P.S.G., Grillner, S. et al. (Ed.) (1997) *Neurons, Networks and Motor Behavior*, Poggio, T.A. Cambridge, MA, The MIT Press.

Turrigiano, G.G. and Selverston, A.I. (1989) Cholecystokinin-like peptide is a modulator of a crustacean central pattern generator. 9: 2486–2501.

Turrigiano, G.G. and Selverston, A.I. (1990) A cholecystokinin-like hormone activates a feeding-related neural circuit in lobster. *Nature*, 344: 866–868.

M.D. Binder (Ed.)
Progress in Brain Research, Vol 123
© 1999 Elsevier Science BV. All rights reserved.

CHAPTER 23

Central pattern generators and interphyletic awareness

Paul S.G. Stein*

Department of Biology, Washington University, St. Louis, MO 63130, USA

Introduction

Central pattern generators (CPGs) have been extensively studied in the last four decades of the 20th century. The 60s were marked by key experimental support for the CPG concept in invertebrate motor neuroscience. An important 1965 Society for Experimental Biology conference emphasized invertebrate contributions; its conference volume introduced new preparations to a wider audience (Hughes, 1966). Breakthroughs with major impact on CPG research occurred as well in mammalian motor neuroscience in the 60s. In that decade, however, papers on invertebrate preparations rarely cited important mammalian work, and vice versa. In the 70s, key international conferences (1973 in Edmonton; 1975 in Valley Forge) provided a venue for investigators working with one species to meet each other and be aware of the important contributions of those working on other species. The associated conference volumes extended the influence of those meetings to a wider audience (R.B. Stein et al., 1973; Herman et al., 1976). 'Interphyletic awareness' is the term introduced by Professor Douglas G. Stuart to describe the interactions among investigators working on one species with those working on other species (Stuart, 1985). The 80s were marked by an expansion of work with non-mammalian vertebrates in addition to excellent progress with invertebrate and mammalian preparations. Key meetings in the 80s (1982

Society for Experimental Biology; 1985 in Stockholm) followed the tradition of the 70s meetings and solidified the interactions among investigators working on different preparations. Associated conference volumes again played a key role in transmitting new perspectives to a larger audience (Roberts and Roberts, 1983; Grillner et al., 1986a). The concept of CPG modulation flourished in the 90s, to a large extent based upon invertebrate experiments; this concept influenced workers studying vertebrate preparations. Major conferences served as venues for important interactions among investigators studying invertebrates, lower vertebrates, and mammals (1995 in Tucson; 1998 in New York; 1998 in Tucson). Their associated conference volumes communicate the contents of these meetings to a wider audience (P.S.G. Stein et al., 1997; Kiehn et al., 1998; Binder, this volume).

This chapter reviews my perspective of CPG research in both invertebrates and vertebrates in the last 40 years. Contributions from many investigators from a set of conferences and their volumes serve as benchmarks. Noted are changes in points of view concerning CPGs that were held by the investigators in the field. Interphyletic awareness is the focus of the chapter – in particular, the influences of experimental results obtained in one preparation on hypotheses and experimental designs in other preparations. These influences were important for many investigators; I discuss examples from my own work that illustrate how interphyletic awareness can modify an investigator's research program. This chapter is not comprehensive: space constraints do not permit the

---

*Corresponding author. Tel.: 314–935–6824; Fax: 314–935–4432; e-mail: stein@biology.wustl.edu

discussion of many excellent and important contributions.

This volume edited by Marc Binder honors Professor Douglas G. Stuart, a strong advocate of interphyletic awareness. He helped organize many conferences; he was a co-organizer of three of the conferences described above and a co-editor of their associated volumes (Herman et al., 1976; Grillner et al., 1986a; P.S.G. Stein et al., 1997). He wrote many influential reviews; several of these include important commentary on pattern generation (Wetzel and Stuart, 1976; Stuart, 1985; Hasan and Stuart, 1988; Callister et al., 1995; Stuart and McDonagh, 1998). This chapter joins the other chapters of this volume in honoring Professor Douglas G. Stuart's important contributions to motor neuroscience.

The central patterning of motor behavior and its modulation by movement-related sensory feedback

Specific motor patterns of motoneuron and muscle activation occur during behavior. The motor pattern that is produced during the behavior of an intact organism is generated by the 'motor pattern generator' or MPG, a collection of body cells including neurons, muscles, and skeletal cells (Dean and Cruse, 1995). Those aspects of the motor pattern that are preserved in the absence of movement-related sensory feedback are termed the 'central motor pattern'. In some experimental preparations, the central motor pattern is an excellent replica of the motor pattern produced in the presence of movement-related sensory feedback (Delcomyn, 1980; Stein, 1984). The central neuronal circuit responsible for generating the central motor pattern in these preparations is termed the 'central pattern generator' or CPG. The cells of the CPG are strictly neuronal and are a subset of the cells of the MPG. The CPG does not include the other cell types of the MPG, the body cells of the mechanical apparatus, e.g. muscle and skeleton. Some investigators have made excellent progress in studies that focus on CPGs. This chapter describes aspects of this progress.

Three different experimental strategies have been used to demonstrate the existence of a CPG: (1) de-

afferentation, (2) de-efferentation, and (3) in vitro. All three strategies initially require the characterization of the motor pattern during movement in the presence of movement-related sensory feedback. Following this characterization, movement-related sensory feedback is removed and the central motor pattern is recorded. In the de-afferentation strategy, axons of all sensory neurons carrying movement-related sensory feedback are transected and their feedback blocked. For vertebrate limbs, this involves transection of all dorsal roots carrying movement-related sensory information (e.g. Stein and Grossman, 1980). In the de-efferentation strategy, the synaptic connection between motoneurons and skeletal muscles is chemically blocked by an antagonist of the transmitter at the neuromuscular postsynaptic receptor. In a vertebrate, this involves use of antagonists of the nicotinic acetylcholine receptor, e.g. curare or gallamine (e.g. Edgerton et al., 1976; Stein et al., 1986, 1998; Stein and Smith, 1997). In some types of preparations using the in vitro strategy, all or some of the nervous system is removed from the organism and placed in a bath of physiological saline. In these types of in vitro preparations, all movement is prevented since no muscles are present in the experimental bath (Kiehn et al., 1997; Cazalets et al., 1998; Kiehn and Kjaerulff, 1998; Schmidt et al., 1998). In each situation, activity of the appropriate motoneurons must be recorded and the central motor pattern compared to the motor pattern during motor behavior in the intact organism. The motor patterns recorded in the de-efferentation and in the in vitro preparations are often termed 'fictive' motor patterns since they are produced in the absence of actual movements.

In some preparations that demonstrate the existence of a central motor pattern, the pattern occurs spontaneously and is expressed without specific stimulation. In other preparations, the nervous system must be activated properly to generate a central motor pattern that is an excellent replica of the motor pattern during movement. Activation can be accomplished by electrical stimulation of specific sites in the nervous system, by natural stimulation of sensory neurons that do not carry movement-related sensory information, and/or by chemical stimulation of the nervous system.

Movement-related sensory feedback exerts powerful influences on the neurons of the CPG. This feedback is absolutely critical in the performance of adaptive behavior. One role of the feedback is to measure the mechanical properties of the organism and its interactions with the environment; these measurements are required for the survival of the organism and its species (Wilson, 1972). In order to study the natural activation patterns of sensory neurons, central neuronal circuits as well as the peripheral neurons and the mechanical apparatus must be present. The motor pattern generator or MPG includes central and peripheral neurons as well as the cells of the mechanical apparatus. For some questions it is critical to study the entire MPG in an intact, behaving organism; some investigators have made excellent progress with such a focus. Others have made excellent progress by focusing on reduced MPG preparations that include some central neurons, some peripheral neurons, and some elements of the mechanical apparatus. The reader is directed elsewhere for outstanding discussions of MPGs and sensory modulations of CPGs (Dean and Cruse, 1995; Pearson and Ramirez, 1997; Chiel and Beer, 1997).

CPG research in the 1960s

Invertebrate motor control

The 60s were marked by strong experimental support in invertebrates for the concept of the central pattern generator. Many of the experimentalists whose work in the 60s placed the CPG concept on firm ground were present at the 1965 Society for Experimental Biology Symposium on 'Nervous and Hormonal Mechanisms of Integration' that was held in St. Andrews; their contributions comprise the Symposium volume (Hughes, 1966). My doctoral mentors Donald Kennedy and Donald Wilson and my postdoctoral mentor Theodore H. Bullock contributed to the meeting and the volume. I did not attend this Symposium but was influenced by the volume and my mentors' reports of the meeting. Notable in this decade were demonstrations of the central activity patterns for crustacean cardiac ganglion and stomatogastric ganglion (Maynard, 1966), locust flight (Wilson, 1966), crustacean swimmerets (Ikeda and

Wiersma, 1964; Wiersma and Ikeda, 1964), and crustacean abdominal posture (Kennedy et al., 1966). Wilson (1966, p. 199) asserted that these demonstrations settled long-standing controversies concerning sensory vs. central control of movement. He argued that "There are now conclusive studies of cases of central nervous rhythms which can produce adaptive behavioural outputs without special sensory inflow. On the other hand, no one denies the importance of reflexes in the initiation or regulation of motor outflow". Wilson's point of view is held by many investigators who study CPGs.

Motor patterns were produced in each of these different preparations. In some preparations, there was spontaneous production of motor output (Ikeda and Wiersma, 1964; Maynard, 1966). In other preparations, strategies were developed to activate motor activity. Wilson (1966) activated locust flight after removal of movement-related sensory feedback by stimulation with constant velocity wind on the locust's head; he termed this non-movement-related sensory input a 'tonic' input to distinguish it from the 'phasic' movement-related sensory input from the wings that was removed in some of his preparations. Wiersma and Ikeda (1964) demonstrated that constant-frequency electrical stimulation of specific central axons (termed command fibers or command neurons) could activate coordinated swimmeret motor patterns in preparations that did not show spontaneous activity. Kennedy et al. (1966) demonstrated command neurons for abdominal postural motor patterns. Maynard (1966) also used constant-frequency electrical stimulation of the stomatogastric nerve to activate stomatogastric motor patterns. In all these preparations, the neuronal circuits generated excellent motor patterns.

A key contribution of the invertebrate work of the 60s was the demonstration of the existence of the central pattern generator. Which neurons were members of the CPG and how these CPGs worked became foci of work that followed. In the 60s, many investigators believed that if all the neurons of a CPG could be identified and their synaptic connections characterized (termed the 'circuit diagram'), then an 'understanding' of how that CPG worked could be achieved.

A major contribution of the 60s invertebrate work was the recognition that, during a study of the neuronal circuit responsible for a motor behavior, it was critical to have that neuronal circuit activated and producing the motor pattern associated with that behavior. This research strategy contrasted with an alternate point of view held in the 60s by some neuroscientists studying mammalian motor systems (e.g. Eccles et al., 1967) in which circuits such as spinal cord or cerebellum were studied in quiescent preparations in the absence of motor patterns similar to those during actual behavior.

My doctoral studies in the 60s focused on the neuronal mechanisms responsible for interlimb coupling during rhythmic swimmeret movements of the crayfish (Stein, 1971). I shared with others who studied invertebrates the hope that invertebrate research was leading to new points of view that would also be relevant to those studying vertebrate systems. At the end of the 60s, however, few investigators studying vertebrate systems were familar with invertebrate work.

Vertebrate motor control

Two important preparations demonstrating activation of cat locomotor rhythms were developed in the 60s. They influenced how mammalian locomotor control was studied in later decades.

First, there was the discovery in Moscow that electrical stimulation of a site in the midbrain termed the mesencephalic locomotor region (MLR) could elicit locomotion in a mesencephalic cat (Shik et al., 1966; see review by Stuart and McDonaugh, 1998). Low intensity stimulation could evoke a walk; higher intensity stimulation could evoke a trot; still higher intensity stimulation could evoke a gallop. The work of Shik, Severin, and Orlovsky was largely unknown in the West in the 60s and was hardly discussed in Western journal articles until Engberg and Lundberg (1969). Members of the Moscow school started publishing in Western journals in the 70s and their work eventually became more widely known. For a thorough account of the results of the Moscow School, see Shik and Orlovsky (1976), Orlovsky and Shik (1976), and Arshavsky et al. (1986).

The results of Shik et al. (1966) were very interesting and I wanted to learn more about the preparation. At the First Annual Society for Neuroscience Meeting in 1971, I spoke with Dr. Edward Evarts, a neuroscientist who pioneered single-unit recordings from primate cerebral cortex during motor tasks; he had visited Moscow and witnessed the MLR preparation. He stated that the results were robust. His positive statements about the preparation played a role in my switch in the 70s from studying invertebrate motor control in crayfish to studying vertebrate motor control in turtle.

Second, there was the discovery in Sweden that electrical stimulation of afferents in specific hindlimb nerves in a spinal cat chemically modulated by L-DOPA and Nialamide could elicit a locomotor-like motor rhythm (Jankowska et al., 1967; reviewed by Lundberg, 1981). The working model of Lundberg and his collaborators was that the chemical stimulation had transformed the spinal cord so that it would respond with locomotor-like rhythms in response to brief sensory stimulation. Lundberg's working model was an updated version of the half-center hypothesis initially proposed by Brown (1911). A key component of this hypothesis was that reciprocial inhibition between flexor interneurons and extensor interneurons played a critical role in rhythm generation. The research of Lundberg and his collaborators has served as a strong foundation for subsequent work.

These preparations contributed to a shift in research programs that occurred in later decades for investigators studying mammalian motor rhythms. A consequence of these experimental breakthroughs was the recognition that a reduced system was helpful in revealing underlying neuronal mechanisms and that some strategy was needed to activate neuronal networks for motor rhythms in the reduced system.

CPG research in the 1970s

A dramatic improvement in interphyletic awareness occurred in the 70s. Previously, papers reporting motor patterns in vertebrates cited other vertebrate work and rarely cited papers reporting work in other phyla, and vice versa. Important factors in this change were two influential meetings and their associated volumes, the 1973 Edmonton Meeting on 'Control of Posture and Movement' (R.B. Stein et al., 1973) and the 1975 Valley Forge Meeting on 'Neural Control of Locomotion' (Herman et al., 1976).

The 1973 Edmonton Meeting included a section on 'Control of Locomotion' that discussed both invertebrate preparations (lobster and crayfish swimmerets, Tritonia swimming, crustacean and cockroach walking), and vertebrate preparations (spinal and intact cat locomotion). Davis' article (1973) on lobster swimmerets included a section on 'Comparison with Vertebrate Motor Systems' that highlighted important similarities including the observation that major features of locomotor output are programmed centrally in both invertebrates and cats.

I attended the Edmonton meeting and presented a short paper on the interlimb phase control in crayfish swimmerets (Stein, 1973). At that time, I was still working on crayfish; however, my two graduate students had begun work on vertebrate preparations. Anne Bekoff, co-mentored by Viktor Hamburger and myself, studied the development of motor patterns in the chick embryo hindlimb (Bekoff et al., 1975; Bekoff, 1976). Paul Lennard studied activation of swimming in turtle by electrical stimulation of the dorsolateral funiculus in the midbody spinal cord (Lennard and Stein, 1977). By the mid 70s, I concentrated my own experimental effort on turtle spinal cord control of swimming (Stein, 1978a). One of my goals was to apply the points of view of invertebrate motor research to vertebrate motor systems.

After the Edmonton Meeting, Richard Herman invited me to join him, Sten Grillner, and Douglas Stuart, in organizing the 1975 Valley Forge meeting on 'Neural Control of Locomotion'. Herman chaired the meeting, served as the local coordinator, and was chief editor of the conference volume. Our planning sessions for the Valley Forge meeting were very exciting. We felt that new understandings were about to be reached and structured our meeting to facilitate their development. Our points of view were that there were common problems that needed to be solved during rhythmic motor behaviors, especially locomotion, by a number of different invertebrates and vertebrates, and there were key insights to be gained by comparing how these different organisms solved similar problems. We organized the meeting so that in each section of the meeting, if possible, contributions were included about invertebrate as well as vertebrate preparations. In addition, in some individual contributions (e.g. Pearson and Duysens, 1976; Stein, 1976), there were direct comparisons of invertebrate and vertebrate data. Reviews of this period stressed the importance of comparing invertebrate and vertebrate research (Stein, 1978b) and comparing non-mammalian with mammalian research (Grillner, 1975).

The 1975 Valley Forge meeting marked a turning point in CPG research. The work of the community studying invertebrate CPGs became known to a major segment of the community studying mammalian motor control. In addition, the work of many of those examining cat locomotor control became known to those studying invertebrates. The experimental strategies of some vertebrate studies were similar to those that were successful in the invertebrates, e.g. see Edgerton et al. (1976).

A key to the success of many of the invertebrate preparations in the 70s was the ability of investigators to obtain cellular recordings during the production of motor rhythms while the nervous system was bathed with physiological saline. After the Valley Forge meeting, several investigators turned to non-mammalian vertebrates, e.g. lamprey and tadpole, that offered these technical advantages for studies of CPGs. These became major preparations in the 80s and 90s.

Invertebrate research in the 70s was also at a critical stage. In a large number of organisms, the existence of a CPG for a behavior had been demonstrated (Delcomyn, 1980). Important progress at the cellular level had been achieved in some preparations. Notable at the 1975 Valley Forge meeting was the demonstration of the synaptic connectivity among the neurons of the stomatogastric ganglion (Selverston, 1976). The demonstration of such synaptic connectivity among the neurons of a well characterized neuronal network was a goal of many invertebrate researchers in the 60s. With the achievement of this goal in the 70s, there was a realization that there were many other issues that needed to be studied – a total 'understanding' of the neuronal network had not yet been reached (Selverston, 1980). This led to a reformulation of the types of questions that experimentalists asked in order to understand how CPGs worked.

The members of the Moscow school studying cat CPGs were very productive and many Western scientists had a strong interest in meeting them and hearing them speak. Invitations were extended to several Moscow scientists to attend the Valley Forge meeting, but the political climate in their country prevented their attendance. In the mid and late 70s, the members of the Moscow school turned their attention to the CPG for scratching in cats with an important emphasis on cellular recordings during the production of the scratch motor pattern (for a review, see Arshavsky et al., 1986). Their papers made a very strong case for the technical advantages of scratching as a model behavior. In the late 70s, Valk-Fai and Crowe (1978) reported scratching in spinal turtles with limb movements. My laboratory turned its attention to turtle scratching: spinal immobilized turtles produced excellent fictive scratching (Stein and Grossman, 1980).

The concept of a command neuron fell out of favor with some investigators in the 70s (Kupfermann and Weiss, 1978). My opinion is that it was a major intellectual contribution to demonstrate that focal stimulation of an element or elements of the nervous system can activate a coordinated motor pattern (Stein, 1978c). In particular, constant-frequency focal stimulation of a portion of the nervous system that activates a coordinated motor pattern played a key role in the development of cat locomotion preparations (Shik et al., 1966; Orlovsky and Shik, 1976; Shik and Orlovsky, 1976; Wetzel and Stuart, 1976).

The accomplishments of the 70s in CPG research were many. By the end of the decade, one of the most prominent accomplishments was that points of view of invertebrate CPG research were also held by some of those who studied vertebrate motor rhythms. Strategies of research programs were shared among experimentalists. A result obtained in one preparation served as a stimulus for a proposed hypothesis by an experimentalist studying another preparation (e.g. electrical activation of locomotion in cat by Shik et al., 1966, influenced the work in turtle of Lennard and Stein, 1977, and Stein, 1978a).

CPG research in the 1980s

The 80s were marked by dramatic growth in our understandings of CPGs. Two important meetings brought together a number of investigators studying the properties of CPGs. The first was the 1982 Society for Experimental Biology Symposium on 'Neural Origin of Rhythmic Movements' that was held at the University of Sussex (Roberts and Roberts, 1983). The second was the 1985 Conference on 'Neurobiology of Vertebrate Locomotion' that was held in Stockholm (Grillner et al., 1986a).

One of the foci of the 1982 meeting was the excellent progress in invertebrate motor control. Selverston et al. (1983) described important progress in stomatogastric ganglion research stimulated, in part, by the discovery of the 'fill/kill' technique that allowed selective lesioning of specific elements of a neural circuit; a new generation of questions could now be asked and new levels of understanding reached. Getting (1983) presented major portions of a circuit for Tritonia swimming. One of his major contributions was the emphasis he put on the importance of multiaction synaptic potentials, postsynaptic potentials whose amplitude and sign varied as a function of the recent history of presynaptic activation. He underscored the importance of kinetic analyses of circuit components by using this information to construct a computational model of the Tritonia swim circuit. The use of computational models is now an important strategy of CPG research (Marder et al., 1997). At the 1985 Stockholm meeting, Getting (1986) summarized existing knowledge about experimental strategies and key results concerning CPG function that had been revealed by invertebrate preparations. He suggested how this knowledge might be used to approach vertebrate motor systems. A key concept proposed by Getting was that of 'building blocks', specific mechanisms that contributed to CPG function. This suggestion has been well received by investigators studying both invertebrate and vertebrate systems: it has become a dominant point of view of many in the field.

An important focus of the 1982 SEB meeting was dramatic progress in several vertebrate preparations – lamprey, tadpole, turtle, and cat. While the planning for the 1982 meeting was in progress, Sten Grillner and I decided that a 1985 Stockholm conference that focused upon progress in vertebrate CPGs would be an excellent addition to the material presented at the 1982 SEB meeting. We invited Douglas Stuart, Hans Forssberg, and Richard Herman to join us in planning the 1985 meeting. Grillner chaired the meeting, served as the local organizer, and was chief editor for the symposium volume. Both the 1982 SEB and the 1985 Stockholm meetings provided opportunities to highlight the major progress in vertebrate CPGs in the 80s.

Several members of the Moscow School were invited to the 1985 Stockholm meeting. Again the politics of the day prevented their attendence. Their manuscripts were published in the symposium volume (Arshavsky and Orlovsky, 1986; Berkinblit et al., 1986; Shik, 1986).

Exciting features of both the 1982 SEB and the 1985 Stockholm meetings were data from the lamprey (Grillner et al., 1983, 1986b; Rovainen, 1983, 1986; see Grillner et al., 1986a for several other lamprey chapters) and tadpole (Roberts et al., 1983, 1986). Lamprey spinal cord was introduced to modern neurophysiology by Rovainen (see Rovainen, 1979, for a description of his work in the 60s and 70s). Margaret Poon worked in Rovainen's laboratory in the mid 70s and discovered that swimming could be activated when D-glutamate was applied to an in vitro preparation of lamprey spinal cord and muscles (Poon, 1980). Application of D-glutamate to the lamprey spinal cord was used by Cohen and Wallen (1980) in the Grillner laboratory to demonstrate that the in vitro lamprey spinal cord could generate a fictive swim motor pattern in the absence of movement. A preparation that allowed examination of neural control of swimming in tadpoles was developed by Roberts and collaborators (Roberts et al., 1983, 1986). Both the lamprey and the tadpole preparations allowed intracellular recordings from motoneurons and interneurons in the spinal cord during the production of the fictive swim motor pattern. These recordings provided strong evidence in both preparations that there was left-right reciprocal inhibition that was similar to the flexor-extensor reciprocal inhibition ('half-center' hypothesis, Lundberg,

1981) proposed for the cat hindlimb. This similarity in the CPG organization served as a stimulus to increase investigators' awareness toward results obtained in different vertebrate preparations.

In both the tadpole and lamprey preparations, direct bath application of neurotransmitter agonists and antagonists to the spinal cord allowed pharmacological exploration of CPG circuitry. The in vitro CPG research in the 80s utilized the dramatic developments in the pharmacology of synaptic transmission, especially with respect to glutamate receptors. In particular, these preparations provided important early evidence in the vertebrates of the multiple actions of a single neurotransmitter, in this case glutamate, on each of several postsynaptic receptors, non-NMDA (now AMPA/kainate) receptors and NMDA receptors (Grillner et al., 1986b; Roberts et al., 1986). Multiaction synapses had already been shown to be a key feature of the invertebrate Tritonia swim CPG (Getting, 1983, 1986); the discovery of vertebrate multiaction synapses was an important generalization.

Major progress with scratching in limbed vertebrates was also reported at the 1982 SEB and the 1985 Stockholm meetings. At the 1982 SEB meeting, I presented an overview of scratching in frog (also termed wiping), turtle, and cat (Stein, 1983). Tactile stimulation of specific sites on the body surface to activate scratching produced excellent motor patterns. Studies of scratching allowed the examination of motor pattern selection in reduced preparations. At the 1985 meeting, I focused on studies of turtle scratching that emphasized the importance of the different forms (= motor strategies) that are produced by spinal cord CPGs (Stein et al., 1986). Berkinblit et al. (1986) discussed a model for the aiming phase of frog wiping. Arshavsky and Orlovsky (1986) presented unit recordings from several different classes of interneurons during fictive scratching in the cat.

Major progress with cat CPGs occurred in the 80s. A number of laboratories studied fictive stepping as well as fictive scratching in the cat. Grillner (1981) proposed a significant variation of the Brown–Lundberg half-center hypothesis. Grillner suggested that a 'unit burst generator' controlled each direction of movement for each joint of the cat hindlimb. He suggested that, for each joint, there was reciprocal inhibition between a flexor unit burst generator and an extensor unit burst generator; he postulated that a unit burst generator could be rhythmogenic even during quiescence of its antagonist unit burst generator. Important progress was made on brainstem mechanisms for activating and modulating stepping (Jordan, 1983, 1986; Mori et al., 1983; Mori and Ohta, 1986; Shik, 1986). In addition, important new information about the spinal circuits in cat involved in motor rhythm generation was reported at both the 1982 and the 1985 meetings (Perret, 1983, 1986; Arshavsky and Orlovsky, 1986; see Grillner et al., 1986a for several other chapters discussing cat motor rhythms).

In the 80s, there was a general consensus among those studying CPGs that major progress could be made by the community of scientists studying a selected group of key preparations. Each preparation had distinct experimental advantages and was therefore amenable to answering specific types of questions. The use of an array of preparations thus yielded the best insights into general features of CPG function. By the end of the 80s, there was an appreciation that there may be a set of biological solutions for each particular problem of organization. While each particular biological solution may differ, there was agreement that there are important shared building blocks used in each of these solutions (Getting, 1986).

CPG research in the 1990s

The 90s were marked by deeper insights into each of a set of model CPG systems. There was a greater appreciation of the possibility that a given CPG network could be adjusted and modulated to produce a complex set of motor patterns and behaviors. To highlight the progress in the 90s, Sten Grillner, Allen Selverston, Douglas Stuart and I organized the 1995 Tucson meeting on 'Neurons, Networks, and Motor Behavior' (P.S.G. Stein et al., 1997) to examine CPG research in both invertebrates and vertebrates since the 1982 SEB and the 1985 Stockholm meetings. Douglas Stuart was the local organizer in Tucson. I chaired the meeting and was the chief editor of the symposium volume. In

order to emphasize the important interactions between those who studied invertebrates and those who studied vertebrates, we used the strategy that had been successful at the 1975 Valley Forge meeting. We organized sessions around specific problems, e.g. modulation and reconfiguration, and asked speakers studying invertebrate preparations as well as those studying vertebrate preparations to contribute to each of the sessions.

We expanded this strategy in the organization of the symposium volume (Stein et al., 1997) by requesting some pairs or trios of speakers to write about a general problem and to synthesize insights from invertebrates as well as vertebrates, e.g. Weeks and McEwen (1997) discuss hormonal reconfiguration of neuronal circuits, and Pearson and Ramirez (1997) discuss sensory modulation. In other cases, we asked groups of speakers to summarize issues for a wide variety of specific organisms such as lower vertebrates and mammals, e.g. Kiehn et al. (1997) discuss spinal CPG organization, and Sillar et al. (1997) discuss modulation of spinal circuits. Many of the chapters of Stein et al. (1997) support the assertion that, in the 90s, interphyletic awareness is a key element of CPG studies (see also Pearson, 1993).

In planning the 1995 Tucson meeting, we were struck by changes in perspectives that had occurred since the 1975 Valley Forge meeting. In the 70s, motor behavior investigators were just beginning to accept the concept that the nervous system had to be activated in order to study the neuronal control of motor behavior. In the 90s, this was a generally accepted experimental strategy. In the 70s, many investigators were content if their system was producing one particular motor behavior; only a few investigators were interested in studying each of several behaviors. In the 90s, many investigators were interested in how the nervous system could produce each of a set of motor patterns, e.g. forward vs. backward stepping in cat and the several forms of scratching in turtle (Stein and Smith, 1997).

The 90s were marked by political changes as well. Several members of the Moscow School attended the 1995 Tucson meeting (Yuri Arshavsky, Tatiana Deliagina, Anatol Feldman, Grigori Orlovsky, and Yuri Panchin). Deliagina and Panchin were speakers at the meeting. Arshavsky, Deliagina, Orlovsky, and Panchin were co-authors of chapters in the symposium volume (Macpherson et al., 1997; Selverston et al., 1997).

Neuromodulation was a most important concept that gained general acceptance in the 90s. Early evidence for this concept was obtained in invertebrate preparations, in particular the stomatogastric ganglion (Harris-Warrick and Marder, 1991; Harris-Warrick et al., 1997). In the 60s and 70s, some investigators believed that each specific network could generate one and only one type of motor output. A new concept started in the 80s and received strong support in the 90s: each specific neuronal network could be modulated into each of several configurations – each configuration could produce a specific type of motor behavior. Key mechanisms for neuromodulation are the specific actions of individual molecules, e.g. transmitters or hormones, on parameters that characterize membrane channels and receptors. Neuromodulation is now an important concept not only for invertebrate systems (Harris-Warrick et al., 1997; Kupfermann et al., 1997) but also for vertebrate systems (Sillar et al., 1997).

The 1998 New York meeting on 'Neuronal Mechanisms Responsible for Locomotor Activity' at the New York Academy of Sciences (Kiehn et al., 1998) continued in the tradition of earlier meetings. Important progress in key preparations in both invertebrates and vertebrates was presented. For example, Katz (1998) extended the concept of modulation to include intrinsic modulation and presented support for intrinsic modulation in the Tritonia swim CPG. Hultborn et al. (1998) reviewed the status of support for the half-center hypothesis of cat stepping. Kiehn and Kjaerulff (1998) emphasized key features of organization of the neuronal circuitry responsible for motor rhythm organization in limbed vertebrates with a special emphasis on the distribution of CPG elements in the lumbosacral enlargement. Stein et al. (1998) presented evidence for the modular organization of scratch CPGs in turtles. We demonstrated that hip flexor rhythms can be expressed even during hip extensor quiescence; reciprocal inhibition between flexor and extensor centers may not be the sole mechanism for rhythmogenesis. The general con-

sensus of the meeting was that the field had achieved important understandings about the nature of CPGs and, with this progress, there were new questions about CPG function that required answers.

An important new preparation in the 90s was the in vitro neonatal rat preparation (Kiehn et al., 1997; Cazalets et al., 1998; Kiehn and Kjaerulff, 1998; Schmidt et al., 1998). Chemical stimulation of the in vitro neonatal rat spinal cord elicits a locomotor-like pattern with rhythmic alternation between flexors and extensors of each hindlimb and between left and right hindlimb homologous motoneurons. Interphyletic awareness of the important progress of in vitro preparations in both invertebrates and vertebrates served as a key stimulus for the development of the in vitro neonatal rat preparation. In turn, this preparation is likely to reveal many cellular mechanisms for CPG function in mammals.

The 1998 Tucson Meeting on 'Peripheral and Spinal Mechanisms in the Neural Control of Movement' was organized to honor the contributions of Douglas Stuart to the field of neuronal control of movement. This meeting, organized by Marc Binder and Jennifer McDonagh with suggestions from Douglas Stuart, emphasized the importance of interphyletic awareness. Attention was paid not only to the cat and human, but also to the rat, turtle, newt, lamprey, and arthropods. The chapters of this volume edited by Binder provide further support for the key role played by interphyletic awareness.

There was major progress in the 90s in CPG research in many different preparations. It is beyond the scope of this chapter to summarize all this work. The chapters of Stein et al. (1997), Kiehn et al. (1998), and Binder (this volume) provide excellent summaries.

Summary

Our understandings of how neuronal networks organized as central pattern generators generate motor behavior have greatly increased in the last 40 years. In the 60s, many investigators studying invertebrate motor behaviors were not aware of the work of those studying vertebrate motor behaviors, and vice versa. In the 70s, key conferences provided venues for important interactions among investigators working on preparations in different species. These interactions, termed interphyletic awareness, continued in the 80s and 90s at major conferences and played important roles in the development of our understandings of central pattern generators for motor behavior in these decades.

Acknowledgements

Research in the author's laboratory is supported by NIH Grant NS–30786 to PSGS. I thank the many colleagues, some named in this chapter and others not named due to space limitations, who influenced the progress in the field of CPG research in the past 40 years. I especially wish to thank Professor Douglas G. Stuart for many outstanding interactions. I thank Gammon Earhart and Sarah Siegel for editorial comments.

References

Arshavsky, Y.I. and Orlovsky, G.N. (1986) Role of the cerebellum in the control of rhythmic movements. In: S. Grillner, P.S.G. Stein, D.G. Stuart, H. Forssberg and R.M. Herman (Eds), *Neurobiology of Vertebrate Locomotion*, Macmillan Press, London, pp. 677–689.

Arshavsky, Y.I., Gelfand, I.M. and Orlovsky, G.N. (1986) *Cerebellum and Rhythmical Movements*, Springer-Verlag, Berlin.

Bekoff, A. (1976) Ontogeny of leg motor output in the chick embryo: a neural analysis. *Brain Res.*, 106: 271–291.

Bekoff, A., Stein, P.S.G. and Hamburger, V. (1975) Coordinated motor output in the hindlimb of the 7-day chick embryo. *Proc. Natl. Acad. Sci. USA*, 72: 1245–1248.

Berkinblit, M.B., Gelfand, I.M. and Feldman, A.G. (1986) A model for the aiming phase of the wiping reflex. In: S. Grillner, P.S.G. Stein, D.G. Stuart, H. Forssberg and R.M. Herman (Eds), *Neurobiology of Vertebrate Locomotion*, Macmillan, Hampshire, pp. 217–227.

Binder, M.D. (Ed.) (this volume) Peripheral and Spinal Mechanisms in the Neural Control of Movement. Progress in Brain Research, volume 123, Elsevier, Amsterdam.

Brown, T.G. (1911) The intrinsic factors in the act of progression in the mammal. *Proc. R. Soc. Lond. Biol.*, 84: 308–319.

Callister, R.J., Laidlaw, D.H. and Stuart, D.G. (1995) A commentary on the segmental motor system of the turtle: implications for the study of its cellular mechanisms and interactions. *J. Morphol.*, 225: 213–227.

Cazalets, J.-R., Bertrand, S., Sqalli-Houssaini, Y. and Clarac, F. (1998) GABAergic control of spinal locomotor networks in the neonatal rat. *Ann. NY Acad. Sci.*, 860: 168–180.

Chiel, H.J. and Beer, R.D. (1997) The brain has a body: adaptive behavior emerges from interactions of nervous system, body and environment. *Trends Neurosci.*, 20: 553–557.

Cohen, A.H. and Wallen, P. (1980) The neuronal correlate of locomotion in fish. 'Fictive swimming' induced in an in vitro preparation of the lamprey spinal cord. *Exp. Brain Res.*, 41: 11–18.

Davis, W.J. (1973) Neuronal organization and ontogeny in the lobster swimmeret system. In: R.B. Stein, K.G. Pearson, R.S. Smith and J.B. Redford (Eds), *Control of Posture and Locomotion*, Plenum Press, New York, pp. 437–455.

Dean, J. and Cruse, H. (1995) Motor pattern generation. In: M.A. Arbib (Ed.), *The Handbook of Brain Theory and Neural Networks*, MIT Press, Cambridge, pp. 600–605.

Delcomyn, F. (1980) Neural basis of rhythmic behavior in animals. *Science*, 210: 492–498.

Eccles, J.C., Ito, M. and Szentagothai, J. (1967) *The Cerebellum as a Neuronal Machine*, Springer-Verlag, Berlin.

Edgerton, V.R., Grillner, S., Sjostrom, A. and Zangger, P. (1976) Central generation of locomotion in vertebrates. In: R.M. Herman, S. Grillner, P.S.G. Stein and D.G. Stuart (Eds), *Neural Control of Locomotion*, Plenum Press, New York, pp. 439–464.

Engberg, I. and Lundberg, A. (1969) An electromyographic analysis of muscular activity in the hindlimb of the cat during unrestrained locomotion. *Acta Physiol. Scand.*, 75: 614–630.

Getting, P.A. (1983) Neural control of swimming in *Tritonia*. *Symp. Soc. Exp. Biol.*, 37: 89–128.

Getting, P.A. (1986) Understanding central pattern generators: insights gained from the study of invertebrate systems. In: S. Grillner, P.S.G. Stein, D.G. Stuart, H. Forssberg and R.M. Herman (Eds), *Neurobiology of Vertebrate Locomotion*, Macmillan Press, London, pp. 231–244.

Grillner, S. (1975) Locomotion in vertebrates: central mechanisms and reflex interaction. *Physiol. Rev.*, 55: 247–304.

Grillner, S. (1981) Control of locomotion in bipeds, tetrapods, and fish. In: V.B. Brooks (Ed.), *Handbook of Physiology, Sect. 1, The Nervous System, Vol. 2, Motor Control*, American Physiological Society, Bethesda, Maryland, pp. 1179–1236.

Grillner, S., Wallen, P., McClellan, A., Sigvardt, K., Williams, T. and Feldman, J. (1983) The neural generation of locomotion in the lamprey: an incomplete account. *Symp. Soc. Exp. Biol.*, 37: 285–303.

Grillner, S., Stein, P.S.G., Stuart, D.G., Forssberg, H. and Herman, R.M. (Eds) (1986a) *Neurobiology of Vertebrate Locomotion*, Macmillan Press, London.

Grillner, S., Brodin, L., Sigvardt, K. and Dale, N. (1986b) On the spinal network generating locomotion in the lamprey: transmitters, membrane properties and circuitry. In: S. Grillner, P.S.G. Stein, D.G. Stuart, H. Forssberg and R.M. Herman (Eds), *Neurobiology of Vertebrate Locomotion*, Macmillan, London, pp. 335–362.

Harris-Warrick, R.M. and Marder, E. (1991) Modulation of neural networks for behavior. *Annu. Rev. Neurosci.*, 14: 39–57.

Harris-Warrick, R.M., Baro, D.J., Coniglio, L.M., Johnson, B.R., Levini, R.M., Peck, J.H. and Zhang, B. (1997) Chemical modulation of crustacean stomatogastric pattern generator networks. In: P.S.G. Stein, S. Grillner, A.I. Selverston and D.G. Stuart (Eds), *Neurons, Networks, and Motor Behavior*, MIT Press, Cambridge, pp. 209–215.

Hasan, Z. and Stuart, D.G. (1988) Animal solutions to problems of movement control: the role of proprioceptors. *Annu. Rev. Neurosci.*, 11: 199–223.

Herman, R.M., Grillner, S., Stein, P.S.G. and Stuart, D.G. (Eds) (1976) *Neural Control of Locomotion*, Plenum Press, New York.

Hughes, G.M. (Ed.) (1966) *Nervous and Hormonal Mechanisms of Integration. Symposium of the Society for Experimental Biology Number XX*, Cambridge University Press, Cambridge.

Hultborn, H., Conway, B.A., Gossard, J.-P., Brownstone, R., Fedirchuk, B., Schomburg, E.D., Enriquez-Denton, M. and Perreault, M.-C. (1998) How do we approach the locomotor network in the mammalian spinal cord? *Ann. NY Acad. Sci.*, 860: 70–82.

Ikeda, K. and Wiersma, C.A.G. (1964) Autogenic rhythmicity in the abdominal ganglia of the crayfish: the control of swimmeret movements. *Comp. Biochem. Physiol.*, 12: 107–115.

Jankowska, E., Jukes, M.G.M., Lund, S. and Lundberg, A. (1967) The effect of DOPA on the spinal cord. 5. Reciprocal organization of pathways transmitting excitatory action to alpha motoneurones of flexors and extensors. *Acta Physiol. Scand.*, 70: 369–388.

Jordan, L.M. (1983) Factors determining motoneuron rhythmicity during fictive locomotion. *Symp. Soc. Exp. Biol.*, 37: 423–444.

Jordan, L.M. (1986) Initiation of locomotion from the mammalian brainstem. In: S. Grillner, P.S.G. Stein, D.G. Stuart, H. Forssberg and R.M. Herman (Eds), *Neurobiology of Vertebrate Locomotion*, Macmillan Press, London, pp. 21–37.

Katz, P.S. (1998) Neuromodulation intrinsic to the central pattern generator for escape swimming in *Tritonia*. *Ann. NY Acad. Sci.*, 860: 181–188.

Kennedy, D., Evoy, W.H. and Fields, H.L. (1966) The unit basis of some crustacean reflexes. *Symp. Soc. Exp. Biol.*, 20: 75–109.

Kiehn, O. and Kjaerulff, O. (1998) Distribution of central pattern generators for rhythmic motor outputs in the spinal cord of limbed vertebrates. *Ann. NY Acad. Sci.*, 860: 110–129.

Kiehn, O., Hounsgaard, J. and Sillar, K.T. (1997) Basic building blocks of vertebrate spinal central pattern generators. In: P.S.G. Stein, S. Grillner, A.I. Selverston and D.G. Stuart (Eds), *Neurons, Networks, and Motor Behavior*, MIT Press, Cambridge, MA, pp. 47–59.

Kiehn, O., Harris-Warrick, R.M., Jordan, L.M., Hultborn, H. and Kudo, N. (Eds) (1998) *Neuronal Mechanisms for Generating Locomotor Activity. Annals of the New York Academy of Sciences Volume 860*, New York Academy of Sciences, New York.

Kupfermann, I. and Weiss, K.R. (1978) The command neuron concept. *Behav. Brain Sciences*, 1: 3–39.

Kupfermann, I., Brezina, V., Cropper, E.C., Deodhar, D., Probst, W.C., Rosen, S.C., Vilim, F.S. and Weiss, K.R. (1997) Reconfiguration of the peripheral plant during various forms of feeding behaviors in the mollusc *Aplysia*. In: P.S.G. Stein, S. Grillner, A.I. Selverston and D.G. Stuart (Eds), *Neurons, Networks, and Motor Behavior*, MIT Press, Cambridge, pp. 217–222.

Lennard, P.R. and Stein, P.S.G. (1977) Swimming movements elicited by electrical stimulation of turtle spinal cord. I. Low-spinal and intact preparations. *J. Neurophysiol.*, 40: 768–778.

Lundberg, A. (1981) Half-centres revisited. *Adv. Physiol. Sci.*, 1: 155–167.

Macpherson, J.M., Deliagina, T.G. and Orlovsky, G.N. (1997) Control of body orientation and equilibrium in vertebrates. In: P.S.G. Stein, S. Grillner, A.I. Selverston and D.G. Stuart (Eds), *Neurons, Networks, and Motor Behavior*, MIT Press, Cambridge, MA, pp. 257–267.

Marder, E., Kopell, N. and Sigvardt, K. (1997) How computation aids in understanding biological networks. In: P.S.G. Stein, S. Grillner, A.I. Selverston and D.G. Stuart (Eds), *Neurons, Networks, and Motor Behavior*, MIT Press, Cambridge, pp. 139–149.

Maynard, D.M. (1966) Integration in crustacean ganglia. *Symp. Soc. Exp. Biol.*, 20: 111–149.

Mori, S. and Ohta, Y. (1986) Interaction of posture and locomotion and initiation of locomotion in decerebrate cats and freely moving intact cats. In: S. Grillner, P.S.G. Stein, D.G. Stuart, H. Forssberg and R.M. Herman (Eds), *Neurobiology of Vertebrate Locomotion*, Macmillan Press, London, pp. 55–71.

Mori, S., Kawahara, K. and Sakamoto, T. (1983) Supraspinal aspects of locomotion in the mesencephalic cat. *Symp. Soc. Exp. Biol.*, 37: 445–468.

Orlovsky, G.N. and Shik, M.L. (1976) Control of locomotion: a neurophysiological analysis of the cat locomotor system. In: R. Porter (Ed.), *Neurophysiology II, Vol. 10, International Review of Physiology*, University Park Press, Baltimore, pp. 291–317.

Pearson, K.G. (1993) Common principles of motor control in vertebrates and invertebrates. *Ann. Rev. Neurosci.*, 16: 265–297.

Pearson, K.G. and Duysens, J. (1976) Function of segmental reflexes in the control of stepping in cockroaches and cats. In: R.M. Herman, S. Grillner, P.S.G. Stein and D.G. Stuart (Eds), *Neural Control of Locomotion*, Plenum Press, New York, pp. 519–537.

Pearson, K.G. and Ramirez, J.M. (1997) Sensory modulation of pattern-generating circuits. In: P.S.G. Stein, S. Grillner, A.I. Selverston and D.G. Stuart (Eds), *Neurons, Networks, and Motor Behavior*, MIT Press, Cambridge, pp. 225–235.

270

Perret, C. (1983) Centrally generated pattern of motoneuron activity during locomotion in the cat. *Symp. Soc. Exp. Biol.*, 37: 405–422.

Perret, C. (1986) Synaptic influences contributing to the pattern of limb motoneuron activity during fictive locomotion in the cat. In: S. Grillner, P.S.G. Stein, D.G. Stuart, H. Forssberg and R.M. Herman (Eds), *Neurobiology of Vertebrate Locomotion*, Macmillan Press, London, pp. 173–184.

Poon, M.L.T. (1980) Induction of swimming in lamprey by L-DOPA and amino acids. *J. Comp. Physiol.*, 136: 337–344.

Roberts, A. and Roberts, B.L. (Eds) (1983) *Neural Origin of Rhythmic Movements. Symposium of the Society for Experimental Biology Number XXXVII*, Cambridge University Press, Cambridge.

Roberts, A., Soffe, S.R., Clarke, J.D.W. and Dale, N. (1983) Initiation and control of swimming in amphibian embryos. *Symp. Soc. Exp. Biol.*, 37: 261–284.

Roberts, A., Soffe, S.R. and Dale, N. (1986) Spinal interneurones and swimming in frog embryos. In: S. Grillner, P.S.G. Stein, D.G. Stuart, H. Forssberg and R.M. Herman (Eds), *Neurobiology of Vertebrate Locomotion*, Macmillan Press, London, pp. 279–306.

Rovainen, C.M. (1979) Neurobiology of lampreys. *Physiol. Rev.*, 59: 1007–1077.

Rovainen, C.M. (1983) Identified interneurons in the lamprey spinal cord and their roles in fictive swimming. *Symp. Soc. Exp. Biol.*, 37: 305–330.

Rovainen, C.M. (1986) The contributions of multisegmental interneurons to the longitudinal coordination of fictive swimming in the lamprey. In: S. Grillner, P.S.G. Stein, D.G. Stuart, H. Forssberg and R.M. Herman (Eds), *Neurobiology of Vertebrate Locomotion*, Macmillan, London, pp. 353–370.

Schmidt, B.J., Hochman, S. and MacLean, J.N. (1998) NMDA receptor-mediated oscillatory properties: potential role in rhythm generation in the mammalian spinal cord. *Ann. NY Acad. Sci.*, 860: 189–202.

Selverston, A.I. (1976) Neuronal mechanisms for rhythmic motor pattern generation in a simple system. In: R.M. Herman, S. Grillner, P.S.G. Stein and D.G. Stuart (Eds), *Neural Control of Locomotion*, Plenum Press, New York, pp. 377–399.

Selverston, A.I. (1980) Are central pattern generators understandable? *Behav. Brain Sciences*, 3: 535–571.

Selverston, A.I., Miller, J.P. and Wadepuhl, M. (1983) Cooperative mechanisms for the production of rhythmic movements. *Symp. Soc. Exp. Biol.*, 37: 55–87.

Selverston, A.I., Panchin, Y.V., Arshavsky, Y.I. and Orlovsky, G.N. (1997) Shared features of invertebrate central pattern generators. In: P.S.G. Stein, S. Grillner, A.I. Selverston and D.G. Stuart (Eds), *Neurons, Networks, and Motor Behavior*, MIT Press, Cambridge, MA, pp. 105–117.

Shik, M.L. (1986) An hypothesis on the bulbospinal locomotor column. In: S. Grillner, P.S.G. Stein, D.G. Stuart, H. Forssberg and R.M. Herman (Eds), *Neurobiology of Vertebrate Locomotion*, Macmillan Press, London, pp. 39–49.

Shik, M.L. and Orlovsky, G.N. (1976) Neurophysiology of locomotor automatism. *Physiol. Rev.*, 56: 465–501.

Shik, M.L., Severin, F.V. and Orlovsky, G.N. (1966) Control of walking and running by means of electrical stimulation of the midbrain. *Biophysics*, 11: 756–765.

Sillar, K.T., Kiehn, O. and Kudo, N. (1997) Chemical modulation of vertebrate motor circuits. In: P.S.G. Stein, S. Grillner, A.I. Selverston and D.G. Stuart (Eds), *Neurons, Networks, and Motor Behavior*, MIT Press, Cambridge, pp. 183–193.

Stein, P.S.G. (1971) Intersegmental coordination of swimmeret motoneuron activity in crayfish. *J. Neurophysiol.*, 34: 310–318.

Stein, P.S.G. (1973) The relationship of interlimb phase to oscillator activity gradients in crayfish. In: R.B. Stein, K.G. Pearson, R.S. Smith and J.B. Redford (Eds), *Control of Posture and Locomotion*, Plenum Press, New York, pp. 621–623.

Stein, P.S.G. (1976) Mechanisms of interlimb phase control. In: R.M. Herman, S. Grillner, P.S.G. Stein and D.G. Stuart (Eds), *Neural Control of Locomotion*, Plenum Press, New York, pp. 465–487.

Stein, P.S.G. (1978a) Swimming movements elicited by electrical stimulation of the turtle spinal cord: the high spinal preparation. *J. Comp. Physiol.*, 124: 203–210.

Stein, P.S.G. (1978b) Motor systems, with specific reference to the control of locomotion. *Annu. Rev. Neurosci.*, 1: 61–81.

Stein, P.S.G. (1978c) Defense of the Wiersma-Kennedy concept of the command neuron. *Behav. Brain Sciences*, 1: 33–34.

Stein, P.S.G. (1983) The vertebrate scratch reflex. *Symp. Soc. Exp. Biol.*, 37: 383–403.

Stein, P.S.G. (1984) Central pattern generators in the spinal cord. In: R.A. Davidoff (Ed.), *Handbook of the Spinal Cord, Vols. 2 and 3: Anatomy and Physiology*, Marcel Dekker, New York, pp. 647–672.

Stein, P.S.G. and Grossman, M.L. (1980) Central program for scratch reflex in turtle. *J. Comp. Physiol.*, 140: 287–294.

Stein, P.S.G. and Smith, J.L. (1997) Neural and biomechanical control strategies for different forms of vertebrate hindlimb motor tasks. In: P.S.G. Stein, S. Grillner, A.I. Selverston and D.G. Stuart (Eds), *Neurons, Networks, and Motor Behavior*, MIT Press, Cambridge, MA, pp. 61–73.

Stein, P.S.G., Mortin, L.I. and Robertson, G.A. (1986) The forms of a task and their blends. In: S. Grillner, P.S.G. Stein, D.G. Stuart, H. Forssberg and R.M. Herman (Eds), *Neurobiology of Vertebrate Locomotion*, Macmillan Press, London, pp. 201–216.

Stein, P.S.G., Grillner, S., Selverston, A.I. and Stuart, D.G. (Eds) (1997) *Neurons, Networks, and Motor Behavior*, MIT Press, Cambridge, MA.

Stein, P.S.G., McCullough, M.L. and Currie, S.N. (1998) Spinal motor patterns in the turtle. *Ann. NY Acad. Sci.*, 860: 142–154.

Stein, R.B., Pearson, K.G., Smith, R.S. and Redford, J.B. (Eds) (1973) *Control of Posture and Locomotion*, Plenum Press, New York.

Stuart, D.G. (1985) Summary and challenge for future work. In: P.S.G. Stein (Ed.), *Motor Control: From Movement Trajectories to Neural Mechanisms. 1985 Short Course Syllabus*, Society for Neuroscience, Washington, pp. 95–105.

Stuart, D.G. and McDonagh, J.C. (1998) Reflections on a Bernsteinian approach to systems neuroscience: the controlled locomotion of high-decerebrate cats. In: M. Latash (Ed.), *Progress in Motor Control: Bernstein's Traditions in Movement Studies, Vol. 1*, Human Kinetics, Champaign, IL, pp. 21–49.

Valk-Fai, T. and Crowe, A. (1978) Analyses of reflex movements in the hind limbs of the terrapin *Pseudemys scripta elegans. J. Comp. Physiol.*, 125: 351–357.

Weeks, J.C. and McEwen, B.S. (1997) Modulation of neural circuits by steroid hormones in rodent and insect model systems. In: P.S.G. Stein, S. Grillner, A.I. Selverston and D.G. Stuart (Eds), *Neurons, Networks, and Motor Behavior*, MIT Press, Cambridge, pp. 195–207.

Wetzel, M.C. and Stuart, D.G. (1976) Ensemble characteristics of cat locomotion and its neural control. *Prog. Neurobiol.*, 7: 1–98.

Wiersma, C.A.G. and Ikeda, K. (1964) Interneurons commanding swimmeret movements in the crayfish, *Procambarus clarkii* (Girard). *Comp. Biochem. Physiol.*, 12: 509–525.

Wilson, D.M. (1966) Central nervous mechanisms for the generation of rhythmic behavior in arthropods. *Symp. Soc. Exp. Biol.*, 20: 199–228.

Wilson, D.M. (1972) Genetic and sensory mechanisms for locomotion and orientation in animals. *Am. Sci.*, 60: 358–365.

M.D. Binder (Ed.)
Progress in Brain Research, Vol 123
© 1999 Elsevier Science BV. All rights reserved.

CHAPTER 24

A brain region in insects that supervises walking

Nicholas J. Strausfeld*

Arizona Research Laboratories Division of Neurobiology, University of Arizona, Tucson, AZ 85721, USA

Introduction

Central pattern generator circuits provide rhythmic patterns of activity amongst connected neurons that mediate walking (see Cruse et al., 1995). Local perturbations, such as irregularities in ground height, are relayed to central pattern generators by feedback from many thousands of mechano-receptors. This sensory information is integrated locally by spiking and non-spiking local inter-neurons that control and maintain patterned firing amongst motor neurons. Local circuits integrate information about leg position, allowing compensatory adjustments at the leg joints for maintaining posture and gait (Burrows and Laurent, 1989). In many insect species, local sensory afferents and the thoracic nervous system could alone maintain forward locomotion (see Yellman et al., 1997). Already in the last century, French physiologists demonstrated that after severing connections between the brain and thoracic ganglia, certain insects maintain coordinated limb movements (Faivre, 1857). However, goal-directed locomotion, that is walking towards selected features of the sensory surround, involves plurisegmental inter-neurons that carry information about sensory events occurring around the animal and about the position of the stimulus. Movement away from a stimulus source often involves specialized escape pathways that are mediated by rapidly conducting giant interneurons. These directly receive sensory affer-

*Corresponding author. Tel.: 001 520 621 8382;
Fax: 001 520 621 8282;
e-mail: flybrain@neurobio.arizona.edu

ents and act directly on segmental motor circuits to initiate escape turns away from a noxious event (Ritzmann, 1993).

Circuits underlying locomotion towards a stimulus source appear to be more complexly organized than those mediating escape behavior. Descending neurons that relay information from the brain to thoracic ganglia have several discrete dendritic domains in the brain, which usually receive sensory inputs indirectly via ensembles of interneurons. In addition, many descending neurons that supply leg motor circuits also receive connections from a prominent mid-line neuropil, called the central complex (Williams, 1975; Kanzaki et al., 1991; Muller et al., 1997). This chapter will outline some of the known properties of this center and speculate about the significance of its structure. To date, behavioral genetics, electrophysiology, and comparative anatomy all suggest that the central complex plays a cerebellar-like role in controlling forward locomotion, change of direction, and other limb actions. However, before considering the central complex itself, it is important to outline the segmental organization of the insect brain and to emphasize the unique position of the central complex within the three preoral ganglia.

The insect forebrain is distinct from thoracic ganglia and shares homology with vertebrate forebrain

The insect brain consists of six neuromeres, each corresponding to a segment of the head. Three neuromeres (the proto- deuto- and tritocerebra) lie dorsally above the eosophagus and are fused into a single mass that is connected to three suboesophageal neuromeres, which are also fused. Paired nerve cords carrying the axons of descending neurons connect the brain with segmental ganglia in the thorax and abdomen. The thorax has three ganglia, one per segment. Each contains motor neuron-interneuron circuits controlling neck muscles, direct and indirect flight muscles, and muscles of the legs and body wall. Other elements of thoracic motor circuits include the terminals of sensory afferents from the same and adjacent segments. These terminate on local interneurons. Plurisegmental interneurons link the left and right halves of each ganglion, and link motor circuits between segments. Local and plurisegmental neuron circuits provide instructions to motor neurons (see Burrows, 1996).

In the brain, all but the most rostral neuromere have features that are reminiscent of organization in segmental ganglia: the deuto- and tritocerebra and neuromeres of the suboesophageal ganglion all receive sensory afferents onto local interneurons and provide motor axons to muscles. The deuto- and tritocerebrum receive afferents from mechanoreceptors, taste receptors, and olfactory receptors on the antennae. Their motor neurons terminate on muscles in the head and neck. The suboesophageal ganglia receive sensory inputs from head mechanoreceptors and gustatory receptors from the mouthparts. Their motor neurons mainly supply mouthparts and neck muscles. Only the most frontal neuromere, the protocerebrum, neither contains motor neurons nor receives sensory inputs – if one discounts the optic lobes, whose segmental identities are still open to question. Like the craniate forebrain, the protocerebrum possesses neuropils that have no homologues in caudal segments.

The possibility that vertebrate and arthropod nervous systems have deep commonalties, such as segmental homology, is suggested by studies of orthologous gene expression (Hartmann and Reichert, 1998). In vertebrates, homeotic genes determine rostro-caudal patterning and segmental identity of the hindbrain and spinal cord. Maps of the rostro-caudal expression of homeotic genes in the *Drosophila* central nervous system, from the level of the labial neuromere in the suboesophageal ganglion towards the abdomen, show the order of expression to be almost identical with the anteroposterior expression of orthologous homeotic genes in mammals (Hirth et al., 1998). Brain areas performing similar functions in mammals and insects may require similar wiring encoded by similarly controlled gene ensembles. For example, the *Drosophila D-MEF2* gene, which is expressed in early embryogenesis and later in developing Kenyon cells of the mushroom bodies, is homologous to the murine *MEF2* gene expressed in neurons of the developing cortex, midbrain, hypothalamus, hippocampus, and hindbrain (Schulz et al., 1996). A comparison between the protocerebrum and forebrain may be justified because of their analogous segmental positions and because genes that are necessary for development of the protocerebrum are homologous and interchangeable with genes that are expressed in mammalian forebrain (Leuzinger et al., 1998). The protocerebrum's development requires the expression of the fruitfly's (*Drosophila*) homeobox gene orthodenticle (*otd*). This gene shares sequence homology with the murine homeobox gene *Otx 1* and *Otx 2* (Nagao et al., 1998), of which *Otx 1* is involved in corticogenesis (Acampora et al., 1999). Protocerebral development does not occur in fruitflies that cannot express *otd* (Hirth et al., 1995). However, development is rescued if murine *Otx* cDNA (Leuzinger et al., 1998) is expressed in the fly embryo. Likewise, mice that are deficient in the *Otx 1* gene also have cortical developmental defects but corticogenesis in *Otx 1* deficient mice can be rescued by expression of *Drosophila otd* cDNA (Acampora et al., 1998).

As in the mammalian forebrain, the protocerebrum consists of many discrete nuclei or centers, each of which is composed of a characteristic arrangement of neurons. So far, only very few of these centers have been described in any detail. The best known are the paired mushroom bodies, which were first identified by Dujardin in 1850. Because of their prominence in social insects Dujardin believed these neuropils to mediate functions that attest to the apparent intelligence of eusocial insects. Received theories about the integrative functions mediated by mushroom bodies include their possible role in learning and memory. They are also involved in higher olfactory processing and in cockroaches they have been implicated in the acquisition of place memory (Mizunami et al., 1998). The mushroom bodies also appear to mediate context-dependent sensory integration and they possibly determine what features of the environment are behaviorally relevant for subsequent processing by deeper protocerebral neuropils (Heisenberg, 1998; Ito et al., 1998). Whatever the function of the mushroom bodies (and possibly all the described functions may be represented in the mushroom bodies of certain species) these centers have a characteristic organization. This is based on many thousands of minute nerve cells whose parallel axons form two or more lobes and whose dendrites receive inputs from olfactory and visual interneurons. Parallel axons, which are modulated by olfactory and visual cues, serve as local interneurons between multimodal afferents in the mushroom body lobes and the dendrites of efferent neurons projecting from the lobes to other regions of the protocerebrum (Li and Strausfeld, 1999). Many of these regions supply subsequent interneurons to the mid-line neuropils of the central complex.

Central complex neuropils

All insects, and even collembolans, possess central complexes (Strausfeld, 1998). In neopteran insects these centers originate embryonically from amongst neuroblasts of the protocerebrum (Boyan and Williams, 1997). Central complexes consist of an arrangement of mid-line neuropils that have the same basic pattern of connections and architecture in all species so far examined (Williams, 1975; Strausfeld, 1976; Hanesch et al., 1989). The most obvious component of the central complex, and the one that can reach the greatest cellular elaboration, is an unpaired midline neuropil called the fan-shaped body (Fig. 1A, B). This lies immediately behind and is connected to another anterior mid-line neuropil called the ellipsoid body. In most insects, this region consists of a mound- or arch-like neuropil (Fig. 1A), but in flies the arch curves into a complete torus.

Both the fan-shaped body and the ellipsoid body are supplied by afferents (Fig. 2A) that originate from many of the higher order sensory neuropils of

the protocerebrum, some of which are also supplied by neurons originating in the mushroom bodies. Afferents to the central complex end in the fan-shaped and ellipsoid bodies as comb- or fan-like arborizations, the branches of which are iso-morphically distributed between 2 and 6 (depending on the species) discrete modular sub-units each side of the mid-line (Fig. 2B). Modules are also defined by the distribution of neuropeptides or transmitter substances, such as proctoline (Fig. 2D). The fan-shaped body and ellipsoid body also supply efferents, many of which terminate in one or more subdivsions of the lateral accessory lobes (Fig. 2C). This neuropil is important to further considerations because it also receives collateral dendrites belonging to descending neurons that supply thoracic motor circuits.

Each module is supplied by connections from a posterior mid-line neuropil called the protocerebral bridge, which links the left and right protocerebral hemispheres (Fig. 1A). The bridge is composed of girder-like arrangements of rod shaped terminals that extend across it from the protocerebral lobes (Fig. 1A). These terminals belong to interneurons whose dendrites are situated in regions of the medial deutocerebrum supplied by terminals of ascending neurons that originate in thoracic ganglia (Fig. 3). In the protocerebral bridge between 16 and 20 groups of small compact dendritic trees intersect the terminal fibers and segment the bridge into discrete subunits (Fig. 3).

Dendritic trees in the bridge provide a dramatic pattern of axon projections between the bridge and the fan-shaped body (Fig. 1A, panels 2, 3; Fig, 1B, panel 2; Fig. 3). The bridge provides each module of the fan-shaped body with converging terminals that represent two different locations across the bridge. In species where the entire bridge is segmented into 8 + 8 subunits, pairing is highly ordered such that the most lateral segment on the left side of the protocerebral bridge is represented by its axon terminal in the most lateral module of the left side of the fan-shaped body. The same module also receives terminals from the most medial segment of dendrites in the right side of the bridge (Fig. 2A). This pairing is continued across the fan-shaped body: the second module in the left side of the fan-shaped body receives terminals from

276

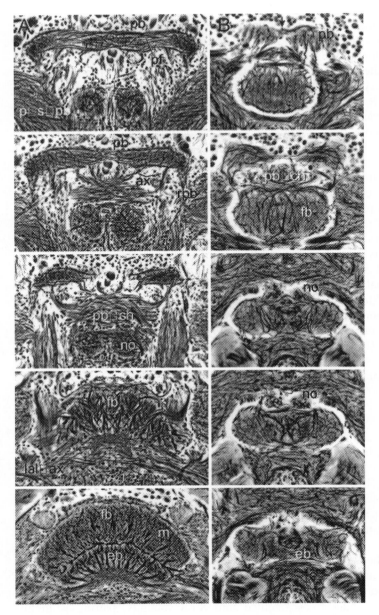

Fig. 1. A. The central complex of the paper wasp *Polistes castaniacolor*: Top panel: the protocerebral bridge (pb) containing many parallel fibers (pf) crossing it from the roots of the bridge (r pb) at the posterior superior protocerebrum (p s pr). The segmental arrangements of dendrites intersecting the parallel fibers provides axons (ax; second panel) that contribute to a chiasmal redistribution (pb ch; third panel) of their terminals in modules (m) of the fan-shaped and ellipsoid bodies (fb, eb; third, fourth panels). In *Polistes*, the noduli (no) lie posterior to the two mid-line neuropils. Axons to the lateral accessory lobes (lal ax) extend laterally from the base of fan-shaped and ellipsoid bodies. B. The central complex of the backswimmer *Notonecta glauca*. The protocerebral bridge (pb; top panel) is almost split at the mid-line (arrow). Nevertheless, axons from dendrites in its lateral parts project forward via a chiasma into the fan-shaped body (second panel). The noduli (no) are small, compared with those of *Polistes*, and the ellipsoid body (eb; bottom panel) is reduced to a vestige.

the second segment of the left side of the bridge and the seventh segment of the right side of the bridge, and so on as described in Fig. 3A. Thus, segments in the left and right sides of the protocerebral bridge are distributively represented in all the modules across the fan-shaped body. Axons from the bridge extend forwards through the fan-shaped body into modules of the ellipsoid body. Axons then invade a pair of ball-like structures, called the noduli, that lie beneath or behind the fan-shaped body. In the cockroach *Periplaneta*, the neuropil of each nodulus is arranged as a mantel and core. The mantel mainly receives axons from the same side of the fan-shaped body; the core receives axons from the other side of the fan-shaped body.

The role of the central complex in motor control

The functional significance of this elaborate organization is not yet known but there is enough anatomical and behavioral data to warrant speculation. Recordings from neurons supplying the fan-shaped and ellipsoid bodies from the protocerebrum demonstrate their sensitivity to multimodal stimuli (Homberg, 1985; Milde, 1988), a feature that correlates with their neuropils of origin, which are supplied by sensory interneurons. Studies on ellipsoid body neurons in the locust suggest that certain afferents are fine-tuned to the balance of sensory inputs each side of the head. For example, in locusts afferents to the ellipsoid body from medial neuropils supplied from the visual system carry information about the angles of sky polarization (Vitzhum et al., 1997). The locust central body also incorporates activity label (H3–2-deoxyglucose) during visual stimulation with moving gratings suggesting that a variety of visual cues are represented in it (Bausenwein et al., 1994). It is unlikely, however, that this is its main property. The large and highly modular central bodies of blind insects such as soldier ants demonstrate that

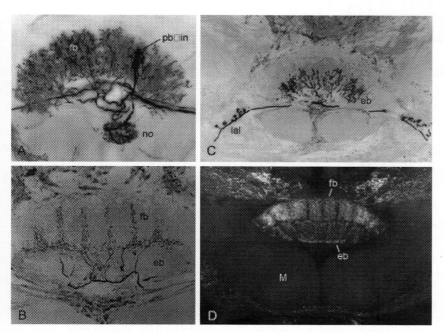

Fig. 2. A. Golgi-impregnated terminal supplying the fan-shaped body of the cockroach *Periplaneta americana*, also showing part of an interneuron (pb in) originating from the segment 3 of the bridge. A prolongation of its axon reaches the ipsilateral nodulus where it terminates in the mantel. B. In *Periplaneta*, the fan-shaped body comprises eight modules. This dye-filled terminal sends boutons between the modules and between the fan-shaped and ellipsoid bodies. C. A pair of efferent neurons from the ellipsoid body send axons over and in front of the mushroom bodies' medial lobes (M) to the lateral accessory lobes (lal). D. Distribution of proctoline in the eight modules of the fan-shaped and ellipsoid bodies.

278

these structures cannot be involved mainly in visual functions (Gronenberg, personal communication).

The most important studies to date on the behavioral significance of the central complex are those by Roland Strauss and his colleagues, whose studies on the walking behavior of *Drosophila* mutants provide important insights into the control function of this brain region.

In normal *Drosophila* as in many other insects, the stride length of the legs depends on the frequency of stepping. When the frequency of steps is high, and the stepping periods low, the strides are proportionally larger than when the frequency is low (Strauss and Heisenberg, 1990). However, in

mutants where the protocerebral bridge is disrupted stride lengths are almost independent of the step frequency. At low frequencies, short strides lengths are approximately the same as in normal flies at low frequency but at high frequencies step length hardly changes in the mutant and remains short (Strauss et al., 1993). Three genetically independent mutant strains, all having various protocerebral bridge defects, have substantiated the protocerebral bridge's role of optimizing step lengths and walking speed (Leng and Strauss, 1997). However, the protocerebral bridge is not involved in timing or in maintaining the basic rhythm of stepping since the timing of swing phases and the dependency of the

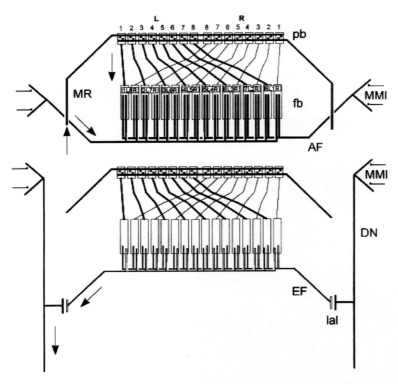

Fig. 3. Modular organization of the central complex. Top: ascending axons are thought to report motor performance (motor reporters MR) to the protocerebral bridge (pb). For simplicity only one MR is shown each side of the brain. MR terminals span the bridge and provide presynaptic sites to segmentally organized dendrites of neurons that send axons to the fan-shaped (fb) and ellipsoid bodies. These axons are arranged so that non-equivalent segments converge in modules of the fan-shaped body (ellipsoid body omitted for simplicity). The 1st segment of one side of the bridge converges with the 8th segment of the other; the 2nd with the 7th, 3rd with the 6th, and so on. Thus the two halves of the bridge representationally overlap in the mid-line neuropil. Modules in the fan-shaped body receive afferent inputs (AF) that are themselves supplied by multimodal sensory inputs onto their dendrites in the protocerebrum (MMI). Lower: Efferent neurons, with dendrites distributed amongst the modules, send axons to the lateral accessory lobe (lal) where they contact branches of descending neurons (DN) that also receive multimodal sensory inputs. Arrows indicate the direction of information flow.

swing phase duration on the frequency of stepping (fast frequencies mean short swing phases and vice versa) is the same in the wild type as in the mutant. This suggests that the basic rhythm of stepping is autonomous to the thoracic ganglia.

A further deficiency seen in flies with abnormal protocerebral bridges is during turning in goal directed walking. In wild-type *Drosophila*, smooth curves are accomplished by reducing the step lengths on the inside of the curve (Fig. 4A). This also occurs in *no-bridge* mutants, even though the dependency of stride lengths on the stepping period is drastically altered (Leng and Strauss, 1997). Thus in *no-bridge* mutants, steps are generally smaller than in wild-type (Fig. 4B; see Wannek and Strauss, 1998). Whereas normal flies reduce the lengths of their strides by shortening the swing phases of the inner legs, in mutants the swing speed is reduced by the legs on the inside of the curve. Whereas normal flies reduce the lengths of their strides by shortening the swing phases of the inner

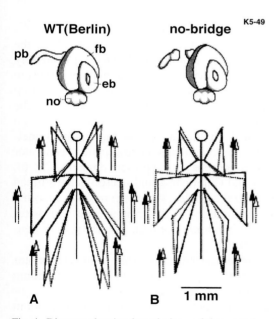

Fig. 4. Diagram showing lateral views of the central complex of normal (A) and mutant (B) *Drosophila*. In wild-type *Drosophila*, smooth curves are achieved by reducing step lengths on the inside of the curve (filled arrows, A). In *no-bridge* mutants, steps are generally smaller than in wild type and differences of step length during turning are abnormally small (from Strauss, 1996; by permission of the author).

legs, in mutants the swing speed is reduced by the legs on the inside of the curve. A mutant flies is unable to place its legs appropriately during a goal-directed turn and as a consequence stumbles over its own feet. Such episodes occur intermittently (Fig. 5; see Straus et al., 1992).

There is additional evidence that the central complex supervises the execution of walking and that it detects and compensates left-right differences in the motor performance of thoracic circuits controlling leg movements. This evidence derives from experiments that use other genetic defects of central body neuropils, some disrupting only the fan-shaped and ellipsoid bodies, others disrupting the bridge as well. In the walking impaired mutant *C31*, for example, the fan-shaped body, ellipsoid body, and the noduli all suffer anatomical defects that suggest disruption of connections between the left and right side of the central complex (Strauss and Trinath, 1996). Although there is some evidence that genes that cause abnormalities in the central complex may have pleiotropic effects (Varnam et al., 1997), the central complex behavioral phenotype can be confirmed using mosaic analysis. This permits a defective gene to be recognizably expressed in patches of tissue, such as in parts of the head, but not in the thorax. Flies walk straight if they possess a normal brain and normal central complex even though their thorax is mutant. Flies walk straight if they possess a normal brain and normal central complex even though their thorax is unilaterally mutant. The intact central complex is thought to compensate for the differences in performance of the body sides. Mosaic flies with a defective brain and central complex and a unilaterally defective body continuously turn in the direction of the defective body side even in the presence of attractice cues (Strauss and Heisenberg, 1993; Strauss and Trinath, 1996).

How does the neuroarchitecture of the bridge relate to studies on *Drosophila* behavior? Clearly, the central complex needs to be intact across its width in order for normal as well as goal directed walking to occur. The convergence in each module of pairs of axons from each side of the protocerebral bridge suggests a mechanism for comparing different strengths of inputs amongst dendritic trees across the bridge. Although each

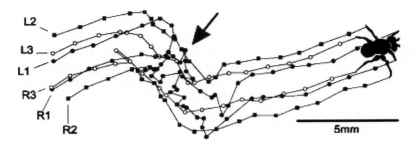

L2
L3
L1
R3
R1
R2

5mm

Fig. 5. Reconstruction of a sequence of steps during an attempt by a mutant fly to execute a smooth turn. Normal flies reduce stride length by shortening the swing phases of the inner legs. Mutants reduce swing speed by the legs on the inside of the curve. A turning mutant literally stumbles over its own feet (from Strauss et al., 1992; with permission of the author).

tree appears to be morphologically equivalent to its neighbor, each tree is unique with respect to its interaction with afferents that enter the bridge from its sides and extend through them. Each pair of bridge neurons ending in a module has a pair of unique identifiers in the bridge (Fig. 3). For example, the 3rd module in the left side of the fan-shaped body is supplied by the 3rd dendritic segment of the left half of the bridge and the 6th dendritic segment of the right half of the bridge. A signal initiated across the bridge from the left side of the brain will reach the dendritic segment on the left side before and possibly with less attenuation than the dendritic tree on the right side.

It is suggested that terminals spanning the bridge report motor activity. When the insect walks forward in a straight line symmetric motor activity is reported symmetrically across the bridge. Outputs from the bridge to the modules on the left side of the fan-shaped body will balance outputs to modules on the right side. In this model, any imbalance between the left and right leg motors, as in a deviation from a straight line, would be reported by ascending interneurons and would asymmetrically weight outputs from across the bridge. Projections from the bridge to the modules of the fan-shaped body may serve to assess quantitative differences between reported leg motor activity, such as forward swing, of the left and right side of the body.

If the central complex supervises walking, as Strauss's experiments suggest, then the complex must also make decisions about the relative weights of sensory cues each side of the body and on this basis determine the direction of walking. This function is likely to involve multimodal afferents that originate from higher sensory regions of the protocerebrum and terminate as fan-shaped arbors in the fan-shaped body and/or ellipsoid body. The observation that some afferents to the ellipsoid body relay accurate information about the angle of polarized light perceived by the two compound eyes supports the idea that this region assesses the relative weights of sensory events each side of the mid-line.

A speculative pathway between leg motor circuits and the brain is shown in Fig. 6. Here, the central complex is integrated into a locomotory control circuit devised by Beer and Chiel (1993) in which swing is generated by a central pattern generator that receives feedback from sensors in the legs. The Beer and Chiel model is equipped with a symmetrical command neuron that initiates metachronal activity amongst central pattern generator pacemaker neurons. In the present chimera (Fig. 6), the Beer and Chiel command neuron is substituted by the central complex, which (a) receives reported motor asymmetry to its bridge and (b) gates descending neurons supplying central pattern generator circuits.

It is hypothesized above that segmental motor performance is reported to the bridge by ascending interneurons that monitor the activity of back- or forward swing motor neurons or from receptors in the legs themselves. To provide a desired direction, the fan-shaped and ellipsoid bodies integrate this information with information about the relative weights of multimodal events occurring each side of the head. It is proposed that their connections to the lateral accessory lobes gate descending neurons

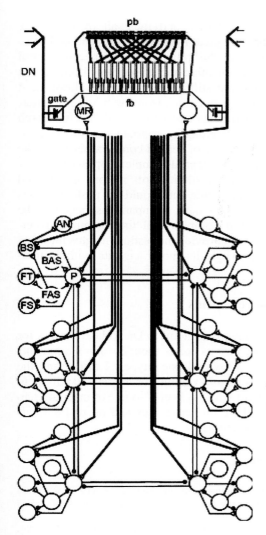

Fig. 6. Modification of a simplified walk generator circuit (from Beer and Chiel, 1993) by the addition of the central complex to substitute for a global command neuron. Abbreviations from the Beer and Chiel model are FT, foot motor neuron; FS and BS, forward and backward swing motor neurons; P, pacemaker neurons; FAS, BAS, forward and backward angle sensors. In the original Beer-Chiel model, a central command neuron inputs to pacemaker neurons. In this modification, a suite of descending neurons (DN; only one pair shown for clarity) substitutes the command neuron. DNs are modulated by instructions from the central complex, via its efferents to the lateral accessory lobe. Inputs to the protocerebral bridge report motor actions. Here ascending neurons (AN) are envisaged as monitoring activity in the backward swing motor neurons, themselves locally modulated by forward angle sensors. ANs relay information in the brain to motor reporter neurons (MR) supplying the bridge.

that modifying stride length and stepping frequency. Two lines of evidence support this. Gating of descending neurons has been recorded in freely walking crickets where the sensory responses and outputs of these cells is dependent on the behavioral context in which the sensory stimulus is presented (Staudacher and Schildberger, 1998). In locusts, tonic excitation of descending neurones that have branches in the lateral accessory lobes corresponds to the duration of flight while neurons linking the central complex to the lateral accessory lobes show different activity during and after flight (Homberg, 1994). While these results do not address the role of the central complex and lateral accessory lobes in walking, they do suggest collaboration between central complex efferents and descending neurons.

Evidence that the central complex is crucial to locomotor actions also comes from experiments in which the neural ablation agent, tetanus toxin, can be expressed in identified neurons of specific *Drosophila* enhancer trap lines (Martin et al., 1999). Two types of neurons targeted are those linking the superior medial protocerebrum with the superior arch and fan-shaped body, and neurons linking the protocerebral bridge to the ellipsoid body and noduli. In both cases, their ablation leads to a profound decrease in locomotory activity.

Central complexes in insects that swim or cling

Central complex neuropils are readily identifiable across insect taxa. Although there is no fused protocerebral bridge in primitive thysanurah insects, such as the firebrat *Thermobia*, nevertheless three columnar mid-line neuropils can be distinguished whose intrinsic neuroarchitecture is little different from mid-line neuropils in more recently evolved taxa, such as the brachyceran Diptera. This contrasts with the brains of most malacostracan crustaceans in which midline columnar neuropils are, at most, subtle. The exception is in certain eumalacostracans that have invaded land, such as the fast moving and highly maneuverable isopod *Ligia occidentalis*, which lives on the shore above the high tide line. Its brain possesses a protocerebral bridge connected by chiasmal arrangement of axons to a columnar neuropil that is architecturally reminiscent of the insect ellipsoid body (Strausfeld, 1998).

Comparisons amongst pterygote species suggest that the central complex is most elaborate in those taxa that use their legs for goal directed walking and running, and for dexterous limb actions, such as grooming, grasping, seizing, manipulating, and building. One of the most spectacular examples of an elaborate and isomorphically constructed central complex is in polistine wasps (Fig. 1A). In contrast, species that use their legs mainly for grasping possess discontinuous protocerebral bridges. They have fewer modules in the fan-shaped and ellipsoid bodies, both of which may be reduced in volume. The association of the central complex in limb movements is also suggested by its relative development in larval holometabolous insects. In larvae that lack legs, the central complex is rudimentary or undeveloped. In larvae that actively walk using their thoracic legs, like the mealworm *Tenebrio molitor*, the central complex appears early in development and elaborates its modular organization throughout larval life (Wegerhoff and Breidbach, 1988).

The role of the central complex in mediating asymmetries in limb movements is strongly suggested by aquatic insects that use their legs for rowing. The hemipteran *Notonecta glauca* uses its first two leg pairs for grasping prey and the metathoracic (3rd) leg pair for propulsion. This species is not able to walk well, and most locomotory actions are swimming actions, driven by symmetric movements of the last leg pair. The central complex of *Notonecta* is quite small and much simplified in comparison to those insects that walk. The protocerebral bridge is split into two halves with most terminals restricted to one half of the bridge only. Its noduli are greatly reduced, as is its ellipsoid body. The fan-shaped body contains large modules only laterally (Fig. 1B). A related species, *Gerris* (the water strider) uses symmetrical rowing movements of all its leg pairs. Its protocerebral bridge is vestigial, completely divided at the mid-line, and there is no discernible ellipsoid body. In *Gerris*, sculling is accomplished by symmetric movements of the left and right limb pairs working conjointly. This contrasts to the exploratory walking and running of insects such as

cockroaches, wasps, and flies, all of which are hallmarked by great maneuverability and agility.

Studies on the relationships between central complex organization and taxonomic differences in locomotion are still in their infancy. However, it seems that such comparisons will suggest interesting experiments and will provide useful search images for designing appropriate stimuli for intracellular recording of central complex neurons. The evolution of the central complex appears to correspond to the evolution of motor agility and dexterity. And while one should not push analogies too far and too hard, comparisons between the insect central complex and the mammalian cerebellum could provide interesting insights into how a brain provides its motor circuits with instructions.

Acknowledgements

I am particularly grateful to Dr. Roland Strauss for discussing various points about *Drosophila* mutants and their behavioral phenotypes. I also thank the organizers of this volume for a splendid tribute to Doug Stuart who has been a source of inspiration to those working on vertebrates and on real animals with exoskeletons.

References

Acampora D, Gulisano, M. and Simeone, A. (1999) *Otx* genes and the genetic control of brain morphogenesis. *Mol. Cell Neurosci.*, 13: 1–7.

Bausenwein, B., Muller, N.R. and Heisenberg, M. (1994) Behavior-dependent activity labeling in the central complex of *Drosophila* during controlled visual stimulation. *J. Comp. Neurol.*, 340: 255–268.

Beer, R. and Chiel, H.J. (1993) Simulations of cockroach locomotion and escape. In: R.D. Beer, R.E. Ritzmann and T. McKenna (Eds), *Biological Neural Networks in Invertebrate Neuroethology and Robotics*, Academic Press, N.Y. pp. 267–285.

Boyan, G.S. and Williams, J.L.D. (1997) Embryonic development of the pars intercerebralis central complex of the grasshopper. *Dev. Genes Evol.*, 207: 317–329.

Burrows, M. (1996) The neurobiology of an insect brain. Oxford U.P.

Burrows, M. and Laurent, G. (1989) Reflex circuits and the control of movement. In: R. Durbin, C. Miall and G. Mitchison (Eds), *The Computing Neuron*, Addison Wesley. Wokingham. pp. 224–261.

Cruse, H., Bartling, C., Dreifert, M., Schmitz, J., Brunn, D.E., Dean, J. and Kindermann, T. (1995) Walking – a complex behavior controlled by simple networks. *Adapt. Behav.*, 3: 385–418.

Dujardin, F. (1850) Memoire sur le systéme nerveux des Insectes. *Ann. Sci. Natl. Zool.*, 14: 195–206.

Faivre, E. 1857. Du cerveau des dytisques considéré dans ses rapports avec la locomotion. *Ann. Sci. Nat (Zool.)*, 8: 245–274.

Hanesch, U., Fischbach, K.F. and Heisenberg, M. (1989) Neuronal architecture of the central complex in *Drosophila melanogaster*. *Cell Tissue Res.*, 257: 343–366.

Hartmann, B. and Reichert, H. (1998) The genetics of embryonic brain development in *Drosophila*. *Mol. Cell Neurosci.*, 12: 194–205.

Heisenberg, M. (1998) What do the mushroom bodies do for the insect brain? *Learn. Mem.*, 5: 1–10,.

Hirth, F., Hartmann, B. and Reichert, H. (1998) Homeotic gene action in embryonic brain development of *Drosophila*. *Development*, 125: 1579–1589.

Hirth F, Therianos, S., Loop, T., Gehring, W.J., Reichert, H. and Furukubo-Tokunaga, K. (1995) Developmental defects in brain segmentation caused by mutations of the homeobox genes orthodenticle and empty spiracles in *Drosophila*. *Neuron*, 15: 769–778.

Homberg, U. (1985) Interneurones of the central complex in the bee brain (*Apis mellifera*, L). *J. Insect Physiol.*, 31: 251–257.

Homberg, U. (1994) Flight-correlated activity changes in neurons of the lateral accessory lobes in the brain of the locust *Schistocerca gregaria*. *J. Comp. Physiol.*, 175: 597–610.

Ito, K., Suzuki, K., Estes, P., Ramaswami, M., Yamamoto, D. and Strausfeld, N.J. (1998) The Organization of extrinsic neurons and their implications in the functional roles of the mushroom bodies of *Drosophila melanogaster* Meigen. *Learn. Mem.*, 5: 52–75.

Kanzaki, R., Arbas, E.A. and Hildebrand, J.G. (1991) Physiology and morphology of descending neurons in pheromone-processing olfactory pathways in the male moth *Manduca sexta*. *J. Comp. Physiol.* (A), 169: 1–14.

Leng, S. and Strauss, R. (1997) Impaired step lengths common to three unrelated *Drosophila* mutant lines with common brain defects confirm the involvement of the protocerebral bridge in optimizing walking speed. In: W. Elsner and H. Wässle (Eds), *Proc. 25th Göttingen Neurobiol. Conf.* Vol. II, Thieme, Stuttgart, 294.

Leuzinger, S., Hirth, F., Gerlich, D., Acampora, D., Simeone, A., Gehring, W.J., Finkelstein, R., Furukubo-Tokunaga, K. and Reichert, H. (1998) Equivalence of the fly orthodenticle gene and the human OTX genes in embryonic brain development of *Drosophila*. *Development*, 125: 1703–1710.

Li, Y.-S. and Strausfeld, N.J. (1999) Multimodal efferent and recurrent neurons in the medial lobes of cockroach mushroom bodies. *J. Comp. Neurol.*, 409: 647–663.

Martin, J.-R., Raabe, T. and Heisenberg, M. (1999) Central complex substructures are required for the maintenance of

locomotory activity in *Drosophila melanogaster. J. Comp. Physiol. A.*, 185: 277–288.

Milde, J.J. (1988) Visual responses of interneurones in the posterior median protocerebrum and the central complex of the honey bee *Apis mellifera. J. Insect Physiol.*, 34: 427–436.

Mizunami, M., Weibrecht, J.M. and Strausfeld, N.J. (1998) Mushroom bodies of the cockroach: their participtation in place memory. *J. Comp. Neurol.*, 402: 520–537.

Muller, M., Homberg, U. and Kuhn, A. (1997) Neuroarchitecture of the lower division of the central body of the locust (*Schistocerca gregaria*). *Cell Tissue Res.*, 288: 159–176.

Nagao, T., Leuzinger, S., Acampora, D., Simeone, A., Finkelstein, R., Reichert, H. and Furukubo-Tokunaga, K. (1998) Developmental rescue of *Drosophila* cephalic defects by the human Otx genes. *Proc. Nat. Acad. Sci. USA*, 95: 3737–3742.

Ritzmann, R.E. (1993) The neural organization of cockroach escape and its role in context-dependent orientation. In: R.D. Beer, R.E. Ritzmann and T. McKenna (Eds), *Biological Neural Networks in Invertebrate Neuroethology and Robotics*, Academic Press, N.Y. pp. 113–137.

Schulz, R.A., Chromey, C., Lu, M.-F. and Olson, E.N. (1996) Expression of the D-MEF2 transcription factor in the *Drosophila* brain suggests a role in neuronal cell differentiation. *Oncogene*, 12: 1827–1831.

Staudacher, E. and Schildberger, K. (1998) Gating of sensory responses of descending neurons during walking in crickets. *J. Exp. Biol.*, 201: 559–572.

Strausfeld, N.J. (1976) *Atlas of an Insect Brain*, Springer, Heidelberg.

Strausfeld, N.J. (1998) Crustacean – insect relationships: The use of brain characters to derive phylogeny amongst segmented invertebrates. *Brain, Behav. Evolut.*. 52: 186–206.

Strauss, R. and Heisenberg, M. (1990) Coordination of legs during straight walking and turning in *Drosophila melanogaster. J. Comp. Physiol. A*, 167: 403–412.

Strauss, R. and Heisenberg, M. (1993) Higher control center of locomotor behavior in the *Drosophila* brain, *J. Neurosci.*, 13: 1852–1861.

Strauss, R., Hanesch, U., Kinkelin, M., Wolf, R. and Heisenberg, M. (1992) no-bridge of *Drosophila melanogaster* – portrait of a structural brain mutant of the central complex. *J. Neurogen.*, 8: 125–155.

Strauss, R. and Trinath, T. (1996) Is walking in a straight line controlled by the central complex? Evidence from a new *Drosophila* mutant. In: N. Elsner and U.-U. Schitzler (Eds), *Proc. 24th Göttingen Neurobiol. Conf.* Vol. II, Thieme, Stuttgart, 135.

Varnam, C.J., Strauss, R., deBelle, J.S. and Sokolowski, M.B. (1997) Larval behavior of *Drosophila* central complex mutants: interactions between *no bridge*, *foraging*, and *chaser. J. Neurogen.*, 11: 99–115.

Vitzhum, H., Müller, M. and Homberg, U. (1997) Polarization-sensitive interneurons in the central complex of the locust *Schistocerca gergaria*. In: N. Elsner and H. Wässle (Eds),

Proc. 25th Göttingen Neurobiol. Conf. Vol. II, Thieme, Stuttgart, 470.

Wannek, U. and Strauss, R. (1998) How flies perform turns – high resolution statistical analyses in normal and brain-defective *Drosophila melanogaster*. In: N. Elsner and R. Wehner (Eds), *Proc. 26th Göttingen Neurobiol. Conf.* Vol. II, Thieme, Stuttgart, 258.

Wegerhoff, R. and Breidbach, O. (1988) Structure and development of the larval central complex in a holometabolous insect, the beetle *Tenebrio molitor. Cell Tiss. Res.*, 268: 341–358.

Williams, J.L.D. (1975) Anatomical studies of the insect nervous system: a ground plan of the midbrain and an introduction to the central complex in the locust, *Schistocerca gregaria* (Orthoptera). *J. Zool.*, 176: 67–86.

Yellman, C., Tao, H., He, B. and Hirsch, J. (1997) Conserved and sexually dimorphic behavioral responses to biogenic amines in decapitated *Drosophila. PNAS*, 94: 4131–4136.

M.D. Binder (Ed.)
Progress in Brain Research, Vol 123

Behavior of hindbrain neurons during the transition from rest to evoked locomotion in a newt

I. Bar-Gad, I. Kagan and M.L. Shik*

Department of Zoology, G.S. Wise Faculty of Life Sciences, Tel Aviv University, Tel Aviv, 69978, Israel

Introduction

The transition from a resting state to locomotion can be elicited by local electrical stimulation of the midbrain 'locomotor region' (MLR) (Shik et al., 1966). The MLR projects to the spinal cord via hindbrain neurons, at least in mammals (Orlovsky, 1970a). A portion of the hindbrain neurons increases their firing during walking both in the cat and in the rough skin newt (Lowry et al., 1996).

A state transition may arise due to neuronal interaction at the level of the hindbrain when the input from the MLR reaches the threshold for locomotion, similarly to transition between two different rhythmic motor patterns (cf. Green and Soffe, 1996). It can also result due to the shift of individual properties of some neurons or their connections induced by the MLR input.

The aim of this study was to monitor the behavior of hindbrain neurons during the initiation of locomotion. Experiments were performed on rough skin newts. The parameters of the train of stimuli applied to the MLR were near the threshold for locomotion; the latency of movements was about 10 s. This allowed us to record the impulses of single neurons before the motion started. The discharge of a neuron was recorded during one or a few successive trials. If the intensity of stimulation is just threshold for locomotion, one can expect that

mainly those neurons that participate in the initiation of this motor pattern would be affected. Part of this study was reported in abstract form elsewhere (Bar-Gad et al., 1995).

Methods

The spike trains of 44 neurons in the hindbrain of five rough skin newts *Taricha granulosa* were recorded in 10 experiments. The animals had total body length 14 to 17 cm and weighed 12 to 15 g. The animals were immersed in 200 ml of water with 50 mg of MS 222 (Sigma). After 20 min, ice was added. When spontaneous movements as well as tactile reflexes disappeared, a parieto-occipital craniotomy was done. The animals were kept in the refrigerator at 7°C. The first experiment was performed one day after surgery.

The head was fixed while the body was placed in the bath filled with the cool water. The monopolar stimulation was delivered through a microelectrode introduced by a manual micromanipulator under visual guidance. The electrode consisted of a carbon fiber of 7 μm diameter with glass insulation. A train of negative pulses of 1 ms duration with interstimulus intervals from 80 to 120 ms was applied through a constant-current stimulus isolation unit, and the mesencephalic low threshold (3 to 12 μA, 6 μA in an average) point for initiation of locomotion was found. Usually it was located 1–1.5 mm rostral to the caudal border of the tectum, 0.6–0.8 mm from the midline, at a depth

---

*Corresponding author. Tel.: 972-3-6407390; Fax: 972–3–6409403; e-mail: mrkshik@ccsg.tau.ac.il

0.7–1.0 mm below the dorsal surface of the brain. Intervals between successive trials were not less than 2 min.

The action potentials of neurons were recorded extracellularly with a similar microelectrode installed in the ipsilateral hindbrain, 0.2 to 0.5 mm from the midsagittal plane using an independent micromanipulator. Recordings were made during the 10 s period before movements started, when near threshold train was delivered. The action potentials were usually biphasic. The action potential width at half-amplitude was typically about 1 ms in the first wave and nearly 2 ms for the second wave. The output of an AC amplifier, bandpass 0.1 to 5 kHz (A-M Systems) was connected to the Board AT-MIO–16-L–9 (National Instruments). After sampling at 10 kHz and storing the data on the hard disk of the PC, the action potentials of particular neuron were identified off line by the threshold ('window') discriminator and checked by their shape. Usually units with amplitudes three or more times higher than the mean level of noise were recognized. Discriminated spike train and the corresponding train of stimuli were then transformed to point processes. Interstimulus intervals (ISIs) were in the range 60 to 1000 ms, usually 200 or 100 ms. A firing ratio (FR) was defined as ISI/$\mu_c(I)$, where average interimpulse interval $\mu_c(I) = [\Sigma I_k]/n$, $k = 1 \ldots n$, n – number of interimpulse intervals in record.

Results

Direct responses

Action potentials of a neuron whose axon or body was excited by electrical pulse in the midbrain can be recorded at the hindbrain level. These direct responses (11 neurons) had latencies (L) in the range 3 to 15 ms with a standard deviation $\sigma(L)$ from 0.2 to 0.5 ms at FR < 1. The median coincided with mean latency $\mu(L) \pm 0.2$ ms.

In records with long latencies, drift of latency could be observed during stimulation with ISI = 100 ms and sometimes even 200 ms. The value of drift could achieve 2 to 3 ms during 10 s stimulation by threshold current, and σ reached 0.6 ms. Nevertheless fluctuations around the sliding

average remained 0.1 to 0.2 ms (Fig. 1B). Therefore, we considered these as direct responses. Latencies of late direct and early synaptic responses overlapped, but the latter varied in the characteristic span of 2 to 4 ms (Fig. 1C, the early mode).

Direct responses persisted even when responses with longer latency and higher standard deviations could no longer be evoked. The distance between sites of stimulation and recording was 2 to 3 mm, and the conduction velocity was in the range 0.2 to 1.0 m/s. The latency of direct responses remained the same at ISIs 1000 to 60 ms. These responses could be recorded either from the dorsal (granular) or ventral (funicular) layer of the hind brain (Fig. 1A).

Synaptic responses

Non-direct, i.e. synaptic, responses can be subdivided into three groups: time locked to stimuli, non-locked and composite ones. The data presented below are derived from 37 records, each of which contained 17 or more impulses (34 impulses on average). Responses remained unclassified when only a few impulses were generated during 10 s of stimulation.

The response is termed time-locked if the impulses arise in a limited span of ISI and non-locked if they are distributed throughout the ISI. In composite responses, time-locked and non-locked components coexisted. The time-locked component expressed as narrow peak (1.2 to 4 ms wide) in the ISI histogram was defined as a mode. Short (mode < 20 ms) as well as long latency synaptic responses could be recognized among time locked impulses.

Time locked responses

Pure time locked responses occurred in six neurons. All of these neurons were silent. Poststimulus histograms (PSTH) contained both early and late modes, e.g. Fig. 1C, or only the late one as in Fig. 1D, dashed line. In superposition of several histograms, there were two peaks, one at 17 ms, and one at 28 ms. The early responses could alternate with the late ones in the same record. As a rule, the late response arose after those stimuli in the train that did not evoke the early discharge. This suggests that the threshold of firing is enhanced during a certain epoch after discharge.

Composite responses

Composite responses were observed in 13 neurons, five of them with background discharge (BD). Some neurons generated composite responses and either pure time locked or non-locked responses depending on the parameters of stimulation. Fig. 2A shows that the modes persisted throughout the trial, and the deviations in latency were due to the non-locked responses (Fig. 2C) or BD (Fig. 2B). In fact, the mean interimpulse interval $\mu(I)$ during stimulation (Fig. 2D) became larger than it was during BD in this neuron.

Superposition of histograms of composite responses contains a hump between 18 and 31 ms. In individual histograms either narrow peaks or broad humps could occur apart, and the median of latency was usually 10 to 20% shorter than $\mu(L)$. The relative expression of the time-locked and non-locked components was diverse in different neurons, and in the same neuron the proportion of non-locked impulses could be enhanced when ISI was shortened from 200 to 100 ms (Fig. 3A, C).

Early and late firing

The PSTH for pure time-locked responses was commonly bimodal. There was a late time-locked component in composite responses whereas the early mode rarely did.

Huge deviations of latency occurred in the neuron presented in Fig. 4 during stimulation at ISI = 60 ms (A, D), but not at 100 and 200 ms (A–

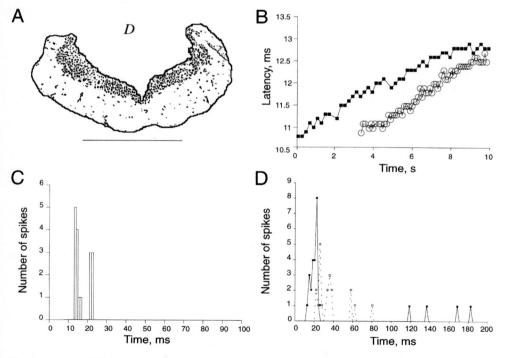

Fig. 1. A: Frontal 10 μm section of the hindbrain (Nissl staining). The bar corresponds to 1 mm. D – dorsal. B: Drift of latency of the direct response in the slow conducting axons. Abscissa indicates time of stimulation, ordinate – latency. Neuron 79A (filled squares) responded to stimuli delivered at ISI = 200 ms, FR = 0.96. Neuron 84A (open circles) fired during stimulation with ISI = 100 ms, FR = 0.97. C, D: Poststimulus histograms of the synaptic responses. Abscissa designates time after stimulus. C: neuron 13A, FR = 0.37, current 3.5 μA, bin 1 ms, only first 100 ms of ISI = 200 ms are presented. D: bin 2 ms. Solid line (black squares): Neuron 64A, ISI = 200 ms, current 6 μA, FR = 0.56. Dashed line (open squares): Neuron 62B, ISI = 100 ms, FR = 0.56.

C). In other neurons, deviations from the normal latency could be observed even at ISI = 200 ms (Fig. 2A–C). These deviations occurred both at low and high FR. Sometimes it was difficult to decide if the late firing was time locked or distributed in ISI (Fig. 1D, solid line, and 3C) or to distinguish uni- and bimodal responses (Fig. 3D).

Nevertheless in 11 records two or even three distinct modes could be identified. The distance between adjacent modes varied from 2 to 12 ms, and the average difference was 5.1 ± 2.2 ms. Together with 12 unimodal records, 38 modes ranged between 12 and 116 ms. Thirty of these modes were less than 33 ms, and their distribution, in turn, included modes at 18, 23 and 28 ms (Fig. 3B). Hence both distances in bimodal histograms and the distribution of modes in records of different neurons indicate that there is a characteristic minimal span near to 5 ms between consecutive latencies. In fact, sometimes there were also the earliest latency responses approximately at 13 ms.

Background discharge and non-locked responses

The distribution of interimpulse intervals in the background discharge (BD) was unimodal and somewhat skewed to the longer intervals, so that usually, the median was less than $\mu(I)$. The duration of I_n was almost independent on the duration of I_{n-1}, and the correlation coefficient was less than 0.2. Typically $\sigma(I)$ was enhanced from 30 to 190 ms when $\mu(I)$ increased from 80 to 250 ms and reached 340 ms at $\mu(I)$ 500 ms. Correspondingly CV(I) increased from 0.4 to 0.7. This relationship, although variable, was common for BD of different neurons, as well as the distinct states of the same neuron (Table 1). The points corresponding to both non-locked and composite responses were inter-mingled with BD points on the plane $[\mu, \sigma]$.

Non locked responses exhibited $\mu(L)$ of about ISI/2 and $\sigma(L)$ of nearly ISI/4. Neurons with BD could show either non-locked or composite responses. Usually, both $\mu(I)$ and $\sigma(I)$ of BD

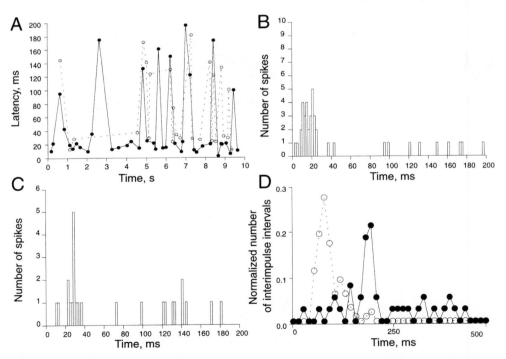

Fig. 2. Composite responses. A: Fluctuations of latency (ordinate) in time course of the trial (abscissa). The same records as in B (solid line, filled circles) and C (dashed line, open circles). B, C: Distribution of impulses throughout ISI = 200 ms, bin = 1 ms. B: Neuron 21A with BD. C: Silent neuron 27A. D: Neuron 21A, normalized histograms (40 bins) of distribution of interimpulse intervals during BD (dashed line, open circles, n = 101) and during stimulation at ISI = 200 ms (solid line, filled circles, n = 42).

diminished during stimulation, but in one neuron $\mu(I)$ decreased while $\sigma(I)$ remained the same. Sometimes $\mu(I)$ remained unchanged whereas $\sigma(I)$ increased. There was also one neuron in which both $\mu(I)$ and $\sigma(I)$ increased when the stimulus train was delivered.

The probability of firing of non-locked responses in silent neurons diminished when the ISI was increased from 200 to 1000 ms. The distribution of interimpulse intervals was similar to that observed during BD of other neurons (Fig. 2D, dashed line). Impulses could be slightly bound to stimuli at the threshold for locomotion, but were distributed in ISI when lower currents were applied. The diminution of the current was followed by a decrease of the firing rate.

Histograms of intervals between impulses in non-locked responses of both silent neurons and neurons with BD were usually unimodal and slightly skewed to the right. Diminished μI during non-locked responses of neurons with BD could remain unrelated to ISI. Distribution of intervals between impulses for the composite response sometimes deviated from the BD pattern.

Rate of stimulation

Three parameters of the train of stimuli effect the threshold for locomotion: the duration of stimulus, the current strength and ISI. They are interchangeable over a certain verge for both initiation of locomotion and single neuron responses. However, the effects of changing the parameters vary for different neurons. The synaptic response of most neurons did not appear at ISI = 1000 or 500 ms, but did appear at ISIs of 200 or 100 ms. To evoke firing at 1000 or 500 ms, it was usually necessary to deliver paired shocks with a 20 or 30 ms-interval between them. A few neurons that responded to single pulses at ISI = 1000 ms increased their FR significantly at ISI = 200 ms (e.g. the silent neuron in Fig. 4B increased its FR by 50% to 0.76). Several neurons generated fewer than 10 impulses

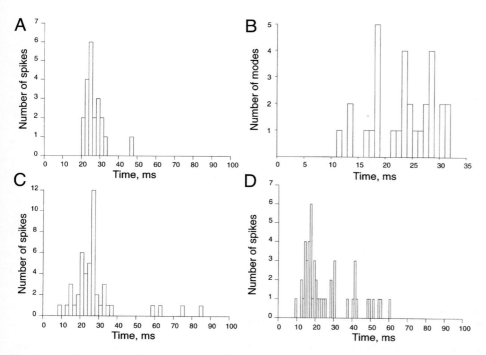

Fig. 3. A, C: Time locked (A) and composite (C) reactions of the same neuron. Distribution of impulses in ISI = 200 ms (A, only first 100 ms are presented) and ISI = 100 ms (C), bin 2 ms. Neuron 64A. B: Histogram of modal latencies <35 ms, bin 1 ms. D: Obscure response: Neuron 86E, distribution of impulses in ISI = 100 ms, bin 1 ms.

during the 10 s stimulation period even at ISI = 200 ms (FR < 0.2). When ISI was diminished from 200 to 100 ms, these cells showed increased FR. Frequency potentiation was not observed if the neuron has already reached a high FR already at ISI 200 ms.

TABLE 1

Mean interimpulse interval and its CV of the background discharge in four neurons, each being recorded twice

Neuron	Record	$\mu(I)$	CV(I)
21A	21	70	0.21
21A	22	96	0.31
7A	9	205	0.79
7A	7	298	0.87
107A	109	206	0.63
107A	107	424	0.90
14A	17	348	0.51
14A	14	356	0.46

A neuron could display pure time locked responses to weak pulses at ISI = 200 ms, and add non-locked component when the current or stimulus frequency was increased (Fig. 1D, solid line). One neuron generated impulses time locked to stimuli at ISI = 200, 100 and 60 ms. The earliest latency mode shifted to the right (Fig. 4B–D) in this cell. In the latter record, a non-locked component appeared as well.

Stimulation that was subthreshold for locomotion commonly evoked the time-locked responses in neurons with low FR. When the stimulus train reached the threshold, non-locked component developed, both FR and $\mu(L)$ increased, and $\sigma(L)$ was enhanced. The behavior of almost every neuron had its peculiarities. For example, one silent neuron did not respond to single pulses of 4 μA delivered with ISI = 200 ms. An increase in the current to 5 μA was followed by an increased FR and a shortening of $\mu(L)$. The average latency and FR almost did not change when pulses 5 μA were

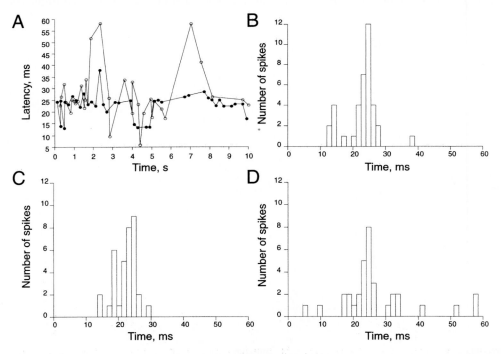

Fig. 4. Latency of the response to stimuli 3.4 μA applied at ISI = 200, 100 or 60 ms. A: Neuron 98A: Fluctuations of latency (ordinate, ms) during a train {abscissa, s} at ISI = 200 ms (filled circles) and 60 ms (open circles). B-D: Distribution of impulses throughout ISI: the first 60 ms are shown. Responses at ISI = 200 ms (B) and 100 ms (C) were pure time locked, and it became a composite one at ISI = 60 ms (D), FR = 0.76, 0.35, and 0.20, respectively.

applied with ISI either 200 or 100 ms (Fig. 3A,C). Late impulses appeared at ISI 200 ms when current pulses 6 μA were delivered (Fig. 1D, solid line).

The reproducibility of the neurons' responses seems to be an individual feature of neuronal behavior. A few neurons gave similar responses even though the ISI or stimulus current was altered. In contrast, some neurons did not retain either their FR or latency and σ(L) even in two consecutive trials under the same conditions of stimulation.

Time course of firing

The time course of firing during 10 s of repetitive stimulation was stable in a portion of cells while the rate was augmenting or decrementing in others. Most of augmenting neurons produced 6 to 9 impulses in the first 2 s, while decrementing neurons started mainly from 3 to 6 spikes (Fig. 5A). The difference between the number of impulses produced by augmenting and decrementing neurons grew during the trial twice, although the time course of firing in individual records was almost never monotonic.

The average, normalized time course of firing for the whole population of neurons was uniform, but activity augmented in most of records of non-locked responses, while time locked responses occurred usually with decrement. The time course of firing also depended on strength of stimulation. Four consecutive trials are shown in Fig. 5B at

currents 8, 7, 6 and 5 μA. The first response was the composite, others were of the non-locked type. At the two highest currents, the number of impulses produced in the last 2 s of the trial was larger than in the first 2 s. The two lower currents were subthreshold for locomotion, and the firing was rather stable during period of stimulation. Sometimes the rate of BD during stimulation or the FR of time-locked impulses in the silent neuron was cyclically modulated with a period of 4 to 5 s.

Discussion

Polysynaptic propagation of the input volley

The earliest latency of synaptic responses was 13 ms after the stimulus, although characteristic modes occurred at 18, 23 and 28 ms. This suggests that the (minimal) translation time is approximately 5 ms. This estimation is compatible with data on synaptic delay, rise time and a half-width of excitatory postsynaptic potential in amphibians (Babalian and Shapovalov, 1984).

In our experiments near threshold stimuli were used, therefore the translation time was determined by the rise time and half-width of EPSP rather than by the synaptic delay. A similar value was obtained earlier by Matsushima et al. (1989) in a study in which stimuli applied to the optic tectum evoked monosynaptic EPSPs and spikes in the ipsilateral medullary reticular neurons in a toad with minimal

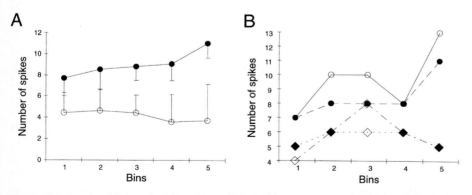

Fig. 5. Time course of firing, abscissa – time, consecutive bins 2 s each. A: 11 records with the output 38 to 51 impulses per 10 s each (filled circles) and 11 records with the total output 17 to 23 impulses (open circles), ordinate – an average number of impulses produced per bin, vertical bars denote σ. B: Neuron 33A, currents 8 (open circles), 7 (filled circles), 6 (filled diamonds) and 5 (open diamonds) μA were applied at ISI = 200 ms. Ordinate indicates number of impulses per bin. Response at 8 μA was composite, others were non-locked reactions.

latencies 2.9 to 3.6 ms and 3.8 to 6.9 ms, respectively. The mean latency of disynaptic EPSPs in cells of nucleus isthmi evoked by stimuli delivered to the optic tract in toads was 16 ± 7 ms (Wu and Wang, 1995).

Since the mode at 13 ms was expressed weaker than later modes and occurred in just a few records, the number of neurons that responded disynaptically was greater than those that responded monosynaptically. This suggests propagation with the coefficient of multiplication > 1 at the second relay. However, the wave-like propagation sharply decrements after 3–4 relays either due to the increased thresholds of neurons that fired in the initial part of ISI, or to the involvement of inhibitory neurons (cf. McLean et al., 1995). In other cases, the activity does not cease but rather becomes asynchronous, in particular if the train achieves the threshold of locomotion.

State transition

Neurons with various rates of BD can coexist at rest because of the paucity of active neurons and their weak interactions. During the transition from rest to locomotion, the neurons must be unified to a certain degree. Perhaps neurons with both decrementing, time-locked responses and augmenting, composite and non-locked responses participate in the transition. The first neurons may start, and those with composite responses then continue processing the input from the 'locomotor region'. Non-synchronized firing of reticulospinal neurons can elicit locomotion without spasticity. The propagation and transformation of synchronous input into this output is executed through polysynaptic interactions between hindbrain neurons.

The state transition means that certain change in the parameters of the input must alter the rules of its processing. Stimulus train applied to the MLR confers on the system the rhythm that might be close to the intrinsic rhythm of a portion of the neurons or neuronal circuits with the corresponding BD. Even if the neurons were silent this input is sufficient to change their average membrane potential slightly, and they will be recruited.

An ample number of medullary neurons discharging at 2 to 7 impulses per second may be

necessary to activate the spinal generation of locomotor movements (their characteristic cycle duration ranges between 1 to 5 s). The input neurons and some remote ones in the hindbrain produce impulses that are locked to stimuli when the near-threshold train is applied to MLR. This is a 'laboratory phenomenon' and does not develop under natural conditions of initiation of locomotion. Even when stimuli are applied to one site and all the directly excited neurons fire simultaneously, only a portion of the hindbrain neurons gives synaptic responses that are time-locked to stimuli.

Comparison with the cat

Subthreshold, repetitive stimuli delivered to two different 'locomotor sites' in the feline brain stem together can elicit locomotion, and they can do so whether applied in phase or out of phase (Selionov and Shik, 1991). This suggests that the time-locked responses can be at least partially replaced by responses of other types.

Near threshold (for locomotion) stimulation of MLR evokes EPSPs or short latency impulses only in a small portion of medullary neurons. Most of sensitive neurons give di- or polysynaptic responses both in turtle (Kazennikov et al., 1980) and in cat (Selionov and Shik, 1991), and portion of neurons generate impulses non-locked to stimuli. Frequency potentiation is a prominent feature of the responses of medullary neurons to near threshold stimuli applied to the MLR both in the cat and in the newt. The potentiation is expressed at lower frequency in some neurons than in others. Frequency potentiation enhances the efficiency of weak, distributed input (Selionov and Shik, 1992). Both non-locked reactions and locomotion arise only when the frequency of stimulation is sufficiently high.

Many reticulospinal neurons give off collaterals at the bulbar level both in mammals (Mitani et al., 1988) and in fishes (Metcalfe et al., 1986; Lee et al., 1993). Therefore, these neurons as well as the propriobulbar ones can contribute to interaction at the level of the hindbrain (Kimmel et al., 1985; McCarley et al., 1987). The diversity of the behaviors of hindbrain neurons during the transition between rest and locomotion may be related to the broad inventory of motor patterns that can arise during stimulation of MLR in urodele (Shik, 1997). There is a wide distribution of properties of individual hindbrain neurons (Rouse et al., 1998; Serafin et al., 1996). Various neurons receive non-identical inputs from different brain stem centers (Shik and Selionov, 1992). Many reticulospinal neurons exhibit stepping rhythm as soon as it arises (Orlovsky, 1970b).

Functional implications

Our data reveal the diversity of the behavior of hindbrain neurons during the transition from rest to locomotion. This diversity can depend on both the individual properties and the position of a neuron in the hindbrain network, in particular on its functional distance from MLR input.

There is a short pathway from MLR to the spinal cord via the reticulospinal neurons (Orlovsky, 1970a). But during the transition period, at least when the threshold train is applied, the processing of the MLR input occurs in the hindbrain. At ISI time scale, multiplication and synchronous translation is executed up to 3–4 relays. Then the wave-like propagation abruptly ceases or transforms into asynchronous activity provided that the train exceeded the threshold. Non-locked firing of these neurons must be transmitted to the spinal cord to elicit locomotion that is not complicated by spasticity.

During the transition epoch, the portion of neurons with composite and non-locked response increases in relation to those with time locked responses, and their firing rates increase. Both the changes in the manner of firing and shift of the latency of the response were observed. We shall report on these and related events in the next communication.

Excitation of a certain number of medial reticulospinal neurons is necessary to activate the spinal locomotor generator from MLR. But the hindbrain is not just a relay station: there is an essential interaction of its neurons, which results in recruiting the reticulospinal neurons appropriate for induction of locomotion rather then postural, scratching or other movements.

Summary

Trains of electrical stimuli were delivered to the mesencephalic 'locomotor region' in the rough skin newt. The current (3–12 mcA) and the inter-stimulus interval (100 to 200 ms) were adjusted so that locomotion arose in approximately 10 s, or so that the train remained subthreshold for initiation of locomotion. Impulses of single neurons in the hindbrain were recorded during the transition period from rest to locomotion. Time-locked synaptic responses were bi- or unimodal with typical latencies close to 18, 23 or 28 ms, and weak irregular mode near 13 ms.

Impulses that were not locked to the stimuli arose in some silent neurons, and the rate of firing of neurons with background discharge was sometimes enhanced. Composite responses consisted of both time-locked component and impulses distributed throughout the interstimulus interval. The data suggest that short-lived, wave-like propagation of the input volley ceases or is transformed into asynchronous activity after three or four translations. The latter variant could occur if the train reached the threshold for initiation of locomotion. The asynchronous activity persisted throughout interstimulus interval and could coexist with time-locked impulses.

Some neurons generated only a few impulses, while others remained active from beginning to end of the train. These active neurons could either spike at a steady rate, or decrement or augment their rate of firing during the train. The time course of their activity was related to the initial rate of firing. The augmenting type of firing in a subset of neurons may arise due to the interaction of neurons with unstable, steady state and decrementing activity.

Acknowledgments

We thank Prof. Y. Yarom for his help in the arrangement of the experimental set up and the data acquisition. This research was supported by the National Institute for Psychobiology in Israel.

294

List of abbreviations

BD	background discharge
CV	coefficient of variation
EPSP	excitatory postsynaptic potential
FR	firing ratio
I	interimpulse interval
ISI	interstimulus interval
L	latency
MLR	midbrain 'locomotor region'

References

Babalian, A.L. and Shapovalov, A.I. (1984) Synaptic actions produced by individual ventrolateral tract fibres in frog lumbar motoneurones. *Exp. Brain Res.*, 54: 551–563.

Bar-Gad, I., Kagan, I. and Shik, M. (1995) Responses of single neurons in the hindbrain of the newt to threshold repetitive stimulation of the mesencephalic 'locomotor region'. *Israel J. Med. Sci.*, 31: 762.

Green, C.S. and Soffe, S.R. (1996) Transitions between two different motor patterns in *Xenopus* embryos. *J. Comp. Physiol. A*, 178: 279–291.

Kazennikov, O.V., Selionov, V.A. and Shik, M.L., Yakovleva G.V. (1980) The rhombencephalic 'locomotor region' in turtle. *Neirofiziologia*, 12: 382–390.

Kimmel, C.B., Metcalfe, W.K. and Schabtach, E. (1985) T reticular interneurons: a class of serially repeating cells in the zebrafish hindbrain. *J. Comp. Neurol.*, 233: 365–376.

Lee, R.K.K., Eaton, R.C. and Zottoli, S.J. (1993) Segmental arrangement of reticulospinal neurons in the goldfish hindbrain. *J. Comp. Neurol.*, 329: 539–556.

Lowry, C.A., Rose, J.D. and Moore, F.L. (1996) Corticotropin-releasing factor enhances locomotion and medullary neuronal firing in an amphibian. *Horm. Behav.*, 30: 50–59.

McCarley, R.W., Ito, K. and Rodrigo-Angulo, M.L. (1987) Physiological studies of brain stem reticular connectivity. II. Responses of mPRF neurons to stimulation of mesencephalic and contralateral pontine reticular formation. *Brain Res.*, 409: 111–127.

McLean, H.A., Perry, S.F. and Remmers, J.E. (1995) Two regions in the isolated brainstem of the frog that modulate respiratory related activity. *J. Comp. Physiol. A*, 177: 135–144.

Matsushima, T., Satou, M. and Ueda, K. (1989) Medullary reticular neurons in the Japanese toad: morphologies and excitatory inputs from the optic tectum. *J. Comp. Physiol. A*, 166: 7–22.

Metcalfe, W.K., Mendelson, B. and Kimmel, C.B. (1986) Segmental homologies among reticulospinal neurons in the hindbrain of the zebrafish larva. *J. Comp. Neurol.*, 251: 147–159.

Mitani, A., Ito, K., Mitani, Y. and McCarley, R.W. (1988) Descending projections from the gigantocellular tegmental field in the cat: cells of origin and their brainstem and spinal cord trajectories. *J. Comp. Neurol.*, 268: 546–566.

Orlovsky, G.N. (1970a) Connections of the reticulospinal neurons with the 'locomotor regions' of the brain stem. *Biofizika*, 15: 171–177.

Orlovsky, G.N. (1970b) Work of the reticulospinal neurons during locomotion. *Biofizika*, 15: 728–735.

Rouse, D.T., Quan, X. and McClellan, A.D. (1998) Biophysical properties of descending brain neurons in larval lamprey. *Brain Res.*, 779: 301–308.

Selionov, V.A. and Shik M.L. (1991) Convergence of influences from locomotor points of the midbrain and medulla and from an inhibitory pontine point onto medullary neurons. *Neirofiziologia*, 23: 297–306.

Selionov, V.A. and Shik M.L. (1992) Responses of medullary and spinal neurons to simultaneous stimulation of two locomotor points. *Neirofiziologia*, 24: 471–481.

Serafin, M., Vidal, P.-P. and Muhlethaler M. (1996) Electrophysiological study of nucleus gigantocellularis neurons in Guinea-pig brainstem slices. *Neuroscience*, 73: 797–805.

Shik, M.L. (1997) Locomotor patterns elicited by electrical stimulation of the brain stem in the mudpuppy. *Motor Control*, 1: 354–368.

Shik, M.L. and Selionov, V.A. (1992) Different populations of medullary neurons contributing to the control of locomotion. In: L. Jami, E. Pierrot-Deseilligny and D. Zytnicki (Eds), *Muscle afferents and Spinal Control of Movement*, Pergamon, Oxford, pp. 447–451.

Shik, M.L., Severin, F.V. and Orlovsky, G.N. (1966) Control of walking and running by electrical stimulation of the midbrain. *Biofizika*, 11: 659–666.

Wu, G.-Y. and Wang, S.-R. (1995) Excitatory and inhibitory transmission from the optic tectum to nucleus isthmi and its vicinity in amphibians. *Brain Behav. Evol.*, 46: 43–49.

SECTION VII

Spinal interneurons and pattern generation

M.D. Binder (Ed.)
Progress in Brain Research, Vol 123
© 1999 Elsevier Science BV. All rights reserved.

CHAPTER 26

On the cellular bases of vertebrate locomotion

Sten Grillner* and Peter Wallén

Nobel Institute for Neurophysiology, Department of Neuroscience, Karolinska Institutet, SE–171 77, Stockholm, Sweden

Introduction

In this chapter we review some of the main developments since the beginning of the 70s in our understanding of the neural control of vertebrate locomotion, with particular emphasis on the cellular bases of the control mechanisms as studied in the lamprey model system.

The ability of the spinal cord circuitry to generate a detailed locomotor pattern is being addressed, as is the significant influence from sensory, movement-related feedback on the final motor output. The neuronal mechanisms underlying these general characteristics of locomotor control is then further discussed for the lamprey, in which isolated brainstem-spinal cord preparations have been utilized for detailed cellular analyses.

Mathematical modeling and computer simulations have been used extensively in this analysis, which has not only confirmed that the proposed network can account for the different experimental findings but has also been instrumental in gaining insight into the functional significance of several cellular properties. Using a neuro-mechanical model of the body of the lamprey, and also a hydro-mechanical model of the surrounding water, it has furthermore been possible to simulate the actual locomotor movements, including steering movements to the left or right and also in 3-D.

The control of body orientation has been extensively studied in the lamprey preparation, detailing the role of vestibular and visual sensory input, and a conceptual model for the control strategy used to maintain the normal, dorsal side up position has been proposed. As a further step in the analysis of vertebrate locomotor behavior, investigations of the mechanisms underlying goal-directed locomotion have been initiated. Thus, an in vitro preparation has been developed in which "fictive turning" behavior can be elicited. Along the same lines, the mechanisms underlying the initiation of goal-directed locomotion by visual and olfactory stimuli are being investigated. Also in this context, the role of the forebrain with the striatum-basal ganglia is being studied, thereby initiating investigations of a higher level control of locomotor behavior in the lamprey model.

Nostalgia

I (SG) met Douglas Stuart for the first time at the IUPS Conference of Physiology in Munich in 1971. It was an intense first encounter in a German pub, Douglas was filled with enthusiasm and information about the extraordinary locomotor ability of the wild Arizona cats and about how their muscle receptors were activated during ordinary movements. I on my part was on my way back from a period working together with Mark Shik and Grigori Orlovsky in Moscow and had a lot to tell about the neural control of locomotion in the decerebrate cat. This experimental model had been developed in Russia and it was just being acknowledged in the West – the papers were only available in English translation from Russian. During the next few years a number of papers were to appear

*Corresponding author. Tel.: (46) 8 728 69 00; Fax: (46) 8 34 95 44; e-mail: sten.grillner@neuro.ki.se

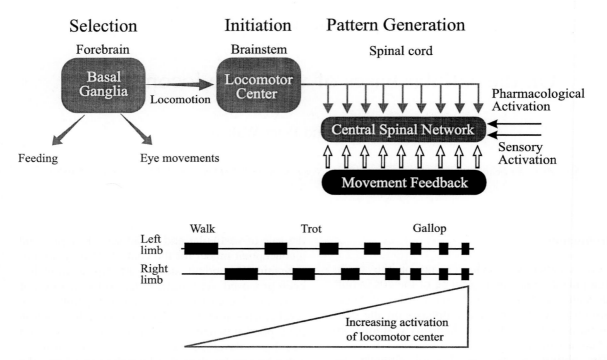

Fig. 1. General control strategy for vertebrate locomotion. Locomotion is initiated by an increased activity in reticulospinal neurons of the brainstem locomotor center, which activates the central spinal network, which in turn produces the locomotor pattern in close interaction with sensory feedback. With increased activation of the locomotor center the speed of locomotion will also increase. In quadrupeds this also leads to a shift in interlimb coordination, from walk to trot and then to gallop. The basal ganglia exert a tonic inhibitory influence on different motor centers. Once a pattern of motor behavior is selected the inhibition is released, allowing in this case the locomotor center in the brainstem to be activated. Experimentally, locomotion can also be elicited pharmacologically by administration of excitatory amino acid agonists and by sensory input.

in international journals by Orlovsky, Arshavsky and colleagues. Since then we have interacted in many different ways over the years although we have never collaborated scientifically. We co-organized three different symposia on locomotion in 1975, 1985 and 1995 together with Paul Stein and in different combinations with Richard Herman and Al Selverston. We will soon start to plan the 2005 meeting. In this chapter we will discuss a few pertinent topics within the area of locomotor control that has been of interest to me and I believe also to Doug.

The 70s – the basic organization of the neural locomotor system

During the 70s the focus was on the cat locomotor system. Goslow et al. (1973) described the locomotor movements in the full natural range from slow

walk to trot and fast gallop. This was important since it showed that during slow walk there was ample time for a sensory control of the different phases of the step cycle. On the other hand during the fastest gallop there was not sufficient time to exert an effective feedback within the different sub-phases of the support phase and the fast compensation to perturbations had to rely on muscle properties (Grillner 1972). Goslow et al.'s (1973) study was crucial, since it provided information about the limits of the neuro-mechanical system. By using the decerebrate preparation that can be made to locomote by stimulation of the brainstem locomotor areas (cf. Fig. 1), Shik et al. (1966) and Orlovsky (1970, 1972 a, b) showed that the different descending pathways from the brain-stem (vestibulo-, rubro- and reticulospinal) were phasically active. This activity was driven from cerebellar purkinje cells that in turn were modulated by different spinocerebellar pathways providing sensory information from the moving limb as well as efference copy information from different components of the locomotor networks in the spinal cord (Arshavsky et al., 1972).

The decerebrate preparation also allowed investigators to make acute lesions and study the effect on the locomotor control directly after the intervention. It was thus shown that the pattern of muscle activity in the hind limbs could remain unchanged, although more susceptible to perturbations, after transection of all sensory afferents from the limb (Grillner and Zangger, 1975, 1984; Grillner, 1979). The long standing question of whether the spinal cord, without descending brainstem control, could coordinate not only alternating limb movements (Brown, 1911; Sherrington, 1910; Lundberg, 1969) but also a detailed motor pattern to the different limb muscles was addressed (Grillner and Zangger, 1975). Indeed spinal cats could walk on the treadmill and adapt to the belt speed and change from the alternating gait of walk and trot to the in-phase pattern of gallop (Grillner, 1973; Forssberg et al., 1980). The adaptation to the speed of the treadmill belt requires a sensory control of the spinal circuits coordinating locomotion (cf. Fig. 1). It turned out that afferents influenced by hip position could affect the duration of the support phase and also influence the initiation of the swing phase when the limb was extended (Grillner and Rossignol, 1978). Similarly it was shown that afferents influenced by the load on the muscles activated during the support phase could play a prominent role in determining when the swing phase can be initiated (Duysens and Pearson, 1980).

Since the 1970s we have thus had a good grasp of the basic features of the neural control system underlying mammalian locomotion. Since then a number of important studies have been performed on the sensory control of the limb in a number of laboratories including those of Pearson, McCrea, Rossignol, Edgerton and Hultborn, which we are not going to summarize here. Others, like Jordan and colleagues and Mori, have focused on the brainstem organization for initiation of locomotion. With regard to our own work we try to understand

the cellular bases of the pattern generating network underlying locomotion. We were soon frustrated over this formidable task which required that we should be able to define which interneurons are part of the network, and how they connect to each other by inhibitory and excitatory synapses and function together (Edgerton et al., 1976).

Next step – vertebrate in vitro preparations

As the complexity of this control system is daunting, a number of investigators found that it was important to look for alternative experimental models, if one were to achieve the goal of understanding the cellular mechanisms of the neuronal networks responsible for this motor behaviour. As much information gathered demonstrating that the basic organization of the locomotor control system was designed in a similar way in all vertebrates, a solution to the experimental problem was to find a simpler animal model with fewer neurons and which was more amenable to experimentation. Despite the attractiveness of many invertebrate systems, a vertebrate model was obviously required with the same basic neural organization as in mammals. Alan Roberts and his colleagues opted for the frog embryo stage 36/37, Paul Stein for the turtle spinal cord and somewhat later a neonatal rat spinal cord preparation was developed in the laboratories of Kudo, Garcia-Rill and Feldman. We on our side chose the lamprey nervous system, which holds a strategic place in the evolution of vertebrates. Cyclostomes evolved before fishes around 450 million years ago and have remained comparatively unchanged since then. Moreover the isolated lamprey brainstem – spinal cord can be maintained in vitro over several days (Fig. 2A; Rovainen, 1974), which facilitates the analyses of circuitry, membrane properties, receptors and alike which is information required to comprehend a network. The other important factor is that the locomotor circuitry could be activated in this isolated nervous system, which is another precondition for a meaningful analysis of a given network (see Grillner et al., 1998).

The lamprey model

By stimulation in the locomotor areas of the lamprey brainstem, locomotor like activity could be

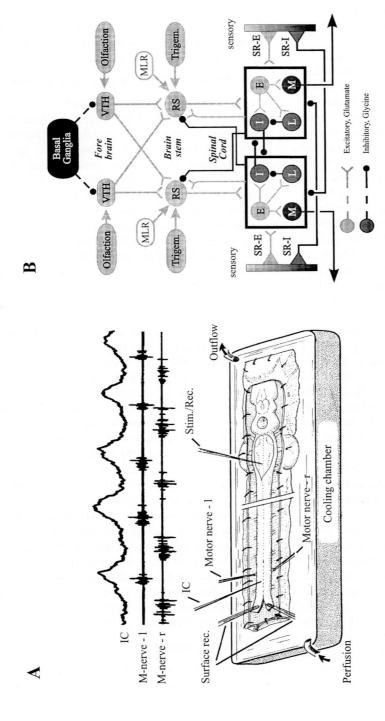

Fig. 2. A: In vitro preparation of the lamprey CNS. The isolated brainstem-spinal cord of the lamprey can be maintained alive for several days in an experimental chamber that is kept cold (4–7 °C) and continuously perfused with physiological solution. The motor pattern underlying locomotion can be produced by stimulating the brainstem locomotor centers or by adding glutamate receptor agonists to the perfusion medium. The motor activity can be recorded in the ventral roots (motor nerves) that normally activate the musculature on the left (l) and right (r) sides. The activity in single or pairs of cells can be recorded intracellularly with microelectrodes (IC). An intracellular record (IC) of a network neuron with subthreshold membrane potential oscillations is shown above together with the alternating motor activity in the ventral roots on the left and right sides. B: Locomotor network of the lamprey. Schematic representation of the forebrain, brainstem and spinal components of the neural circuitry that generates rhythmic locomotor activity. All neuron symbols denote populations rather than single cells. The reticulospinal (RS), glutamatergic neurons excite all classes of spinal interneurons and motoneurons. The excitatory interneurons (E) excite all types of spinal neurons on the ipsilateral side, i.e. the inhibitory glycinergic interneurons (I) that cross the midline to inhibit all neuron types on the contralateral side, the lateral interneurons (L) that inhibit I interneurons, and motoneurons (M). The stretch receptor neurons are of two types; one excitatory (SR-E) which excites ipsilateral neurons and one inhibitory (SR-I) which crosses the midline to inhibit contralateral neurons. RS neurons receive excitatory synaptic input from cutaneous afferents (Trigem.), the mesencephalic locomotor region (MLR) and from the ventral thalamus (VTH), which in turn receives input from the basal ganglia.

elicited in the spinal cord (McClellan and Grillner, 1984). The alternating segmental burst activity is coordinated along the spinal cord, generally with a rostro-caudal phase lag, which corresponds to the coordination in the swimming lamprey in which an undulatory wave pushes the animal forward through the water (cf. Grillner, 1974; Wallén and Williams, 1984). Also in the isolated spinal cord locomotor coordination can be elicited by elevating the excitability of the spinal cord by administering excitatory amino acid receptor agonists like NMDA, kainate, AMPA, and D-glutamate to the bath (Fig. 2A; Cohen and Wallén, 1980; Grillner et al., 1981b; Brodin et al., 1985; cf. Poon, 1980). Pharmacological analyses indicated that the network essentially depends on excitatory glutamatergic, and inhibitory glycinergic synaptic transmission (Grillner and Wallén, 1980; Brodin and Grillner, 1985). In addition a number of modulatory transmitters modify neuronal and thereby network activity, which will be dealt with separately below.

Brainstem–spinal cord circuitry. The spinal cord networks are thus responsible for the motor pattern produced. They are activated from the brainstem via reticulospinal axons (Fig. 2B) that excite spinal excitatory and inhibitory interneurons and motoneurons via both NMDA and AMPA/kainate receptors. The reticulospinal system thus drives the spinal cord networks and determines the level of activity in a burst range from 0.2 to 10 Hz. The excitatory spinal interneurons have ipsilateral axons and excite motoneurons, inhibitory interneurons with ipsilateral and contralateral axons. In a simplified manner, the ipsilateral excitatory interneurons excite all types of cells on the same side of the spinal cord, while the inhibitory cells provide inhibition of the neurons on the contralateral side (Fig. 2B; Buchanan and Grillner, 1987, 1988; Buchanan, 1982; Parker and Grillner, 1998, 1999 and unpublished). The network produces one half cycle of excitation in motorneurons and interneurons of one side followed by one half cycle of inhibition when the contralateral side is active (Russell and Wallén, 1983). Using biophysically realistic modeling it has been shown that pools of model interneurons, with similar proper-

ties to those found experimentally, can produce the alternating motor pattern (see below; Hellgren et al., 1992).

Importance of cellular properties for the pattern generation. Not only the connectivity but also the membrane properties of different cell types are of critical importance. Calcium currents as well as the activation of calcium dependent potassium channels (K_{Ca}) have a key role. The post-spike afterhyperpolarization is the main determinant of the frequency regulation including frequency adaptation in all network neurons (Fig. 3A; El Manira et al., 1994). During network activity the short range spike frequency adaptation is one important factor. In most cases only a few spikes are generated within each burst. K_{Ca} currents are also important in relation to other processes that cause increased Ca^{2+} levels in the dendrites or cell body. These include the activation of NMDA receptors which give rise to plateau-like depolarizations (Fig. 3C; Wallén and Grillner, 1987). The termination of these plateaus are caused by the activation of K_{Ca} currents (Fig. 3B, C), and presumably also by an activation of low voltage activated Ca^{2+} currents (Matsushima et al., 1993). These lamprey neurons express Ca^{2+} channels of the N subtype, which mainly are responsible for the activation of K_{Ca} channels of the afterhyperpolarization and for the synaptic transmission (El Manira and Bussières, 1997; Wikström and El Manira, 1998; El Manira et al., 1994). L-channels are less abundant and contribute, however, to the NMDA induced plateau depolarizations.

Sensory control of the spinal locomotor network. The isolated spinal cord can thus produce a reasonably well co-ordinated motor pattern without any movement related feedback. During normal swimming, the laterally directed undulatory movements will activate stretch receptors on one side and unload the corresponding receptors on the contralateral side at a given moment in time. The activation of the stretch receptors influences the spinal network and can, depending on peripheral events, change the timing and the duration of the locomotor bursts.

The stretch receptors are located in the very lateral part of the flattened spinal cord and will be

302

stretched or unloaded with the corresponding body segments (Grillner et al., 1984). They are of two types, one with an ipsilateral axon that is excitatory and activates the spinal pattern network on the same side while the other type has a crossed axon and inhibits the neurons on the opposite side (Viana di Prisco et al., 1990). These neurons provide a sensory overlay on the central spinal network (Fig. 2B). In the normally moving lamprey they are always activated as an integral part of the control system. An illustration of the strength of the sensory feedback system is the following experiment (Fig. 4). If the dissected spinal cord is left on the notochord with surrounding connective tissue, the spinal cord can be activated to produce the locomotor pattern with NMDA. If part of the spinal cord/notochord is fixed to the bottom of a Sylgard chamber, while the other free part is moved back and forth simulating locomotor movements, the burst activity will become entrained by the imposed movement. If it has a faster frequency than the resting burst rate (without movement) the motor activity will become entrained within a certain range. Similarly if the frequency of the imposed movement is lower than the rest rate, it will also become entrained. The phase relation between

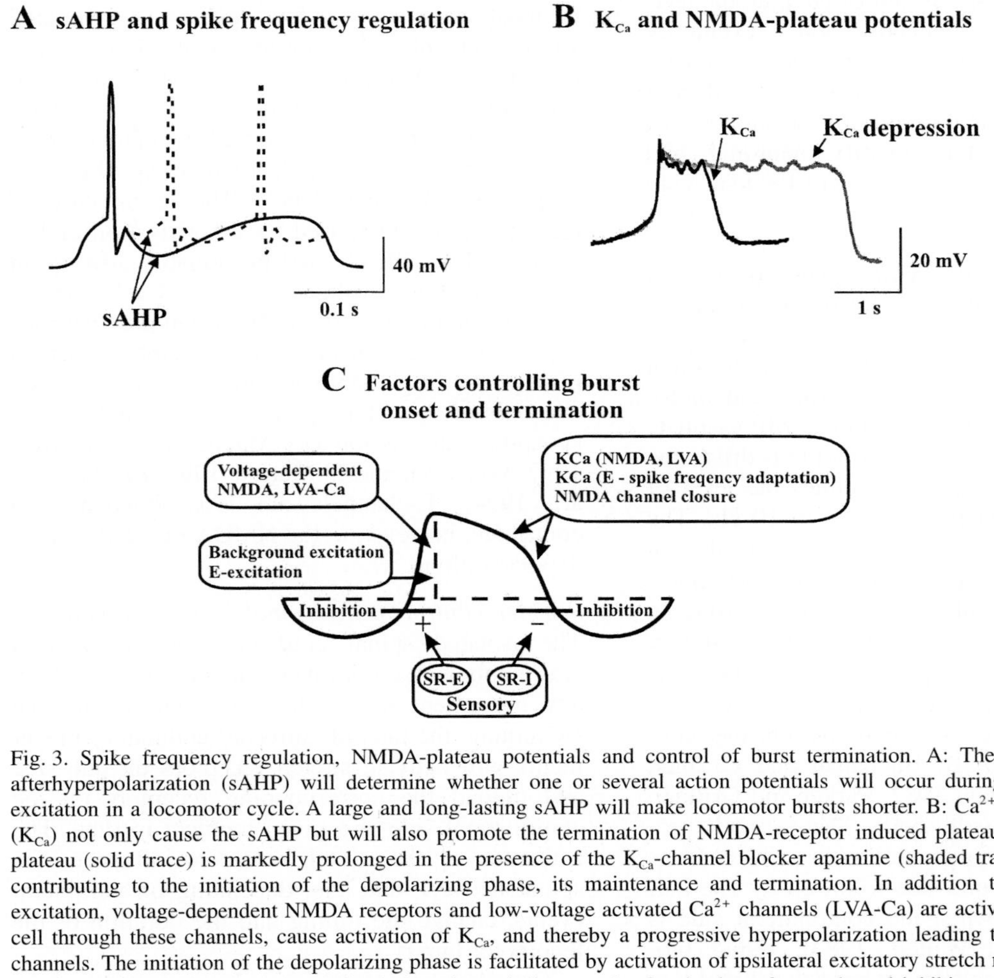

A sAHP and spike frequency regulation

B K_{Ca} and NMDA-plateau potentials

C Factors controlling burst onset and termination

Fig. 3. Spike frequency regulation, NMDA-plateau potentials and control of burst termination. A: The amplitude of the slow afterhyperpolarization (sAHP) will determine whether one or several action potentials will occur during the phase of synaptic excitation in a locomotor cycle. A large and long-lasting sAHP will make locomotor bursts shorter. B: Ca^{2+}-dependent K^+ channels (K_{Ca}) not only cause the sAHP but will also promote the termination of NMDA-receptor induced plateau potentials. The control plateau (solid trace) is markedly prolonged in the presence of the K_{Ca}-channel blocker apamine (shaded trace). C: Different factors contributing to the initiation of the depolarizing phase, its maintenance and termination. In addition to conventional synaptic excitation, voltage-dependent NMDA receptors and low-voltage activated Ca^{2+} channels (LVA-Ca) are activated. Ca^{2+} will enter the cell through these channels, cause activation of K_{Ca}, and thereby a progressive hyperpolarization leading to closure of the NMDA channels. The initiation of the depolarizing phase is facilitated by activation of ipsilateral excitatory stretch receptor neurons (SR-E), while the termination of the depolarized phase is partially a result of activation of contralateral inhibitory stretch receptor neurons (SR-I).

imposed movement and locomotor burst is such that the lower the burst rate, the earlier in the movement cycle the burst will occur (Grillner et al., 1981a; McClellan and Sigvardt, 1988).

Modeling on the cellular, network and behavior levels. In order to evaluate the experimental data which indeed is very extensive, it was important to utilize mathematical modeling on a cellular and network level, as an interactive analysis tool. So many interactive processes operate in parallel, at the cell and network level, that it is virtually impossible to intuitively deduce the net outcome. We therefore modelled each type of neuron (Fig. 5A) with voltage dependent Na^+, K^+ and Ca^{2+} currents of different subtypes, using Hodgkin–Huxley formalism (Ekeberg et al., 1991, Tegnér et al., 1997). Moreover, K_{Ca} channels activated by the Ca^{2+} entry during the action potential are responsible for the post-spike afterhyperpolarization. The latter is a major determinant of frequency regulation in these cells. Each type of neuron was assigned its specific characteristics with for instance the appropriate input resistance within a

certain range. It had five different compartments, axon hillock, soma and three dendritic compartments, each of which could be given different properties. These model neurons behaved on simulated current injections as their biological counterparts; they were subsequently equipped with conductance increase EPSPs and IPSPs (Cl^- equilibrium potential). In addition voltage dependent NMDA channels were simulated (Ekeberg et al., 1991; Brodin et al., 1991; Tråvén et al., 1993). The inhibitory synapses were placed closer to the soma and the excitatory ones more distally as indicated by the biology; subsequently the inhibitory and excitatory neurons of the network were connected in a similar way to that established experimentally. Simulation of segmental networks driven from the brainstem could produce alternating burst activity in populations of model neurons of each cell type as referred to above (Fig. 5B).

The burst rate produced by the segmental network could cover the normal biological frequency range. The properties of the NMDA channels were of particular importance for maintaining regular burst activity in a lower frequency

Sensory entrainment of CPG

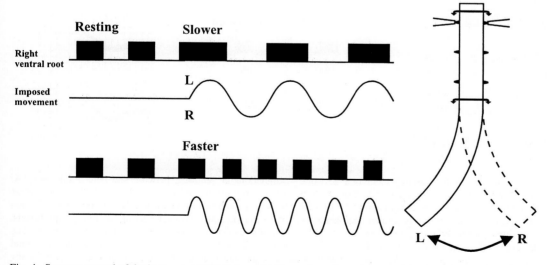

Fig. 4. Sensory control of the locomotor CPG. Schematic illustration of entrainment of the central pattern-generating network evoked by imposed lateral movements of the isolated spinal cord preparation, mimicking swimming movements. Imposed movement to the left (L) and right (R) sides is depicted by the trace below the burst activity pattern in a ventral root on the right side. The centrally generated rhythm can be entrained to follow burst rates above as well as below the resting burst rate.

304

range; including low voltage activated Ca^{2+} channels in the network model could also promote a more distinct burst pattern (Wallén et al., 1992; Hellgren et al., 1992; Tråvén et al., 1993; Tegnér et al., 1997). By simulating a number of segments along the spinal cord, an intersegmental lag from rostral to caudal could be produced (Fig. 5C; Wadden et al., 1997). The simulations show that with the available information on interneurons and their connectivity and membrane properties we can

largely account for the output of the locomotor network, at least to a first approximation.

Ekeberg et al. (1995) simulated the visco-elastic properties of the muscle segments along the spinal cord and constructed a mechanical model of the body controlled by a neuronal network similar to the one just described. By also including the viscous properties of water, the simulated lamprey could be made to swim through the simulated water with seemingly normal movements (Fig. 5D);

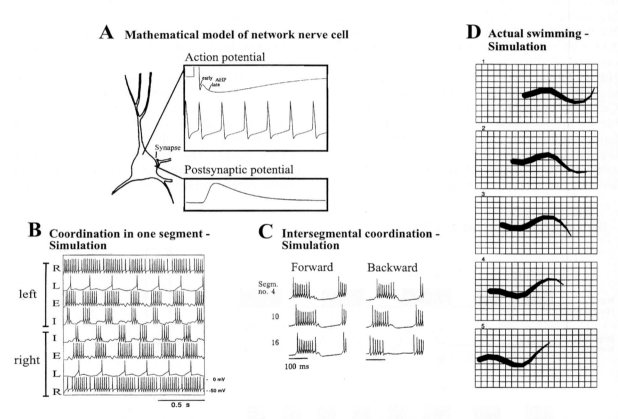

Fig. 5. Mathematical modelling of the lamprey locomotor network – simulations at neuronal, network and behavioral levels. A: Neurons of the network were simulated in a realistic fashion, with the different voltage-dependent (Na^+, K^+, Ca^{2+}), Ca^{2+}-dependent K^+ channels, and ligand-gated channels (AMPA/kainate, NMDA, glycine). Action potentials with early and late afterhyperpolarization (AHP), and spike frequency adaptation, can be simulated, together with postsynaptic potentials occurring in different compartments. B: Simulation of the segmental network using a pool of excitatory (E) and inhibitory (I) interneurons and lateral (L) interneurons. The activity is driven by excitatory reticulospinal neurons (R). Activity on the left and right sides alternates. C: Pattern of intersegmental coordination, produced by a simulated network of 60 segments. This circuitry will produce a rostro-caudal phase lag along the simulated spinal cord, and this lag can be reversed if the excitability is increased in the caudal end, which results in backward locomotion. D: Simulation of actual swimming movements using a neuro-mechanical model. Frames show steady-state swimming at 4 Hz, resulting from tonic excitation of the network, with the model lamprey moving forwards at a speed of 0.73 m/s. Time interval between frames is 50 ms. (modified from Grillner et al., 1995).

moreover, by increasing the activity of the reticulo-spinal drive signals unilaterally, the 'fictive animal' could be made to turn left or right.

A further elaboration of the model myotome into a ventral and a dorsal compartment, allowed a separate control of these two parts, and thereby swimming movements with a superimposed steering in 3-D (Ekeberg et al., 1995; see Grillner, 1996).

Control of body orientation

During locomotion through the water volume, fishes and lampreys must be able to continuously orient their body in relation to the gravity field and to external cues. The control of body orientation has been extensively studied in the lamprey (Orlovsky et al., 1992; Deliagina et al., 1992a, b). Figure 6 (1) depicts in a schematic form the principal control strategy; if the normal, dorsal side up orientation becomes disturbed, sensory input from the vestibular apparatus on either side excite contralateral groups of reticulospinal neurons, which in turn elicit a corrective motor response. For

instance, if the animal is tilted towards the right side, the right side vestibular afferents will excite the left side reticulospinal neurons, which will result in a motor response towards the left back to the upright position. In this way, the control system will assure that the body position will always be restored to an equilibrium point at 0 degrees tilt angle (i.e. dorsal side up; Fig. 6 (2)) Grillner et al., 1995).

Other external cues may, however, influence the equilibrium point and thereby the resulting body orientation. In the lamprey the 'dorsal light response' manifests itself in an inclination of the body with the dorsal, darker side tilted towards the light, which is presumed to have a survival value. This response has been analyzed using the control scheme for body orientation (Ullén et al., 1996; Grillner et al., 1995; Fig. 6 (3)). When light from one side hits, e.g. the right eye, excitation of the right side reticulospinal neurons will cause a motor response towards the right side, in the direction towards the light (Fig. 6 (1)). This extra excitation of the right side reticulospinal neurons will shift the

Control of body orientation

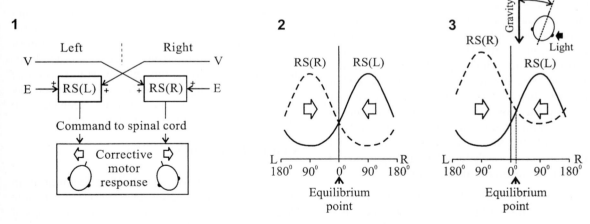

Fig. 6. Control of body orientation in lamprey – Conceptual model of the roll-control system. 1: Vestibular input (V) preferentially excites contralateral RS neurons, while input from the eyes (E) excites ipsilateral neurons. The two subdivisions (left and right) of the reticulospinal system produce reciprocal effects in the spinal cord, resulting in rotation (roll) of the animal in opposite directions. 2: Characteristics of the roll control system. The two subdivisions of the reticulospinal system, driven by vestibular inputs, are activated upon opposite roll tilts. Rotatory effects are elicited in opposite directions (arrows). The two curves intersect at the equilibrium point (here at 0°, dorsal side up position) of the roll-control system. 3: Influence of visual input–Dorsal light response. When light hits the right eye, the right side of the reticulospinal system is further excited, resulting in a shift of the corresponding curve. This, in turn, results in a shift of the equilibrium point to the right, i.e. towards the light source (modified from Grillner et al., 1995).

corresponding response curve upwards (Fig. 6 (3)), which in turn will cause a shift of the equilibrium point towards the light source. To summarize, this control scheme for body orientation in the lamprey can account for the observed behavior of the swimming animal, also after unilateral labyrinthectomy and/or removal of visual input on one side (Deliagina, 1997).

Goal-directed locomotion

The above has dealt with neural control of the basic propulsive synergy and of the body orientation during locomotion, mainly in lamprey. A natural next step in the analysis is to understand the processes that are used to decide when and where to locomote, and how to avoid obstacles on the way. We obviously know much less about these issues, but both in the lamprey and in mammals these mechanisms start to become unraveled.

Fictive steering in the lamprey. If the skin of the head or the trigeminal nerve is stimulated in the intact lamprey during locomotion, it will make a turning movement and swim away from the side of the stimulation (McClellan, 1984; Ullén et al., 1998). Similarly, a trigeminal stimulation in the isolated brainstem–spinal cord preparation during rhythmic locomotor activity will induce a turning motor pattern recorded as ventral root activity along the spinal cord (Ullén et al., 1998 and unpublished). The reticulospinal neurons in the middle rhombencephalic nuclei, and to a somewhat lesser extent the posterior nuclei, become further activated on the side towards which the animal is 'turning' as compared to the contralateral side. The possible contribution of the large propriospinal lateral interneurons with fast descending axons is particularly interesting in this context.

Olfactory and visual stimuli elicit locomotor activity. Olfactory stimuli, like substances present in fish skin, are very effective in inducing locomotor activity in the intact lamprey (Kleerekoper, 1963); similarly strong light makes the lamprey swim in a direction away from the stimulus. Both collaterals of the optic tract and mitral cells from the olfactory bulb project to the ventral thalamus (Fig. 7; Thompson et al., 1998), a nucleus that contains

descending glutamatergic fibers projecting to reticulospinal cells in the caudal brainstem (El Manira et al., 1997). Stimulation of the ventral thalamus elicits locomotor activity in the spinal cord. It therefore seems likely that behaviorally relevant locomotion can be elicited via an oligosynaptic linkage from the receptors via the forebrain and brainstem to the spinal cord (Fig. 7), although contributions via more complex pathways may also be important.

We know rather little about the overall function of the forebrain in the lamprey. One system that is important in this context is striatum and associated structures (Fig. 7). The lamprey striatum has the same neuronal components with spiny GABAergic neurons, and an extensive dopamine input from the corresponding areas as in mammals (Pombal et al., 1997a, b). The different types of inputs present are, with regard to immunohistochemical markers also very similar, indicating that the overall neural organization of the striatum is phylogenetically ancient. GABAergic striatal neurons in turn project to an area in the ventrolateral pallium, which contains GABAergic neurons, which in turn project to the ventral thalamus. These GABAergic neurons are thought to correspond to the mammalian pallidum. If so, one may in analogy expect these neurons to have a high level of resting activity and to exert a tonic control over the ventral thalamus. They could then exert a gate control; inhibition of ventrolateral pallium from striatum would disinhibit the ventral thalamus, which would facilitate the induction of locomotion from different sensory stimuli. This could be an important mechanism to control locomotor behavior, if demonstrated!

Concluding remarks

The neural mechanisms controlling locomotion in vertebrates are now being revealed in considerable detail on the cellular level in in vitro preparations of lower vertebrates like the lamprey and the frog embryo. It is very likely that these findings are of general significance, and thus that similar, albeit more complex, principal cellular and network solutions are to be found in other vertebrates. This assumption rests upon the fact that the basic organization of the control system is similar among

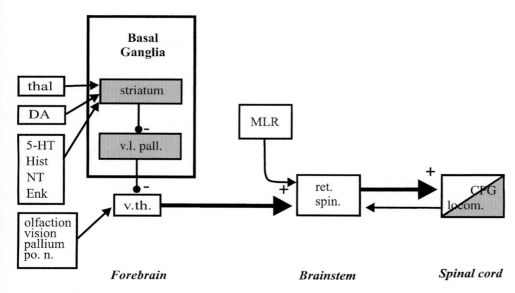

Forebrain   *Brainstem*   *Spinal cord*

Fig. 7. Forebrain and brainstem structures important for initiation of locomotion in lamprey. The striatum of the basal ganglia receives dopaminergic, serotonergic, histaminergic and peptidergic inputs, as well as input from thalamus and telencephalon. GABAergic striatal neurons project to ventrolateral pallium, which in turn sends GABAergic projections to ventral thalamus. This nucleus also receives olfactory and visual input, and projects to the brainstem where reticulospinal neurons are excited. In addition to this diencephalic locomotor control, the brainstem MLR area also may initiate locomotion by exciting reticulospinal neurons. The brainstem reticulospinal neurons will then in turn activate the spinal locomotor network.

all studied vertebrate species. The pioneering investigations made in the 70s, using primarily the cat preparation and where the work of Doug Stuart forms an essential part, constitutes the platform from which the characterization of the general organization of vertebrate locomotor control has originated.

References

Arshavsky, Yu. I., Berkinblit, M.B., Fukson, O.I., Gelfand, I.M. and Orlovsky, G.N. (1972) Origin of modulation in neurones of the ventral spinocerebellar tract during locomotion. *Brain Res.*, 43: 276–279.

Brodin, L., Grillner, S. and Rovainen, C.M. (1985) NMDA, kainate and quisqualate receptors and the generation of fictive locomotion in the lamprey spinal cord. *Brain Res.*, 325: 302–306.

Brodin, L. and Grillner, S. (1985) The role of putative excitatory amino acid neurotransmitters in the initiation of locomotion in the lamprey spinal cord. I. The effects of excitatory amino acid antagonists. *Brain Res.*, 360: 139–148.

Brodin L., Tråvén, H.G., Lansner, A., Wallén, P., Ekeberg, Ö. and Grillner, S. (1991) Computer simulations of *N*-methyl-D-Aspartate (NMDA) receptor induced membrane properties in a neuron model. *J. Neurophysiol.*, 66: 473–484.

Brown. T.G. (1911) The intrinsic factors in the act of progression in the mammal. *Proc. R. Soc. B.*, 84: 308–319.

Buchanan, J.T. (1982) identification of interneurons with contralateral, caudal axons in the lamprey spinal cord: synaptic interactions and morphology. *J. Neurophysiol.*, 47: 961–975.

Buchanan, J.T. and Grillner, S. (1987) Newly identified 'glutamate interneurons' and their role in locomotion in the lamprey spinal cord. *Science*, 236: 312–314.

Buchanan, J.T. and Grillner, S. (1988) A new class of small inhibitory interneurones in the lamprey spinal cord. *Brain Res.*, 438: 404–407.

Cohen, A.H. and Wallén, P. (1980) The neural correlate of locomotion in fish: 'fictive swimming' induced in an in vitro preparation of the lamprey spinal cord. *Exp. Brain Res.*, 41: 11–18.

Deliagina, T. (1997) Vestibular compensation in lampreys: impairment and recovery of equilibrium control during locomotion. *J. Exp. Biol.*, 200: 1459–1471.

Deliagina, T., Orlovsky, G., Grillner, S. and Wallén, P. (1992a) Vestibular control of swimming in lamprey: 2. Characteristics of spatial sensitivity of reticulospinal neurons. *Exp. Brain Res.*, 90: 489–498.

Deliagina, T., Orlovsky, G., Grillner, S. and Wallén, P. (1992b) Vestibular control of swimming in lamprey: 3. Activity of vestibular afferents. Convergence of vestibular inputs on reticulospinal neurons. *Exp. Brain Res.*, 90: 499–507.

308

Duysens J.D. and Pearson, K.G. (1980) Inhibition of flexor burst generation by loading ankle extensor muscles in walking cats. *Brain Res.*, 187: 321–332.

Edgerton, V.R. et al. (1976) Central generation of locomotion in vertebrates. In: R. Herman, S. Grillner, P. Stein and D. Stuart (Eds). *Neural Control of Locomotion.* Plenum Press, New York. pp. 181–201.

Ekeberg, Ö., Wallén, P., Lansner, A., Tråvén, H., Brodin, L. and Grillner, S. (1991) A computer based model for realistic simulations of neural networks. I. The single neuron and synaptic interaction. *Biol. Cybernet.*, 65: 81–90.

Ekeberg, Ö., Lansner, A. and Grillner, S. (1995) The neural control of fish swimming studied through numerical simulations, *Adapt. Behav.*, 3: 363–384.

El Manira, A. and Bussières N. (1997) Calcium channel subtypes in lamprey sensory and motor neurons. *J. Neurophysiol.*, 78: 1334–1340.

El Manira, A., Tegnér, J. and Grillner, S. (1994) Calcium-dependent potassium channels play a critical role for burst termination in the locomotor network in lamprey. *J. Neurophysiol.*, 72: 1852–1861.

El Manira, A., Pombal, M.A. and Grillner, S. (1997) Diencephalic projection to reticulospinal neurons involved in the initiation of locomotion in adult lampreys *Lampetra fluviatilis. J. Comp. Neurol.*, 389: 603–616.

Forssberg, H., Grillner, S., Halbertsma, J. and Rossignol, S. (1980) The locomotion of the low spinal cat. II. Interlimb coordination. *Acta Physiol. Scand.*, 108: 283–295).

Goslow, G.E. Jr, Reinking, R.M. and Stuart, D.G. (1973) The cat step cycle: hind limb joint angles and muscle lengths during unrestrained locomotion. *J. Morphol.* 141: 1–41.

Grillner, S. (1972) The role of muscle stiffness in meeting the changing postural and locomotor requirements for force development by the ankle extensors. *Acta Physiol. Scand.* 86: 92–108.

Grillner, S. (1973) Locomotion in the spinal cat. In: R.B. Stein, K.G. Pearson, R.S. Smith and J.B. Redford (Eds). *Control of posture and Locomotion*, Plenum Press, New York, pp. 515–535.

Grillner, S. (1974) On the generation of locomotion in the spinal dogfish. *Exp. Brain Res.* 20: 459–470.

Grillner, S. (1979) On the central generation of locomotion in the low spinal cat. *Exp. Brain Res.* 34: 241–261.

Grillner, S., Ekeberg, Ö., El Manira, A., Lansner, A., Parker, D., Tegnér, J. and Wallén, P. (1998) Intrinsic function of a neuronal network – a vertebrate central pattern generator. *Brain Res. Rev.*, 26: 184–197.

Grillner, S., Williams, T. and Lagerbäck, P.Å., (1984) The edgecell, a possible intraspinal mechanoreceptor. *Science*, 223: 500–503.

Grillner, S. (1996) Neural networks for vertebrate locomotion. *Scientific American.*, January. 64–69.

Grillner, S., McClellean, A. and Perret, C. (1981a) Entrainment of the spinal pattern generators for swimming by mechanosensitive elements in the lamprey spinal cord in vitro. *Brain Res.*, 217: 380–6.

Grillner, S., McClellan, A., Sigvardt, K., Wallén, P. and Wilén, M. (1981b) Activation of NMDA-receptors elicits 'fictive locomotion' in lamprey spinal cord in vitro. *Acta Physiol. Scand.*, 113: 549–551.

Grillner, S. and Rossignol, S. (1978) On the initiation of the swing phase of locomotion in chronic spinal cats. *Brain Res.*, 146: 269–277.

Grillner, S. and Zangger, P. (1975) How detailed is the central pattern generator for locomotion in the cat? *Brain Res.*, 88: 367–371.

Grillner, S. and Zangger, P. (1984) The effect of dorsal root transection on the efferent motor pattern in the cat's hindlimb during locomotion. *Acta Physiol. Scand.*, 120. 393–405.

Grillner, S. and Wallén, P. (1980) Does the central pattern generation for locomotion in the lamprey depend on glycine inhibition? *Acta Physiol. Scand.*, 110: 103–105.

Grillner, S., Deliagina, T., Ekeberg, Ö., El Manira, A., Hill, R.H., Lanser, A., Orlovsky, G.N. and Wallén, P. (1995) Neural networks that co-ordinate locomotion and body orientation in lamprey. *Trends Neurosc.*, 18: 270–279.

Hellgren, J., Grillner, S. and Lansner, A. (1992) Computer simulation of the segmental neural network generating locomotion in lamprey by using populations of network interneurons. *Biol. Cybern.*, 68: 1–13.

Kleerekoper, H. (1963) Role of olfaction in the orientation of *petromyzon marinus.* I. Response to a single amine in prey's body odor. *Physiol. Zool.*, 36: 347–360.

Matsushima, T. et al. (1993) GABA$_B$ receptor activation causes a depression of low- and high-voltage-activated Ca^{2+} currents, postinhibitory rebound, and postspike afterhyperpolarisation in lamprey neurons. *J. Neurophysiol.*, 70 (6): 2606–2619.

Lundberg, A. (1969) The excitatory control of the Ia inhibitory pathway. In: P. Andersen, J.K.S. Jansen, (Eds), *Excitatory Synaptic Mechanisms*, pp 333–340. Oslo: Universitetsforlaget.

McClellan, A. (1984) Descending control and sensory gating of 'fictive' swimming and turning responses elicited in an vitro preparation of the lamprey brainstem/spinal cord. *Brain Res.*, 302: 151–162.

McClellan, A. and Grillner, S. (1984) Activation of 'fictive' swimming by electrical microstimulation of 'locomotor command regions' in the brainstem of the lamprey. *Brain Res.*, 300: 357–361.

McClellan, A.D. and Sigvardt, K.A. (1988) Features of entrainment of spinal pattern generators for locomotor activity in the lamprey spinal cord. *J. Neurosci.*, 8: 133–145.

Orlovsky, G.N. (1970) Activity of reticulospinal neurones during locomotion. *Biophysics.*, 15: 761–771.

Orlovsky, G.N. (1972a) Activity of rubrospinal neurons during locomotion. *Brain Res.*, 46: 99–112.

Orlovsky, G.N. (1972b) Activity of vestibulospinal neurons during locomotion. *Brain Res.*, 46: 85–98.

Orlovsky. G., Deliagina, T. and Wallén, P. (1992) Vestibular control of swimming in lamprey: 1. Responses of reticulospinal neurons to roll and pitch. *Exp. Brain Res.*, 90: 479–488.

Parker, D. and Grillner, S. (1998) Cellular and synaptic modulation underlying substance P-mediated plasticity of the lamprey locomotor network. *J. Neurosci.*, 18(19): 8095–8110.

Parker, D. and Grillner, S. (1999) Activity-dependent metaplasticity of inhibitory and excitatory synaptic transmission in the lamprey spinal cord locomotor network. *J. Neurosci.*, 19(5): 1647–1656.

Pombal, M.A., El Manira, A. and Grillner, S. (1997a) Afferents of the lamprey striatum with special reference to the dopaminergic system: a combined tracing and immunohistochemical study. *J. Comp. Neurol.*, 386: 71–91.

Pombal, M.A., El Manira, A. and Grillner, S. (1997b) Organization of the lamprey striatum – transmitters and projections. *Brain Res.*, 766: 249–254.

Poon, M.L.T. (1980) Induction of swimming in lamprey by L-DOPA and amino acids. *J. Comp. Physiol.*, 136: 337–344.

Rovainen, C.M. (1974) Synaptic interactions of identified nerve cells in the spinal cord of the sea lamprey. *J. Comp. Neurol.*, 154: 189–206.

Russell, D.F. and Wallén, P. (1983) On the control of myotomal motoneurones during 'fictive swimming' in the lamprey spinal cord in vitro. *Acta Physiol Scand.*, 117: 161–170.

Sherrington. C.S. (1910) Flexion-reflex of the limb, crossed extension-reflex, and reflex stepping and standing. *J. Physiol.*, 40: 28–121.

Shik, M.L. et al. (1966) Control of walking and running by means of electrical stimulation of the mid-brain. *Biophysics*, 11: 756–765.

Tegnér, J., Hellgren-Kotaleski, J., Lansner, A. and Grillner, S. (1997) Low-voltage-activated calcium channels in the lamprey locomotor network: simulation and experiment. *J. Neurophysiol.*, 77: 1795–1812.

Thompson, R.H., Pombal, M.A., El Manira, A. and Grillner, S. (1998) Forebrain circuitry underlying goal-directed behavior in the lamprey. *Eur. Conf. Comp. Neurobiol. Abstr.*, 2.

Tråvén, H., Brodin, L., Lansner, A., Ekeberg, Ö., Wallén, P. and Grillner, S. (1993) Computer simulations of NMDA and non-NMDA mediated synaptic drive – sensory and supraspinal modulation of neurons and small networks. *J. Neurophysiol.* 70 (2): 695–709.

Ullén, F., Deliagina, T.G., Orlovsky, G.N. and Grillner, S. (1996) Visual potentiation of vestibular responses in lamprey reticulospinal neurons. *Eur. J. Neurosc.*, 8: 2298–2307.

Ullén, F., Fagerstedt, P., Ekeberg, Ö., Lansner, A., Orlovsky, G.N. and Grillner, S. (1998) Lateral turns in the lamprey. II. The brain stem descending command system – computer modeling and lesion studies. *Soc. Neurosci.*, Abstr. 1156.

Viana di Prisco, G., Wallén, P. and Grillner, S. (1990) Synaptic effects of intraspinal stretch receptor neurons mediating movement-related feedback during locomotion. *Brain Res.*, 530: 161–166.

Wadden, T., Hellgren, J., Lansner, A. and Grillner, S. (1997) Intersegmental coordination in the lamprey: simulations using a network model without segmental boundaries. *Biol. Cybern.*, 76: 1–9.

Wallén, P. and Grillner, S. (1987) N-Methyl-D-Aspartate receptor-induced, inherent oscillatory activity in neurons active during locomotion in the lamprey. *J. Neurosci.*, 7: 2745–2755.

Wallén, P. and Williams, T. (1984) Fictive lomotion in the lamprey spinal cord 'in vitro' compared with swimming in the intact and spinal animal. *J. Physiol.*, 347: 325–329.

Wallén, P., Ekeberg, Ö., Lansner, A., Brodin, L., Tråvén, H. and Grillner, S. (1992). A computer based model for realistic simulations of neural networks. II. The segmental network generating locomotor rhythmicity in the lamprey. *J. Neurophysiol.*, 68: 1939–1950.

Wikström, M.A. and El Manira, A. (1998) Calcium influx through N- and P/Q-type channels activate apamin-sensitive calcium-dependent potassium channels generating the late afterhyperpolarization in lamprey spinal neurons. *Eur. J. Neurosci.*, Vol 10, pp. 1528–1532.

M.D. Binder (Ed.)
Progress in Brain Research, Vol 123

CHAPTER 27

The roles of spinal interneurons and motoneurons in the lamprey locomotor network

James T. Buchanan*

Department of Biology, Marquette University, PO Box 1881, Milwaukee, WI 53201–1881, USA

Introduction

The nervous system of the lamprey, a primitive vertebrate fish, is a relatively simple and convenient adult preparation for investigating the neuronal basis for locomotor behavior. This chapter will provide a brief overview of some of the cellular mechanisms underlying fictive locomotion in the lamprey. Experiments aimed at assessing the minimal spinal substrate required for fictive swimming will be presented, including the number of segments required and whether commissural interneurons are necessary for rhythm generation. The morphology and activities of motoneurons and interneurons involved in fictive locomotion will be shown, and some information about how their electrophysiological properties change when the spinal cord goes from quiescence to an active state. Finally, the existence of feedback interactions from motoneurons to spinal neurons and the possible role for these interactions on network function will be discussed.

Fictive swimming

The isolated lamprey spinal cord generates rhythmic ventral root bursting upon bath application of an excitatory amino acid (Cohen and Wallén, 1980). The pattern of this rhythmic activity closely resembles electromyographic activity recorded in

*Corresponding author. Tel.: 414–288–1482; Fax: 414–288–7357; e-mail: james.buchanan@marquette.edu

the intact swimming lamprey and is therefore called fictive swimming (Wallén and Williams, 1984). As shown in Fig. 1A, extracellular recordings of ventral roots from preparations consisting typically of 8 to 12 spinal segments reveal rhythmic bursts of action potentials with stable cycle periods, generally in the range of 0.3 to 2 s, depending on the concentration of the excitatory amino acid (Brodin et al., 1985). Ventral roots on opposite sides of the spinal cord burst in alternation, and ventral roots on the same side exhibit a rostral-to-caudal propagation of bursting activity along the spinal cord (Fig. 1B). The latency between burst onsets is scaled to cycle period so that over a wide range of cycle periods, the delay of the bursts in more caudal ventral roots is a constant fraction of the cycle period, about 1% of a cycle period per segment (Matsushima and Grillner, 1992). Since there are about 120 segments in the lamprey spinal cord, the consequence of this phase lag constancy for the swimming lamprey is that about one swim cycle is maintained over the length of the lamprey body for a wide range of swimming frequencies (Wallén and Williams, 1984). At the level of network organization within the spinal cord, phase lag constancy means that the propagation velocity of burst activity increases with swim frequency, and therefore, axonal propagation velocity alone cannot account for the rostral-to-caudal phase relationships.

In addition to the isolated spinal cord preparation in which fictive swimming is induced by bath

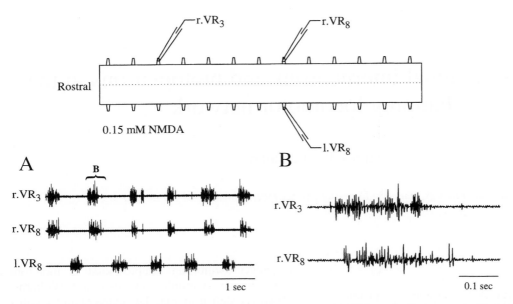

Fig. 1. Fictive swimming in the isolated lamprey spinal cord preparation. Schematic diagram at top illustrates a length of isolated spinal cord consisting of 12 segments and with three ventral root recordings (r.VR$_3$ = third ventral root from the rostral end on the right side). A: rhythmic bursting in the ventral roots elicited with bath-application of 0.15 mM N-methyl-D-aspartate (NMDA). B: an expanded portion of the recording as indicated in A to illustrate the delay of bursts in more caudal ventral roots.

application of an excitatory amino acid, fictive swimming can also be observed in the brainstem-spinal cord preparation without the addition of an excitatory amino acid. In this preparation, a brief electrical stimulus to the spinal cord or to a cranial nerve can elicit episodes of fictive swimming lasting several seconds (McClellan and Grillner, 1984).

Minimum substrate for rhythm generation

The locomotor network is distributed throughout the length of the spinal cord since spinal segments taken from any rostral-caudal level of the spinal cord will exhibit stable rhythmic activity in the presence of NMDA. It has been generally assumed that the locomotor network is segmentally organized such that each spinal segment contains a unit rhythm generator and that these segmental oscillators are coupled to produce the appropriate phase relationships for rostral-to-caudal propagation. While as few as four segments have been documented to exhibit fictive swimming (Cohen and Wallén, 1980), the relationship between the number

of segments and rhythmicity has not been demonstrated.

To address the question of the minimal substrate for rhythm generation, one can reduce the number of segments and assess the presence and quality of the remaining rhythmic activity. There is a clear deterioration in the quality of rhythmic activity as the number of segments is reduced (Fig. 2A$_1$). To quantify this deterioration, an autocorrelation was performed on the event times of the action potentials in the ventral root bursts. The amplitude of the second peak of the autocorrelation provides a measure of rhythm quality (Fig. 2A$_2$). A plot of this measure of rhythmic quality versus the number of segments demonstrates the progressive deterioration in the rhythm as the number of segments is reduced (Fig. 2B). Rhythm quality is not compromised until the number of segments falls below about eight. Alternating rhythmic activity persists in two-segment preparations, but when reduced to a single segment, the activity is either completely abolished or it becomes sporadic and non-rhythmic. Thus, it may be more accurate to describe it as a continuous neuronal network

313

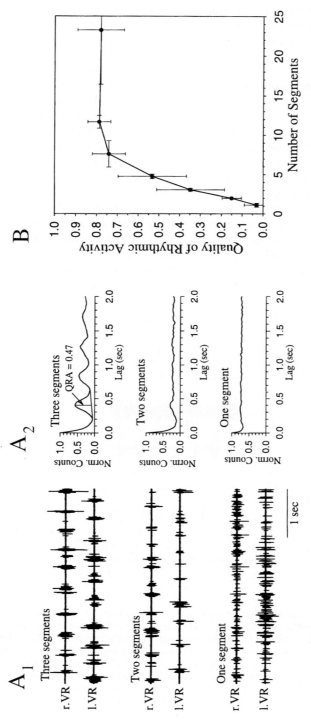

Fig. 2. Relationship of the number of spinal segments to the quality of rhythmic activity of fictive swimming. A_1: ventral root recordings on opposite sides of the spinal cord in a preparation that was progressively reduced from 3 segments to 1 segment. Rhythmic alternating bursting was apparent at lengths of 3 and 2 segments but not when the preparation was reduced to a single segment. A_2: autocorrelations of the event times of action potentials in the raw ventral root recordings of A_1. A measure of rhythm quality (Quality of Rhythmic Activity or QRA) is the amplitude of the second peak of the autocorrelation function as shown in the top autocorrelation. B: plot of the rhythm quality versus the number of segments in the spinal cord preparation. Each point is the average of four to eight experimental preparations.

distributed throughout the spinal cord which requires at least eight spinal segments for full rhythm regularity and a minimum of two segments for detectable, though highly degraded, rhythmic activity.

Necessity for commissural interneurons

As described above, the basic swim rhythm is an alternation between the two sides of the spinal cord, indicating a role for commissural interneurons in pattern formation. One can suggest two possible levels of involvement of commissural interneurons. In the first case, they would not be necessary for rhythm generation but would serve to coordinate an alternating phase relationship between autonomous oscillators located on the two sides of the spinal cord (Cohen and Harris-Warrick, 1984; Hagevik and McClellan, 1994). In the second case, the commissural interneurons would be necessary for

rhythm generation so that the rhythm-generating network would span the midline (Buchanan and McPherson, 1995). As a test of these two possibilities, one can make cuts along the midline of the isolated spinal cord (Fig. 3). If one end of the spinal cord is split partially so that a region of intact cord remains, then bath-application of N-methyl-D-aspartate (NMDA) results in rhythmic activity in both the intact region and in the split regions (Fig. 3A). The quality of the rhythmic activity in the split region is poorer than in the intact region, and there is a progressive fall in rhythm quality in ventral roots located at greater distances from the intact region. After isolating the split regions from the intact cord, the rhythmic activity of fictive swimming is always lost in the isolated hemicord (Fig. 3B). This result can be seen both in the raw ventral root recordings (compare Fig. 3A_2 and 3B_2) and in the autocorrelations done on the event times of the action potentials (compare Fig. 3A_3 and 3B_3).

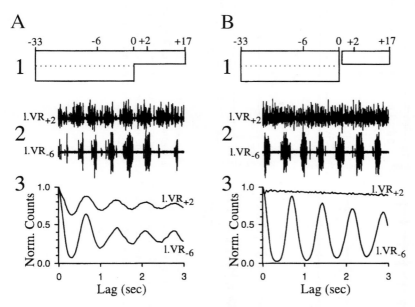

Fig. 3. The effect of removing commissural interneuron inputs on fictive swimming. A_1: in a 50-segment length of spinal cord, the midline was cut for 17 segments at the rostral end, and the right split region was removed. A_2: ventral root recordings were made from a segment in the split region (l.VR$_{+2}$, i.e. on the left side and two segments from the beginning of the midline cut in the split region) and from a segment in the intact region of spinal cord (l.VR$_{-6}$, i.e. left side and six segments from the beginning of the cut in the intact region). Rhythmic activity was still present in the split region. A_3: the rhythmic activity of the two ventral roots is shown in autocorrelations of the spike event times. B_1: the split region of cord was detached from the intact region by making a transverse cut. B_2: the ventral root recording in the isolated left hemicord was no longer rhythmic while the rhythmic activity of the intact cord improved. B_3: these changes in rhythmic activity after the cut were confirmed in the autocorrelations (figure adapted from Buchanan, 1999).

These experiments support the second hypothesis that the commissural interneuron outputs to the opposite side of the cord are necessary for rhythm generation (Buchanan, 1999). In the embryonic *Xenopus* tadpole, commissural interneurons are not necessary for rhythm generation (Kahn and Roberts, 1982; Soffe, 1989). The lamprey also has some capability for bursting in the absence of reciprocal inhibition. The output synapses of CC interneurons have been shown to be blocked by strychnine (Buchanan, 1982; McPherson et al., 1994), and in the presence of strychnine, rhythmic ventral root bursting can be observed (Cohen and Harris-Warrick, 1984; Alford and Williams, 1989).

Spinal neurons

Several classes of spinal nerve cells have been characterized in the lamprey spinal cord. Drawings of the cell classes that show the most membrane potential activity during fictive swimming are shown in Fig. 4A. These include motoneurons and three classes of interneurons: lateral interneurons, CC interneurons, and excitatory interneurons. The lateral interneurons (LIN) are large inhibitory cells located on the lateral edge of the column of cell bodies. They have ipsilateral, descending axons that extend up to 50 segments (Rovainen, 1974). The CC interneurons are commissural interneurons

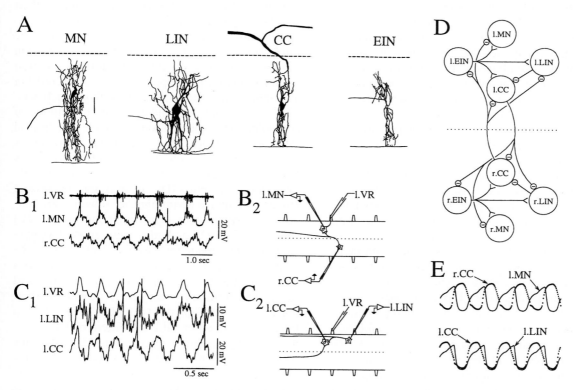

Fig. 4. Lamprey spinal neurons, their morphology, activity during swimming, and connectivity. A: representative drawings of four classes of lamprey spinal neurons. MN = motoneuron; LIN = lateral interneuron; CC = CC interneuron (commissural interneurons with caudally directed axon); EIN = excitatory interneuron. Calibration bar applies to all four cells = 100 μm. Dashed line = midline of spinal cord, and caudal is in the leftward direction. B$_1$: membrane potential activities of a motoneuron and a CC interneuron recorded during fictive swimming in a brainstem/spinal cord preparation. B$_2$: the relative positions of the cells of B$_1$. This CC interneuron inhibited the contralateral motoneuron. C$_1$: membrane potential activities of a lateral interneuron and a CC interneuron during fictive swimming in a brainstem/spinal cord preparation. C$_2$: the relative positions of the cells of C$_1$. The lateral interneuron inhibited the CC interneuron. D: summary of the synaptic interactions demonstrated between the four cell types shown in A. E: activities of cells in connectionist-style modeling of the network shown in D. The top trace shows a CC interneuron and motoneuron on opposite sides as in B$_1$. The bottom trace shows a CC interneuron and a lateral interneuron on the same side as in C$_1$.

with small- to medium-sized cell bodies, and they often have both caudally- and rostrally-directed axonal branches (Buchanan, 1982). The excitatory interneurons (EIN) have small cell bodies with ipsilateral axons (Buchanan et al., 1989).

Intracellular microelectrode recordings of these cells during fictive swimming have been carried out both in the isolated spinal cord (Buchanan and Cohen, 1982) and in brainstem-spinal cord preparations (Buchanan and Kasicki, 1995). The membrane potential activities are similar in the two types of preparations, which lends support to the conclusion that the isolated spinal cord preparation provides a reasonable representation of the neuronal correlate of swimming activity.

Examples of the membrane potential activities observed in spinal neurons during fictive swimming in the brainstem-spinal cord preparation are shown in Fig. 4B, C. Simultaneous recordings of a motoneuron and a CC interneuron located on opposite sides of the spinal cord and in adjacent segments is shown in Fig. 4B. During fictive swimming, the cells exhibited oscillating membrane potentials in which the depolarizations were generally in phase with the nearby ipsilateral ventral root bursts and the repolarizations occurred when the ipsilateral ventral roots were silent. Because the cells were located on opposite sides of the cord (Fig. 4B$_2$), the membrane potential oscillations of the motoneuron and the CC interneuron were active in antiphase (Fig. 4B$_1$). The CC interneuron made inhibitory synaptic contact with the contralateral motoneuron, which is one of the common synaptic output targets of CC interneurons (Fig. 4D) (Buchanan, 1982). Thus, when CC interneurons fire action potentials, the timing is such that the resulting inhibitory postsynaptic potentials (ipsps) contribute to the repolarizing phases of the motoneuron membrane potential oscillations. Simultaneous recordings of a lateral interneuron and a CC interneuron during fictive swimming in a brainstem-spinal cord preparation is shown in Fig. 4C. These two cells were located on the same side of the spinal cord less than one segment apart (Fig. 4C$_2$). Again, the cells exhibited oscillating membrane potentials, and their depolarizations were in phase with the ipsilateral ventral root bursts. However, close inspection of the records in Fig. 4C$_1$ reveals a slight

difference in the timings of the two cells, such that the CC interneuron is phase advanced compared to the lateral interneuron. This 10 to 15% phase advance of CC interneurons compared to other nearby cell types is a consistent finding in both the isolated spinal cord preparation (Buchanan and Cohen, 1982) and in the brainstem-spinal cord preparation (Buchanan and Kasicki, 1995). This may be explained by the synaptic inputs to CC interneurons as shown with paired intracellular recordings: lateral interneurons commonly make inhibitory synaptic contacts upon nearby, ipsilateral CC interneurons (Fig. 4D) (Buchanan, 1982). Thus, the lateral interneurons provide a feedforward inhibition of the CC interneurons, terminating their depolarizing phase earlier than other cell types.

A summary of the most common synaptic interactions among the cells of Fig. 4A is shown in Fig. 4D. The CC interneurons not only inhibit motoneurons on the opposite side of the cord but also inhibit the other cell types shown (Buchanan, 1982), and the CC interneuron inhibition of contralateral CC interneurons results in a reciprocal inhibitory network. The excitatory interneurons excite ipsilateral motoneurons and interneurons (Buchanan et al., 1989). The pattern of synaptic interactions of Fig. 4D can account for several features of fictive swimming as shown with connectionist-style computer modeling (Fig. 4E) (Buchanan, 1992) and also with more biophysically-detailed modeling (Wallén et al., 1992). The reciprocal inhibitory network between populations of CC interneurons on opposite sides of the cord forms the core of a rhythm generator with alternating activity between the two sides (Fig. 4E, top traces). The feedforward inhibition of CC interneurons by lateral interneurons allows this reciprocal inhibitory network to oscillate by providing a mechanism for burst termination of the CC interneurons. Thus, when the lateral interneurons begin to fire action potentials during ipsilateral activity, they inhibit the CC interneurons, which removes their inhibition of cells on the opposite side and allowing them to become active. This early inhibition of the CC interneurons also produces a slight phase advance in the CC interneurons compared to other nearby, ipsilateral neurons as observed in the modeling (Fig. 4E, bottom traces) and experimentally (Fig. 4C). While the connectionist-style modeling of Fig. 4E requires lateral interneurons for rhythmic activity, other mechanisms can be invoked in more biophysically-detailed modeling, such as accumulation of calcium-activated potassium currents in the CC interneurons (El Manira et al., 1994).

Not only can the network of Fig. 4D account for alternating rhythmic activity and the phase advance of CC interneurons, it can also account for phase coupling. As shown by Williams (1992), the network of Fig. 4D can be coupled by the spread of synaptic connections from the network neurons to adjacent networks. With adjustment of synaptic weights, a chain of these networks can be made to show phase lag constancy over a range of oscillation frequencies (Williams, 1992).

Changes in electrophysiological properties during fictive swimming

As in other systems, the cellular electrophysiological properties of lamprey spinal neurons play an important role in the generation of the swim rhythm and in its modulation. While a characterization of the electrophysiological properties of lamprey spinal neurons has been done in the quiescent, non-swimming state (Buchanan, 1993), there has not been a systematic examination of how these properties change as the neurons go from a quiescent state into swimming activity. There is evidence in other vertebrate preparations that neuronal properties do change dramatically during fictive locomotion (Brownstone et al., 1992). Thus, a more complete understanding of the cellular and synaptic basis of rhythm generation in the lamprey will require a characterization of how the electrophysiological and synaptic properties of spinal neurons change as the network goes from the quiescent state to swimming. Knowledge of these electrophysiological and synaptic properties will also be needed to understand the roles of neuromodulators in producing these alterations during fictive swimming.

An example of the type of electrophysiological changes that can occur in spinal neurons when the network goes from quiescence to activity is shown in Fig. 5. In this example, an intracellular microelectrode recording was made from a myotomal motoneuron before and during bath perfusion of D-glutamate to induce fictive swimming (Fig. 5B). A comparison was made between action potentials elicited antidromically in the quiescent state versus action potentials occurring as a result of swimming activity (Fig. 5C). The membrane potential just preceding the action potential was several millivolts more depolarized during fictive swimming, yet the fast upswing, peak, and rapid repolarization of the action potential were unchanged. The most dramatic difference between the action potentials was a reduction of the slow post-spike afterhyperpolarization (AHP) during swimming activity compared to rest. The decrease in the slow AHP amplitude is likely due to a reduction of the underlying conductance, which is an apamin-sensitive calcium-activated conductance (Meer and Buchanan, 1992), because it occurred in spite of an increase in driving force as the motoneuron depolarized.

To determine whether this swimming-associated decrease in the slow AHP had a functional consequence on the input–output relationship of the cell, suprathreshold depolarizing current pulses were injected into the motoneuron. As shown in Fig. 5D, the motoneuron fired more spikes during a current pulse during swimming compared to rest, and the slope of the frequency-current (F–I) relationship was increased (Fig. 5E). This shift in the F–I relationship is similar to that observed after application of apamin (Meer and Buchanan, 1992; Hill et al., 1992). A possible mechanism for the reduction of the slow AHP may be the release of serotonin and/or dopamine. Both serotonergic and dopaminergic cells are present in the lamprey spinal cord (Van Dongen et al., 1985; McPherson and Kemnitz, 1994; Schotland et al., 1995), and application of either serotonin or dopamine reduces the slow AHP of motoneurons (McPherson and Kemnitz, 1994; Schotland et al., 1995; Wikström et al., 1995; Kemnitz, 1997). In cat motoneurons, a similar reduction in the slow AHP occurs during fictive locomotion, yet the slope of the F–I relationship decreases so that firing frequency of the cell becomes less sensitive to changes in input current (Brownstone et al., 1992). This result suggests that other factors also contribute to firing frequency regulation. Other electrophysiological

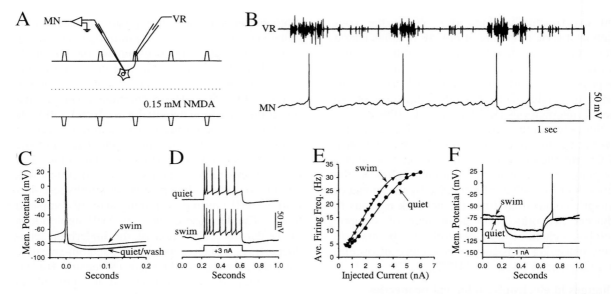

Fig. 5. Changes in electrophysiological properties with fictive swimming. A: schematic diagram of an intracellular recording from a motoneuron during fictive swimming induced with 0.5 mM D-glutamate. B: sample of ventral root bursting and the intracellular membrane potential activity of the motoneuron. C: averages of action potentials occurring before fictive swimming in a quiescent spinal cord, during fictive swimming, and then after the glutamate was washed off the preparation. The membrane potential just preceding the action potential was depolarized about 10 mV during swimming and the amplitude of the slow post-spike afterhyperpolarization was reduced by about 50%. D: a depolarizing current injection of 3 nA produced more action potentials with shorter interspike intervals during fictive swimming compared to the quiescent cord. E: the relationship between average firing frequency and the injected current showed a greater slope during fictive swim compared to the quiet cord. F: during fictive swimming, a hyperpolarizing current pulse initiated a post-inhibitory rebound spike upon termination of the pulse, but the same current pulse did not induce a spike in the quiescent preparation.

changes have also been observed in lamprey spinal cord such as an increased tendency to show post-inhibitory rebound when the cell is depolarized (Fig. 5F).

Motoneuron feedback

In lamprey, motoneurons have been considered to be only output elements with no feedback to the locomotor network (Wallén and Lansner, 1984). Motoneurons are clearly not passive elements with no involvement in shaping the final pattern as it has been shown that they exhibit membrane potential oscillations in the presence of NMDA and tetrodotoxin (Grillner and Wallén, 1985; Wallén and Grillner, 1987). These oscillations are not due to spike-mediated synaptic transmission nor are they likely due to non-spiking synaptic interactions because their cycle periods can be easily shifted with current injection into a single neuron (Wallén and Grillner, 1985). The oscillations are due to the

voltage-dependent properties of the NMDA receptors in combination with other ion channels. However, motoneurons have not been thought to have feedback synaptic connections to the locomotor network. This conclusion was based on ventral root stimulation experiments during fictive swimming, which showed no effect on the burst pattern of other ventral roots (Wallén and Lansner, 1984).

Recently, we have begun looking more closely at the possibility of feedback interactions of motoneurons to spinal neurons (Buchanan et al., 1998). One approach has been to examine whether acetylcholine affects the swimming rhythm when applied to the bath, which would be expected if the cholinergic motoneurons had feedback connections to the locomotor network. As shown in Fig. 6A, bath application of acetylcholine decreases the cycle period of fictive swimming, and nicotinic antagonists reduce this action. The decrease in cycle period is also seen with the application of

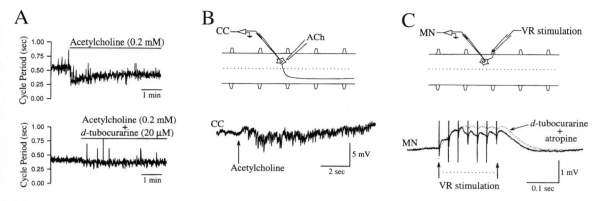

Fig. 6. Evidence for cholinergic input to the swim network and for motoneuron feedback connections in lamprey. A: bath application of acetylcholine produced shortening of cycle periods in fictive swimming induced by NMDA (top trace) and this action of acetylcholine was mostly blocked by nicotinic antagonists (bottom trace). B: local application of acetylcholine to the surface of the spinal cord, while recording intracellularly from a CC interneuron in normal physiological solution, evoked a barrage of hyperpolarizing postsynaptic potentials suggesting that local interneurons that inhibited the CC interneuron were strongly excited by the acetylcholine. C: electrical stimulation of a ventral root at a current level just below antidromic threshold for an intracellularly-recorded motoneuron produced depolarizing potentials in the motoneuron. During a train of ventral root pulses, the potentials summated and hyperpolarizing potentials appeared after the third stimulus. Cholinergic antagonists blocked these hyperpolarizing potentials.

nicotine and to a lesser extent with oxotremorine, a muscarinic cholinergic agonist. Local application of acetylcholine generally produces a depolarization of motoneurons and interneurons in the presence of tetrodotoxin. In the example of Fig. 6B, acetylcholine was applied locally to a CC interneuron in normal physiological solution, without tetrodotoxin. At first, the cell began to depolarize in response to the acetylcholine but then received a barrage of inhibitory psps. This observation suggests that near the CC interneuron, there are cells strongly excited by the acetylcholine and these are inhibitory to the CC interneuron. Possibly, then, motoneuron axons could excite these local inhibitory interneurons by the release of acetylcholine, and the interneurons would in turn inhibit nearby neurons.

If motoneurons provide feedback interactions, then one should be able to antidromically stimulate a ventral root and evoke responses in nerve cells located in the same ipsilateral segment. Such interactions do exist as demonstrated in Fig. 6C. In this experiment, an intracellularly-recorded motoneuron was identified by antidromic stimulation of the ventral root. When the stimulation intensity was reduced below the spike threshold for the moto-

neuron, a small depolarizing potential remained. Stimulation of the ventral root with a train of seven stimuli summated these depolarizing psps, but beginning with the third stimulus, a hyperpolarizing psp was superimposed on the depolarizing responses. Cholinergic antagonists blocked this hyperpolarizing response (Fig. 6C). Presumably, when the ventral root stimulation was reduced below threshold for the axon of the recorded motoneuron, some of the motoneuron axons within the root were still being antidromically activated. Perhaps then these antidromic spikes produced synaptic release of acetylcholine, which then excited local inhibitory interneurons. These interneurons in turn inhibited the motoneuron, in a Renshaw-like feedback inhibition (Windhorst, 1996). The depolarizing psps seen with antidromic stimulation persist in zero calcium solution suggesting that they are mediated electrotonically. Functionally, the inhibitory interneurons may be performing a role similar to that proposed for the lateral interneurons in terminating activity on one side of the cord, allowing the reciprocally inhibitory network to oscillate. Feedback interactions of motoneurons have also been demonstrated in the embryonic *Xenopus* tadpole spinal cord and are

320

thought to contribute to the generation of locomotor activity in that preparation (Perrins and Roberts, 1995).

Summary

The isolated lamprey spinal cord offers a relatively simple and convenient adult preparation in which to investigate how nerve cells generate behavior and in particular the rhythmic motor patterns of locomotion. Nerve cell classes can be identified and their cellular and synaptic properties characterized, and a simple model based on demonstrated synaptic connectivity can account for major aspects of fictive swimming. Clearly, however, much remains to be learned. In particular, the properties of the spinal neurons have been shown to change during swimming activity but relatively little is known about how these changes occur or the effects that these changes have upon the activities of the network. In addition, much remains to be learned about the cell types and their synaptic interactions as demonstrated here with the newly discovered feedback connections from motoneurons, which have not been previously taken into account in modeling of the lamprey locomotor network.

Acknowledgement

The author's research has been sponsored in part by NIH grants NS28369 and NS35725.

List of abbreviations

AHP	afterhyperpolarization
CC	interneurons with contralaterally and caudally directed axon
EIN	excitatory interneuron
F–I	spike frequency vs. current relationship
LIN	lateral interneuron
MN	motoneuron
NMDA	N-methyl-D-Aspartate

References

Alford, S. and Williams, T.L. (1989) Endogenous activation of glycine and NMDA receptors in lamprey spinal cord during fictive locomotion. *J. Neurosci.*, 9: 2792–2800.

Brodin, L., Grillner, S. and Rovainen, C.M. (1985) *N*-methyl-D-aspartate (NMDA), kainate and quisqualate receptors and the generation of fictive locomotion in the lamprey spinal cord. *Brain Res.*, 325: 302–306.

Brownstone, R.M., Jordan, L.M., Kriellars, D.J., Noga, B.R. and Shefchyk, S.J. (1992) On the regulation of repetitive firing in lumbar motoneurons during fictive locomotion in the cat. *Brain Res.*, 90: 441–455.

Buchanan, J.T. (1982) Identification of interneurons with contralateral, caudal axons in the lamprey spinal cord: synaptic interactions and morphology. *J. Neurophysiol.*, 47: 961–975.

Buchanan, J.T. (1992) Neural network simulation of coupled locomotor oscillators in the lamprey spinal cord. *Biol. Cybern.*, 66: 367–374.

Buchanan, J.T. (1993) The electrophysiological properties of identified classes of lamprey spinal neurons. *J. Neurophysiol.*, 70: 2313–2325.

Buchanan, J.T. (1999) Commissural interneurons in rhythm generation and intersegmental coupling in the lamprey spinal cord. *J. Neurophysiol.*, 81: 2037–2045.

Buchanan, J.T. and Cohen, A.H. (1982) Activities of identified interneurons, motoneurons, and muscle fibers during fictive swimming in the lamprey and effects of reticulospinal and dorsal cell stimulation. *J. Neurophysiol.*, 47: 948–960.

Buchanan, J.T., Grillner, S., Cullheim, S. and Risling, M. (1989) Identification of excitatory interneurons contributing to generation of locomotion in lamprey: structure, pharmacology, and function. *J. Neurophysiol.*, 62: 59–69.

Buchanan, J.T. and Kasicki, S. (1995) Activities of spinal neurons during brain stem-dependent fictive swimming in lamprey. *J. Neurophysiol.*, 73: 80–87.

Buchanan, J.T., Kasicki, S. and Quinlan, K.A. (1998) Effects of motoneuron stimulation in the lamprey spinal cord. *Soc. Neurosci. Abstr.*, 24: 1666.

Buchanan, J.T. and McPherson, D.R. (1995) The neuronal network for locomotion in the lamprey spinal cord: evidence for the involvement of commissural interneurons. *J. Physiol. Paris*, 89: 221–234.

Cohen, A.H. and Harris-Warrick, R.M. (1984) Strychnine eliminates alternating motor output during fictive locomotion in the lamprey. *Brain Res.*, 293: 164–167.

Cohen, A.H. and Wallén, P. (1980) The neuronal correlate of locomotion in fish. 'Fictive swimming' induced in an in vitro preparation of the lamprey spinal cord. *Exp. Brain Res.*, 41: 11–18.

El Manira, A., Tegner, J. and Grillner, S. (1994) Calcium-dependent potassium channels play a critical role for burst termination in the locomotor network in lamprey. *J. Neurophysiol.*, 72: 1852–1861.

Grillner, S. and Wallén, P. (1985) The ionic mechanisms underlying NMDA receptor induced, TTX-resistant membrane potential oscillations in lamprey neurones active during locomotion. *Neurosci. Lett.*, 60: 289–294.

Hagevik, A. and McClellan, A.D. (1994) Coupling of spinal locomotor networks in larval lamprey revealed by receptor blockers for inhibitory amino acids: neurophysiology and computer modeling. *J. Neurophysiol.*, 72: 1810–1829.

Hill, R., Matsushima, T., Schotland, J. and Grillner, S. (1992) Apamin blocks the slow AHP in lamprey and delays termination of locomotor bursts. *NeuroReport*, 30: 943–945.

Kahn, J.A. and Roberts, A. (1982) Experiments on the central pattern generator for swimming in amphibian embryos. *Phil. Trans. R. Soc. Lond. B.*, 296: 229–243.

Kemnitz, C.P. (1997) Dopaminergic modulation of spinal neurons and synaptic potentials in the lamprey spinal cord. *J. Neurophysiol.*, 77: 289–298.

Matsushima, T. and Grillner, S. (1992) Neural mechanisms of intersegmental coordination in lamprey: local excitability changes modify the phase coupling along the spinal cord. *J. Neurophysiol.*, 67: 373–388.

McClellan, A.D. and Grillner, S. (1984) Activation of 'fictive swimming' by electrical microstimulation of brainstem locomotor regions in an in vitro preparation of the lamprey central nervous system. *Brain Res.*, 300: 357–361.

McPherson, D.R., Buchanan, J.T. and Kasicki, S. (1994) Effects of strychnine on fictive swimming in the lamprey: evidence for glycinergic inhibition, discrepancies with model predictions, and novel modulatory rhythms. *J. Comp. Physiol. A*, 175: 311–321.

McPherson, D.R. and Kemnitz, C.P. (1994) Modulation of lamprey fictive swimming and motoneuron physiology by dopamine, and its immunocytochemical localization in the spinal cord. *Neurosci. Lett.*, 166: 23–26.

Meer, D.P. and Buchanan, J.T. (1992) Apamin reduces the late afterhyperpolarization of lamprey spinal neurons, with little effect on fictive swimming. *Neurosci. Lett.*, 143: 1–4.

Perrins, R. and Roberts, A. (1995) Cholinergic contribution to excitation in a spinal locomotor central pattern generator in Xenopus embryos. *J. Neurophysiol.*, 73: 1013–1019.

Rovainen, C.M. (1974) Synaptic interactions of identified nerve cells in the spinal cord of the sea lamprey. *J. Comp. Neurol.*, 154: 189–206.

Schotland, J., Shupliakov, O., Wikström, M., Brodin, L., Srinivasan, M., You, Z.-B., Herrera-Marschitz, M., Zhang, W., Hökfelt, T. and Grillner, S. (1995) Control of lamprey locomotor neurons by colocalized monoamine transmitters. *Nature*, 374: 266–268.

Soffe, S.R. (1989) Roles of glycinergic inhibition and *N*-methyl-D-aspartate receptor-mediated excitation in the locomotor rhythmicity of one half of the *Xenopus* embryo CNS. *Euro. J. Neurosci.*, 1: 561–571.

Van Dongen, P.A.M., Hökfelt, T., Grillner, S., Verhofstad, A.A.J., Steinbusch, H.W.M., Cuello, A.C. and Terenius, L. (1985) Immunohistochemical demonstration of some putative neurotransmitters in the lamprey spinal cord and spinal ganglia. 5-hydroxytryptamine-, tachykinin-, and neuropeptide Y-immunoreactive neurons and fibers. *J. Comp. Neurol.*, 234: 501–522.

Wallén, P., Ekeberg, Ö., Lansner, A., Brodin, L., Tråvén, H. and Grillner, S. (1992) A computer-based model for realistic simulations of neural networks. II. The segmental network generating locomotor rhythmicity in the lamprey. *J. Neurophysiol.*, 68: 1939–1950.

Wallén, P. and Grillner, S. (1985) The effect of current passage on *N*-methyl-D-aspartate-induced, tetrodotoxin-resistant membrane potential oscillations in lamprey neurons active during locomotion. *Neurosci. Lett.*, 56: 87–93.

Wallén, P. and Grillner, S. (1987) *N*-methyl-D-aspartate receptor-induced, inherent oscillatory activity in neurons active during fictive locomotion in the lamprey. *J. Neurosci.*, 7: 2745–2755.

Wallén, P. and Lansner, A. (1984) Do the motoneurones constitute a part of the spinal network generating the swimming rhythm in the lamprey? *J. Exp. Biol.*, 113: 493–497.

Wallén, P. and Williams, T.L. (1984) Fictive locomotion in the lamprey spinal cord in vitro compared with swimming in the intact and spinal animal. *J. Physiol. (Lond.)*, 347: 225–239.

Wikström, M., Hill, R., Hellgren, J. and Grillner S. (1995) The action of 5-HT on calcium-dependent potassium channels and on the spinal locomotor network in the lamprey is mediated by 5-HT$_{1A}$-like receptors. *Brain Res.*, 678: 191–199.

Williams, T.L. (1992) Phase coupling by synaptic spread in chains of coupled neuronal oscillators. *Science*, 258: 662–665.

Windhorst, U. (1996) On the role of recurrent inhibitory feedback in motor control. *Prog. Neurobiol.*, 49: 517–587.

M.D. Binder (Ed.)
Progress in Brain Research, Vol 123
© 1999 Elsevier Science BV. All rights reserved.

CHAPTER 28

Primate spinal interneurons: muscle fields and response properties during voluntary movement

E.E. Fetz,* S.I. Perlmutter, Y. Prut and M. A. Maier

Department of Physiology and Biophysics and Regional Primate Research Center, University of Washington, Seattle, WA 98195, USA

Introduction

Our current view of the functions of spinal interneurons in generating voluntary movements is based largely on inferences from observations in anesthetized, immobilized animals. Previous studies have elucidated the convergent inputs to interneurons from afferent fibers and from descending tracts (for reviews see Baldissera et al., 1981; Jankowska, 1992). Still, little is known about two crucial properties that are essential to understanding the functions of segmental neurons in movements: their activity patterns during normal voluntary limb movements and their output effects on the agonist muscles. These two properties together provide significant information about how the activity of spinal neurons contributes to muscle activity. Similar studies have elucidated the response patterns and the output effects of supraspinal premotor (PreM) neurons in the motor cortex and red nucleus (reviews: Cheney et al., 1988; Fetz et al., 1989) and dorsal root afferent fibers (Flament et al., 1992). This paper summarizes results of comparable experiments with interneurons in the cervical spinal cord.

To elucidate the role of segmental neurons in voluntary movement, we applied the techniques previously used to investigate supraspinal PreM

cells. Spike-triggered averages (STAs) of muscle activity during active movement have revealed output connections of neurons in the motor cortex and red nucleus to alpha-motoneurons (Fetz and Cheney, 1980; Lemon et al., 1986; Mewes and Cheney, 1991). The activities of these corticomotoneuronal (CM) and rubromotoneuronal (RM) cells during the performance of a simple ramp-and-hold motor task exhibit characteristic discharge patterns that provide insight into the control of dynamic and static components of force (Cheney and Fetz, 1980; Buys et al., 1986; Cheney et al., 1988; Fetz et al., 1989; Mewes and Cheney, 1994). Here, we describe properties of primate segmental interneurons during a similar step-tracking task. Information on the discharge pattern and post-spike effects of interneurons enables us to contrast the relative contributions of supraspinal and segmental PreM neurons to voluntary muscle activity.

The methods for recording activity of units in the cervical spinal cord with movable tungsten microelectrodes have been described elsewhere (Perlmutter et al., 1998). Electromyographic (EMG) activity from wrist and digit flexor and extensor muscles was recorded with multi-stranded wires implanted trans- or subcutaneously. During recording sessions the monkeys made ramp-and-hold torque responses of the wrist in an isometric step-tracking task.

STAs of full-wave rectified EMG activity (Fetz and Cheney, 1980) were computed to identify

*Corresponding author. Tel.: (206) 543–4839; Fax: (206) 685–0305; e-mail: fetz@u.washington.edu

correlational linkages with muscles. PreM-INs produced a post-spike effect in EMG, defined as a change in the level of the averaged EMG activity beginning at least 3.5 ms after the trigger spike (from the minimal latency of post-stimulus effects evoked by single-pulse microstimuli delivered through the spinal recording electrode). PreM-INs could produce either post-spike facilitation (PSF) or post-spike suppression (PSS) or both. The cell's muscle field was defined as the set of muscles exhibiting post-spike effects (after elimination of potentially redundant recordings via electrical cross-talk). In some cases, changes in the level of averaged EMG activity started before or near the trigger point. These early changes could be due only to synchronous activity in other PreM units that fired before the triggering neuron and were termed synchrony effects.

Response patterns of the units during ramp-and-hold torque trajectories were determined from averages aligned at onset of the torque ramps. These response averages included time histograms of the unit activity, averages of rectified EMG activity, and the isometric torque.

Output effects from spinal interneurons

Activity of 575 neurons was recorded in the C6-T1 spinal segments in three macaques while they performed isometric flexion-extension torques about the wrist. These cells were encountered throughout the gray matter, but most were in the intermediate and ventral laminae. Twenty-nine neurons were identified as motoneurons, on the basis of their low firing rates, non-zero recruitment threshold, and depth from the cord dorsum. STAs of unrectified EMGs from these motoneurons often revealed characteristic motor unit profiles in a single forearm muscle after a few hundred triggers. Their response patterns during this task resembled those of peripherally recorded motor units documented more extensively in a previous study (Palmer and Fetz, 1985).

One hundred interneurons exhibited PSF or PSS in at least one muscle beginning at latencies of ≥ 3.5 ms and were classified as premotor interneurons (PreM-INs). In addition, 32 interneurons exhibited synchrony effects without identifiable post-spike effects in any of the recorded muscles (classified as Sy-INs). (25 of the 100 PreM-INs also showed superimposed synchrony and post-spike effects.) Most of the interneurons (414 of 575) showed no spike-related changes and were called unidentified interneurons (U-INs).

Figure 1 shows the STAs and response averages for an excitatory PreM-IN, estimated to reside in lamina VII of the caudal C_8 segment. This PreM-IN discharged tonically during static torques in both directions, with a higher rate during flexion, as shown by the response average (right). This neuron produced PSF in both the pronator teres (PT) and flexor carpi ulnaris (FCU) muscle (left). Of the 100 PreM-INs, 82% showed PSF of target muscles, either in isolation (as in Fig. 1) or superimposed on synchrony facilitation. The mean onset latency of the PSF was 7.3 ms ($n = 137$). The average mean percent increase of PSF above baseline (after synchrony was discounted) was 4.6%.

An inhibitory PreM-IN in segment C_8 is shown in Fig. 2. The STAs reveal PSS in two of the co-activated flexor muscles, flexor carpi radialis (FCR) and FCU. This cell also fired while the monkey generated both flexion and extension torques, with a higher level of activity during the flexion hold than during extension. A transient pause accompanied the dynamic transitions between extension and flexion holds. Fourteen (14%) of the PreM-INs showed only PSS of target muscles. The mean latency of the PSS was 8.5 ms ($n = 24$) and the average mean percent decrease relative to baseline was 4.2%. An additional 4 PreM-INs showed reciprocal effects: PSF of some muscles and PSS of their antagonists.

Surprisingly, post-spike and synchrony effects were about twice as common in flexor muscles as in extensors: 58% of PreM-INs had post-spike effects in flexor muscles only, while 29% had effects in extensors alone and 11% had effects in both. These proportions were similar for both PSF and PSS.

The number of muscles affected by PreM-INs was relatively restricted. Sixty-four of the 100 PreM-INs had post-spike effects in only one of the recorded muscles; the rest had larger muscle fields. On average, post-spike effects were distributed to 33% of the independent co-active muscles (after eliminating potentially redundant recordings). The PreM-INs with divergent post-spike effects in more than one muscle typically affected either flexor or extensor muscles, but not both (25/36 = 69%).

Response patterns and output effects of spinal interneurons

Most of the PreM-INs showed tonic or phasic-tonic activity associated with the ramp-and-hold torque trajectory in their preferred direction. Figure 3 summarizes the responses of various classes of spinal neurons, and also shows the patterns of other PreM cells in their preferred direction. All populations included phasic, tonic and phasic-tonic cells, in varying proportions. Interestingly, the relative proportions of response patterns were generally similar among the three groups of interneurons, indicating no clear preferential patterns for those with functional linkages to muscles.

In contrast to CM cells, afferent PreM fibers and motor units, only one-fourth of the interneurons were active for one direction of movement only. Most of the interneurons were activated more during movements in their preferred direction, but also had some activity during movement in the opposite direction.

A basic functional question concerns the relationship between the post-spike output effects of a PreM-IN and its response patterns relative to its target muscles. These relations are tabulated in Fig. 4, which shows the distribution of post-spike effects to 'agonist' muscles, activated in the cell's preferred direction, and to the 'antagonist' muscles. For some PreM-INs this relationship was totally 'congruent': the postspike effects and activation patterns were functionally completely consistent with simple reciprocal control of flexion/extension movements. Such was the case for the 24 PreM-INs that facilitated agonist muscles and fired only when these muscles were active (Fig. 4). All the other PreM-INs had more 'complex' relations: they showed some degree of 'inappropriate' activity, in which the postspike effect would seem counterproductive. The circled numbers in Fig. 4 indicate interneurons that had postspike effects that were partially consistent with their activation – for example, those that facilitated agonist muscles but were also active during antagonist muscle activity. The cells denoted by triangles had largely paradoxical relations. For example, the inhibitory IN in Fig. 2 increased its activity more during flexion torques and produced PSS in flexor muscles. A few PreM-INs had a steady discharge rate that was not

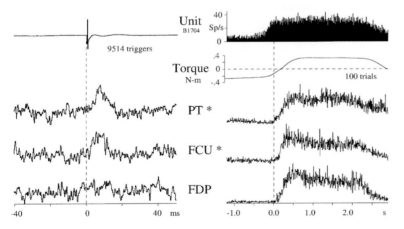

Fig. 1. STAs and response averages of a facilitatory PreM-IN located in lamina VII of caudal C8. The STAs (left) show the triggering action potential (top) and average of rectified EMG in 3 independently recorded co-active muscles. Asterisks indicate muscles with significant post-spike effects. The STAs are plotted with the variances in baseline activity normalized to the STA of the muscle with the largest post-spike effect (PT). The average activity of the neuron during flexion torques is shown in the top right, above the average torque trajectory (positive torque in flexion, negative torque in extension) and average responses of the co-active muscles. This neuron exhibited tonic firing during static torques in both directions, with higher rates for flexion. (From Perlmutter et al., 1998).

modulated during alternating flexion and extension torques, similar to the previously reported unmodulated RM cells (Mewes and Cheney, 1991).

Functional classes of interneurons

These studies have documented the response properties and output effects of segmental interneurons during voluntary motor responses in the primate. Of course, they immediately raise questions about the identity of these interneurons, as conventionally defined by criteria used in acute experiments. Unfortunately, our ability to evoke reflex responses in awake monkeys was limited by our desire to maintain unit isolation and to avoid aversive stimulation. Although our interneurons were not identified in terms of the classical reflex categories, their responses during movement and their output effects on muscles are two important features

relevant to understanding spinal control of voluntary movement. Moreover, these two properties were also characterized in other populations of PreM neurons under similar experimental conditions, allowing us to compare the functional properties of spinal and supraspinal PreM populations.

Comparison of post-spike effects of PreM neurons

The post-spike effects of PreM neurons are probably mediated by a monosynaptic linkage to motoneurons (Cope et al., 1987) although polysynaptic relays could also contribute, as previously discussed (Watt et al., 1976; Fetz and Cheney, 1980; Perlmutter et al., 1998). The onset latencies of post-spike effects from different PreM populations are generally consistent with the differences

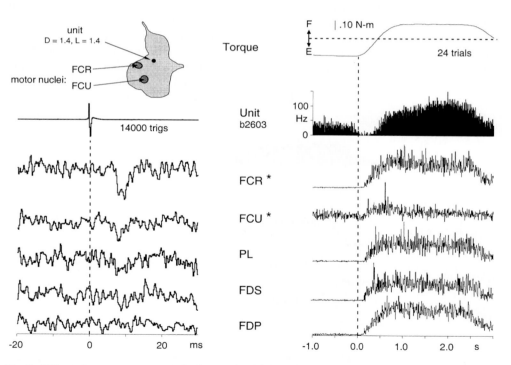

Fig. 2. STAs and response averages of a flexor-related inhibitory PreM-IN. This neuron produced significant postspike suppression in the FCR and FCU muscles (asterisks), in the STA of rectified EMG activity (left). The weak suppressions seen in PL and FDS were not statistically significant. The cell's location was estimated on the basis of microelectrode coordinates (inset). For the locations of cervical motoneuron pools, see Jenny and Inukai (1983). The response average (right) shows higher activity during flexion than extension and a pause during dynamic transition in torque direction. (From Fetz et al., 1996).

Response Type		Population							
		CM	RM	DRG	PreM-IN	Sy-IN	U-IN	MU	
	Phasic-Tonic	48%	46%	21%	39%	23%	37%	22%	
	Tonic	28	8	52	38	53	37	41	
	Phasic	2	20	27	14	13	19	4	
	Phasic-Ramp	10	0	0	2	0	1	0	
	Ramp	6	0	0	1	3	1	0	
	Decrementing	5	3	0	4	0	5	33	
	Unmodulated	0	23	0	3	7	–	0	
0.5 s	Torque N =	211	61	29	96	30	387	114	

PreM Cells

Fig. 3. Summary of response patterns in the preferred direction for different populations of neurons during generation of flexion and extension torques at the wrist. Examples of each pattern are illustrated on left, and schematic of populations on right. Proportions are given for corticomotoneuronal (CM; Fetz et al., 1989) and rubromotoneuronal cells (RM; Mewes and Cheney, 1991), premotor afferents in dorsal root ganglia (DRG; Flament et al., 1992), spinal premotor interneurons (PreM-IN), spinal unidentified interneurons (U-IN), spinal interneurons with synchrony effects (Sy-IN) and motor neurons (MU) (Maier et al., 1998). The latter combines motor unit data from Palmer and Fetz (1985) with putative motoneurons from present study. Unmodulated U-INs are not included because they were not studied systematically and their proportion could be made arbitrarily large.

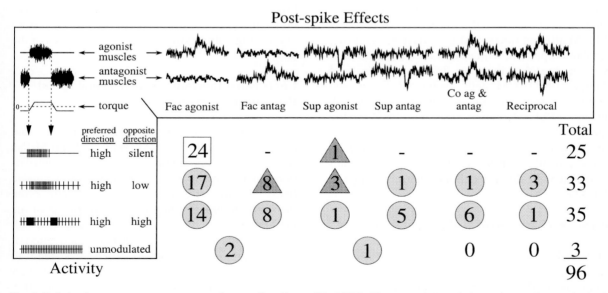

Fig. 4. Relation between response patterns and post-spike effects of PreM-INs. The neuron's 'agonist' muscles are those active in the cell's preferred direction, the direction of torque for which the neuron has the largest increase in activity. Fac, facilitatory effects; Sup, suppressive effects; dashed lines, connections that are not detectable by spike-triggered averaging; agonist and antagonist are not defined for unmodulated neurons. Square, circles and triangles indicate increasing incongruity between response pattern and post-spike effects. (From Perlmutter et al., 1998).

in conduction times, as discussed in more detail elsewhere (Fetz et al., 1989; Perlmutter et al., 1998). The magnitude of the PSF, as quantified by the mean change as a percentage of the pre-trigger baseline EMG activity, was generally similar across populations. Excitatory PreM-INs produced PSFs that were comparable in magnitude to those produced by CM cells (Kasser and Cheney, 1985) and by afferents in the dorsal root ganglion (DRG) (Flament et al., 1992), and slightly larger than those produced by RM cells (Mewes and Cheney, 1991). On the other hand, post-spike suppressions produced by spinal PreM-INs had a shorter mean latency and a larger mean amplitude than those produced by CM (Kasser and Cheney, 1985) and RM cells (Mewes and Cheney, 1991). This suggests that suppressive PreM-INs were probably last-order inhibitory interneurons.

The muscle fields of PreM-INs (expressed as the proportion of independent muscle recordings exhibiting post-spike effects) was slightly smaller than those of CM and RM cells. More than half of the PreM-INs affected only a single target muscle. The fact that PreM-INs facilitated flexor muscles about twice as often as extensor muscles was unique among the PreM populations. Flexors and extensors were facilitated by nearly equal numbers of PreM afferent fibers. RM cells have the opposite distribution pattern, with effects seen more often in extensor muscles than in flexors (Mewes and Cheney, 1991). CM cells facilitated flexor and extensor muscles in similar proportions, although the largest PSFs were in extensor muscles (Fetz and Cheney, 1980). This suggests that certain muscles are preferentially controlled from supraspinal inputs and others from segmental inputs, a result consistent with the intracellular data of Clough et al. (1968).

Discharge characteristics of premotor neurons

While PSF identifies the target muscles affected by the PreM neurons, the neuron's effect on target motoneurons during active movement is proportional to its discharge rate. Comparing the discharge patterns of populations of PreM neurons and motor units in their preferred direction (Fig. 3) shows that all include phasic, tonic and phasic-tonic neurons. The other response patterns appeared in specific subsets of the PreM groups. A remarkable difference is the degree to which the neurons fired in the non-preferred direction. All motor units and CM cells and most PreM DRG afferents were strictly unidirectional. In contrast, all RM cells and most spinal interneurons showed bidirectional activity. Thus, many interneurons that produced PSFs in primary flexor or extensor muscles continued to fire when their target motor units became silent.

The combined inputs from all PreM populations to forearm muscle motoneurons during the wrist task were dominated by tonic and phasic response components. The tonic discharge pattern most accurately reflects the torque trajectory itself and the level of tonic discharge has been proportional to torque for the CM, RM and PreM-IN populations (Cheney and Fetz et al., 1980; Mewes and Cheney, 1994; Maier et al., 1998). Phasic discharges prior to the onset of movement in PreM cells could contribute to rapid activation of motoneurons. Other patterns of activity also were observed during step-tracking, which could provide additional types of control over the motoneurons. Rubral and spinal PreM neurons with steady, unmodulated bidirectional discharge apparently provide an excitatory bias during both flexion and extension phases of the task.

Contrasting functions of cortical and spinal PreM neurons in movement

The differences in the response properties and projection patterns of CM cells and PreM-INs suggest corresponding differences in their contributions to reciprocal wrist movements. The muscle fields of CM cells were larger, and more often involved reciprocal inhibition of antagonists of the facilitated target muscles, indicating that CM cell activity tends to produce a coordinated activation of muscle groups. In contrast, PreM-INs tend to facilitate or suppress specific muscles. On the other hand, the activation of CM cells was more specific: CM cells fired with flexion or extension, but not both, whereas most spinal interneurons were bidirectionally active. This suggests that CM cells are activated under relatively particular movement conditions, while spinal PreM-INs are recruited more generally, with excitatory and inhibitory interneurons coactivated in an overlapping fashion. Thus CM cells represent more explicitly a pattern of coordinated muscle activity, while spinal interneurons tend to affect particular muscles.

Delay period activity in interneurons

To investigate the possible involvement of spinal interneurons in early stages of movement preparation we recorded their activity in two monkeys performing an instructed delay task (Prut et al., 1998, 1999). Again, the monkeys controlled a cursor position by isometric flexion/extension torques about the wrist. Trials included a rest period (cursor held in a central target zone corresponding to zero torque), an instructed delay period (initiated by a transient cue that indicated the direction of the next movement and terminated by a go signal that indicated the time to begin the movement), and an active torque hold period (when the monkey acquired the remembered target). Many spinal interneurons (123/394 = 31%) showed significant delay period modulation (SDM) relative to the precue rest period – in the absence of any sensory input or motor output. There was no detectable low-level EMG activity during the delay. For some interneurons the change in firing rate during the instructed delay was in the same direction as the activity change during the subsequent movement, as would be expected if a cell's preparatory activity were simply a subthreshold version of its movement-related activity. However for most interneurons this was not the case. Some showed changes specifically in the delay, but not during movement, and many were modulated during movement without SDM. In addition, for 39% of the interneurons that showed changes in both, firing rates during the delay and torque periods were modulated in the opposite direction (i.e. increase vs. decrease). Two-thirds of interneurons with SDM were inhibited during the delay, irrespective of the direction of change of firing rates during movement. These results indicate that preparation for movement involves extensive modulation of spinal interneurons that cannot be predicted from their responses during active move-

ment. Thus, spinal circuitry is involved in the earliest stages of movement preparation, in a manner similar to motor and premotor cortical areas. Indeed, this set-related activity appears to involve widely distributed neural mechanisms.

The activity of spinal interneurons during an instructed delay period suggests that spinal interneurons can be involved in additional functions beyond simple peripheral sensory or motor events. During the delay interval, after the instructional cue and before the go signal, the changes in IN activity reflect more subtle computations than simple subthreshold changes in the direction required for the upcoming movement. In terms of motor preparation, these changes can be understood as reflecting two overlapping processes: a subthreshold preparation for the required movement, superimposed on a general inhibition of overt expression of this activity until the go signal. These first observations of spinal cord neurons in behaving animal raise the intriguing possibility that other 'higher-order' representations might be found at the spinal level, indicating that cognitive processes could be widely distributed.

Acknowledgements

We thank J. Garlid and L. Shupe for their expert technical assistance and K. Elias for editorial assistance. This study was supported by NIH grants NS12542, NS09189 and RR00166, American Paralysis Association grants PB1–9402 & PBR2–9502, and the Swiss Science Foundation.

List of abbreviations

IN	interneuron
CM	corticomotoneuronal
RM	rubromotoneuronal
STA	Spike-triggered average
PreM	premotor
EMG	electromyographic
PreM-IN	premotor interneuron
PSF	post-spike facilitation
PSS	post-spike suppression
Sy-IN	synchrony interneuron
U-IN	unidentified interneuron
PT	pronator teres

330

FCU   flexor carpi ulnaris
FCR   flexor carpi radialis
DRG   dorsal root ganglion
SDM   significant delay period modulation

References

Baldissera, F., Hultborn, H. and Illert, M. (1981) Integration in spinal neuronal systems. In: *Handbook of Physiology*, Sect. 1, 2: 509–595.

Buys, E.J., Lemon, R.N., Mantel, G.W.H. and Muir, R.B. (1986) Selective facilitation of different hand muscles by single corticospinal neurones in the conscious monkey. *J. Physiol. (Lond.)*, 381: 529–549.

Cheney, P.D. and Fetz, E.E. (1980) Functional classes of primate corticomotoneuronal cells and their relation to active force. *J. Neurophysiol.*, 44: 773–791.

Cheney, P.D., Mewes, K. and Fetz, E.E. (1988) Encoding of motor parameters by corticomotoneuronal (CM) and rubromotoneuronal (RM) cells producing postspike facilitation of forelimb muscles in the behaving monkey. *Behav. Brain Res.*, 28: 181–191.

Clough, J.F.M., Kernell, D. and Phillips, C.G. (1968) The distribution of monosynaptic excitation from the pyramidal tract and from primary spindle afferents to motoneurons of the baboon's hand and forearm. *J. Physiol. (Lond.)*, 198: 145–166.

Cope, T.C., Fetz, E.E. and Matsumura, M. (1987) Cross-correlation assessment of synaptic strength of single Ia fibre connections with triceps surae motoneurons in cats. *J. Physiol. (Lond.)*, 390: 161–188.

Fetz, E.E. and Cheney, P.D. (1980) Postspike facilitation of forelimb muscle activity by primate corticomotoneuronal cells. *J. Neurophysiol.*, 44: 751–772.

Fetz, E.E., Cheney, P.D., Mewes, K. and Palmer, S. (1989) Control of forelimb muscle activity by populations of corticomotoneuronal and rubromotoneuronal cells. *Progr. Brain Res.*, 80: 437–449.

Fetz, E.E., Perlmutter, S., Maier, M, Flament, D. and Fortier, P.A. (1996) Response patterns and post-spike effects of premotor neurons in cervical spinal cord of behaving monkeys. *Can. J. Physiol. Pharmacol.*, 74:531–546.

Flament, D., Fortier, P.A. and Fetz, E.E. (1992) Response patterns and post-spike effects of peripheral afferents in dorsal root ganglia of behaving monkeys. *J. Neurophysiol.*, 67: 875–889.

Jankowska, E. (1992) Interneuronal relay in spinal pathways from proprioceptors. *Progr. Neurobiol.*, 38: 335–378.

Jenny, A.B. and Inukai, J. (1983) Principles of motor organization of the monkey cervical spinal cord. *J. Neurosci.*, 3: 567–575.

Kasser, R.J. and Cheney, P.D. (1985) Characteristics of corticomotoneuronal postspike facilitation and reciprocal suppression of EMG activity in the monkey. *J. Neurophysiol.*, 53: 959–978.

Lemon, R.N., Mantel, G.W. and Muir, R.B. (1986) Corticospinal facilitation of hand muscles during voluntary movement in the conscious monkey. *J. Physiol. (Lond.)*, 381: 497–527.

Maier, M.A., Perlmutter, S.I. and Fetz, E.E. (1998) Response patterns and force relations of monkey spinal interneurons during active wrist movement. *J. Neurophysiol.*, 80: 2495–2513.

Mewes, K. and Cheney, P.D. (1991) Facilitation and suppression of wrist and digit muscles from single rubromotoneuronal cells in the awake monkey. *J. Neurophysiol.*, 66: 1965–1977.

Mewes, K. and Cheney, P.D. (1994) Primate rubromotoneuronal cells: parametric relations and contribution to wrist movement. *J. Neurophysiol.*, 72: 14–30.

Palmer, S.S. and Fetz, E.E. (1985) Discharge properties of primate forearm motor units during isometric muscle activity. *J. Neurophysiol.*, 54: 1178–1193.

Perlmutter, S.I., Maier, M.A. and Fetz, E.E. (1998) Activity and output linkages of spinal premotor interneurons during voluntary wrist movements in the monkey. *J. Neurophysiol.*, 80: 2475–2494.

Prut, Y., Perlmutter, S.I. and Fetz, E.E (1998) Activity of spinal interneurons during premovement delay period in primates. *Soc. Neurosci.*, Abstracts, 24: 918.

Prut, Y. and Fetz, E.E. (1999) Primate spinal interneurons show pre-movement instructed delay activity. *Nature*, 401: 590–594.

Watt, D.G.D., Stauffer, E.K., Taylor, A., Reinking, R.M. and Stuart, D.G. (1976) Analysis of muscle receptor connections by spike-triggered averaging. I. Spindle primary and tendon organ afferents. *J. Neurophysiol.*, 39: 1375–1392.

M.D. Binder (Ed.)
Progress in Brain Research, Vol 123
© 1999 Elsevier Science BV. All rights reserved.

CHAPTER 29

Correlations between neurograms and locomotor drive potentials in motoneurons during fictive locomotion: implications for the organization of locomotor commands

Thomas M. Hamm,* Tamara V. Trank and Vladimir V. Turkin

Division of Neurobiology, Barrow Neurological Institute, St. Joseph's Hospital and Medical Center, Phoenix, AZ 85015, USA

Introduction

An excitatory postsynaptic potential increases the probability that a neuron will discharge, and this effect can be seen in the peaks of a crosscorrelation, or peristimulus time histogram (e.g. Moore et al., 1970; Sears and Stagg, 1976; Kirkwood and Sears, 1982; Cope et al., 1987; Powers and Binder, Chapter 7, this volume). This correlational approach is recognized as a powerful experimental tool, for it can provide insight into the synaptic organization of neurons whose synaptic inputs cannot readily be observed. We have utilized this approach to investigate the organization of synaptic inputs to motoneuron pools during locomotion.

Several proposals have been made regarding the organization of spinal neurons responsible for locomotor activity patterns, dating from Graham Brown's half-center hypothesis (Brown, 1911). However, patterns of locomotion can be more detailed than strict alternation between flexors and extensors even in immobilized or deafferented preparations. Based on observations of locomotion in reduced preparations or intact animals, proposals for complex organizations of spinal locomotor pattern generators have been forwarded (e.g. Grillner, 1981; Smith et al., 1998). A critical factor in

distinguishing between different models of spinal pattern generators is the synaptic input received by different motor nuclei. Motor nuclei which are controlled by the same element of the pattern generator should share common synaptic input during locomotion, either from branched premotor neurons or from synchronized sets of interneurons. Consequently, motor nuclei whose activities are correlated can be identified as those that are controlled by the same element of the pattern generator.

Detecting correlations in aggregate recordings of motoneuron activity with coherence functions

Correlations between the activities of different motoneuron pools can be assessed using coherence functions and aggregate measures of pool activity like electroneurograms (ENGs) or electromyograms (EMGs). The amplitude of rectified EMGs and ENGs is determined in part by the number of active motor units and their rate of discharge (e.g. Fuglevand et al., 1993). Because synaptic input influences the discharge of motoneurons that contribute to these signals, fluctuations in amplitude of a rectified ENG or EMG should represent the pattern of synaptic input to the motoneuron pool. Accordingly, rectified EMGs have been used to reveal the presence of projections from central

---
*Corresponding author. Tel.: 602–406–3731; Fax: 602–406–4172; e-mail: thamm@mha.chw.edu

neurons to spinal motoneurons during task performance (e.g. Fetz and Cheney, 1980). Hoffer et al. (1987) found evidence that rectified EMGs provide an accurate representation of the synaptic drive to a motoneuron pool at frequencies of 30 Hz and below. If higher frequencies are accurately represented as well in rectified signals, then information about common synaptic input to motoneuron pools during locomotion should be available from correlations between the rectified ENGs of different muscle nerves.

Coherence functions (Rosenberg et al., 1989) provide an alternative approach to correlation techniques in the time domain. The coherence function gives a measure of correlation between two signals as a function of frequency, varying from a value of 0 for no correlation to a value of 1 for a perfect correlation. It has been suggested that the coherence function provides some information about the frequency of discharge of the neurons that provide the common input to the motoneurons whose activity is correlated (Farmer et al., 1993).

Previous studies in this laboratory utilized coherence functions to detect correlations between the activity of motor pools during fictive locomotion in decerebrate cats, using rectified ENGs as measures of locomotor activity. Data from these studies revealed correlations between the extensors of the hip and ankle, and between these extensors and the bifunctional semitendinosus (St) and posterior biceps femoris (PBF) when they are coactive with extensors (Hamm and McCurdy, 1996). Based on this analysis, we concluded that motor pools of hip and ankle extensors and some bifunctional muscles like St receive similar locomotor commands. Similar conclusions have been made regarding locomotor signals to flexor motor pools, again based on coherence analysis of pairs of rectified ENGs (Turkin and Hamm, 1996).

Correlations between locomotor drive potentials and motor pool activity during fictive locomotion

A limitation of the work just cited is the uncertainty that arises from the use of rectified signals. How well the rectified signal represents the synaptic input to the motoneuron pools at higher frequencies

is uncertain, and the nonlinear process of rectification introduces harmonics that likely corrupt the information about the frequencies of synaptic input potentially available from the coherence spectra. To address these difficulties, we have made intracellular recordings from motoneurons during fictive locomotion, obtaining recordings of locomotor drive potentials (LDPs) as a direct measure of the synaptic input to individual motoneurons for comparison to the rectified neurograms. The LDPs were recorded intracellularly from motoneurons during fictive locomotion induced by stimulation of the mesencephalic locomotor region (MLR; Shik et al., 1966). Recordings were made with microelectrodes filled with 2 M K acetate and QX314 to block action potentials. This report gives examples of findings which are characteristic of recordings from 41 motoneurons obtained in 10 experiments. ENGs were recorded from sectioned muscle nerves with bipolar electrodes. Coherence functions were determined from data segments in which the contributing ENGs exhibited motor activity.

Coherence functions between LDPs and rectified neurograms confirm the correlations observed between pairs of ENGs. Figure 1 shows coherence functions between an LDP and the rectified ENGs of extensor motor pools, and the coherence functions for the corresponding pairs of ENGs. Partial coherence functions are shown in these and subsequent figures. Stimulating the MLR to produce fictive locomotion produces EPSPs in motoneurons (Shefchyk and Jordan, 1985) and provides a synchronizing input. However, partial coherence functions measure the correlation between two signals after removal of the linear contribution of a common signal to their correlations (Rosenberg et al., 1998). They have been used in this study to determine the correlations between neural signals produced by spinal pattern generating circuits independently of the contribution of the MLR stimulus.

The top of Fig. 1 shows that coherence functions between the ENGs of FHL and ABF or MG have significant correlation peaks through much of the spectrum. In these figures it is important to distinguish the correlations produced by moment-to-moment fluctuation in the synaptic input to the motoneuron pools from those produced by low-frequency modulation; that is, the modulation of neurogram activity and the cyclic changes in locomotor drive produced by the alternating excitation and inhibition of the locomotor drive. To estimate the contribution of this modulation to correlations evident in the coherence functions, LDPs were passed through a high-pass digital filter having a corner frequency of 16 Hz. This procedure removed the primary depolarizing-hyperpolarizing component of the LDPs, leaving the synaptic noise in the LDP (not shown). This finding indicates that the components in the coherence function above 15–20 Hz represent correlations produced by moment-to-moment fluctuations in synaptic input. Disregarding the correlations at these lower frequencies in Fig. 1, significant peaks are evident in

the range of 50 to 100–150 Hz and above, frequencies clearly above the range in which coherence can be expected from the common modulation associated with the flexor and extensor phases of locomotion. These coherence spectra suggest that motor nuclei of the hip extensor, ABF, the ankle extensor, MG, and the ankle extensor and digit plantar flexor, FHL, receive common synaptic input during fictive locomotion.

This conclusion is supported by the partial coherence functions at the bottom of the figure. In both cases, significant coherence peaks can be seen from 60 to 110–130 Hz between the LDP of a FHL motoneuron and the two ENGs. The frequency range is more limited, and the coherence peaks are smaller than in the coherence functions between

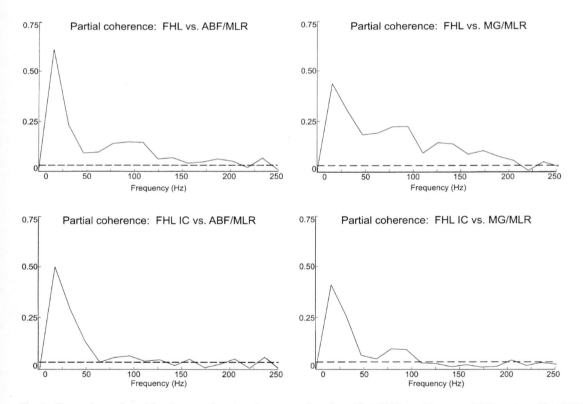

Fig. 1. Comparison of partial coherence functions between pairs of rectified ENGs and between LDPs and rectified ENGs during fictive locomotion. The figures at the top demonstrate correlations between the neurogram activity of flexor hallucis longus (FHL) and the activities of anterior biceps femoris (ABF) and medial gastrocnemius (MG). The figures at the bottom show the corresponding correlations between the locomotor drive potential in a FHL motoneuron, recorded intracellularly (FHL IC) and the neurogram activities in ABF and MG. The dashed lines in this and subsequent figures show 99% confidence limits.

neurograms. These findings are consistent with the expectation that some peaks in the coherence functions between neurograms may reflect harmonics of processes that occur at lower frequencies, rather than synaptic events. They are also consistent with the greater sensitivity expected from coherence functions computed from pairs of aggregate recordings, like neurograms, in comparison to coherence functions between unitary and aggregate recordings (Christakos, 1997).

Figure 2 shows a similar comparison for pools active during the flexor phase of the fictive step cycle. The coherence functions between neurograms show evidence for common signals to the bifunctional muscle PBF, the ankle flexor TA, and the ankle abductor PerL. Again, coherence spectra between the LDP of a PBF motoneuron and the TA and PerL neurograms confirm the presence of significant coherence peaks over a range from 30 to 100 Hz. These data suggest that motor nuclei active during the flexion phase of locomotion share common locomotor drive signals, even though they innervate muscles with actions at different joints, as do motor nuclei of the principal extensors.

Correlations between inhibitory locomotor drive and activity of antagonists

Recordings of the LDP also provide the opportunity to examine the relationship between the

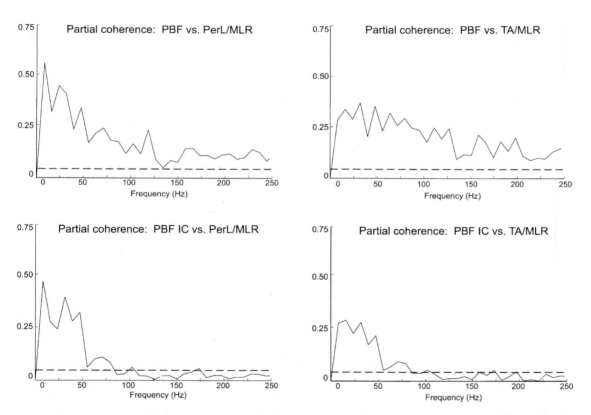

Fig. 2. Comparison of partial coherence functions between pairs of rectified ENGs and between LDPs and rectified ENGs during fictive locomotion. The figures at the top demonstrate correlations between the neurogram activity of posterior biceps femoris (PBF) and the activities of peroneus longus (PerL) and tibialis anterior (TA). The figures at the bottom show the corresponding correlations between the locomotor drive potential in a PBF motoneuron, recorded intracellularly (PBF IC) and the neurogram activities in PerL and TA.

inhibitory synaptic input to a motor pool during its inactive phase of the step cycle and the activity of its antagonists. Work by Perret (1983) and Jordan (1983) have shown that the inactive phase of an LDP in a motoneuron is a synaptic hyperpolarization, rather than the absence of excitatory input. If the interneurons that produce this inhibition share any input with motor pools that are active during this phase of locomotion, then correlations should be evident between the LDP hyperpolarization and the rectified ENGs of antagonists. Figure 3 shows an example of locomotion and corresponding coherence functions between the LDP of an MG motoneuron and the LGS and PerL neurograms. The function at the top, with LGS, was computed from data collected when this MG motoneuron was depolarized. The function shown at the bottom, with PerL, was computed from data collected when

this motoneuron was hyperpolarized. Significant coherence peaks are evident in the MG–LGS coherence function. A significant peak is also observed in coherence spectrum between the MG LDP and the neurogram activity of PerL. Comparison of the phase of these coherence functions (not shown) revealed a difference of approximately 180° over the frequency range with significant correlations; the phase of the coherence function between the MG LDP and the PerL ENG was consistent with a negative correlation plus conduction delay. These findings suggest that this MG motoneuron received inhibition from interneurons that receive common input from sources that also project to motor pools active during the flexion phase of locomotion. Similar findings during the hyperpolarizing phase of the LDP in other motoneurons suggest that interneurons that mediate the

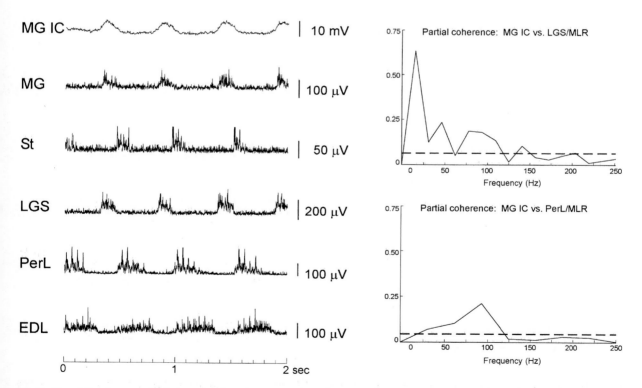

Fig. 3. Correlation between the hyperpolarizing phase of a LDP and the activity of an antagonist. A sample of fictive locomotion is shown at the left with a LDP recorded from a MG motoneuron (MG IC). Partial coherence functions demonstrate correlations between the LDP and the rectified neurogram of lateral gastrocnemius-soleus (LGS) during the depolarizing phase of the LDP (upper right), and between the LDP and the rectified neurogram of PerL during the hyperpolarizing phase of the LDP (lower right).

hyperpolarizing phase of the LDP are driven by locomotor drive that is also directed to antagonist motor nuclei.

Motor nuclei subject to independent locomotor commands

While the previous two figures demonstrate that motor pools innervating different joints share some synaptic input during fictive locomotion, not all motor nuclei receive these common synaptic inputs. Figure 4 shows an example of fictive locomotion that includes the activity of the ankle extensor and digit dorsiflexor, EDL. In this episode of locomotion, we recorded the LDP from an EDL motoneuron with neurograms from the EDL and other muscle nerves. The timing of the EDL burst is slightly different from that of TA and PerL, a finding consistent in our data. However, there is a considerable period of overlap. If we examine the partial coherence functions between this EDL LDP and the TA and PerL neurograms for data during this overlap, we find an absence of significant coherence peaks. For comparison, the top right plot

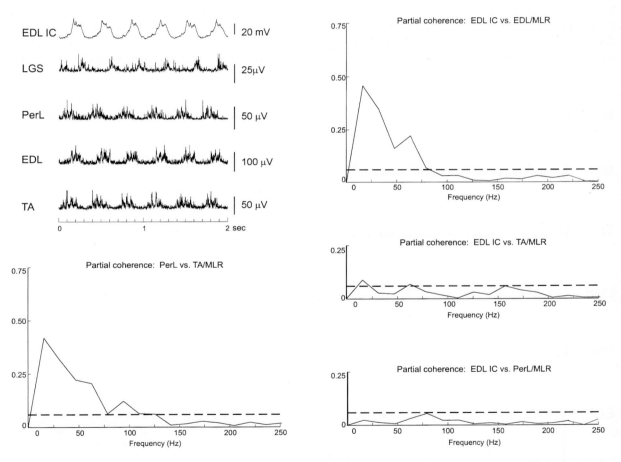

Fig. 4. Lack of correlation between the LDP of an EDL motoneuron and activity in other motor pools. A segment of fictive locomotion is shown at upper left, including the LDP recorded in an extensor digitorum longus motoneuron (EDL IC). The partial coherence functions between this LDP and the rectified ENGs of TA and PerL (lower right) show an absence of correlation, in contrast to the partial coherence functions between the EDL LDP and the rectified ENG of EDL (upper right) and between the rectified ENGs of PerL and TA.

shows the coherence between the LDP of this EDL motoneuron and the activity of the rest of the EDL motor pool, as represented by the rectified neurogram of EDL. This shows a significant coherence peak at higher frequencies between 50–80 Hz, consistent with the expectation that all motoneurons of this pool would share synaptic drive during locomotion. Also shown is the partial coherence between the PerL and TA neurograms during this episode of locomotion, which demonstrates significant coherence from 50–110 Hz, with a pattern roughly similar to that observed within the EDL motor pool.

Correlations were sometimes found between EDL and other nuclei, but they were always weaker than those found between other pairs of coactive motor nuclei. These observations suggest that EDL does not receive the common locomotor commands to the extent that other motor pools do. Based on coherence spectra between neurogram pairs, we have also observed that activity of the digit plantar flexor FDL is poorly correlated with other motoneuron pools. Thus, while most motor pools active in either the extensor or flexor phase of locomotion receive a common locomotor drive, EDL and FDL appear to be subject to a differentiated set of commands.

Summary and conclusions

The patterns of correlation found between motoneuron pools during fictive locomotion are the same whether the coherence functions used to detect the correlations are determined using pairs of rectified ENGs or motoneuron LDPs and rectified ENGs. This finding suggests that the higher frequencies in rectified ENGs (and, perhaps, EMGs) contain information about the synaptic input to motoneurons. Nevertheless, differences between the coherence functions of rectified ENG pairs and those of LDPs and rectified ENGs suggests that this information is distorted by harmonics introduced by rectification.

The activities of many motoneuron pools are correlated during the flexor or extensor phase of fictive locomotion, indicating that they receive common synaptic input from branched presynaptic axons or from pools of interneurons whose activities are synchronized. Similar findings were reported by Bayev (1978), based on temporal correlations. Our results indicate that the investigated motor nuclei, which innervate muscles with actions at the hip, knee and ankle, are subject to a set of common locomotor commands. These commands are also received by inhibitory interneurons that project to the motor nuclei of antagonists, as indicated by the correlations between the hyperpolarizing phase of LDPs and activity in the rectified ENGs of antagonists. This last result is consistent with a modular organization for the spinal locomotor generator, in which one set of interneurons drives a motor pool and the inhibitory interneurons that project to the motor pool's antagonist (Jordan, 1991). However, these results also suggest that the spinal modules for locomotion may not be separable into independent unit-burst generators that produce commands for control of each joint as Grillner (1981) has suggested. Our results are more consistent with a model in which a generator distributes flexor and extensor commands to many motor pools (like the half-center model) with as yet unidentified spinal mechanisms that determine differences in the initiation and termination of activity of individual motor nuclei. Alternatively, the correlations between motor pools that we have observed could be explained by spinal mechanisms that synchronize the activity of unit-burst type generators.

Despite the distribution of common locomotor commands to many functionally diverse motor nuclei, the spinal locomotor pattern generator is differentiated to the extent that some motor nuclei, like EDL and FDL, receive separate locomotor commands. This conclusion is consistent with other observations. EDL and FDL display distinctive, individualized patterns of locomotor activity that may vary in a facultative manner or in different forms of locomotion (O'Donovan et al., 1980; Trank et al., 1996). A recent study has shown that during fictive locomotion EDL and FDL motoneurons receive input from different sets of last-order interneurons than those which project to other motor pools (Degtyarenko et al., 1998). These results suggest that spinal locomotor generators are differentiated for the individualized control of some digit muscles, like FDL and EDL.

338

Acknowledgements

We thank Ms. Tracy Fleming for her excellent technical assistance and Dr. Mitchell Maltenfort for his comments on this manuscript. This work was supported by USPHS grant NS22454 to T. M. Hamm and NS07309 to the Motor Control Neurobiology Training Program at the University of Arizona, Barrow Neurological Institute, and Arizona State University.

List of abbreviations

ABF	Anterior biceps femoris
EDL	Extensor digitorum longus
EMG	Electromyogram
ENG	Electroneurogram
FDL	Flexor digitorum longus
FHL	Flexor hallucis longus
IC	Intracellular
LDP	Locomotor drive potential
LGS	Lateral gastrocnemius – soleus
MG	Medial gastrocnemius
MLR	Mesencephalic locomotor region
PerL	Peroneus longus
PBF	Posterior biceps femoris
St	Semitendinosus
TA	Tibialis anterior

References

Bayev, K.V. (1978) Central locomotor program for the cat's hindlimb. *Neuroscience*, 3: 1081–1092.

Brown, T.G. (1911) The intrinsic factors in the act of progression in the mammal. *Proc. Roy. Soc. B.*, 84: 308–319.

Christakos, C.N. (1997) On the detection and measurement of synchrony in neural populations by coherence analysis. *J. Neurophysiol.*, 78: 3453–3459.

Cope, T.C., Fetz, E.E. and Matsumura, M. (1987) Cross-correlation assessment of synaptic strength of single Ia fibre connections with triceps surae motoneurones in cats. *J. Physiol. (Lond.)*, 390: 161–188.

Degtyarenko, A.M., Simon, E.S. and Burke, R.E. (1998) Locomotor modulation of disynaptic EPSPs from the mesencephalic locomotor region in cat motoneurons. *J. Neurophysiol.*, 80: 3284–3296.

Farmer, S.F., Bremner, F.D., Halliday, D.M., Rosenberg, J.R. and Stephens, J.A. (1993) The frequency content of common synaptic inputs to motoneurones studied during voluntary isometric contraction in man. *J. Physiol. (Lond.)*, 470: 127–155.

Fetz, E.E. and Cheney, P.D. (1980) Postspike facilitation of forelimb muscle activity by primate corticomotoneuronal cells. *J. Neurophysiol.*, 44: 751–772.

Fuglevand, A.J., Winter, D.A. and Patla, A.E. (1993) Models of recruitment and rate coding organization in motor-unit pools. *J. Neurophysiol.*, 70: 2470–2488.

Grillner, S. (1981) Control of locomotion in bipeds, tetrapods, and fish. In: V.B. Brooks (Ed.), *Handbook of Physiology*, Sec. 1, Vol. II, Pt. 2, *The Nervous System: Motor Control*, American Physiological Society, Bethesda, pp. 1179–1236.

Hamm, T.M. and McCurdy, M.L. (1996) The use of coherence spectra to determine common synaptic inputs to motoneurone pools of the cat during fictive locomotion. In: A. Taylor, M.H. Gladden and R. Durbaba (Eds), *Alpha and Gamma Motor Systems*, Plenum, New York, pp. 309–315.

Hoffer, J.A., Sugano, N., Loeb, G.E., Marks, W.B., O'Donovan, M.J. and Pratt, C.A. (1987) Cat hindlimb motoneurons during locomotion. II. Normal activity patterns. *J. Neurophysiol.*, 57: 530–553.

Jordan, L.M. (1983) Factors determining motoneuron rhythmicity during fictive locomotion. In: A. Roberts and B.L. Roberts (Eds), *Neural Origin of Rhythmic Movements. Symposia of the Society for Experimental Biology*, Cambridge University Press, London, pp. 423–444.

Jordan, L.M. (1991) Brainstem and spinal cord mechanisms for the initiation of locomotion. In: M. Shimamura, S. Grillner and V.R. Edgerton (Eds), *Neurobiological Basis of Human Locomotion*, Japan Scientific Societies Press, Tokyo, pp. 3–20.

Kirkwood, P.A. and Sears, T.A. (1982) The effects of single afferent impulses on the probability of firing of external intercostal motoneurones in the cat. *J. Physiol. (Lond.)*, 322: 315–336.

Moore, G.P., Segundo, J.P., Perkel, D.H. and Levitan, H. (1970) Statistical signs of synaptic interaction in neurons. *Biophys. J.*, 10: 876–900.

O'Donovan, M.J., Pinter, M.J., Dum, R.P. and Burke, R.E. (1982) Actions of FDL and FHL muscles in intact cats: functional dissociation between anatomical synergists. *J. Neurophysiol.*, 47: 1126–1143.

Perret, C. (1983) Centrally generated pattern of motoneuron activity during locomotion in the cat. In: A. Roberts and B.L. Roberts (Eds), *Neural Origin of Rhythmic Movements. Symposia of the Society for Experimental Biology*, Cambridge University Press, London, pp. 405–422.

Rosenberg, J.R., Amjad, A.M., Breeze, P., Brillinger, D.R. and Halliday, D.M. (1989) The Fourier approach to the identification of functional coupling between neuronal spike trains. *Prog. Biophys. Molec. Biol.*, 53: 1–31.

Rosenberg, J.R., Halliday, D.M., Breeze, P. and Conway, B.A. (1998) Identification of patterns of neuronal connectivity – partial spectra, partial coherence, and neuronal interactions. *J. Neurosci. Meth.*, 83: 57–72.

Sears, T.A. and Stagg, D. (1976) Short-term synchronization of intercostal motoneurone activity. *J. Physiol. (Lond.)*, 263: 357–381.

Shefchyk, S.J. and Jordan, L.M. (1985) Excitatory and inhibitory postsynaptic potentials in alpha-motoneurons produced during fictive locomotion by stimulation of the mesencephalic locomotor region. *J. Neurophysiol.*, 53: 1345–1355.

Shik, M.L., Severin, F.V. and Orlovskii, G.N. (1966) Control of walking and running by means of electrical stimulation of the mid-brain. *Biophysics*, 11: 659–666.

Smith, J.L., Carlson-Kuhta, P. and Trank, T.V. (1998) Forms of forward quadrupedal locomotion. III. A comparison of posture, hindlimb kinematics, and motor patterns for down-slope and level walking. *J. Neurophysiol.*, 79: 1702–1716.

Trank, T.V., Chen, C. and Smith, J.L. (1996) Forms of forward quadrupedal locomotion. I. A comparison of posture, hindlimb kinematics, and motor patterns for normal and crouched walking. *J. Neurophysiol.*, 76: 2316–2326.

Turkin, V. and Hamm, T.M. (1996) Patterns of synchronization among hindlimb motor nuclei during fictive locomotion in the cat. *Soc. Neurosci.*, Abstr., 22: 1841.

M.D. Binder (Ed.)
Progress in Brain Research, Vol 123

CHAPTER 30

Failure analysis of stepping in adult spinal cats

R. D. de Leon,[1,*] N.J.S. London,[1] R. R. Roy[2] and V. R. Edgerton[1,2]

[1] *Department of Physiological Science, UCLA, Los Angeles, CA 90095, USA*
[2] *Brain Research Institute, UCLA, Los Angeles, CA 90095, USA*

Introduction

Adult cats that receive complete spinal cord transections can regain the ability to perform bipedal hindlimb locomotion on a treadmill (Lovely et al., 1986, 1990; Barbeau and Rossignol, 1987; Belanger et al., 1996; de Leon et al., 1998). Further, locomotor recovery is enhanced by daily training of the hindlimbs on a motorized treadmill (Lovely et al., 1986, 1990; Barbeau and Rossignol, 1987; de Guzman et al., 1991; Hodgson et al., 1994; Belanger et al., 1996; Chau et al., 1998; de Leon et al., 1998). Spinal cats that do not receive treadmill training recover poor locomotor ability relative to step-trained spinal cats (Lovely et al., 1986; de Leon et al., 1998). Non-trained spinal cats stumble frequently and thus are unable to maintain long stepping sequences (de Leon et al., 1998). Deficits in the range of flexion and extension movements performed by a single hindlimb contribute to the poor locomotor performances observed after spinalization. Insufficient flexion of the hindlimb, for instance, results in dragging of the paw during the swing phase of stepping (Belanger et al., 1996; de Leon et al., 1998). As a result, the kinematic pattern during forward movement is disrupted (de Leon et al., 1999a). Training the spinal cats to step enhances the lift of the hindlimb during late swing, thereby allowing the successful execution of a step cycle (de Leon et al., 1999a).

The importance of interlimb coordination in the successful execution of stepping in spinal cats has not been examined thoroughly. Forssberg and colleagues (1980) reported that the hindlimb coordination patterns in cats transected at one or two weeks of age resembled that found in normal animals. The hindlimbs moved in an alternating pattern, i.e. an event in one limb was delayed by half a step cycle with the same event in the contralateral limb, during treadmill locomotion ($< 1.0 \text{ ms}^{-1}$; Forssberg et al., 1980). Similarly, Grillner and Rossignol (1978) demonstrated that the relative movements in the two hindlimbs of spinal cats (transected one or two weeks after birth) tended to occur in predictable patterns. Swing was initiated in one limb when the contralateral limb was either in midstance (walking) or in midswing (galloping) (Grillner and Rossignol, 1978). These findings indicate that sensory information from the contralateral limb plays a role in the generation of ipsilateral limb movements during spinally-mediated locomotion. However, the extent that the coordination between ipsilateral and contralateral limbs impacts the success or failure of spinal cats to execute a step cycle remains unclear.

In the present study, we examined whether the patterns of hindlimb coordination during locomotion in adult cats was altered after the cats received a complete low-thoracic spinal cord transection. In addition, to determine if training improved stepping in spinal cats by normalizing hindlimb coordination, stepping was compared before and after spinalization in spinal cats that received treadmill

*Corresponding author. Tel.: (310) 825–4672; Fax: (310) 206–9184; e-mail: rdeleon@ucla.edu

training and in spinal cats that received no training after spinalization. The present findings demonstrate that abnormal patterns of hindlimb coordination are a major cause of step failures, i.e. stumbling, during stepping in spinal cats. Furthermore, treadmill training improved hindlimb coordination sufficiently to maintain successful stepping, but did not restore the pre-spinal pattern of hindlimb coordination.

Changes in hindlimb coordination after spinalization affect the ability of spinal cats to step

To determine if hindlimb coordination affects the ability to successfully execute stepping after spinalization we examined treadmill locomotion in eight adult female cats before and after they received a complete spinal cord transection (T12–T13; for details see Roy et al., 1992). Four of the cats received daily treadmill training beginning one week after spinalization while the remaining four cats served as spinal, non-trained controls. The ability to perform treadmill stepping was tested 12 weeks after spinalization. The spinal cats that did not receive treadmill training were unable to consistently execute full weight-bearing step cycles. Stepping sequences were only briefly maintained before the hindlimbs stumbled and the hindquarters collapsed (de Leon et al., 1998). The number of steps performed by the non-trained spinal cats declined significantly relative to the number of steps performed before spinalization (Fig. 1).

We analyzed the kinematic patterns in the two hindlimbs before and after spinalization and found that the relative movements of the two hindlimbs changed after the cats were spinal transected. Before spinalization, the hindlimbs moved in an alternating pattern during stepping at a moderate treadmill speed (0.4 ms^{-1}), i.e. swing occurred in the ipsilateral limb while the contralateral limb executed stance. Moreover, there was a consistent order in which ipsilateral swing and contralateral stance were executed. Swing was initiated after the contralateral limb was well into the stance phase of the step cycle (Fig. 2A). This order was observed in all of the pre-spinal step cycles (Fig. 3A).

The pattern of coordination of the two hindlimbs was altered after spinalization. Although a normal order of events was preserved during successfully-executed step cycles, swing began in the ipsilateral limb shortly after the contralateral limb made contact with the treadmill belt (Fig. 2B). A shorter mean interval was measured between the onsets of ipsilateral swing and contralateral stance after (0.11 ± 0.005 s) relative to before spinalization (0.17 ± 0.007 s) in the non-trained spinal cats as well as in the spinal cats that received treadmill training (Fig. 3B). Thus, the period in which the two hindlimbs supported the weight of the hindquarters, i.e. bilateral support, decreased after spinalization (Fig. 2B).

The greatest changes in hindlimb coordination were observed in the failed step cycles of the spinal cats. Ipsilateral swing and contralateral stance began simultaneously (mean interval: 0.02 ± 0.009 s; Fig. 3C). Moreover, in half of the failed step cycles a reversal in the sequence of events

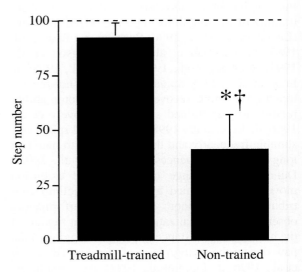

Fig. 1. Performance of bipedal hindlimb stepping on a treadmill following spinalization in treadmill-trained and non-trained cats. The average number of steps performed during 45 s of testing (0.4 ms^{-1}) in four treadmill-trained and four non-trained cats are shown 12 weeks after spinalization. The horizontal line indicates the average number of steps observed during pre-spinalization tests of stepping in the same cats. Bars, standard errors of the mean. * †, significantly different from pre-spinal or treadmill-trained, respectively ($p \leqslant 0.05$).

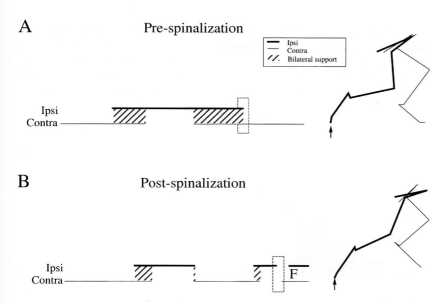

A   Pre-spinalization

Ipsi
Contra

B   Post-spinalization

Ipsi
Contra

Fig. 2. Schematic and stick figure diagrams depicting hindlimb coordination before spinalization (A) and 12 weeks after spinalization (B). In the schematic diagram, stance duration for a sequence of steps is represented by the horizontal lines while swing duration is represented by the area between successive lines. Overlapping lines between the ipsilateral and contralateral limbs represent periods of bilateral support, i.e. both limbs supporting the weight of the body. Stick figures depict the positions of the ipsilateral (thick line) and contralateral (thin lines) hindlimbs during ipsilateral toe off in the cycles that are indicated by boxes in the schematic diagram. Upward arrows, toe off; F, failed step cycle.

occurred, i.e. swing was initiated before the contralateral limb was weight-bearing (see F in Fig. 2B; Fig. 3C). Flexion in the contralateral limb was prolonged at the end of swing and the limb briefly hung in the air (see stick figure in Fig. 2B). Meanwhile, swing in the ipsilateral limb was delayed and the limb was extended beyond the normal range of extension during late stance (see stick figure in Fig. 2B; Fig. 4). When swing eventually was triggered, neither limb was positioned appropriately to support the weight of the hindquarters. The dorsum of the ipsilateral paw dragged forward and the limb collapsed under the weight of the hindquarters (Fig. 5A). Stumbling in this manner occurred in 95% of the failures that were observed during post-spinal stepping in the treadmill-trained and non-trained cats.

Step training improves hindlimb coordination but does not restore gait patterns within the normal range of variability

The treadmill trained spinal cats performed a greater number of full weight-bearing steps than the non-trained spinal cats (Fig. 1) and maintained long (>45 steps) sequences of stepping at moderate treadmill speeds. We examined the coordination of the hindlimbs during stepping sequences in treadmill-trained and non-trained spinal cats to determine if the superior locomotor performance observed in the treadmill-trained spinal cats was due to their ability to perform consistent, well-coordinated movements in the two hindlimbs. In the absence of treadmill training, the coordination of the hindlimbs varied widely when the animals executed a sequence of full weight-bearing stepping. The interval between ipsilateral toe-off and contralateral paw contact was shorter after than before spinalization (Fig. 6A). After the initial step, coordination progressively worsened as the onsets of ipsilateral swing and contralateral stance occurred more synchronously and a step failure occurred when there was a simultaneous onset of swing and stance or when a reversal in the order of events occurred (see F in Fig. 6A).

The treadmill-trained spinal cats exhibited a more normal pattern of hindlimb movement than the non-trained spinal cats (Fig. 6B). However, even in the treadmill-trained spinal cats, the interval between ipsilateral toe-off and contralateral paw contact was often shorter after spinalization and was not consistently maintained during stepping (Fig. 6B). Similar to that observed in the non-trained spinal cats, ipsilateral toe-off and contralateral paw contact occurred close together during some step cycles (see Step cycle 6, Fig. 6B). Occasionally, simultaneous onset or reversal in the

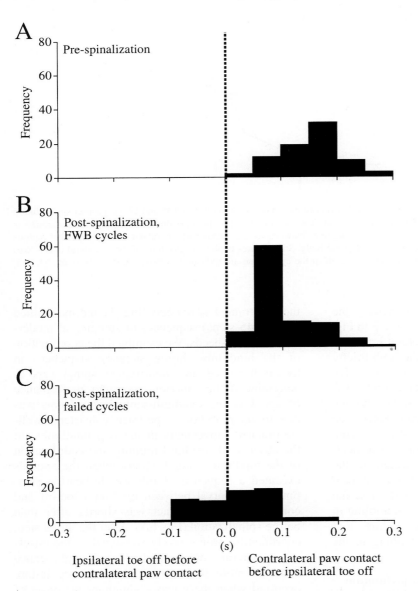

Fig. 3. Histograms of the interval between ipsilateral toe off and contralateral paw contact during pre-spinal (A), post-spinal full weight-bearing (FWB) (B) and post-spinal failed (C) step cycles. The vertical dashed line indicates an interval of 0 s, i.e. simultaneous ipsilateral toe off and contralateral paw contact. Pre-spinal and post-spinal (12 weeks after spinalization) data were collected from eight cats. The number of step cycles was 79, 104 and 68 for the pre-spinal, post-spinal full weight-bearing and post-spinal failed cycles, respectively (8–15 cycles/cat).

345

order of ipsilateral toe-off and contralateral paw contact occurred and the gait was destabilized. Treadmill-trained cats avoided stumbling, however, by flexing the knee and ankle to lift the paw (Fig. 5B). After the initial misstep, hindlimb movements were adjusted to recover stable gait patterns, i.e. longer intervals between ipsilateral toe-off and contralateral paw contact were recovered within

1–2 cycles following a poorly-coordinated step (see Step cycles 6–8, Fig. 6B).

Why do spinal cats stumble when they walk?

The present findings suggest that the coordination of motor pools between the two hindlimbs is important in determining the ability of spinal cats to execute weight-bearing stepping on a treadmill. Previous studies have demonstrated that stepping in spinal cats is disrupted when one hindlimb stumbles during the execution of a step. The cause of the misstep has been attributed most often to an inability to adequately lift the paw during swing causing the paw to drag on the dorsal surface (Eidelberg et al., 1980; Lovely et al., 1986; Robinson and Goldberger, 1986; de Leon et al., 1998). When paw contact occurs on the dorsal rather than the plantar surface of the paw, it is not appropriately positioned for weight support and the

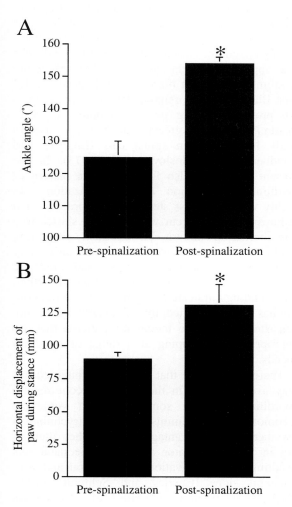

Fig. 4. Ankle angle (A) and paw displacement (B) during stepping before and 12 weeks after spinalization. Ankle angle at toe off and horizontal displacement of the paw from midswing to toe off were measured from 8–10 cycles of full weight-bearing bipedal hindlimb stepping (0.4 ms^{-1}) before and 12 weeks after spinalization. Mean ± standard errors for eight cats are shown. *, significantly different than pre-spinalization ($p \leq 0.01$).

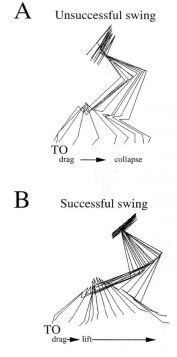

Fig. 5. Stick figure representation of the hindlimb during swing of a collapsed step cycle (A) and a successful step cycle (B) in one spinal cat. The arrow indicates the progression of movement of the limb starting with toe off (TO).

hindquarters collapse (Lovely et al., 1986; de Leon et al., 1998). Based on the present findings, deficits in intralimb movements during stepping in the spinal cat are linked to abnormal coordination patterns in the two hindlimbs. Poorly-coordinated hindlimb movements exacerbate the paw dragging and dorsal stepping which, in turn, disrupts weight-bearing stepping (Fig. 5A). We conclude that step failures in spinal cats occur primarily because the locomotor-generating spinal networks are unable to

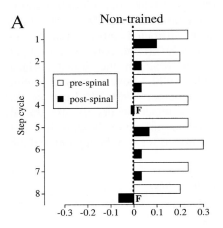

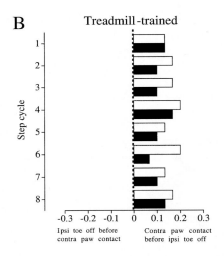

Fig. 6. The interval between ipsilateral toe off and contralateral paw contact during an 8-step sequence in one representative non-trained cat (A) and one representative treadmill-trained cat (B), before (open bars) and 12 weeks after (filled bars) spinalization. The vertical dashed line indicates an interval of 0 s, i.e. simultaneous ipsilateral toe off and contralateral paw contact.

consistently coordinate intralimb and interlimb movements during treadmill-induced locomotion.

Variability in hindlimb coordination has been previously reported to destabilize the locomotor gait of spinal cats (Eidelberg et al., 1980). Gait patterns shifted frequently when spinal kittens stepped at constant treadmill speeds (Grillner, 1973; Forssberg et al., 1980). Within a few step cycles, the patterns changed from alternating hindlimb movements to various forms of in-phase movements, e.g. galloping (Forssberg et al., 1980). Disorganized movements between the hindlimbs also appear to prevent spinal cats from executing hindlimb stepping at high treadmill speeds (> 1.2 m/s; Barbeau and Rossignol, 1987). In-phase gaits are prevalent during normal stepping at faster treadmill speeds, i.e. greater than the speeds used to study locomotion in spinal cats (Engberg and Lundberg, 1969; Goslow et al., 1973). In the present study, we also found that the pattern of hindlimb coordination after spinalization was highly variable across step cycles. Moreover, step failures tended to occur when the gait shifted to a non-alternating pattern. In contrast, alternating hindlimb movements were observed consistently when the cats stepped at slow and moderate treadmill speeds before spinalization. Together, these findings indicate that when supraspinal control has been eliminated, the spinal networks do not consistently generate locomotor patterns that are appropriate for stepping at a range of treadmill speeds.

There is evidence that glycinergic interneurons play a critical role in the ipsilateral-contralateral coordination during some forms of vertebrate locomotion. The administration of strychnine, a glycinergic receptor antagonist, abolishes alternating in vitro locomotor activity in neonatal rats resulting in a coactivation of ipsilateral and contralateral sides (Cowley and Schmidt, 1995). Contralateral rhythmic inhibition of motoneurons during in vitro neonatal rat locomotion also is abolished by strychnine (Kjaerulff and Kiehn, 1997). We have recently examined the effects of strychnine on hindlimb locomotion in adult spinal cats (de Leon et al. 1999b; Edgerton et al., 1997a,b). Strychnine induced weight-bearing hindlimb stepping in spinal cats that were unable to consistently execute stepping prior to the administration of strychnine. Although these findings suggest that the levels of glycinergic inhibition are related to locomotor recovery, it is unclear if the deficits in hindlimb coordination are due to impaired activation of the glycinergic spinal pathways which control ipsilateral and contralateral hindlimb movements.

It is unlikely that step failures were caused by hindlimb muscle fatigue or other properties of the hindlimb musculature. The amount of force that can be generated in the hindlimb muscles of treadmill-trained and non-trained spinal cats is not significantly different, based on muscle mass and twitch and tetanic tension characteristics (Roy and Acosta, 1986; Roy et al., 1991, 1998, 1999). In addition, the non-fatigable properties of the soleus muscle, the primary slow extensor of the ankle, were maintained after spinalization in both the trained and non-trained cats (Roy et al., 1991, 1998). These findings suggest that the inability to produce sufficient levels of force in the muscles was not a factor in determining the frequency of step failures occurring after spinalization. Rather, the ability to successfully execute stepping after spinalization depended on how well the spinal networks were able to activate hindlimb motor pools in correct spatiotemporal patterns.

Novel locomotor strategies to execute stepping after spinalization are acquired with treadmill training

Treadmill training did not fully restore the prespinal pattern of hindlimb coordination during locomotion in the present study. This result is consistent with other findings that some of the characteristics of stepping in intact cats are not regained in spinal cats even after the trained spinal cats have recovered full weight-bearing stepping. For example, drag and lift of the paw during swing persist in spinal cats following years of training (Belanger et al., 1996; de Leon et al., 1998). To overcome drag, treadmill-trained spinal cats exhibit greater than normal levels of flexion during swing (de Leon et al., 1998). Treadmill-trained spinal cats in the present study performed poorly-coordinated step cycles but avoided step failures more often that the non-trained spinal cats by adjusting hindlimb movements to enhance flexion and to recover a stable gait. Thus, rather than recovering normal locomotor kinematics, the spinal networks acquired a novel motor strategy to generate and maintain locomotion in the absence of supraspinal input.

It is likely that the acquisition of novel gait patterns involves the ability of the spinal networks to utilize various sources of sensory input to drive locomotion. Load-related and proprioceptive sensory input are important factors in generating spinal locomotion. Unloading the hindlimb signals the termination of stance in cats and the beginning of the air-borne phase of the step cycle, i.e. the swing phase (Duysens and Pearson, 1980). If, however, the load is prolonged at the end of stance, the initiation of swing is delayed (Duysens and Pearson, 1980). The onset of swing also is determined by the extent that the hip is extended at the end of stance. Flexion is triggered in spinal cats after a critical hip angle (~90 degrees) has been reached (Grillner and Rossignol, 1978). The present findings indicate that contralateral sensory input also contributes to the generation of stepping in spinal cats. For example, prolonging the onset of weight bearing in the contralateral hindlimb delayed the initiation of swing in the ipsilateral limb, even after the ipsilateral limb was extended beyond normal. Thus, it is evident that in order to generate stable locomotor patterns, the spinal networks must interpret multiple sensory inputs and effectively integrate this afferent information with the central programs that control stepping. We conclude that repetitively activating sensory and motor pathways through training enhances the synaptic efficacy within these pathways such that novel strategies are acquired to execute stepping in the absence of supraspinal input.

References

Barbeau, H. and Rossignol, S. (1987) Recovery of locomotion after chronic spinalization in the adult cat. *Brain Res.*, 412: 84–95.
Belanger, M., Drew, T., Provencher, J. and Rossignol, S. (1996) A comparison of treadmill locomotion in adult cats before and after spinal transection. *J. Neurophysiol.* 76: 471–491.

Chau, C., Barbeau, H. and Rossignol, S. (1998) Early locomotor training with clonidine in spinal cats. *J. Neurophysiol.*, 79: 392–409.

Cowley, K.C. and Schmidt, B.J. (1995) Effects of inhibitory amino acid antagonists on reciprocal inhibitory interactions during rhythmic motor activity in the in vitro neonatal rat spinal cord. *J. Neurophysiol.*, 74: 1109–1117.

de Guzman, C.P., Roy, R.R., Hodgson, J.A. and Edgerton, V.R. (1991) Coordination of motor pools controlling the ankle musculature in adult spinal cats during treadmill walking. *Brain Res.*, 555: 202–214.

de Leon, R.D., Hodgson, J.A., Roy, R.R. and Edgerton, V.R. (1998) Locomotor capacity attributable to step training vs. spontaneous recovery following spinalization in cats. *J. Neurophysiol.*, 79: 1329–1340.

de Leon, R.D., Hodgson, J.A., Roy, R.R. and Edgerton, V.R. (1999a) The retention of hindlimb stepping ability in adult spinal cats after the cessation of step training. *J. Neurophysiol.*, 81: 85–94.

de Leon, R.D., Tamaki, H., Hodgson, J.A., Roy, R.R. and Edgerton, V.R. (1999b) Hindlimb locomotor and postural training modulates glycinergic inhibition in the spinal cord of the adult spinal cat. *J. Neurophysiol.*, 82: 359–369.

Duysens, J.D. and Pearson, K.G. (1980) Inhibition of flexor burst generation by loading ankle extensor muscles in walking cats. *Brain Res.*, 187: 321–332.

Eidelberg, E., Story, J.L., Meyer, B.L. and Nystel, J. (1980) Stepping by chronic spinal cats. *Exp. Brain Res.*, 40: 241–246.

Engberg, I. and Lundberg, A. (1969) An electromyographic analysis of muscular activity in the hindlimb of the cat during unrestrained locomotion. *Acta Physiol. Scand.*, 75: 614–630.

Edgerton, V.R., de Leon, R.D., Tillakaratne, N., Recktenwald, M.R., Hodgson, J.A. and Roy, R.R. (1997a) Use-dependent plasticity in spinal stepping and standing. In: F.J. Seil (Ed.), *Advances in Neurology: Neuronal Regeneration, Reorganization and Repair*, Philadelphia, Lippincott-Raven Publishers, pp. 233–247.

Edgerton, V.R., Roy, R.R., de Leon, R., Tillakaratne N. and Hodgson, J.A. (1997b) Does motor learning occur in the spinal cord? *Neuroscientist*, 3: 287–294.

Forssberg, H., Grillner, S., Halbertsma, J. and Rossignol, S. (1980) The locomotion of the low spinal cat. II. Interlimb coordination. *Acta Physiol. Scand.*, 108: 283–295.

Goslow, G.E., Reinking, R.M. and Stuart, D.G. (1973) The cat step cycle: hind limb joint angles and muscle lengths during unrestrained locomotion. *J. Morphol.*, 141: 1–41.

Grillner, S. (1973) Locomotion in the spinal cat. In: R.B. Stein, K.G. Pearson, R.S. Smith and J.B. Redford (Eds), *Control of Posture and Locomotion*, Plenum Press, New York, pp. 515–535.

Grillner, S. and Rossignol, S. (1978) On the initiation of the swing phase of locomotion in chronic spinal cats. *Brain Res.*, 146: 269–277.

Hodgson, J.A., Roy, R.R., de Leon, R., Dobkin, B. and Edgerton, V.R. (1994) Can the mammalian lumbar spinal cord learn a motor task? *Med. Sci. Sports Exerc.*, 26: 1491–1497.

Kjaerulff, O. and Kiehn, O. (1997) Crossed rhythmic synaptic input to motoneurons during selective activation of the contralateral spinal locomotor network. *J. Neurosci.*, 17: 9433–9447.

Lovely, R.G., Gregor, R.G., Roy, R.R. and Edgerton, V.R. (1986) Effects of training on the recovery of full-weight-bearing stepping in the adult spinal cat. *Exp. Neurol.*, 92: 421–435.

Lovely, R.G., Gregor, R.J., Roy, R.R. and Edgerton, V.R. (1990) Weight-bearing hindlimb stepping in treadmill-exercised adult spinal cats. *Brain Res.*, 514: 206–218.

Robinson, G.A. and Goldberger, M.E. (1986) The development and recovery of motor function in spinal cats. I. The infant lesion effect. *Exp. Brain Res.*, 62: 373–386.

Roy, R.R. and Acosta, L. (1986) Fiber type and fiber size changes in selected thigh muscles six months after low thoracic spinal cord transection in adult cats: exercise effects. *Exp. Neurol.*, 92: 675–685.

Roy, R.R., Baldwin, K.M. and Edgerton, V.R. (1991) The plasticity of skeletal muscle: effects of neuromuscular activity. In: J.O. Holloszy (Ed.), *Exercise and Sport Science Reviews*, vol. 19. Baltimore, Williams and Wilkins, pp. 269–312.

Roy, R.R., Hodgson, J.A., Lauretz, S.D., Pierotti, D.J., Gayek, R.J. and Edgerton, V.R. (1992) Chronic spinal cord-injured cats: surgical procedures and management. *Lab. Anim. Sci.*, 42: 335–343.

Roy, R.R., Talmadge, R.J., Hodgson, J.A., Zhong, H., Baldwin, K.M. and Edgerton, V.R. (1998) Training effects on soleus of cats spinal cord transected (T12–13) as adults. *Muscle & Nerve*, 21: 63–71.

Roy, R.R., Talmadge, R.J., Hodgson, J.A., Oishi, Y., Baldwin, K.M. and Edgerton, V.R. (1999) Differential response of fast hindlimb extensor and flexor muscles to exercise in cats spinalized as adults. *Muscle & Nerve*, 22: 230–241.

M.D. Binder (Ed.)
Progress in Brain Research, Vol 123

Locomotor performance and adaptation after partial or complete spinal cord lesions in the cat

S. Rossignol,* T. Drew, E. Brustein and W. Jiang

Centre de recherche en sciences neurologiques, Université de Montréal, Montréal, PQ, Canada

Introduction

Much of our information on the role of various structures of the central nervous system in the regulation of different aspects of locomotion in the cat has come from studies based on micro-stimulation, unit recordings or acute ablations (reviewed in: Shik and Orlovsky, 1976; Grillner, 1981; Armstrong, 1986; Gelfand et al., 1988; Grillner and Dubuc, 1988; Pearson, 1993; Rossignol and Dubuc, 1994; Rossignol, 1996). Less attention has been paid to the performance and functional reorganization of locomotor control after *chronic* lesions of these central structures. In part, this may be because interpretation of the results of such studies is problematic in that it has to take into consideration that the consequences of the lesion on the expression of the remaining functions is a mixture of deficits due to the removed structures as well as to compensation by other structures. Nevertheless, some indication of the degree of compensation can be obtained by comparing the short and long term locomotor performance. In the short term, the deficits represent the uncompensated state and give some indication of the normal role of a given structure in the control of locomotion. Later on, after maximal compensation has

taken place, the remaining permanent behavioral deficits give a fair indication of the essential contributions of the ablated structures as well as the limits of other structures to replace, totally or in part, the function of the missing structures. Such an understanding of how the nervous system optimizes the expression of essential motor functions, such as locomotion, following lesions is important because it sheds light both on the contribution of different structures to the normal control of locomotion as well as on the physiopathological mechanisms responsible for functional recovery.

In this chapter we will summarize the results of our different studies in which the locomotor performance of chronically instrumented cats was documented before and after either partial or complete spinal lesions. We will discuss some of the kinematic and electromyographic (EMG) changes that occur during ordinary treadmill locomotion and will briefly describe how these lesioned cats adapt their locomotion to more demanding situations (slopes, tilts and obstacles). Finally, we will correlate these changes with current knowledge on the function of different supraspinal structures in the control of locomotion obtained from unit recording and microstimulation studies.

Partial spinal lesions

The first section of this review concentrates on the consequences of partial lesions of the ventromedial and ventrolateral funiculi of the spinal cord on the

---
*Corresponding author. Tel.: 514–343–6366 or 6371; Fax: 514–343–6113;
e-mail: rossigno@ere.umontreal.ca;
Internet: http://www.cam.org/ ~ cyrd/CRSN

locomotor capacities of cats and briefly discusses the deficits and functional recovery that were observed in these animals. The deficits observed in these animals are then compared to those seen in cats with partial lesions of the dorsolateral funiculi (DLF); a brief section on the effects of hemisections of the spinal cord is also included; a selected list of references pertaining to different types of partial lesions can be found in Table 1.

Ventral and ventrolateral pathways

The results of partial acute or chronic lesions of the spinal cord suggest a very important role for the ventral and ventrolateral pathways in the control of locomotion (Eidelberg, 1981). Although it was originally claimed that sparing of at least a small part of one ventrolateral quadrant was essential for recovery of locomotion in both cats (Afelt, 1974; Eidelberg et al., 1981a; Contamin, 1983) and monkeys (Eidelberg et al., 1981b), a number of more recent studies have shown that both of these species (cats: Gorska et al., 1990, 1993a, 1993b; Zmyslowski et al., 1993; Bem et al., 1995; Brustein and Rossignol, 1998, 1999; monkeys: Vilensky et al., 1992) can walk quadrupedally even after severe damage to the ventral and ventrolateral pathways at the lower thoracic level (T_{11}–T_{13}). Our recent work (Brustein and Rossignol, 1998, 1999) on chronically implanted cats showed that the locomotor deficits observed after such lesions depend largely

on the size of the lesion and the time of observation after the lesion. With relatively small unilateral or bilateral lesions, cats recuperated quadrupedal locomotion rapidly so that within 1–3 days their locomotor performance, as documented by EMG and kinematic analyses, was largely indistinguishable from that of the pre-lesion period control. However, after large bilateral lesions involving all of the ventral and most of the ventrolateral quadrants, sparing only part of the dorsal columns or the dorsolateral funiculus, there was an initial period, that lasted up to 3–6 weeks, during which cats behaved essentially as complete spinal cats, using their forelimbs to advance and dragging their hindquarters on the ground. Eventually, however, even these cats were capable of voluntarily standing up and walking overground on all four limbs. Nevertheless, the cats with the largest lesions walked very slowly and, because of their lack of stability (see below) were unable to follow treadmill speeds of >0.4 m/s.

An example of the type of deficits produced by these large lesions of the ventral quadrants is shown in Fig. 1, which illustrates one of the better locomotor sequences that was observed in case EB6, which had a large bilateral lesion of the ventromedial and ventrolateral funiculi (Fig. 1C). This cat had a generally more crouched posture than in the intact state as can be appreciated both from the stick figures illustrating the stance phase of locomotion before and after the lesion (Fig. 1A)

TABLE 1

Chronic partial spinal section in cats

Type and level of spiral lesions	References
Various quadrants	(Eidelberg and Stein, 1974; Eidelberg, 1981; Eidelberg et al., 1981a, 1983, 1985; Alstermark et al., 1987)
Ventral and Ventrolateral	(Afelt, 1974; Gorska et al., 1990; Gorska et al., 1993a, b; Zmyslowski et al., 1993; Bem et al., 1995; Brustein and Rossignol, 1998, 1999)
Large lesions of dorsal spinal cord, sparing only some of the ventral quadrants	(Windle et al., 1958; Afelt, 1974; Contamin, 1983; Bem et al., 1995)
Lesions restricted largely to the dorsal columns and dorsolateral funiculi	(Afelt, 1974; English, 1980; English, 1985; Gorska et al., 1993b; Zmylowski et al., 1993; Jiang and Drew, 1996)
Single or serial hemisections	(Kato et al., 1984; Masamichi et al., 1984; Kato et al., 1985; Kato, 1988; Kato, 1989; Kato, 1991; Helgren and Goldberger, 1993)

351

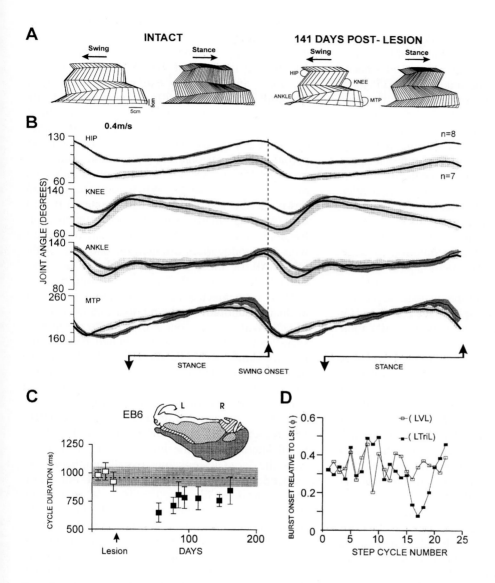

Fig. 1. Kinematics of a cat with a partial lesion of the ventral and ventrolateral quadrants of the spinal cord at T_{13}. A: stick figures of the left hindlimb of the cat during swing and stance before (intact) and 141 days after the lesion. The legs are separated one from the other by a distance proportional to the length of travel of the paw between video fields (16.7ms). B: averaged joint angles from this cat; data are normalized to the average step cycle duration in each condition. The thicker lines illustrate the data obtained following the lesion and the thinner lines those from the intact situation. Shaded regions for each trace indicate the 0.01 level of confidence of the standard error of the mean. C: average step cycle duration of the cat at a speed of 0.4 ms^{-1} on different days before and after the partial lesion. The horizontal dotted line and the shaded rectangle indicate the average step cycle in the control period together with the standard deviation. D: phase of the onset of the left (L) vastus lateralis (VL) and the lateral head of triceps (TriL) with respect to the onset of the left semitendinosus (St) during 25 consecutive step cycles (141 days post-lesion). The transverse section of the spinal cord above part C illustrates the extent of the lesion in this cat; dark gray regions represent severe damage; hatched areas, moderate damage and clear areas, no damage; the dotted region indicates a syrinx.

as well as from the averaged joint angles shown in Fig. 1B. In this latter figure, inspection of the traces shows that there was an increased level of flexion at the hip and knee, both during swing and stance. Changes at the level of the ankle and MTP joint were less evident. This more flexed posture, suggesting that the cats had difficulty in supporting their weight, was observed in all cats in the first few days or weeks following the lesion but only persisted in those animals with the largest lesions. Inspection of Fig. 1B also shows that the interval of confidence of the averaged angles was larger after the lesion, indicating that the locomotion was more variable after the lesion. There was also a decrease in the lateral stability of these cats that could be quantified during overground locomotion as large and variable shifts in the mediolateral ground reaction forces (Brustein et al., 1995). In most cats there was also a decrease in the average step cycle duration for any one given speed (see e.g. Fig. 1C) so that at the same speed, the cats generally took more frequent steps after the lesion.

One of the most evident deficits in these cats was the increase in the variability of the homolateral interlimb coordination. This is shown in Fig. 1D which illustrates the relative phase of onset of the activity in a fore- and hindlimb extensor on the left side with respect to onset of activity in the left hindlimb flexor, semitendinosus (St). This panel illustrates two points. First, there was frequently a large variability between the times of onset of the two illustrated muscles, indicating that the interlimb coupling between the fore- and the hindlimb was very variable. Second, the relative phase of onset of the fore- and hindlimb extensor muscles was, generally, similar indicating that the cats were pacing in contrast to the walking gait (phase of approximately 0.25 between the onset of activity in these same two muscles) that they used prior to the lesion. We have argued that this latter observation may reflect an adaptation by the cat in response to the decreased stability of the locomotion (Brustein and Rossignol, 1998).

When the cats with the larger partial lesions walked uphill on a treadmill inclined at 10° there were major changes in the amplitude of the forelimb elbow extensor muscles to accommodate for the increasing load whereas little change was observed in the hindlimb extensors (Fig. 2B). This is different from the intact cat (Fig. 2A) in which there was only a modest increase (in the order of 10–15%) in the level of the EMG activity of both the fore- and hindlimb extensor muscles. At a treadmill inclination of 20° these increases in the level of EMG activity in the fore- and hindlimb extensor muscles were more obvious in the intact cat (see e.g. Fig. 6A), but the cats with these larger partial spinal lesions of the ventral and ventrolateral funiculi were unable to walk at this level of treadmill inclination. When required to walk downhill, the lesioned cats had greater difficulty than walking uphill. Stumbles were much more frequent and the cats tended to walk diagonally with the hindquarters oriented on one side or the other. All of these cats were able to negotiate obstacles attached to the moving treadmill belt.

HRP was injected below the spinal lesions to evaluate quantitatively the number and distribution of cells with intact axons projecting to the lumbosacral cord. The number of labelled cells in the pontomedullary reticular formation (PMRF) in the three cats with the largest partial lesions accounted for only 5–48% of the number observed in intact control cats (Brustein and Rossignol, 1998). Indeed, as represented in Fig. 3A, while HRP-labelled cells were abundant throughout the PMRF at all lateralities in the intact cat, in the animals with the large lesions the overall numbers were reduced and their distribution modified. For example, in the case illustrated in Figs 3C and D, no neurones were labelled on the left side of the brainstem at a laterality of 1.1 mm from the midline and HRP-labelled neurones were restricted to sections close to the midline (Fig. 3C) or more laterally within the pons (not illustrated). Overall, the total number of HRP-labelled cells found within the left PMRF of this cat was only 7% of the average count obtained from 3 control cats. On the right hand side, HRP-labelled cells were more numerous (Fig. 3D) and the total number was 60% of the average control value. It should be emphasized that even in the cats with the largest lesions, some labelled cells were observed in the PMRF and it is possible that these remaining reticulospinal cells, some of which may descend in the DLF (see Shik, 1983), may very well participate in the

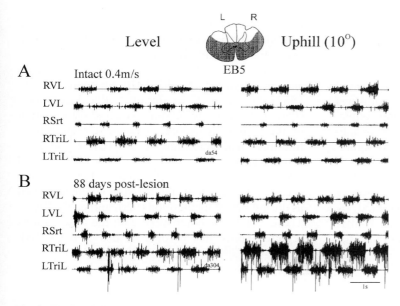

Fig. 2. EMG activity recorded from selected fore- and hindlimb muscles during level walking and during uphill locomotion on a treadmill inclined at 10° before and after a partial spinal lesion of the ventral and ventrolateral funiculi at T_{13}. The gain of each of the EMG traces is identical in each of the illustrated sections. The inset of the spinal cord illustrates the extent of the lesion in this case. Abbreviations: L, left; R, right; Srt, anterior head of sartorius.

locomotor compensation observed. It is unlikely that the vestibulospinal tract played a role in the recovery process as the anatomical examination suggested that few vestibulospinal axons were intact in the cats with the largest lesions.

Rubrospinal cell counts were found to be either normal or decreased in these cats (some of the larger lesions encroached on rubrospinal axons). In most cats, examination of the motor cortex showed that the corticospinal tract was untouched. As illustrated in Fig. 4B, for example, the density of labelled corticospinal cells, even in the cats with the largest lesions, was comparable to that observed in the intact animals (Fig. 4A). Indeed, preliminary evidence suggests that the number of HRP-labelled cells in the motor cortex of some of these cats may have been higher than that observed in control cats (compare e.g. Figs 4A and 4B).

In summary, lesions of the ventral and ventrolateral pathways at the level of T_{11}-T_{13} resulted in an initial incapacity to walk quadrupedally. Eventually, voluntary quadrupedal locomotion was regained in all cats. However, major deficits persisted in those cats with the largest lesions, even

after recovery periods of several months. In particular, the fore- and hindlimb coupling was inconsistent and led to an unstable gait with frequent stumbles which limited the maximal speed to about 0.4 m/s. In addition, there was a loss in the lateral stability of these cats and the limbs were generally more flexed during locomotion suggesting some loss in muscle tonus. Further, the cats had major difficulties adapting to ascending and descending slopes. It is concluded that although the remaining descending pathways can initiate and maintain quadrupedal locomotion they are insufficient to completely compensate for the deficits caused by the lesions.

It is interesting to relate these findings to previous findings on the role of the PMRF in the initiation and control of locomotion. The PMRF has been shown to play a crucial relay role in the initiation of locomotion by stimulation of the Mesencephalic Locomotor Region (MLR) of decerebrate cats as extensively reviewed in (Shik and Orlovsky, 1976; Grillner, 1981; Armstrong, 1986; Rossignol, 1996). Therefore, it is not surprising that with these very large lesions, cats are indeed unable to walk with their hindlimbs for several weeks. The return of voluntary initiation of quadrupedal locomotion was more surprising given the results previously obtained in decerebrate cats (see above). However, it is not totally unexpected since, in the cats described here, other pathways such as the corticospinal pathway and others coursing through the DLF have also been shown to be capable of initiating locomotion (see Rossignol, 1996).

The PMRF also plays a role in the control of posture (Mori, 1987, 1989) as well as in the step by step regulation of locomotion as suggested by recordings and microstimulation of the PMRF. Single unit recordings have shown that the dis-

charge of a proportion of reticulospinal cells is related to the activity of various muscles, including ipsilateral hindlimb flexors and hindlimb extensors in both freely walking, intact (Drew et al., 1986) and decerebrate (Orlovsky, 1970; Shimamura et al., 1982) cats as well as during fictive locomotion (Perreault et al., 1993). Moreover, microstimulation of the PMRF gives rise to coupled responses in forelimbs and hindlimbs at rest (Drew and Rossignol, 1990a; Drew and Rossignol, 1990b) and during real locomotion in the intact (Drew, 1991) or decerebrate cat (Drew and Rossignol, 1984) as well as during fictive locomotion (Perreault et al., 1994). These results are compatible with the observations reported above that chronic lesions of the PMRF

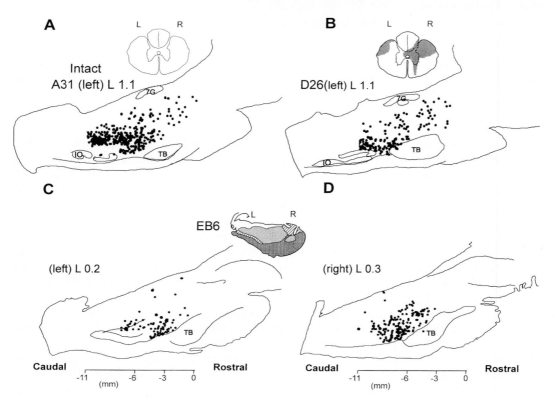

Fig. 3. Number of HRP-labelled cells in the brainstem following injections into the L_2 segment of the spinal cord in an intact cat (A), and following partial lesion of the dorsolateral funiculi (B) or the ventral and ventrolateral funiculi (C,D) at T_{13}. Each tracing represents a single parasagittal section of the brainstem at the laterality (L) indicated and illustrates those HRP-labelled cells (filled circles) that were located rostral to P11 in that section. Data are shown for the left brainstem of cat D26 and for both the left and right brainstem of cat EB6: (414 cells are illustrated in A, 258 in B, 111 in C and 245 in D). Stereotaxic anteroposterior coordinates are shown below C and D. Abbreviations: 7G, genu of the 7th nerve; IO, inferior olive; TB, trapezoid body. Transverse sections of the spinal cord in B and in C and D illustrate the extent of the lesions (shaded areas). Details of the extent of the lesions can be found in the original papers (Jiang and Drew, 1996; Brustein and Rossignol, 1998).

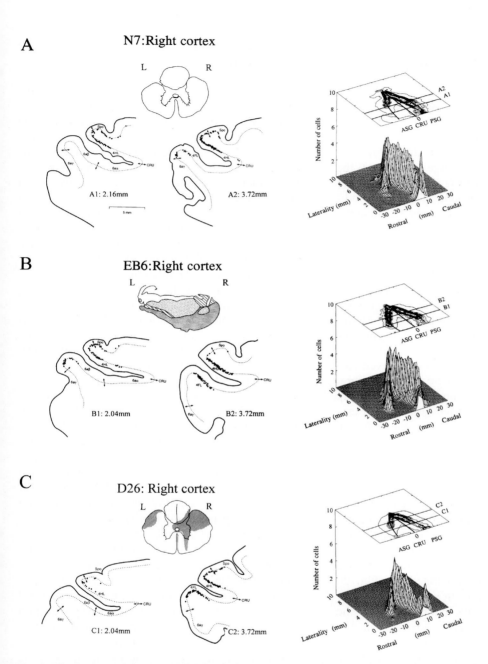

Fig. 4. Distribution and density of HRP-labelled cells observed in the pericruciate cortex following injections into the L_2 segment of the spinal cord in an intact cat (A), and following partial lesion of the ventral and ventrolateral funiculi (B) or dorsolateral funiculi (C) at T_{13}. B, and C, same cats as illustrated in Fig. 3. For each cat we illustrate the labelled cells (filled circles) observed in two representative, parasagittal sections of the cortex, together with a 3-D representation and a contour plot of the overall distribution and density of labelled cells in the cortex. In these latter representations, each histological section has been flattened and the number of cells in each 200 μm section binned. Each section is then positioned according to its laterality from the midline. For details, see Jiang and Drew (1996).

pathways result mainly in an impairment of interlimb coupling, lateral stability and weight support.

Dorsal and dorsolateral pathways

Gorska and her group (Gorska et al., 1993a, b; Zmyslowski et al., 1993; Bem et al., 1995) have shown that even cats with large lesions of the dorsolateral quadrants or of the lateral funiculi are readily able to walk overground. They have indicated that the primary deficits are to be found in the altered structure of the step cycle and particularly in the balance between stance and swing. However, detailed observations of the kinematics and EMG activity in these cats were not performed.

In a recent, quantitative study, large lesions of the dorsolateral funiculus, with and without damage to the dorsal columns (Jiang and Drew, 1996), were also found to lead to only short-term impairments in the ability of the cats to walk on a treadmill. Within a period of 3–10 days, even cats with complete bilateral lesions of the dorsolateral funiculi were able to walk unsupported at speeds up to 0.4 m/s, and over the next few weeks most cats improved to the point that they were able to follow treadmill speeds of $0.8 \, \mathrm{ms}^{-1}$ (the fastest speed tested). Analysis of the kinematics of these cats showed that all of the lesioned cats adopted a slightly crouched gait over the first 2–3 weeks with increased flexion during stance and swing. Subsequently, the kinematics of the cats with the smaller lesions (see e.g. Fig. 4C) recovered close to control levels, while the deficits remained in the two cats with the larger lesions. Sample kinematics for one of these latter cats are illustrated in Fig. 5. Inspection of the stick figures in Fig. 5A, and of the joint angles in Fig. 5B, shows that the angles at the more distal joints (knee, ankle and MTP) in the lesioned cat were generally more flexed during the E2 phase of stance and during swing, although the overall extension of the leg at the end of stance was similar to that observed in the intact cat. On the other hand, contrary to the situation in the cats with the lesions of the ventral quadrants (Fig. 1B), the extension of the hip slightly exceeded that of the intact animal and there was a correspondingly increased step cycle duration in this cat (Fig. 5C).

There was also a change in the intralimb coordination in both the illustrated cat, and in the other animal with a large, bilateral, lesion of the dorsolateral funiculi. As can be seen in Fig. 5B, flexion at the hip, knee and ankle (lines a, b, and c, respectively) occurred almost simultaneously in the lesioned cat. In addition, there was a change in the temporal relationships between the St and the Srt, such that they were both activated simultaneously (rather than the St onset preceding Srt onset, as in the normal cat: not illustrated). Again, this change in temporal relationships was seen in all cats in the first 2–3 weeks and persisted throughout the testing period in the two animals with the largest lesions. This change in intralimb coordination is probably responsible for the paw drag that was equally observed in all cats in the first 2–3 weeks following the lesion and which persisted throughout the testing period in the illustrated cat (Fig. 5D) as well as in the other cat with a large lesion. This paw drag was accompanied by increased flexion of the MTP joint during the swing phase as the paw was dragged along the surface of the treadmill belt (Figs 5A, B, E). In some of the cats there was also a change in interlimb coordination (not illustrated), although this deficit was never as pronounced as in the cats with lesions of the ventrolateral pathways. Contrary to cats with ventrolateral lesions, the two cats with the largest lesions of the dorsolateral funiculi were unable to voluntarily modify their gait sufficiently to avoid hitting obstacles attached to the moving treadmill belt (Drew et al., 1996), even after recovery periods of up to five months.

Also contrary to the cats with the ventral and ventrolateral lesions, these cats with lesions to the dorsolateral funiculi easily adapted their locomotion to the requirements of walking on an inclined plane, and had few difficulties in walking uphill on a treadmill inclined at 20°. As illustrated in Fig. 6A, in intact cats walking at this inclination, there was a clear increase in the level of activity in both the fore- and hindlimb extensor muscles (see also Pierotti et al., 1989; Carlson-Kuhta et al., 1998). After the partial spinal lesions, there were similar increases in the level of activity of both the fore- and hindlimb extensor muscles. Thus, in these cats the remaining descending pathways are capable of producing the requisite postural adaptations.

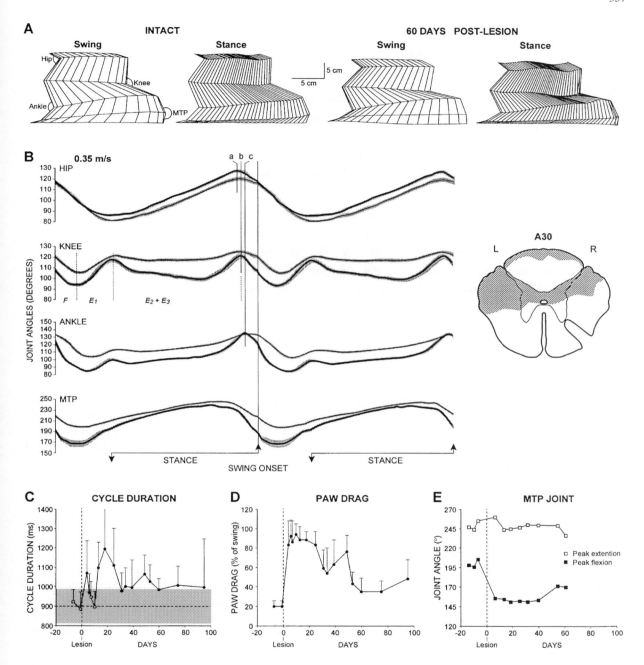

Fig. 5. Kinematics of an intact cat and one with a partial lesion of the dorsolateral funiculi at T_{13} (60 days post-lesion). A, B and C arranged as in Fig. 1. D: extent of the paw drag of this cat following the spinal lesion. Paw drag was measured as the percentage of the hip flexion period (approximating to swing) that the paw remained in contact with the treadmill belt. Note that even in the intact cat, hip flexion begins slightly before the paw is lifted from the treadmill belt. E: Joint angles subtended by the MTP joint of this cat before and after the spinal lesion. (Adapted from Jiang and Drew, 1996).

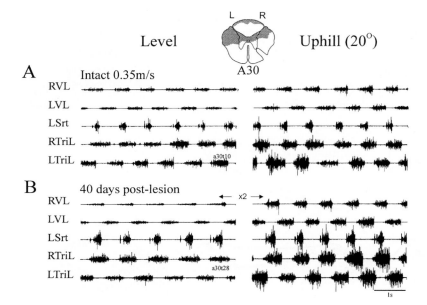

Level　Uphill (20°)

L　R

A30

A　Intact 0.35m/s

RVL

LVL

LSrt

RTriL

LTriL

a30t10

B　40 days post-lesion

RVL

← x2 →

LVL

LSrt

RTriL

LTriL

a30t28

1s

Fig. 6. EMG activity during locomotion with the treadmill inclined at 20°; same cat as illustrated in Fig. 5. Data arranged as for Fig. 2. Note that the gain of the RVL in the post-lesion session was twice that used in the control session.

HRP was also injected caudal to the lesion site in most of the cats used in this study and analysis of the results showed that most cats had varying degrees of damage to the cortico- and rubrospinal tracts, with the two cats showing the most severe deficits having almost complete severance of these two pathways. In the cat with the largest lesion, the results suggested that the corticospinal and the rubrospinal tract were completely transected. In the other cats the interruption of the cortico- and rubrospinal tracts was generally less severe. In the example illustrated in Fig. 4C, the lesion of the spinal cord was asymmetric, being smaller on the left than on the right. This resulted in a slight loss of corticospinal neurones in the right cortex (decreased to 62% of control), particularly in the most medial part of the representation (Fig. 4C) and a more severe loss (decreased to 5% of control) in the left cortex (illustrated in Jiang and Drew, 1996). As might be expected, there was only a slight loss of HRP-labelled neurones in the brainstem in most of these cats. For example, Fig. 3B illustrates that the number of HRP-labelled cells that were observed in a single section of the left

brainstem of cat, D26, 1.1 mm from the mid-line, was only slightly less than that observed in the intact animal. In the cats with larger lesions, there was a more substantial reduction suggesting some interruption of the reticulospinal tracts in the dorsolateral funiculus and, perhaps, some of the ventrolateral component as well.

In summary, small lesions of the dorsolateral funiculi led to rapid recovery of locomotion over a 2–3 week period, and left few long-term deficits. In contrast in the two cats with the larger lesions there were persistent behavioral deficits in locomotion that were reflected both in the kinematics and the EMG recordings. Chief among these was the persistent paw drag that was probably the behavioral expression of the change in the intralimb coordination. There was also a persistent problem in the ability of the cats to make voluntary modifications of gait to step over obstacles. Contrary to the findings in the cats with the lesions of the ventral quadrants, there were no problems with lateral stability, few problems with weight support and only relatively minor changes in the interlimb coordination. Table 2 makes a comparison of the

TABLE 2

Comparison of persistent locomotor deficits in cats after chronic lesions of different parts of the spinal cord

	Dorsal and Dorsolateral	Ventral and Ventrolateral
Quadrupedal walk	Yes	Yes
Paw drag	Yes	No
Lateral stability	Good	Poor
Weight support	Good	Reduced
Intralimb coordination	Abnormal	Normal
Interlimb coordination	Minor changes	Major changes
Adaptation to obstacles and ladder	Poor	Fair to good
Adaptation to speed	Good	Limited
Adaptation to slopes	Good	Poor

main deficits seen in cats with ventral and ventrolateral lesions with those seen in cats with dorsal and dorsolateral lesions.

The deficits observed in these cats with the dorsolateral lesions are compatible with the results obtained from data from other studies. For example, studies in which the motor cortex or the red nucleus has been pharmacologically inactivated during locomotion (Lavoie et al., 1995 and unpublished observations) also show that the cats have deficits in intralimb coordination and exhibit paw drag. Single unit recording studies in walking cats have shown that many pyramidal tract neurones (PTNs) in the motor cortex are rhythmically active (Durelli et al., 1978; Armstrong and Drew, 1984a, b; Palmer et al., 1985). A portion of these discharge preferentially at the transition from stance to swing leading to the suggestion that one of the functions of the motor cortex may be to regulate this critical transition phase (Armstrong and Drew, 1984b). This suggestion is supported by other studies in which unit activity has been recorded from the motor cortex while cats make voluntary gait modifications (Drew, 1988, 1993; Widajewicz et al., 1994). The results from these experiments show that PTNs in the motor cortex increase their discharge frequency during the swing phase of gait modifications and that different groups of PTNs may signal the changes in activity of muscles acting around different joints of the limbs, thus encoding the appropriate intralimb coordination required for the task. Studies from other groups have also reported increases in discharge frequency in PTNs during other tasks in which cats need to exert a fine control over their locomotion (Amos et al., 1990; Beloozerova and Sirota, 1993). The results from microstimulation studies in the decerebrate (Orlovsky 1972) and the intact cat (Rho et al., 1999), showing that motor cortical stimulation at the end of stance may reset the step cycle by initiating a new swing phase, also supports a role for the motor cortex in controlling the relative time of onset of different muscle groups and of the stance to swing transition period.

It was noteworthy that only the cats with the largest lesions, interrupting both the cortico- and rubrospinal tracts showed persistent deficits. This would agree with other reports suggesting that these two pathways have complementary, although not identical functions, in the control of locomotion and other motor behaviors (see e.g. Martin and Ghez, 1988). For example, several other studies have also emphasized that permanent deficits in limb control are only seen when both pathways are interrupted (Kuypers, 1963; Lawrence and Kuypers, 1968; Alstermark et al., 1987). Moreover, work from our laboratory (Lavoie et al., 1997) has shown that cells in the magnocellular region of the red nucleus also increase their discharge frequency during voluntary gait modifications and may play a role in intralimb coordination. However, the results from both these unit recording studies and from the microstimulation studies (Rho et al., 1999) suggest that each of these pathways probably has a unique role to play in the control of locomotion.

Spinal hemisections

Other types of partial lesions have been performed in cats and their consequences documented in various manners, but generally with less quantitative techniques. Work on spinal hemisections has clearly shown the ability of cats to walk with both hindlimbs (Basso et al., 1994; Helgren and Goldberger, 1993). With a second transection performed at the midthoracic level contralaterally to the first section, cats can still regain voluntary locomotor functions overground, albeit with deficits of the fore- and hindlimb coupling (Kato et al., 1984). One month after a longitudinal split of the lumbar cord from L2–3 to L7–S1, cats could stand and walk with bilateral hindlimb coordination suggesting that the interlimb coordination can be assured by descending pathways in the absence of commisural connections (Kato, 1988). With a further unilateral hemisection, it was reported that the isolated spinal cord could eventually produce stepping (Kato, 1989, 1991). The quality of such locomotion, however, needs to be assessed with EMG and kinematic data.

Complete spinal lesions

The above results may help to better understand the recovery and remaining deficits after a complete spinal transection. Table 3 lists a number of studies on cats with complete spinal sections and more complete general reviews can be found in Rossignol (1996; Rossignol et al., 1999). The following section summarizes some of the more salient findings from the work in our laboratory on these spinal cats. These animals were all chronically implanted with electrodes for recording EMG activity, thus facilitating the comparison with the work in the cats with partial spinal lesions. In addition, some of the cats were also implanted with an intrathecal cannula for drug administration (see Rossignol et al., 1999). As in the other studies, locomotor movements and associated EMGs were recorded for a period of approximately one month prior to spinalisation in order to establish baseline values.

Recovery of locomotion

In the first few days following the complete spinal cord transection, the hindquarters needed to be supported by the experimenter and strong cutaneous stimulation needed to be applied to the perineum to induce very small but coordinated steps. Over the next five days or so the locomotion gradually improved but the hindlimbs were generally held extended behind the body and the joint excursions were small compared to the intact cat. The paw was dragged for most of the swing phase and at foot contact landed either on the tip of the toes, or on the dorsum of the paw. By one to two weeks post-lesion, the stance length was increased and the cats began to support the weight of the hindquarters and to place the plantar surface of the paw on the treadmill belt. Nevertheless, the paw drag still persisted for approximately half of the swing phase in most cases. Over the next 3–4

TABLE 3

Chronic complete spinal section in cats

Age of cats	Level of transection	References
Cat-kittens	T12 to L1 & L3	(Shurrager and Dykman, 1951; Freeman, 1952; Forssberg et al., 1980a, b; Smith et al., 1982; Goldberger, 1986; Robinson and Goldberger, 1986b)
Cat-adult	C1 or thoracic	(Ranson and Hinsey, 1930; McCouch, 1947; Kozak and Westerman, 1966; Miller and Van der Meche, 1976; Eidelberg et al., 1980; Zangger, 1981)
Cat-adult	T11-L1	(Sherrington, 1910; Ranson and Hinsey, 1930; Ten Cate, 1962; Kozak and Westerman, 1966; Afelt, 1970; Baker et al., 1984; Goldberger, 1986; Lovely et al. 1986; Robinson and Goldberger, 1986a, b; Barbeau and Rossignol, 1987; Giuliani and Smith, 1987; Rossignol et al., 1989; Lovely et al., 1990; Barbeau and Rossignol, 1991; Edgerton et al., 1991; Roy et al., 1992; Barbeau et al., 1993; Bélanger et al., 1996;Chau et al., 1998; Rossignol et al., 1999)

weeks, the paw was placed ahead of the hip at paw contact, thus further increasing the stance length. Full, but transient, weight support was maintained at this stage and locomotion could be elicited by movement of the belt without using perineal stimulation. The amount of paw drag varied among cats, from practically none to a drag persisting close to 50% of the swing.

The timing of the flexor muscles was somewhat altered after spinalisation. As in the cats with the partial lesions of the dorsolateral funiculi, there was normally a change in the intralimb coordination and activity in the St and the Srt frequently began simultaneously, instead of sequentially as in the intact cat. As for the cats with the lesions of the dorsolateral funiculi, it is postulated that this alteration in flexor coupling (i.e. earlier start of the ankle flexor and more or less synchronous activation of knee and hip flexors) may cause the paw drag observed during the early part of swing.

Although spinal cats had a shorter step cycle than the intact cat at any given speed, both the intact and spinal cats increased their step length when the speed of the treadmill was increased. However, whereas these changes in speed are associated with characteristic increases in extensor muscle amplitude in the intact cat, the changes in EMG activity were much more inconsistent and variable in the spinal cat (Bélanger et al., 1996). These cats with total transections of the spinal cord showed very little adaptation of their posture or EMG pattern when the treadmill slope was changed and the cats were required to walk uphill or downhill (Rossignol et al., 1999).

Conclusions

Comparison of the deficits and the observed recovery in these different preparations leads to several conclusions concerning the capacities of the spinal cord for locomotion and the role of supraspinal and peripheral afferents in modifying the spinal activity. The results from the spinal cats clearly emphasize the capacity of the spinal cord, in isolation from all descending influences to generate a well organized pattern of locomotion. However,

this preparation has a limited ability to maintain an upright position and only poorly adapts its locomotion to changes in speed and treadmill inclination. In these latter situations, it is probable that the adaptations that were observed were due to the influences of modified peripheral afferent feedback. The results from the cats with partial spinal lesions emphasize that even cats with substantial damage to either the dorsolateral or ventrolateral and ventromedial quadrants of the spinal cord are able to recover a remarkably good locomotor capability. There thus seems to be no specific part of the spinal cord white matter which is essential for locomotion in the otherwise intact animal. Further, descending pathways in either funiculus are able to compensate to some extent for the deficits produced by these lesions. However, the results strongly suggest that pathways in the ventrolateral and ventromedial funiculi play a predominant role in the regulation of posture, including lateral stability, and in the control of the interlimb coordination. The descending pathways in the dorsolateral funiculi seem to play their predominant role in regulating intralimb coordination and in mediating the descending commands that are necessary for the appropriate production of voluntary modifications of gait, e.g. to overcome obstacles. The results also demonstrate that even given extensive training, none of the cats with large partial lesions fully recovered to pre-lesion capabilities. As stated in the Introduction, these persistent deficits provide some indication of the essential role of the interrupted pathways, while the compensation that was observed gives an indication of the capacity for the remaining pathways to participate in functional recovery.

Acknowledgements

We would like to thank France Lebel, Janyne Provencher and Natacha de Sylva for their help with these experiments and Daniel Cyr and Claude Gauthier for their preparation of figures. We thank Dr. Elaine Chapman for her comments on this manuscript. Supported by grants from the MRC and NCE.

362

References

Afelt, Z. (1970) Reflex activity in chronic spinal cats. *Acta Neurobiol. Exp.*, 30: 129–144.

Afelt, Z. (1974) Functional significance of ventral descending tracts of the spinal cord in the cat. *Acta Neurobiol. Exp.*, 34: 393–407.

Alstermark, B., Lundberg, A., Pettersson, L.-G., Tantisira, B. and Walkowska, M. (1987) Motor recovery after serial spinal cord lesions of defined descending pathways in cats. *Neurosci. Res.*, 5: 68–73.

Amos, A., Armstrong, D.M. and Marple-Horvat, D.E. (1990) Changes in the discharge patterns of motor cortical neurones associated with volitional changes in stepping in the cat. *Neurosci. Lett.*, 109: 107–112.

Armstrong, D.M. (1986) Supraspinal contributions to the initiation and control of locomotion in the cat. *Prog. Neurobiol.*, 26: 273–361.

Armstrong, D.M. and Drew, T. (1984a) Discharges of pyramidal tract and other motor cortical neurones during locomotion in the cat. *J. Physiol.*, 346: 471–495.

Armstrong, D.M. and Drew, T. (1984b) Locomotor-related neuronal discharges in cat motor cortex compared with peripheral receptive fields and evoked movements. *J.Physiol.*, 346: 497–517.

Baker, L.L., Chandler, S.H. and Goldberg, L.J. (1984) L-Dopa induced locomotor-like activity in ankle flexor and extensor nerves of chronic and acute spinal cats. *Exp. Neurol.*, 86: 515–526.

Barbeau, H., Chau, C. and Rossignol, S. (1993) Noradrenergic agonists and locomotor training affect locomotor recovery after cord transection in adult cats. *Brain Res. Bull.*, 30: 387–393.

Barbeau, H. and Rossignol, S. (1987) Recovery of locomotion after chronic spinalization in the adult cat. *Brain Res.*, 412: 84–95.

Barbeau, H. and Rossignol, S. (1991) Initiation and modulation of the locomotor pattern in the adult chronic spinal cat by noradrenergic, serotonergic and dopaminergic drugs. *Brain Res.*, 546: 250–260.

Basso, D.M., Murray, M. and Goldberger, M.E. (1994) Differential recovery of bipedal and overground locomotion following complete spinal cord hemisection in cats. *Restor. Neurol. Neurosci.*, 7: 95–110.

Bélanger, M., Drew, T., Provencher, J. and Rossignol, S. (1996) A comparison of treadmill locomotion in adult cats before and after spinal transection. *J. Neurophysiol.*, 76: 471–491.

Beloozerova, I.N. and Sirota, M.G. (1993) The role of the motor cortex in the control of accuracy of locomotor movements in the cat. *J. Physiol.*, 461: 1–25.

Bem, T., Gorska, T., Majczynski, H. and Zmyslowski, W. (1995) Different patterns of fore-hindlimb coordination during overground locomotion in cats with ventral and lateral spinal lesions. *Exp. Brain Res.*, 104: 70–80.

Brustein, E., Lavoie, S., Lebel, F., Provencher, J., McFadyen, B. and Rossignol, S. (1995) The recovery of locomotion in adult cats subjected to bilateral lesions of the ventral and ventrolateral spinal quadrants. *Soc. Neurosci. Abstr.*, 21: 420.

Brustein, E. and Rossignol, S. (1998) Recovery of locomotion after ventral and ventrolateral spinal lesions in the cat. I. Deficits and adaptive mechanisms. *J. Neurophysiol.*, 80: 1245–1267.

Brustein, E. and Rossignol, S. (1999) Recovery of locomotion after ventral and ventrolateral spinal lesions in the cat. II. The effects of noradrenergic and serotoninergic drugs. *J. Neurophysiol.*, 81: 1513–1530.

Carlson-Kuhta, P., Trank, T.V. and Smith, J.L. (1998) Forms of forward quadrupedal locomotion. II. A comparison of posture, hindlimb kinematics and motor patterns for upslope and level walking. *J.Neurophysiol.*, 79: 1687–1701.

Chau, C., Barbeau, H. and Rossignol, S. (1998) Early locomotor training with clonidine in spinal cats. *J. Neurophysiol.*, 59: 392–409.

Contamin, F. (1983) Sections médullaires incomplètes et locomotion chez le chat. *Bull. Acad. Nat. Med.*, 167: 727–730.

Drew, T. (1988) Motor cortical cell discharge during voluntary gait modification. *Brain Res.*, 457: 181–187.

Drew, T. (1991) Functional organization within the medullary reticular formation of the intact unanesthetized cat. III. Microstimulation during locomotion. *J. Neurophysiol.*, 66: 919–938.

Drew, T. (1993) Motor cortical activity during voluntary gait modifications in the cat. I. Cells related to the forelimbs. *J.Neurophysiol.*, 70: 179–199.

Drew, T., Dubuc, R. and Rossignol, S. (1986) Discharge patterns of reticulospinal and other reticular neurons in chronic, unrestrained cats walking on a treadmill. *J. Neurophysiol.*, 55: 375–401.

Drew, T., Jiang, W., Kably, B. and Lavoie, S. (1996) Role of the motor cortex in the control of visually triggered gait modifications. *Can. J. Physiol. Pharmacol.*, 74: 426–442.

Drew, T. and Rossignol, S. (1984) Phase-dependent responses evoked in limb muscles by stimulation of medullary reticular formation during locomotion in thalamic cats. *J. Neurophysiol.*, 52: 653–675.

Drew, T. and Rossignol, S. (1990a) Functional organisation within the medullary reticular formation of intact unanaesthetized cat. I. Movements evoked by microstimulation. *J. Neurophysiol.*, 64: 767–781.

Drew, T. and Rossignol, S. (1990b) Functional organisation within the medullary reticular formation of intact unanaesthetized cat. II. Electromyographic activity evoked by microstimulation. *J. Neurophysiol.*, 64: 782–795.

Durelli, L., Schmidt, E.M., McIntosh, J.S. and Bak, M.J. (1978) Single unit chronic recordings from the sensorimotor cortex of unrestrained cats during locomotion. *Exp. Neurol.*, 62: 580–594.

Edgerton, V.R., de Guzman, C.P., Gregor, R.J., Roy, R.R., Hodgson, J.A. and Lovely, R.G. (1991) Trainability of the spinal cord to generate hindlimb stepping patterns in adult spinalized cats. In: M. Shimamura, S. Grillner and V.R.

Edgerton (Eds), *Neurobiological Basis of Human Locomotion*, Tokyo: Japan Scientific Societies Press, pp. 411–423.

Eidelberg, E. (1981) Consequences of spinal cord lesions upon motor function, with special reference to locomotor activity. *Prog. Neurobiol.*, 17: 185–202.

Eidelberg, E. (1983) Loss and recovery of locomotor function after spinal cord lesions in cats and monkeys. In: F.J. Seil (Ed.), *Nerve Organ and Tissue Regeneration: Research Perspectives*, New York: Academic Press, pp. 231–242.

Eidelberg, E., Jones, D.J., Keenan, R.W. and Schwartzman, R.J. (1985) Report from the spinal cord injury research program. *Eur. J. Neurosci.*, 225–234.

Eidelberg, E. and Stein, D.G. (1974) Functional recovery after lesions of the nervous system. *Neurosci. Res. Prog. Bull.*, 12: 191–303.

Eidelberg, E., Story, J.L., Meyer, B.L. and Nystel, J. (1980) Stepping by chronic spinal cats. *Exp. Brain Res.*, 40: 241–246.

Eidelberg, E., Story, J.L., Walden, J.G. and Meyer, B.L. (1981a) Anatomical correlates of return of locomotor function after partial spinal cord lesions in cats. *Exp. Brain Res.*, 42: 81–88.

Eidelberg, E., Walden, J.G. and Nguyen, L.H. (1981b) Locomotor control in macaque monkeys. *Brain*, 104: 647–663.

English, A.W. (1980) Interlimb coordination during stepping in the cat: effects of dorsal column section. *J. Neurophysiol.*, 44: 270–279.

English, A.W. (1985) Interlimb coordination during stepping in the cat. The role of the dorsal spinocerebellar tract. *Exp. Neurol.*, 87: 96–108.

Forssberg, H., Grillner, S. and Halbertsma, J. (1980a) The locomotion of the low spinal cat. I. Coordination within a hindlimb. *Acta Physiol. Scand.*, 108: 269–281.

Forssberg, H., Grillner, S., Halbertsma, J. and Rossignol, S. (1980b) The locomotion of the low spinal cat: II. Interlimb coordination. *Acta Physiol. Scand.*, 108: 283–295.

Freeman, L.W. (1952) Return of function after complete transection of the spinal cord of the rat, cat and dog. *Ann. Surg.*, 136: 193–205.

Gelfand, I.M., Orlovsky, G.N. and Shik, M.L. (1988) Locomotion and scratching in tetrapods. In: A.H. Cohen, S. Rossignol and S. Grillner (Eds), *Neural Control of Rhythmic Movements in Vertebrates*, New York: John Wiley & Sons, pp. 167–199.

Giuliani, C.A. and Smith, J.L. (1987) Stepping behaviors in chronic spinal cats with one hindlimb deafferented. *J. Neurosci.*, 7: 2537–2546.

Goldberger, M.E. (1986) Autonomous spinal motor function and the infant lesion effect. In: M.E. Goldberger, A. Gorio and M. Murray (Eds), *Development and Plasticity of the Mammalian Spinal Cord.Fidia Research Series.*, Padova: Liviana Press, pp. 363–380.

Gorska, T., Bem, T. and Majczynski, H. (1990) Locomotion in cats with ventral spinal lesions: support patterns and duration of support phases during unrestrained walking. *Acta Neurobiol. Exp.*, 50: 191–200.

Gorska, T., Bem, T., Majczynski, H. and Zmyslowski, W. (1993a) Unrestrained walking in cats with partial spinal lesions. *Brain Res. Bull.*, 32: 241–249.

Gorska, T., Majczynski, H., Bem, T. and Zmyslowski, W. (1993b) Hindlimb swing, stance and step relationships during unrestrained walking in cats with lateral funicular lesion. *Acta Neurobiol. Exp.*, 53: 133–142.

Grillner, S. (1981) Control of locomotion in bipeds, tetrapods and fish. In: J.M. Brookhart and V.B. Mountcastle (Eds), *Handbook of Physiology. The Nervous System II.*, Bethesda: American Physiological Society, pp. 1179–1236.

Grillner, S. and Dubuc, R. (1988) Control of locomotion in vertebrates: spinal and supraspinal mechanisms. In: S.G. Waxman (Ed.), *Functional Recovery in Neurological Disease*, New York: Raven Press, pp. 425–453.

Helgren, M.E. and Goldberger, M.E. (1993) The recovery of postural reflexes and locomotion following low thoracic hemisection in adult cats involves compensation by undamaged primary afferent pathways. *Exp. Neurol.*, 123: 17–34.

Jiang, W. and Drew, T. (1996) Effects of bilateral lesions of the dorsolateral funiculi and dorsal columns at the level of the low thoracic spinal cord on the control of locomotion in the adult cat: I. Treadmill walking. *J. Neurophysiol.*, 76: 849–866.

Kato, M. (1988) Longitudinal myelotomy of lumbar spinal cord has little effect on coordinated locomotor activities of bilateral hindlimbs of the chronic cats. *Neurosci. Lett.*, 93: 259–263.

Kato, M. (1989) Chronically isolated lumbar half spinal cord produced by hemisection and longitudinal myelotomy generates locomotor activities of the ipsilateral hindlimb of the cat. *Neurosci. Lett.*, 98: 149–153.

Kato, M. (1991) Chronically isolated lumbar half spinal cord and locomotor activities of the hindlimb. In: M. Shimamura, S. Grillner and V.R. Edgerton (Eds), *Neurobiological Basis of Human Locomotion*, Tokyo: Japan Scientific Societies Press, pp. 407–410.

Kato, M., Murakami, S., Yasuda, K. and Hirayama, H. (1984) Disruption of fore-and hindlimb coordination during overground locomotion in cats with bilateral serial hemisection of the spinal cord. *Neurosci. Res.*, 2: 27–47.

Kato, M., Murakami, S., Hirayama, H. and Hikino, K. (1985) Recovery of postural control following chronic bilateral hemisections at different spinal cord levels in adult cats. *Exp. Neurol.*, 90: 350–364.

Kozak, W. and Westerman, R. (1966) Basic patterns of plastic change in the mammalian nervous system. *Nervous and Hormonal Mechanisms of Integration*. Soc. Exp. Biol. Symp., 20: Cambridge: Cambridge University Press, pp. 509–544.

Kuypers, H.G.J.M. (1963) The organization of the 'motor system'. *Int. J. Neurol.*, 4: 78–91.

Lavoie, S., Martin, J.H. and Drew, T. (1995) Effect of reversible inactivation of the motor cortex on voluntary gait modifications in the cat. *Soc. Neurosci. Abstr.*, 21: 419.

364

Lavoie, S. and Drew, T. (1997) Discharge characteristics of neurones in the red nucleus during voluntary gait modifications in the intact cat. *Soc. Neurosci. Abstr.*, 23: 762.

Lawrence, D.G. and Kuypers, H.G.J.M. (1968) The functional organization of the motor system in the monkey. I. The effects of bilateral pyramidal lesions. *Brain*, 91: 1–15.

Lovely, R.G., Gregor, R.J., Roy, R.R. and Edgerton, V.R. (1986) Effects of training on the recovery of full-weight-bearing stepping in the adult spinal cat. *Exp. Neurol.*, 92: 421–435.

Lovely, R.G., Gregor, R.J., Roy, R.R. and Edgerton, V.R. (1990) Weight-bearing hindlimb stepping in treadmill-exercised adult spinal cat. *Brain Res.*, 514: 206–218.

Martin, J.H. and Ghez, C. (1988) Red nucleus and motor cortex: parallel motor systems for the initiation and control of skilled movement. *Behav. Brain. Res.*, 28: 217–223.

Masamichi, K., Murakami, S., Yasuda, K. and Hirayama, H. (1984) Disrupting of fore- and hindlimb coordination during overground locomotion in cats with bilateral serial hemisection of the spinal cord. *Neurosci. Res.*, 2: 27–47.

McCouch, G.P. (1947) Reflex development in the chronically spinal cat and dog. *J. Neurophysiol.*, 10: 425–428.

Miller, S. and Van der Meche, F.G.A. (1976) Coordinated stepping of all four limbs in the high spinal cat. *Brain Res.*, 109: 395–398.

Mori, S. (1987) Integration of posture and locomotion in acute decerebrate cats and in awake, freely moving cats. *Prog. Neurobiol.*, 28: 161–195.

Mori, S. (1989) Contribution of postural muscle tone to full expression of posture and locomotor movements: multifaceted analyses of its setting brainstem-spinal cord mechanisms in the cat. *Jpn. J. Physiol.*, 39: 785–809.

Orlovsky, G.N. (1970) Work of the reticulo-spinal neurons during locomotion. *Biophys. (USSR)*, 15: 761–771.

Orlovsky, G.N. (1972) The effect of different descending systems on flexor and extensor activity during locomotion. *Brain Res.*, 40: 359–371.

Palmer, C.I., Marks, W.B. and Bak, M.J. (1985) The responses of cat motor cortical units to electrical cutaneous stimulation during locomotion and during lifting, falling and landing. *Exp. Brain. Res.*, 58: 102–116.

Pearson, K.G. (1993) Common principles of motor control in vertebrates and invertebrates. *Ann. Rev. Neurosci.*, 16: 265–297.

Perreault, M.-C., Drew, T. and Rossignol, S. (1993) Activity of medullary reticulospinal neurons during fictive locomotion. *J. Neurophysiol.*, 69: 2232–2247.

Perreault, M.-C., Rossignol, S. and Drew, T. (1994) Microstimulation of the medullary reticular formation during fictive locomotion. *J. Neurophysiol.*, 71: 229–245.

Pierotti, D.J., Roy, R.R., Gregor, R.J. and Edgerton, V.R. (1989) Electromyographic activity of cat hindlimb flexors and extensors during locomotion at varying speeds and inclines. *Brain Res.*, 481: 57–66.

Ranson, S.W. and Hinsey, J.C. (1930) Reflexes in the hind limbs of cats after transection of the spinal cord at various levels. *Am. J. Physiol.*, 94: 471–495.

Rho, M.-J., Lavoie, S. and Drew, T. (1999) Effects of red nucleus microstimulation on the locomotor pattern and timing in the intact cat: a comparison with the motor cortex. *J. Neurophysiol.*, 81: 2297–2315.

Robinson, G.A. and Goldberger, M.E. (1986a) The development and recovery of motor function in spinal cats. I. The infant lesion effect. *Exp. Brain Res.*, 62: 373–386.

Robinson, G.A. and Goldberger, M.E. (1986b) The development and recovery of motor function in spinal cats. II. Pharmacological enhancement of recovery. *Exp. Brain Res.*, 62: 387–400.

Rossignol, S. (1996) Neural control of stereotypic limb movements. In: L.B. Rowell and J.T. Sheperd (Eds), *Handbook of Physiology, Section 12. Exercise: Regulation and Integration of Multiple Systems*. Oxford: American Physiological Society, pp. 173–216.

Rossignol, S., Bélanger, M., Barbeau, H. and Drew, T. (1989) Assessment of locomotor functions in the adult chronic spinal cat. *Conference proceedings: criteria for assessing recovery of function: behavioral methods*, A.P.A. Springfield, N.J., 10–11.

Rossignol, S., Bélanger, M., Chau, C., Giroux, N., Brustein, E., Bouyer, L., Grenier, C.-A., Drew, T., Barbeau, H. and Reader, T.A. (2000) The Spinal Cat. In: R.G. Kalb and S.M. Strittmatter (Eds), *Neurobiology of Spinal Cord Injury*, Humana Press, Totowa, New Jersey, pp. 57–87.

Rossignol, S. and Dubuc, R. (1994) Spinal pattern generation. *Curr. Opin. Neurobiol.*, 4: 894–902.

Roy, R.R., Hodgson, J.A., Lauretz, S.D., Pierotti, D.J., Gayek, R.J. and Edgerton, V.R. (1992) Chronic spinal cord-injured cats: surgical procedures and management. *Laboratory Animal Science*, 42: 335–343.

Sherrington, C.S. (1910) Remarks on the reflex mechanism of the step. *Brain*, 33: 1–25.

Shik, M.L. (1983) Action of the brainstem locomotor region on spinal stepping generators via propriospinal pathways. In: C.C. Kao, R.P. Bunge and P.J. Reier (Eds), *Spinal Cord Reconstruction*, New York: Raven, pp. 421–434.

Shik, M.L. and Orlovsky, G.N. (1976) Neurophysiology of locomotor automatism. *Physiol. Rev.*, 56: 465–500.

Shimamura, M., Kogure, I. and Wada, S.I. (1982) Reticular neuron activities associated with locomotion in thalamic cats. *Brain. Res.*, 231: 51–62.

Shurrager, P.S. and Dykman, R.A. (1951) Walking spinal carnivores. *J. Comp. Physiol. Psychol.*, 44: 252–262.

Smith, J.L., Smith, L.A., Zernicke, R.F. and Hoy, M. (1982) Locomotion in exercised and non-exercised cats cordotomized at two or twelve weeks of age. *Exp. Neurol.*, 76: 393–413.

Ten Cate, J. (1962) Innervation of locomotor movements by the lumbosacral cord in birds and mammals. *J. Exp. Biol.*, 39: 239–242.

Vilensky, J.A., Moore, A.M., Eidelberg, E. and Walden, J.G. (1992) Recovery of locomotion in monkeys with spinal cord lesions. *J. Motor Behav.*, 24: 288–296.

Widajewicz, W., Kably, B. and Drew, T. (1994) Motor cortical activity during voluntary gait modifications in the cat. II. Cells related to the hindlimbs. *J. Neurophysiol.*, 72: 2070–2089.

Windle, W.F., Smart, J.O. and Beers, J.J. (1958) Residual function after subtotal spinal cord transection in adult cats. *Neurology*, 8: 518–521.

Zangger, P. (1981) The effect of 4-aminopyridine on the spinal locomotor rhythm induced by L-Dopa. *Brain Res.*, 215: 211–223.

Zmyslowski, W., Gorska, T., Majczynski, H. and Bem, T. (1993) Hindlimb muscle activity during unrestrained walking in cats with lesions of the lateral funiculi. *Acta Neurobiol. Exp.*, 53: 143–153.

Mechanical properties of neuromuscular systems

M.D. Binder (Ed.)
Progress in Brain Research, Vol 123
© 1999 Elsevier Science BV. All rights reserved.

CHAPTER 32

The role of musculoskeletal mechanics in motor coordination

T. Richard Nichols,[1,*] David C. Lin[2] and Clotilde M.J.I. Huyghues-Despointes[2]

[1]*Department of Physiology, Emory University, Atlanta, GA 30322, USA*
[2]*Department of Neuroscience, University of Florida, Gainesville, FL 32610, USA*

Introduction

Spinal cord physiologists have long appreciated the importance of the mechanical properties of the peripheral motor apparatus in the production of coordinated movement. They have contributed importantly to the literature on muscle physiology in general and in particular on those properties that are expressed during normal motor behavior. The study of muscle and limb mechanics has proceeded along several specific lines of research, including intrinsic mechanics of single muscle fibers and motor units and muscles, muscle architecture, biomechanics of the musculoskeletal system, and kinesiology. In this chapter, we discuss a number of relevant key findings published between 1900 and 1980 that were discovered by researchers primarily interested in spinal mechanisms of motor coordination. We then turn our attention to the more specific subject of the properties of muscle that are dependent upon the history of activation and of prior movements, and the relevance of these properties for motor coordination. For more general coverage on the subjects of muscle and limb mechanics, the reader is referred to the following books, reviews and papers: *Motor unit properties:* (Burke, 1981; Cope and Clark, 1991; Heckman and Sandercock, 1996; Sokoloff et al., 1997); *Intrinsic*

muscle mechanics: (Partridge, 1967; Partridge and Benton, 1981; Houk and Rymer, 1981; Winters and Woo, 1990; Sinkjaer et al., 1992; Heckman and Sandercock, 1996; Brown and Loeb, 1998); *Muscle architecture:* (Sacks and Roy, 1982; Chanaud et al., 1991; Burkholder et al., 1994; Lieber et al., 1997); *Musculoskeletal anatomy and biomechanics:* (Alexander, 1981; Ingen Schenau, 1989; Fowler et al., 1993; Zajac, 1993; Zernicke and Smith, 1996); *Kinesiology:* (Goslow et al., 1973; Rossignol, 1996). In the first half of the twentieth century, investigators of spinal mechanisms studied musculoskeletal organization in relationship to reflex circuits. Sherrington and his coworkers (Creed et al., 1972) recognized that the antagonistic, synergistic, and anti-gravity actions of muscle were important factors in the organization of basic reflex circuits. In addition, Sherrington speculated that biarticular muscles were limited to actions at only one joint through the agency of 'pseud-antagonists' that cancel the actions of the muscle at one joint and promote its actions at the other (Sherrington, 1910). More recently, it has been proposed that biarticular muscles are used to transmit power between joints and enhance interjoint coordination (van Ingen Schenau, 1989). In the 1940s, David Lloyd (1946) defined the myotatic unit concept that provided a direct correspondence between musculoskeletal architecture and neural organization. Synergistic muscle actions were represented by heteronymous projections from group Ia afferents,

---
*Corresponding author. Tel.: (404)727–7406; Fax: (404)727–2648; email: trn@physio.emory.edu

and antagonistic actions by disynaptic inhibition. In this way, the myotatic unit was thought to underlie the patterns of identical innervation of synergists and reciprocal innervation of antagonists for muscles crossing a given joint. Lloyd further speculated that biarticular muscles could be the members of only one myotatic unit, and would mediate mechanical but not neural interactions with the muscles crossing a neighboring joint. These ideas were tested by an extensive series of investigations of afferent projections to motoneurons conducted by Eccles and his coworkers. Considerable variation in the strength of these projections was noted for muscles crossing the feline ankle (Eccles et al., 1957), suggesting that muscles have more complex actions than represented by the myotatic unit concept. In addition, direct violations of the myotatic unit concept were found especially for muscles crossing the knee and hip (Eccles and Lundberg, 1958). For example, monosynaptic connections from some single joint extensor muscles were found to project to the motoneurons of muscles crossing neighboring joints. It was concluded by Eccles and Lundberg that the understanding of connectivity in the spinal cord would depend on further knowledge of the individual actions of muscles, but this line of research was not pursued until later (see Nichols et al., in press). In the late 1950's, the attentions of spinal cord physiologists turned toward a consideration of the intrinsic mechanical properties of active muscle.

The importance of intrinsic properties in muscle and limb mechanics

When an active muscle is stretched in the presence of afferent feedback, the mechanical response consists of contributions from passive structures associated with the muscle, active intrinsic mechanical properties arising from the contractile apparatus, reflex modulation of the firing rates of the active motor units, and reflex recruitment of additional motor units. Granit (1958) showed that the active intrinsic properties probably make a significant contribution to the total response. Granit did not attempt to quantify the relative contributions of intrinsic properties and reflex action partly because the reflex component was subject to

considerable variation. Nonetheless, this paper helped to set the stage for the separation of passive, intrinsic and reflex components of the responses of muscles in situ.

Matthews (1959) improved upon the experiments of Granit in several respects, including the use of a wider range of lengths and a renewed consideration of the significance of activation rate, and in matching to some extent the movement histories of muscles with intact reflex and with direct electrical stimulation. For both reflexive and areflexive muscle, the muscles were slowly and continuously stretched. In qualitative agreement with Granit, Matthews concluded that the increases in active tension of the soleus muscle in response to stretch could not be used to indicate the magnitude of the stretch reflex, because a substantial increase in tension resulted from the intrinsic mechanical properties of previously activated muscle. These two papers were important not only in alerting researchers to the significance of intrinsic properties of muscle, but also to the necessity of characterizing more fully these intrinsic properties under conditions of natural movement or at least intact spinal cord output.

In the next decade, a classic series of papers appeared in which the intrinsic mechanical properties of muscles under many conditions of physiological activation and loading were described (Joyce et al., 1969; Joyce and Rack, 1969; Rack and Westbury, 1969). These papers have been widely quoted and reviewed (Houk and Rymer, 1981), but a recurring theme in these investigations that is relevant to the present discussion is the importance of movement history in determining force output of muscle. The length-tension properties of muscle were initially characterized for different stimulation frequencies using the traditional method of stimulating the muscle at each length (Rack and Westbury, 1969). That is, length changes were made only while the muscle was inactive between trials. Ramp stretches applied to the active muscle at different operating points on this family of curves showed that the muscle is initially much stiffer than predicted by the isometric length-tension curves. Furthermore, the force approaches the values predicted by the isometric curves slowly if at all (Joyce et al., 1969).

These findings underscored the fact that the 'isometric length-tension relationship', as defined above, is not really a relationship at all but a set of disconnected points on the force-length plane. Anytime that a muscle is lengthened or shortened during activation, the force neither follows nor quicky settles to the values predicted by this relationship (Abbott and Aubert, 1952; Edman et al., 1982). Consequently, the slope of the isometric length-tension 'relationship' is not a valid estimate of muscular stiffness for a significant range of muscle lengths. This point can be illustrated by the result that if a muscle is stretched between two points on the 'descending limb' of the isometric length curve, the force actually rises and stays elevated for an extended period of time (Deleze, 1961).

It was also shown that muscles passing through the same length from different initial conditions under isotonic loading generate different forces (Joyce and Rack, 1969). These studies helped to establish that intrinsic mechanical properties are dependent not only on instantaneous length and force but also on prior movement history and therefore behavioral context. It became clear from these investigations that the traditionally described isometric length-tension and force velocity relationships do not constitute a comprehensive description of the mechanical behavior of muscle and therefore any model based solely on these relationships would be inadequate to account for natural behavior. In addition, it was argued by Rack (1970) on the basis of this work that the instantaneous mechanical response of muscle would serve to provide the initial resistance of the muscle to a mechanical disturbance before any reflex activity could act to govern the mechanical response. Therefore, intrinsic mechanical properties were shown to be important not only 'behind the scenes' in the mechanical behavior of the integrated system, but also dictated the initial responses of the body (along with global mechanical properties such as inertia) to mechanical disturbances. These results also revealed a unique design feature of muscle. When a muscle is constrained isometrically, as occurs during the maintenance of steady posture, the muscle exhibits a particularly high stiffness for small amplitudes of stretch (Rack and Westbury, 1974). This initially high stiffness is commonly referred to as *short range stiffness*. The short range is followed by a *yield* in muscular stiffness that is particularly pronounced in slow twitch fibers that exhibit a high short-range stiffness (Malamud et al., 1996).

The possibility raised by Granit and Matthews, that intrinsic mechanical properties of muscle could contribute substantially to the responses of reflexly controlled muscles, was extended in a seminal paper by Grillner (1972). Grillner measured the firing rates of motor units in feline triceps surae muscles during locomotion and activated these muscles at similar rates electrically. He then applied slow, continous stretches to the muscles and measured the force output. After transforming these force-length properties by the geometry of the hindlimb, Grillner concluded that the intrinsic stiffness of the triceps surae would be sufficient to account for the ability of the cat to resist postural disturbances. Although Grillner did not deny the possible participation of reflex activation in setting the stiffness of limb, he claimed to show that intrinsic properties could account for postural stability. He argued further that intrinsic properties would be even more important during locomotion when reflex delays would preclude the participation of neural mechanisms of posture. Grillner was justified in computing muscular stiffness from his experiments since he did use, like Matthews, continuous stretches of activated muscle rather than a length series of isometric forces. He also employed rapid stretches and observed the short-range stiffness described by Rack and colleagues (Joyce et al., 1969).

The relative contributions of reflex activity and intrinsic mechanical properties to the mechanical responses of muscles were evaluated for conditions approximating steady posture by Nichols and Houk in the early 1970s (Nichols and Houk, 1976; Cope et al., 1994). This work was undertaken to test the hypothesis (Stiffness Hypothesis) that the stretch reflex regulates the stiffness of muscle to provide more spring-like behavior than is exhibited by the intrinsic properties alone. In order to estimate the appropriate intrinsic properties more closely than Matthews or Granit, transient responses of muscles electrically stimulated or activated by intact spinal cord output without feedback were employed. Similar movement histories for muscles with and without feedback were preserved, and physiologically realistic length inputs were used. For a wide range of initial forces and velocities of stretch, reflexly generated force blended nearly seamlessly with the initial mechanical response of the muscle to provide a more spring-like response. The contribution of intrinsic properties increased with background force (Houk and Rymer, 1981; Hoffer and Andreassen, 1981; Nichols, 1987; Toft et al., 1991), and the contribution of those motor units recruited by the stretch reflex decreased with background force leading to a reduced dependence of total stiffness on force. In answer to Grillner's argument, the reflex activity provides for a substantial response at low forces where intrinsic muscular stiffness is also small. Similar results have been obtained from human subjects (Carter et al., 1990; Sinkjaer, 1997).

The foregoing review features the influence of previous length history and operating conditions on the mechanical behavior of muscle. The pattern of action potentials transmitted to a muscle also have a profound effect on the force-generating capability of the muscle. By inserting a single extra stimulating pulse at the beginning of an otherwise constant train of stimuli that leads to a subfused contraction, the subsequent force output of the muscle is enhanced dramatically (Burke et al., 1976). This phenomenon has become known as a 'catch-like' property. In addition, muscles can become potentiated after continuous stimulation (Brown and Loeb, 1998; Sinkjaer et al., 1992) by a steady train of impulses, and this effect is particularly prominent for type II muscle (Brown and Loeb, 1998). The bases of these two types of potentiation are not fully understood. However, it is clear that the force output of a muscle is influenced by activation as well as length history.

These studies indicated that both intrinsic properties and the stretch reflex contribute importantly to the net mechanical properties of muscle, but they left open the question of the relative contributions of these two components during ongoing locomotion. The studies of Rack and his coworkers suggested that the mechanical behavior of muscle would be quite different under conditions of posture and locomotion due to the influence of length history. Furthermore, these differences would likely be reflected in the mechanical behavior of extrafusal as well as intrafusal muscle and, therefore both intrinsic and reflex components of the responses of muscles (Gregory et al., 1987). Short latency reflexes are apparently important for normal coordination during locomotion (Nichols et al., in press), but the manner in which these components are altered by a change in behavioral state did not become clear until more recently.

The influence of movement history on intrinsic mechanical properties

As discussed in the previous section, the dependence of the mechanical behavior of muscle on prior movement and activation history has been the subject of active research for many decades and continues to be the focus of intense research. It is timely to discuss this aspect of muscle physiology because the adaptive properties of the entire motor system presently occupy center stage in research devoted to normal and pathological mechanisms of coordination. Although neural mechanisms in the spinal cord are subject to modification on the basis of behavioral context, the mechanics of both extrafusal and intrafusal muscle can also change adaptively in relation to motor task due to differences in prior movement and activation history. Therefore, the admittedly complex mechanisms of neuronal plasticity cannot account entirely for the ability of the motor system to rapidly adjust to changing behavioral demands.

The purpose of this section is to present recent experimental data showing that the intrinsic properties of both extrafusal and intrafusal fibers are modified by movement history. The consequent effects on intrinsic and reflex components are twofold. First, the properties of the composite muscle-reflex system remain spring-like, but the magnitude of stiffness changes as a function of history or behavioral context. Second, in the case of inertial loads where oscillations are likely, the neuromuscular system initially presents high stiffness to stabilize position and then decreases stiffness to damp out subsequent oscillations. This appropriate sequence of mechanical properties for

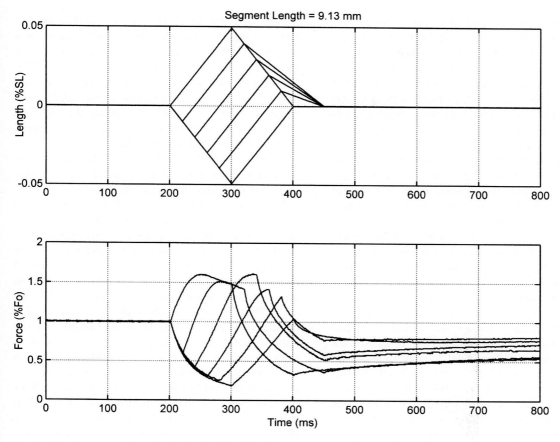

Fig. 1. Data from a cat soleus single muscle fiber. The fiber segment was shortened by 1, 2, 3, 4 and 5% of the segment length (SL) at a velocity of 0.5 SL/s. After the shortening, the fiber was immediately subjected to the test perturbation of a stretch of 5% of the SL at a velocity of 0.5 SL/s.

stabilizing posture occurs without the need for a feedback system with 'gain scheduling', where feedback gains are varied to produce an optimal response according to a complex algorithm or lookup table.

Movement history effects on intrinsic mechanical properties of muscle

Muscle mechanical properties have been characterized at the single muscle fiber and whole muscle levels. A common finding at all these levels is that the properties are generally viscoelastic, and linear and nonlinear behavior can be exhibited under different conditions. However, these behaviors are usually elicited while the muscle is initially iso-

metric, and the generality of these results to conditions of prior movement is not known. Recent data have shown that preceding length changes often determine the intrinsic mechanical properties.

Single muscle fiber studies have most often focused on the steady-state mechanical properties, namely the force-length and force-velocity relationships, when the fiber is initially isometric. However, the history-dependent properties of muscle can be most readily appreciated from an analysis of responses to transient mechanical perturbations. For example, a constant velocity shortening was imposed on a fiber prior to the stretch perturbation (Fig. 1; see Huyghues-Despointes, 1998). The impact of the prior shortening on two important transient properties, short-range stiffness and yielding, was twofold. First, although the absolute short-range stiffness and the force immediately preceding the stretch (initial force) both declined, the stiffness decreased less than the initial force. Second, the short range was extended so that the yield occurred at a longer length change than following the isometric condition. The extent of the linear range depended upon the magnitude of the prior shortening (Huyghues-Despointes, 1998).

Experiments on areflexive, whole muscle have also demonstrated the influence of movement history. The effects of prior shortening on mechanical properties of the homogeneous cat soleus muscle were similar to those observed for single fibers (Huyghes-Despointes, 1998). Prior lengthenings imposed on the whole muscle also decreased initial muscle stiffness to subsequent perturbations (Lin and Rymer, 1993). A comparison of the muscle's mechanical response fitted with a linear viscoelastic model showed that stiffness values were substantially greater during the initial stretch of the muscle from its isometric state than during the continuous random perturbations which followed (Kirsch et al., 1994). In all these experiments, the measured stiffness after prior length changes, for both shortenings and lengthenings, is less compared to the stiffness measured from an isometric condition.

Movement history effects on stretch reflex responses

The response to stretch of muscle spindles, the key receptors of the stretch reflex, has been deduced from primary afferent recordings in reduced animal preparations. In anesthetized cats, history dependent afferent responses have been shown by briefly stimulating the ventral roots innervating the soleus muscle while the muscle was at a long length, and then shortening the muscle before application of the test stretch (Gregory et al., 1986; Proske et al., 1992). The initial afferent response in this protocol was reduced compared to the response while the muscle was kept isometric before the test stretch. It was postulated that prior shortening causes the cross-bridges of the intrafusal muscle fibers to go slack, and this slack must be taken up before the

spindle is sensitive to stretch. In another experimental paradigm, length changes in the form of a triangular waveform were imposed on the soleus muscle in decerebrate cats (Houk et al., 1992). Recordings from primary spindle endings showed that the initial burst in response to the stretch was reduced in the second stretch compared to the first stretch, which started from the isometric condition. It was hypothesized that the initial stretch causes a yield in the intrafusal fibers, causing them to be more compliant in subsequent stretches and reducing the overall sensitivity of the spindle.

In human studies, the electromyographic (EMG) signal from a muscle has been used to infer that the stretch reflex gain is decreased by prior movement. At the human ankle, prior movement reduced the reflex gain in the ankle extensor muscles, measured by the amount of short-latency EMG and torque increase to a stretch perturbation (Stein and Kearney, 1995). In addition, the reflex gain was graded by the amplitude of the prior movement. At the human distal thumb joint, the application of a torque impulse caused a larger EMG response in the flexor pollicis longus (FPL) muscle during the first cycle of oscillation than in the second cycle of oscillation for similar amplitudes of stretch (Lin and Rymer, 1997). It should be noted that changes in synaptic gain at the motoneuron cannot be ruled out as the cause of the reflex gain variations. However, the parallel findings of the primary afferent studies and of the human EMG studies strongly suggest that the source of the movement related EMG response changes is found at the level of the muscle spindle.

In summary, the studies in both reduced animal preparations and humans concur that the stretch reflex gain is dependent on movement history. More specifically, it is likely that prior movement, either in the shortening or lengthening direction, decreases the subsequent spindle response to stretch in proportion to the amplitude of the prior movement.

Movement history effects on the neuromuscular response

The experimental data presented thus far have independently shown that both the intrinsic force

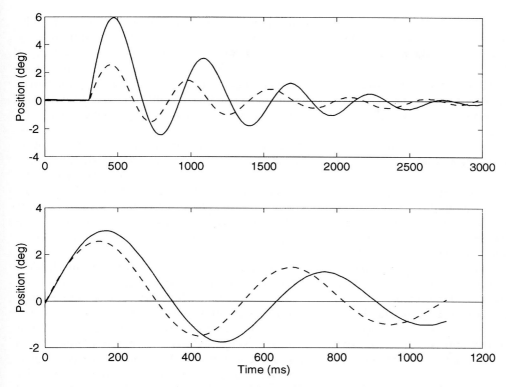

Fig. 2. The oscillations which occur when a torque impulse is applied to an inertial load coupled to the distal thumb joint. The two different impulse magnitudes produced similar velocities for the start of the first cycle of one trial (dashed) and the second cycle of the other trial (solid). The bottom figure shows the first and second cycles aligned in time. The frequency of the second cycle is much less than that of the first cycle, implying that the stiffness had decreased due to the prior movement.

generating properties of muscle and the muscle spindle response to stretch vary with movement history. Although it appears likely that the mechanical properties of neuromuscular system (muscle with reflex activation) should also be movement history dependent, the resulting properties are still not easily predicted.

A length change paradigm in which a shortening movement prior to the test stretch was used as in the single fiber and areflexive whole muscle experiments, was imposed upon reflexively active soleus muscles in decerebrate cats (Huyghes-Despointes, 1998). Instead of the yield-like behavior which progressively diminished as the shortening amplitude increased (Fig. 1), the stretch reflex gain was modulated in order to maintain a linear stiffness response throughout the duration of the stretch perturbation. Thus, although the intrinsic muscle mechanical properties depended upon

the amount of prior shortening, the reflex activation changed in a parallel fashion to produce a net response that resembled a linear stiffness whenever the stretch was imposed.

In order to describe the ability of the neuromuscular system to damp out oscillations, torque impulses of varying magnitudes were applied to an inertial load coupled to the human distal thumb joint (Lin and Rymer, 1997). With the subject given the 'do not intervene' instruction, the FPL muscle, which was initially active, provided viscoelastic properties to counteract the impulse and gave rise to damped oscillations due to the interactions with the inertial load (Fig. 2). As shown in Fig. 2, for some trials with different impulse magnitudes, the first cycle of oscillation had an initial velocity comparable to the velocity at the start of a second cycle of oscillation for another trial. The striking feature of this comparison is that the frequency of oscillation was less for the second cycle of oscillation, implying that the stiffness had decreased in comparison to that which was exhibited when the muscle was initially isometric. This result is consistent with the previously discussed study which also showed a reduction in neuromuscular stiffness due to the prior movement.

Functional significance of movement history dependent neuromuscular properties

The dependence of intrinsic muscle properties on prior movement, as shown in Fig. 1, could be problematic for the neural control system because force response to a given length change can vary dramatically. However, this potential problem is attenuated by the parallel changes in spindle properties, which act in concert to manifest a linear stiffness. Although the magnitude of the stiffness will vary with the movement history, the stability of the musculoskeletal system is preserved because the neuromuscular system still acts like a passive mechanical element ('passivity' constraint, see Hogan, 1990).

The functional significance of movement history dependence for the maintenance of posture can be realized from the experiments with torque impulses applied to an inertial load coupled to the neuromuscular system. Posture often requires that the initial position be maintained and that any velocity transients be damped out. Unfortunately, the viscoelasticity provided by the neuromuscular system interacts with the limb inertia, and the combination often gives rise to oscillations whenever there is an external disturbance.

In mechanical systems with linear viscoelastic elements, the 'optimal' parameter values are set by a compromise between the elasticity (maintains position but causes oscillations) and the viscosity (damps out oscillations but provides no restoration of position). On the other hand, since the neuromuscular system behaves nonlinearly due to the movement history dependence, this compromise may be unneccessary.

The stiffness of the neuromuscular system when it is isometric (pre-perturbation) is high. Immediately following the perturbation, the high stiffness acts to limit the excursion and return the

limb inertia back to its posture position quickly. The kinetic energy of the inertia will subsequently cause an overshoot in initial position, resulting in oscillations. However, the decrease in stiffness of the neuromuscular system due to the prior movement indicates that the intrinsic muscle viscosity has a greater relative role in determining its mechanical properties. The result is that the behavior becomes more characteristic of an overdamped system (see Fig. 2). In summary, the movement dependent properties sequence the mechanical properties during the oscillations following a perturbation, such that initially, position is maintained by high stiffness but subsequently, the oscillations are damped out by the greater relative contribution of muscle viscosity.

This time-varying presentation of mechanical properties is similar to a feedback system with 'gain scheduling', where the gain of the feedback loops (i.e. position and velocity) are varied in time to provide a desired response (Tzafestas, 1993). It has been suggested that the neuromuscular system has the capability of behaving similarly because gamma motoneurons control spindle sensitivity (Prochazka, 1989). However, the experimental evidence presented here demonstrates that previous length changes also automatically modulate the properties of muscle and spindle. Thus, 'gain scheduling' can be achieved by the appropriate dependence of peripheral properties on movement history, instead of a descending, time-varying neural command. The dependence of mechanical properties on movement history is an excellent reason why intrinsic peripheral properties must be integrated into our understanding of the neural control mechanisms of the spinal cord.

Acknowledgement

This work was supported by NIH grants HD32571 and NS20855

References

Abbott, B.C. and Aubert, X.M. (1952) The force exerted by active striated muscle during and after change of length. *J. Physiol.*, 117: 77–86.

Alexander, R. McN. (1981) Mechanics of skeleton and tendon. In: V.B. Brooks, (Ed.), *Handbook of Physiology, Section 1:*

The Nervous System. Volume II. Motor Control, Part 1. American Physiological Society, Bethesda, pp. 17–42.

Brown, I.E. and Loeb, G.E. (1998) Post-activation potentiation- a clue for simplifying models of muscle dynamics. *Amer. Zool.*, 38:743–754.

Burke, R.E. (1981) Motor units: anatomy, physiology, and functional organization. In: V.B. Brooks, (Ed.), *Handbook of Physiology*, Section 1: *The Nervous System*. Bethesda: American Physiological Society, Bethesda, pp. 345–422.

Burke, R.E., Rudomin, P. and Zajac, F.E. (1976) The effect of activation history on tension production by individual muscle units. *Brain Res.*, 109: 515–529.

Burkholder, T.J., Fingado, B., Baron, S. and Lieber, R.L. (1994) Relationship between muscle fiber types and sizes and muscle architectural properties in the mouse hindlimb. *J. Morph.*, 221: 177–190.

Carter, R.R., Crago, P. E. and Keith, M.W. (1990) Stiffness regulation by reflex action in the normal human hand. *J. Neurophysiol.*, 64: 105–118.

Chanaud, C.M., Pratt, C.A. and Loeb, G.E. (1991) Functionally complex muscles of the cat hindlimb II. Mechanical and architectural heterogeneity within the biceps femoris. *Exp. Brain Res.*, 85: 257–270.

Cope, T.C., Bonasera, S.J. and Nichols, T.R. (1994) Reinner- vated muscles fail to produce stretch reflexes. *J. Neurophysiol.*, 71: 817–820.

Cope, T.C. and Clark, B.D. (1991) Motor-unit recruitment in the decerebrate cat: several unit properties are equally good predictors of order. *J. Neurophysiol.*, 66: 1127–1138.

Creed, R.S., Denny-Brown, D., Eccles, J.C., Liddell, E.G.T. and Sherrington, C.S. (1972) *Reflex Activity of the Spinal Cord*, (Lloyd, D.P.C., annotations) Oxford, London, 1972.

Délèze, J.B. (1961) The mechanical properties of the semi- tendinosus muscle of lengths greater than its length in the body. *J. Physiol.*, 158: 154–164.

Eccles, J.C., Eccles, R.M. and Lundberg, A. (1957) The convergence of monosynaptic excitatory afferents on to many different species of alpha motoneurons. *J. Physiol.*, 137: 22–50.

Eccles, R.M. and Lundberg, A. (1958) Integrative pattern of Ia synaptic actions on motoneurons of hip and knee muscles. *J. Physiol.*, 144: 271–298.

Edman, K.A.P., Elzinga, G. and Noble, M.I.M. (1982) Residual force enhancement after stretch of contractiong frog single muscle fibres. *J. General Physiol.*, 80: 769–784.

Fowler, E.G., Gregor, R.J., Hodgson, J.A. and Roy, R.R. (1993) Relationship between ankle muscle and joint kinetics during the stance phase of locomotion in the cat. *J. Biomechanics*, 26: 465–483.

Goslow, G.E. Reinking, R.M. and Stuart, D.G. (1973) The cat step cycle hind limb joint angles and muscle lengths during unrestrained locomotion. *J. Morph.*, 141: 1–42.

Granit, R. (1958) Neuromuscular interaction in postural tone of the cat's isometric soleus muscle. *J. Physiol.*, 143: 387–402.

Gregory, J.E., Morgan, D.L. and Proske, U. (1986) Aftereffects in the responses of cat muscle spindles. *J.Neurophysiol.*, 56: 451–461.

Gregory, J.E., Morgan, D.L. and Proske, U. (1987) Changes in size of stretch reflex of cat and man attributed to aftereffects in muscle spindles. *J.Neurophysiol.*, 58: 628–640.

Grillner, S.(1972) The role of muscle stiffness in meeting the changing postural and locomotor requirements force devel- opment by the ankle extensors. *Acta Physiol. Scand.*, 86: 92–108.

Heckman, C.J. and Sandercock, T. G. (1996) From motor unit to whole muscle properties during locomotor movements. *Exer. Sport Sci. Rev.*, 24: 109–133.

Hoffer, J.A. and Andreassen, S. (1981) Regulation of soleus muscle stiffness in premammillary cat intrinsic and reflex components. *J. Neurophysiol.*, 45: 267–285.

Hogan, N. (1990) Mechanical impedance of single- and multi- articular systems. In: J.M. Winters and S.L-Y Woo, (Eds), *Multiple Muscle Systems. Biomechanics and Movement Organization*, Springer-Verlag, New York, pp. 149–164.

Houk, J.C. and Rymer, W.Z. (1981) Neural control of muscle length and tension. In: V.B. Brooks, (Ed.), *Handbook of Physiology*; v. Section 1, *The Nervous System*; Volume II, *Motor Control*, Part 1, American Physiological Society Bethesda, pp. 257–323.

Houk, J.C., Rymer, W.Z. and Crago, P.E. (1991) Responses of muscle spindle receptors to transitions in stretch velocity. In: L. Jami, E. Pierrot-Deseilligny and D. Zytnicki, (Eds), *Muscle Afferents and Spinal Control of Movement*, Perga- mon, Oxford, pp. 53–61.

Huyghues-Despointes, C.M.J.I. (1998) Effects of Movement History on the Intrinsic Properties and the Neural Regulation of Feline Skeletal Muscle. Ph.D. Dissertation, Emory University, Atlanta.

Ingen Schenau, G.J. van. (1989) From rotation to translation: constraints on multi-joint movements and the unique action of bi-articular muscles. *Hum. Mov. Sci.*, 8:301–337.

Joyce, G. C. and Rack, P.M.H. (1969) Isotonic lengthening and shortening movements of cat soleus muscle. *J. Physiol.*, 204: 475–491.

Joyce, G.C., Rack, P.M.H. and Westbury, D.R. (1969) The mechanical properties of cat soleus muscle during controlled lengthening and shortening movements. *J. Physiol.*, 204: 461–474.

Kirsch, R.F., Boskov, D. and Rymer, W.Z. (1994) Muscle stiffness during transient and continuous movements of cat muscle: perturbation characteristics and physiological rele- vance. *IEEE Trans. Biomed. Eng.*, 41: 758–770.

Lieber, R.L., Ljung, B-O. and Friden, J. (1997) Intraoperative sarcomere length measurements reveal differential design of human wrist extensor muscles. *J. Exp. Biol.*, 200: 19–25.

Lin, D.C. and Rymer, W.Z. (1993) Mechanical properties of cat soleus muscle elicited by sequential ramp stretches: implica- tions for control of muscle. *J. Neurophysiol.*, 70: 997–1008.

Lin, D.C. and Rymer, W.Z. (1997) Nonlinear dampling properties of the human muscle/reflex system with inertial loads. *Soc. Neurosci.*, Abstr. 23: 763.

Lloyd, D.P.C. (1946) Integrative pattern of excitation and inhibition in two-neuron reflex arcs. *J. Neurophysiol.*, 9: 439–444.

378

Malamud, J.G., Godt, R.E. and Nichols, T.R. (1996) Relationship between short-range stiffness and yielding in type-identified, chemically skinned muscle fibers from the cat triceps surae muscles. *J. Neurophysiol.*, 76: 2280–2289.

Matthews, P.B.C. (1959) The dependence of tension upon extension in the stretch reflex of the soleus muscle of the decerebrate cat. *J. Physiol.*, 147: 521–546.

Nichols, T.R. (1987) The regulation of muscle stiffness: implications for the control of limb stiffness. In: P. Marconnet, (Ed.), *Medicine and Sport Science*, v. 26, *Muscular Function in Exercise and Training*, Karger, Basel, pp. 36–47.

Nichols, T.R., Cope, T.C. and Abelew, T.A. Rapid spinal mechanisms of Motor Coordination. *Exerc. Sports Sci. Rev.*, 27: 255–284.

Nichols, T.R. and Houk, J.C. (1976) The improvement in linearity and regulation of stiffness that results from action of the stretch reflex. *J. Neurophysiol.*, 39: 119–142.

Partridge, L.D. (1967) Intrinsic feedback factors producing inertial compensation in muscle. *Biophy J.*, 7: 853–863.

Partridge, L.D. and Benton, L.A. (1981) Muscle, the motor. In: V.B. Brooks, (Ed.), *Handbook of Physiology*, Section 1, *The Nervous System*; Volume II, *Motor Control*, Part 1, American Physiological Society, Bethesda, pp. 43–106.

Prochazka, A. (1989) Sensorimotor gain control: a basic strategy of motor systems? *Prog. Neurobiol.*, 33: 281–307.

Proske, U; Morgan, D.L. and Gregory, J.E. (1992) Muscle history dependence of responses to stretch of primarry and secondary endings of cat soleus muscle spindles. *J. Physiology.*, 445: 81–95.

Rack, P.M.H. (1970) The significance of mechanical properties of muscle in the reflex control of posture. In: P. Andersen and J.K.S. Jansen, (Eds), *Excitatory Synaptic Mechanisms*, Oslo: Universitetsforlaget, Oslo, pp. 317–321.

Rack, P.M.H. and Westbury, D.R. (1969) The effects of length and stimulus rate on tension in the isometric cat soleus muscle. *J. Physiol.*, 204: 443–460.

Rack, P.M.H. and Westbury, D.R. (1974) The short range stiffness of active mammalian muscle and its effect on mechanical properties. *J. Physiol.*, 240: 331–350.

Rossignol, S. (1996) Neural Control of stereotypic limb movements. In: L.B. Rowell and J.T. Shepherd, (Eds), *Handbook of Physiology*. Section 12: *Exercise: Regulation and Integration of Multiple Systems*, Oxford, New York, pp. 173–216.

Sacks, R.D. and Roy, R.R. (1982) Architecture of the hind limb muscles of cvats: functional significance. *J. Morph.*, 173: 185–195.

Sherrington, C.S. (1910) Flexion-reflex of the limb crossed extenison-reflex and reflex stepping and standing. *J. Physiol.*, 40: 28–121.

Sinkjaer, T. (1997) Muscle, reflex and central components in the control of the ankle joint in healthy and spastic man. *Acta Neurol. Scand.*, 96 (Suppl.): 1–28.

Sinkjaer, T., Gantchev, N. and Arendt-Nielsen, L. (1992) Mechanical properties of human ankle extensors after muscle potentiation. *Electroenceph. clin. Neurophysiol.*, 85: 412–418.

Sokoloff, A.J., Cope, T.C., Nichols, T.R. and English, A. W. (1997) Directions of torques produced about the ankle joint by cat medial gastrocnemius motor units. *Mot. Contr.*, 1: 340–353.

Stein, R.B. and Kearney, R.E. (1995) Nonlinear behavior of muscle reflexes at the human ankle joint. *J. Neurophysiol.*, 73: 65–72.

Toft, E., Sinkjer, T., Andreassen, S. and Larsen, K. (1991) Mechanical and electromyographic responses to stretch of human ankle extensors. *J. Neurophysiol.*, 65: 4102–1410.

Tzafestas, S.G. (1993) *Applied Control*. New York: Marcel Dekker.

Winters, J.M. and Woo, S.L-Y. (Eds), *Multiple Muscle Systems*. Biomechanics and Movement Organization. New York: Springer-Verlag; 1990.

Zajac, F.E. (1993) Muscle coordination of movement: a perspective. *J. Biomech.*, 26: 109–124.

Zernicke, R.F. and Smith, J.L. (1996) Biomechanical insights into neural control of movement. In: L.B. Rowell and J.T. Shepherd, (Eds), *Handbook of Physiology*. Section 12: *Exercise: Regulation and Integration of Multiple Systems*. Oxford, New York, pp. 293–332.

M.D. Binder (Ed.)
Progress in Brain Research, Vol 123
© 1999 Elsevier Science BV. All rights reserved.

CHAPTER 33

Kinematic redundancy

Z. Hasan* and J.S. Thomas

College of Health and Human Development Sciences, University of Illinois at Chicago, Chicago, IL 60612, USA

At this stage in our knowledge of the segmental motor-control system, we think that it is particularly important to identify [the] functional components and the conditions under which they may be used in concert or in some degree of separation.

D. G. Stuart et al. (1988)

Introduction

It is often the case that a movement task can be accomplished by choosing any one of many different ways of apportioning motions to various segments of the body and limbs. For example, one can touch one's nose with a fingertip using many different orientations of the upper arm, and correspondingly, different orientations of the other segments of the arm and the fingers. The question then arises as to how the central nervous system (CNS) chooses the orientations. Does it do so based upon fixed rules, or does it vary capriciously the apportionment of segmental motions from one attempt to the next? If indeed there are rules, which at least to some extent govern the relative involvement of the various segments, do the rules take into account the initial state, desired speed of performance, loading, or other experimentally manipulable quantities? Do the rules vary across individual subjects? And if so, are the rules idiosyncratic to each subject, or do they depend to some extent on anthropometric parameters, gender, or training?

*Corresponding author. Tel.: 312-996-1504; Fax: 312-996-4583; e-mail: zhasan@uic.edu

Surprisingly, rather limited attention has been paid to these issues in the motor-control literature, though they would appear to be of fundamental importance.

When the requirements of a task fall short of specifying uniquely the needed excursions of all the available segments, the extent of this falling short can be judged by comparing the number of task parameters with the number of available kinematic degrees of freedom (DOFs). The DOFs for any unconstrained, rigid object in 3-dimensional space are six in number, three of which are translational and three rotational. When considering several – say, N – linked segments of the body, however, the DOFs number less than 6N, because the segments are constrained translationally by being joined to each other, and the joints are not always of the ball-and-socket type that allows three rotational DOFs. The DOFs of the upper arm and forearm segments, for example, do not add up to 12. Specifically, if one assumes no translational motions of the glenohumeral joint, the upper arm has only three DOFs (which can be characterized, for example, by upper arm flexion/extension, abduction/adduction, and internal/external rotation), and the forearm adds only two DOFs (flexion/extension, and pronation/supination), for a total of five DOFs. If a task required the wrist to touch a target (i.e. a specified point in 3-dimensional space), we would have five DOFs available to perform the task, whereas only three variables specify the target position. Because three equations cannot provide a unique solution when there are five unknowns, there are many different ways of choosing the five kinematic variables so as to accomplish this task. In fact, there are infinitely many ways, because each of the kinematic variables is a continuous variable. In general, for most tasks performed ordinarily, the requirements imposed by the task are few enough to allow considerable leeway in choosing the kinematic variables. The leeway is often seen as stemming from redundant DOFs – though one could, with equal justification, describe them as abundant rather than redundant. This embarrassment of riches is seen as posing for the CNS the problem of how to resolve the redundancy, which is the so-called degrees-of-freedom problem of Bernstein, acknowledged routinely in the literature but not often addressed experimentally.

Here we review, albeit cursorily, some recent ideas that have been advanced in the literature addressing the resolution of kinematic redundancy, and then we present some of our preliminary findings concerning rules governing the motions of the legs, trunk, and arm for reaching movements of the hand to targets that necessitate trunk bending. Throughout, we focus on the selection of the combination of joint rotations, i.e. on the resolution of redundancy at the kinematic level, not on the selection of muscles and motor units, which can add another layer of redundancy to the problem of movement control (Gielen et al., 1998).

Some recent ideas

Many of the ideas pertaining to the resolution of kinematic redundancy can be subsumed under one of two general approaches: In one we posit that the angular excursions at the joints are, in some sense, minimized, and in the other approach we posit constraining relationships among the joint angles, in analogy with Donders' law of eye movements. We now consider some specific proposals based on these approaches, as well as some that address the kinetic variables.

Approach based on minimizing angular excursions

The underlying idea is that the CNS attempts to minimize changes in joint angles from the initial posture to the final posture. Commonly assumed is the minimization of the sum of the squares; in other words, one chooses the angular excursions such that the task requirements are fulfilled, and the sum of the squares of the excursions is minimized[1]. The sum, therefore, can be considered a 'cost' of the movement. The final angles predicted on the basis of this procedure will, in general, depend on the initial angles at the starting configuration.

Cruse and Brüwer (1987) studied slow, comfortable, horizontal-plane movements of the arm involved in moving the tip of a pointer attached to the hand. Because the movements were confined to a plane, the tip position could be specified by two coordinates, and the arm had three DOFs (angles at the shoulder, elbow, and wrist); thus there was one redundant DOF. They tried to account for their observations concerning joint angles as well as path of the pointer tip in terms of a model in which the minimization was performed incrementally throughout the movement rather than only at the end. What was found to be necessary, however, was the minimization not simply of the sum of the squares of the angular changes, but of these squares weighted by certain functions of the joint angles thought to represent the level of discomfort experienced at different angles. In addition, in order to account for nonstraight paths in certain situations, an additional cost was included corresponding to a mass-spring model. The composite model then provided a good qualitative fit for the time-course

---

[1] Another way of stating this is to start with the 'Jacobian' matrix that allows the determination of, say, change in position of the distal end effector when the incremental changes in the joint angles are given as a column vector. This matrix is not a square one – it has more columns than rows – because there are more joint angles than parameters specifying the target position. If one now wishes to find how much the angles need to be altered when the desired incremental shift in position of the distal tip is specified, the inverse of the matrix needs to be determined. A non-square matrix has an infinite number of inverse matrices, but a generalized 'Moore–Penrose' inverse can be found (Pellionisz, 1985) by methods of matrix algebra, for which the sum of the squares of the angular changes is minimized. Repetition of this procedure can provide the initial-to-final excursions.

data. As for the final configuration, Cruse et al. (1993) found it to be virtually independent of the starting configuration (though this was not the case when an additional DOF was included). The final configuration followed from the relationships between discomfort and angle at each joint; the discomfort functions, moreover, varied from one subject to another, introducing a certain degree of subject dependence. Clearly, then, the simple idea of minimizing the sum of squares of the excursions is insufficient for accounting for the data, but can play some role. The reason for this insufficiency, according to Cruse et al. (1993), lies in the shallowness of the minimum. In other words, there are joint configurations that, strictly speaking, do not minimize the cost, and therefore are not picked as minima, but nevertheless entail almost as low a cost as the true minimum. A subject who adopts one of these configurations with marginally more than the minimum cost, contradicts the minimum cost hypothesis, but only in the strict sense.

Lacquaniti and Maioli (1994b) provide a more severe argument against the minimization of the sum of the squares of the excursions. They had observed earlier that the three joint angles of a cat's limb measured in various postural states of the animal, when plotted as points in a 3-dimensional joint space, are not scattered randomly in the joint space, but lie on a plane in this space. The authors calculated where the joint angles would lie in the 3-dimensional space if they were obtained as solutions of the sum-of-squares cost minimization problem, for various assumed initial and final endpoint positions within the observed range. It was found that these points would indeed lie in a plane, but one that was nearly orthogonal to the plane that was actually observed. The authors note that the minimization of the sum of the squares of joint excursions ensures that the limb orientation (e.g. the direction of the line joining the hip to the foot) is highly sensitive to changes in joint angles, whereas the observed planar relationship among the angles is such that the effect of the covarying joint angle changes on limb orientation is small. Although this conclusion is based on postural data rather than data that address movement planning, it appears that minimization of joint angle excursions is not necessarily desirable, as it leads to highly sensitive dependence of the limb orientation on the joint angles.

Rosenbaum et al. (1995) have proposed a scheme in which the cost is determined only partly by the joint excursions, which they consider a travel cost, and partly by the straight-line distance to the goal, which they consider spatial cost. The subject is assumed to have access to a large number of pre-stored postures, selected presumably on the basis of prior learning, which he/she can evaluate in terms of their effectiveness as possible goal postures, and then adopt a weighted sum of these possible postures. To simulate this process, the authors posit a number of possible goal postures, and assign to each a weight, in inverse relationship to the total cost associated with the posture; they then compute an average posture using these weights. Thus, the procedure computes a combination from among pre-stored postures, attempting to reduce travel and spatial costs. Vaughan et al. (1998) applied this procedure to account for the final configurations obtained in experiments on seated human subjects reaching with three DOFs (free hip, shoulder, and elbow) for targets placed in a parasagittal plane. The authors chose 665 different a priori stored postures, and by iterative adjustment of four free parameters for each subject, obtained 'reasonably good' fits to the final configurations of each of the four subjects for the twelve target positions. The model accounted for 96% or more of the variance of the observed joint angles. The model has the biological plausibility of starting from a set of postures that might have been learned previously, rather than trying to solve a mathematical problem from scratch. But it is sobering to consider the amount of computation it takes to account for the final orientations of just three segments.

Approach based on interrelationships among the degrees of freedom

This approach is based on an analogy with the well-known Donders' law, established for eye movements (Tweed and Vilis, 1990). Specifically, although the eyeball has three DOFs, it is observed that when shifting the line of sight voluntarily, the specification of the left/right and up/down angles of shift results in a certain torsional rotation of the eyeball that cannot be controlled independently. Therefore, only two variables need to be specified in voluntary movement of the eyeball, which are sufficient to determine its three DOFs. In other words, the three DOFs are constrained by one equation. Donders' law implies that the final values of the angles when the target is achieved are not influenced by the initial values at the starting position.

The idea that the human hand obeys Donders' law has been supported experimentally, at least when the arm is outstretched in the final, pointing position in 3-dimensional space, and thus the hand has three DOFs. Two of the three DOFs predict the third (Straumann et al., 1991; Hore et al., 1992). When data from pointing experiments in which the arm is not necessarily outstretched in the final position are included, however, some violations of Donders' law are revealed (Gielen et al., 1997b). It is interesting to note that adherence to or violation of Donders' law has significant implications for determining the curvature of the trajectory of movement for targets in different locations (Gielen et al., 1997a, b). Thus, the view that straightness of the path in Cartesian or joint-space coordinates implies planning in those coordinates is problematic (cf. Haggard et al., 1995; Desmurget et al., 1995).

During human walking a large number of kinematic variables can be recorded, and probed for any underlying interrelationships. Mah et al. (1994) examined the relationships among eight kinematic variables, corresponding to the sagittal- and frontal-plane orientations of the foot, shank, thigh, and trunk. During unperturbed walking as well as in the presence of obstacles, they found that all eight time series could be reconstructed as linear combinations of only three functions of time ('principal components,' PCs), which together accounted for at least 91% of the variance in the data. These conclusions were arrived at by the use of Principal Component Analysis, a technique for reducing the dimensionality of a data set in which there are a number of interrelated variables (Jolliffe, 1986). Mah et al. (1994) interpreted the waveform of the first principal component (PC_1) as representing a pendular motion of the leg, the second principal

component (PC_2) as representing hip and ankle flexion, and the third principal component (PC_3) as frontal-plane foot rotation. Irrespective of this interpretation, however, one can conclude that because eight variables were captured quite well as linear combinations of only three, there must be five relationships that are somehow imposed amongst the eight variables. Which of these relationships are mechanical in origin and which are neural, remains to be elucidated. Mah et al. (1994) also examined the altered kinematics in the presence of a brace on one knee, and, remarkably, the time course of PC_1 was quite similar in this situation to that in free walking.

Similarly, Borghese et al. (1996) report that when the sagittal-plane orientations of the foot, shank, and thigh are plotted against each other in a 3-dimensional plot during the gait cycle, the data remain essentially confined to a particular plane. This planar covariation, which was observed at different speeds of locomotion, attests to a specific relationship among the three variables, i.e. an equation relating the three, which remains valid throughout the gait cycle.

As alluded to earlier, a planar covariation is also observed when ankle, knee, and hip angles are plotted against each other in a 3-dimensional plot using data obtained from cats standing freely on a platform with various degrees of tilt, and also in the presence of certain loads applied to the animals (Lacquaniti and Maioli, 1994a). The plane in which the data lie, moreover, is almost the same for different animals, despite the fact that the distribution of data within the plane varies from one animal to another. This latter conclusion is based on a PC analysis, performed not on the time courses of the variables, but on the static values of the variables. The PC_1 and PC_2, which define the plane of covariation, represent two mutually orthogonal directions in the plane; magnitude scalings of PC_1 provide the best fit for the data, and scalings of PC_2 are the best fit of the residual variation. What is remarkable is that the vectors PC_1 and PC_2 were quite different for different cats (Lacquaniti and Maioli, 1994b), which indicates individual or idiosyncratic differences, yet the plane in which PC_1 and PC_2 lie was practically the same for all cats studied, which indicates a certain abstract

383

similarity in the way the kinematic redundancy problem is solved by different cats.

The PC analysis technique has also been utilized to ferret out kinematic synergies in grasping various familiar objects with the hand. Santello et al. (1998) recorded the 15 joint angles of the fingers and the thumb under static conditions, and found that the interrelationships among the 15 DOFs were so strong that for every subject just the first two PCs could account for at least 80% of the variance. The hand postures corresponding to these PCs, however, were not interpretable in terms of conventional descriptions such as the precision and power grips. Principal components are seldom easy to interpret; their value lies perhaps in alerting the investigator to the relationships hidden in the data.

Soechting et al. (1995) tested directly the expectation from Donders' law that in the final position the posture, i.e. the segment orientations, should depend only on that position, and not on the starting position. Seated subjects reached for targets placed in 3-dimensional space, starting from a wide range of initial hand positions. Four DOFs (three at the shoulder and one at the elbow) served to define the posture of the arm. The authors found that the final posture changed when the initial position of the hand was altered, which shows a violation of Donders' law. Moreover, no obvious pattern emerged concerning the dependence of final orientations on initial orientations; the final orientations chosen by the subjects did not appear to correspond to the minimization of the excursions either.

One can conclude that in limb movement the starting position does affect the final posture, unlike Donders' law for eye movement, but, in conformity with Donders' law, certain interrelationships (constraining equations) are observed among the kinematic variables. Of course, if one confines attention to data pertaining to a small range of task variables, one is likely to find some relationships among the measured quantities, which may or may not be interpretable in intuitive terms, or generalizable to other tasks. Nevertheless, an empirical description of these relationships would appear to be a prerequisite for investigations into the mechanisms for the resolution of kinematic redundancy. In a later section we will present another such empirical description of relationships among kinematic variables, observed in the context of reaching movements performed from a standing position.

Approach based on kinetic variables

The preceding approaches were based on consideration of kinematic variables alone. We now turn to the kinetic variables – forces, moments, work, and related quantities – underlying a movement, and the question of whether the minimization of some of these may be consistent with the observations concerning the resolution of kinematic redundancy.

Soechting et al. (1995), in the paper cited earlier, noted that the mechanical work required to accelerate about an axis with a low moment of inertia is small compared to what is required for a different axis, and that subjects indeed prefer rotations about the low inertia axis. The authors proposed, therefore, that it is the minimization of work (summed across the DOFs) that governs the resolution of redundancy. To test this hypothesis quantitatively, the authors ignored the work done against gravity, and, because the work done in accelerating and decelerating adds up to zero, they calculated the peak work involved in moving between actual starting and final positions. They repeated this calculation for different assumed final postures, all of which corresponded to the same final position. With certain simplifying assumptions concerning the trajectory (viz. temporally coincident peak angular velocities, with the peak magnitudes being proportional to the angular excursions), they found that the values of the final angles that minimized peak work during movement were highly correlated with the final angles obtained from data spanning a wide range of initial and final positions. This supports the minimum work hypothesis. Although the simplifying assumptions made about possible trajectories, as well as the neglect of gravitational work, remain questionable, perhaps the test of the hypothesis is relatively insensitive to these assumptions.

A different attempt, aimed at predicting static postures based on kinetic variables, was made by Dysart and Woldstad (1996). Human subjects held a weight in both hands, at each of four different, specified hand positions. The authors measured under static conditions the sagittal-plane angles the subject adopted at five joints: ankle, knee, hip, shoulder, and elbow. The optimality criterion that best fit these data was one which, subject to certain constraints including postural stability, minimized the sum of the absolute values of the moments at the five joints. Even the best fit, however, was quite discrepant from the observations, and was "not within an acceptable margin of error."

None of the optimality criteria discussed so far have provided a clear and general answer to the question of how kinematic redundancy is resolved, although the various approaches have provided some pointers. As we mentioned earlier, an unabashedly empirical approach to the issue, in which one tries to discern any interrelationships among the kinematic variables, may be a useful first step before one tackles the question of how to interpret such relationships.

Some observations on segmental motions for reaching from a standing position

We examined the motions of the shank, thigh, pelvis, trunk (i.e. thoracic spine), upper arm, and forearm segments when standing subjects reached with their right hand for various targets placed in front of them in a parasagittal plane that passed through the right shoulder. A Selspot motion-analysis system was used for kinematic recording; we placed a pair of active markers on each of the six segments enumerated above. The rotations of the six segments in the parasagittal plane, from initial to final, comprised the six variables on which we focused attention. The starting position was not varied: The subject stood erect with the arms vertical. Four target positions were employed, one at shoulder height at a distance of 90% of the arm's length, and three that necessitated forward bending of the trunk. The target positions were chosen based upon the anthropometrics. For example, the target labeled 60° was placed in the parasagittal plane such that if the subject were to flex by 60° at the hip, and flex the shoulder by 90°, keeping all other joint angles unchanged, the hand would touch the target; likewise for the 30° and 15° targets. Note that the subject never actually performed these

particular trunk and shoulder flexions; the targets were defined in the manner described so as to factor out the effect of anthropometric differences among the subjects[2]. For each target position, the subject performed three movement trials at each of three different speeds: one self selected, one faster and one slower than the self selected speed. Eight subjects were tested, four of each gender. We report here on a total of 288 movement trials (eight subjects × four targets × three speeds × three repetitions).

The question we asked was whether the changes in orientation, $\Delta\phi$, of each of the six segments had some relationship(s) among them, which was valid across different subjects, target positions, speeds of movement, and trial repetition. To answer this question, principal component (PC) analysis was performed on the six measured variables, $\Delta\phi$, including all 288 movement trials. The results of this analysis yielded the PCs, given below, as combinations of the unit changes (say, one degree), u, in the $\Delta\phi$s. The subscripts of u identify the segment: *sh* for shank, *th* for thigh, *pl* for pelvis, *tr* for trunk, *ua* for upper arm, and *fa* for forearm. (Each $\Delta\phi$ was defind as positive for counterclockwise rotation as seen from the right of the subject. The coefficients for each PC are scaled so that the sum of their squares equals the eigenvalue.)

$$PC_1 = (+0.201u_{sh}, -0.528u_{th}, +0.872u_{pl}, +0.954u_{tr}, +0.919u_{ua}, +0.910u_{fa})$$

$$PC_2 = (-.965u_{sh}, +0.823u_{th}, +0.326u_{pl}, +0.090u_{tr}, +0.170u_{ua}, +0.112u_{fa})$$

$$PC_3 = (+0.087u_{sh}, +0.154u_{th}, -0.310u_{pl}, -0.170u_{tr}, +0.214u_{ua}, +0.330u_{fa})$$

$$PC_4 = (+0.020u_{sh}, +0.035u_{th}, +0.031u_{pl}, +0.051u_{tr}, -0.283u_{ua}, +0.217u_{fa})$$

---

[2] A similar procedure for target placement was employed in earlier experiments reported by Thomas et al. (1998). However, we tested a different group of subjects than those studied by Thomas et al. (1998), and, unlike the earlier study, we used direct measures of shank and thigh orientations; we also had subjects stand barefoot rather than in gym shoes.

$$PC_5 = (+0.081u_{sh}, +0.036u_{th}, +0.192u_{pl},$$
$$-0.210u_{tr}, +0.013u_{ua}, +0.026u_{fa})$$

$$PC_6 = (+0.121u_{sh}, +0.134u_{th}, +0.013u_{pl},$$
$$+0.076u_{tr}, +0.005u_{ua}, -0.046u_{fa})$$

The variance accounted for by PC_1 was 61.1%, and the cumulative variance accounted for by inclusion of successive PCs was 90.5%, 95.6%, 97.8%, 99.3%, and 100%. The first two PCs are able to account for much of the variance, which means that if the 288 measurements were plotted as points in 6-dimensional space, of which the six $\Delta\phi$s were the coordinates, then the data points would lie close to a 2-dimensional plane in the 6-dimensional space, rather than be scattered throughout the space. This plane would be defined by the mutually orthogonal PC_1 and PC_2 vectors.

Because it is not possible to show in a diagram the distribution of data points in 6-dimensional space, we have chosen to depict it in a 3-dimensional diagram, whose coordinate axes correspond to the directions of PC_1, PC_2, and PC_3. Figure 1 shows the 288 data points plotted in this fashion, as seen from two different perspectives. The plane formed by the directions of PC_1 and PC_2 is also shown, its position along the third axis being the mean value along that axis. As one would have surmised from the variance accounted for, the large majority of data points lie close to the plane. If all the points were precisely in the plane, one could rigorously conclude the following: In the task we employed, only two quantities (corresponding to the scalings of PC_1 and PC_2) need to be specified for every movement trial. These two quantities may depend in some yet-to-be-described way on the target location, the desired speed of movement, the trial number, and the identity of the subject, including the gender (cf. Thomas et al., 1998). But once the two quantities are specified, the excursions for all six DOFs follow unequivocally from them.

To put it differently, the six $\Delta\phi$s were found to be interrelated, being constrained by four equations. The four constraints on the six $\Delta\phi$s can be obtained simply by equating PC_3 through PC_6 to zero in the equations given above, considering that these PCs account for little of the variance in the data. Thus, there is a certain commonality across subjects, speeds, and target locations in how the redundancy is resolved. This commonality is expressed here in abstract terms, but one can attempt to interpret, at least broadly, the implications of PC_3 through PC_6 being zero. In the equation for PC_6 the largest coefficients are those for the shank and the thigh, and these coefficients have the same sign. For PC_6 to be near zero, therefore, the shank and the thigh would be expected to rotate in opposite directions; in other words, ankle plantarflexion would be coupled with knee extension, and ankle dorsiflexion with knee flexion. (Which of the two strategies is chosen may depend on the subject, the speed, the target, or may vary from trial to trial, but the coupling revealed here between shank and thigh excursions would remain valid.) Equating PC_5 to zero, and again focusing on the two coefficients with the largest absolute values, the pelvis and the trunk would be expected to be coupled so as to rotate in the same direction. The equation for PC_4 similarly suggests upper and forearm motions to occur in the same direction. Equating PC_3 to zero is more difficult to interpret, because several coefficients are comparably large and therefore the constraint involves several segments. It is noteworthy that the requirement that the center of mass lie within the base of support would have given us only one constraint, instead of the four constraints we obtained from the data. These four constraints, taken together, not only fulfill the base-of-support requirement, they also demonstrate additional couplings among the segmental motions.

Conclusions

A number of different ideas have been proposed in the literature about the resolution of kinematic redundancy. We have briefly reviewed some of them here. Few ideas based on kinetics have been advanced, most proposals being rooted in kinematic variables. We have divided the latter proposals into two categories, those based on minimizing angular excursions, and those based on an analogy with Donders' law for eye movement. The latter approach, which posits the existence of constraining relationships among the kinematic variables, appears promising, despite the demonstration that Donders' law is not fully applicable to

386

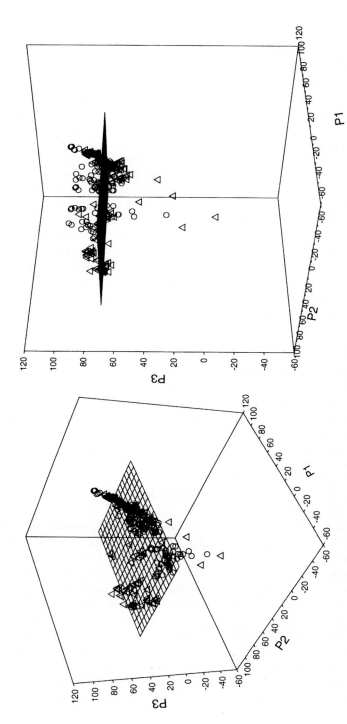

Fig. 1. Two views of the 3-dimensional space defined by the first three principal components (PCs). The PCs were derived from the data on angular excursions of six segments, viz. shank, thigh, pelvis, trunk, upper arm, and forearm. (The axes P1, P2, P3 represent the first three PCs, with scaling that makes each a unit vector in the 6-dimensional space of angular excursions.) The 288 data points shown here were derived from segmental rotations, as described in the text. Circles are for female subjects, and triangles for male subjects. The plane defined by the directions of the first two PCs is shown in both views; it is positioned along the third axis at the mean value of that variable. Most of the points are clustered near the plane, demonstrating that the first two PCs account for much of the variance in the data.

limb movements. Empirical descriptions of inter-relationships among kinematic variables have been advanced, mostly in terms of principal component analyses. This type of analysis, however, results in abstract conclusions that can be difficult to interpret. We have adopted this approach in studying the changes in orientation of the segments of the leg, trunk, and arm in the context of reaching with the hand for targets that necessitate forward bending of the trunk. We found certain commonalities across subjects, speeds, target positions, and trial sequence. These commonalities were expressed as couplings of segmental rotations. Our analysis does not answer the question of how segmental rotations are chosen individually, but makes explicit the rules whereby they are interrelated. It remains to be seen whether similar relationships manifest themselves in widely different tasks, or whether they are specific to the reaching movements we studied. These and similar findings could provide the testing ground for theories concerning the resolution of kinematic redundancy.

References

Borghese, N.A., Bianchi, L. and Lacquaniti, F. (1996) Kinematic determinants of human locomotion. *J. Physiol.*, 494.3: 863–879.

Cruse, H. and Brüwer, M. (1987) The human arm as a redundant manipulator: the control of path and joint angles. *Biol. Cybern.*, 57: 137–144.

Cruse, H., Brüwer, M. and Dean, J. (1993) Control of three- and four-joint arm movement: strategies for a manipulator with redundant degrees of freedom. *J. Mot. Behav.*, 25: 131–139.

Desmurget, M., Prablanc, C., Rossetti, Y., Arzi, M., Paulignan, Y., Urquizar, C. and Mignot, J.-C. (1995) Postural and synergic control for three-dimensional movements of reaching and grasping. *J. Neurophysiol.*, 74: 905–910.

Dysart, M.J. and Woldstad, J.C. (1996) Posture prediction for static sagittal-plane lifting. *J. Biomech.*, 29: 1393–1397.

Gielen, C.C.A.M., van Bolhuis, B. and Vrijenhoek, E. (1998) On the number of degrees of freedom in biological limbs. In: M.L. Latash (Ed.), *Progress in Motor Control: Bernstein's Traditions in Movement Studies*, Human Kinetics, Champaign, pp. 173–190.

Gielen, C.C.A.M., Vrijenhoek, E.J. and Flash, T. (1997a) Principles for the control of kinematically redundant limbs. In: M. Fetter, H. Misslisch and D. Tweed (Eds), *Three-Dimensional Kinematics of Eye-, Head-, and Limb-Movements*, Harwood Academic Publishers, Chur, Switzerland, pp. 285–297.

Gielen, C.C.A.M., Vrijenhoek, E.J., Flash, T. and Neggers, S.F.W. (1997b) Arm position constraints during pointing and reaching in 3-D space. *J. Neurophysiol.*, 78: 660–673.

Haggard, P., Hutchinson, K. and Stein, J. (1995) Patterns of coordinated multi-joint movement. *Exp. Brain Res.*, 107: 254–266.

Hore, J., Watts, S. and Vilis, T. (1992) Constraints on arm position when pointing in three dimensions: Donders' law and the Fick gimbal strategy. *J. Neurophysiol.*, 68: 374–383.

Jolliffe, I.T. (1986) *Principal Component Analysis*. Springer-Verlag, New York.

Lacquaniti, F. and Maioli, C. (1994a) Independent control of limb position and contact forces in cat posture. *J. Neurophysiol.*, 72: 1476–1495.

Lacquaniti, F. and Maioli, C. (1994b) Coordinate transformations in the control of cat posture. *J. Neurophysiol.*, 72: 1496–1515.

Mah, C.D., Hulliger, M., Lee, R.G. and O'Callaghan, I.S. (1994) Quantitative analysis of human movement synergies: constructive pattern analysis for gait. *J. Mot. Behav.*, 26: 83–102.

Pellionisz, A. (1985) Tensor network theory of the metaorganization of functional geometries in the central nervous system. *Neuroscience*, 16: 245–273.

Rosenbaum, D.A., Loukopoulos, L.D., Meulenbroek, R.G.J., Vaughan, J. and Engelbrecht, S.E. (1995) Planning reaches by evaluating stored postures. *Psych. Rev.*, 102: 28–67.

Santello, M., Flanders, M. and Soechting. J.F. (1998) Postural hand synergies for tool use. *J. Neurosci.*, 18: 10105–10115.

Soechting, J.F., Buneo, C.A., Herrmann, U. and Flanders, M. (1995) Moving effortlessly in three dimensions: does Donders' law apply to arm movement? *J. Neurosci.*, 15: 6271–6280.

Straumann, D., Haslwanter, T., Hepp-Reymond, M.-C. and Hepp, K. (1991) Listing's law for eye, head and arm movements and their synergistic control. *Exp. Brain Res.*, 86: 209–215.

Stuart, D.G., Hamm, T.M. and Vanden Noven, S. (1988) Partitioning of monosynaptic Ia EPSP connections with motoneurons according to neuromuscular topography: generality and functional implications. *Prog. Neurobiol.*, 30: 437–447.

Thomas, J.S., Corcos, D.M. and Hasan, Z. (1998) The influence of gender on spine, hip, knee, and ankle motions during a reaching task. *J. Mot. Behav.*, 30: 98–103.

Tweed, D. and Vilis, T. (1990) Geometric relations of eye position and velocity vectors during saccades. *Vision Res.*, 30: 111–127.

Vaughan, J., Rosenbaum, D.A., Harp, C.J., Loukopoulos, L.D. and Engelbrecht, S. (1998) Finding final postures. *J. Mot. Behav.*, 30: 273–284.

M.D. Binder (Ed.)
Progress in Brain Research, Vol 123
© 1999 Elsevier Science BV. All rights reserved.

CHAPTER 34

Task- and age-dependent variations in steadiness

Roger M. Enoka,* Rebecca A. Burnett, Andrew E. Graves, Kurt W. Kornatz and Douglass H. Laidlaw

Department of Kinesiology and Applied Physiology, University of Colorado at Boulder, Boulder, CO 80309-0354, USA

Introduction

Human aging is typically accompanied by a loss of muscle mass and an associated decrease in muscle strength (Narici et al., 1991; Aniansson et al., 1992). The muscle atrophy appears to be caused by the death of motor neurons in the spinal cord (Campbell et al., 1973; Tomlinson and Irving, 1977) and to preferentially involve the motor neurons that innervate the histochemically defined type IIb muscle fibers (Lexell et al., 1988; Kadhiresan et al., 1996). Surviving motor neurons, however, are able to develop axonal sprouts and reinnervate some of the abandoned muscle fibers (Campbell et al., 1973; Kanda and Hashizume, 1989; Masakado et al., 1994; Kadhiresan et al., 1996). The net result of this reorganization is a reduction in the number of motor units in a muscle but an increase in the innervation ratio of the motor neurons that do remain.

According to the Size Principle (Henneman, 1957), the order in which motor units are recruited progresses from the smallest to the largest motor neuron as we grade the force that a muscle exerts. In this scheme, differences in motor neuron size, and those properties that covary with size, are the major determinants in the spinal cord control of muscle force (Binder and Mendell, 1990; Cope and Pinter, 1995). Therefore, disturbances in the rela-

*Corresponding author. Tel.: (303) 492-7232; Fax: (303) 492-6778; e-mail: enoka@stripe.colorado.edu

tive size of motor units within a population, such as the reorganization that occurs with aging, may have significant consequences for the ability of humans to perform tasks requiring subtle variations in the force exerted by muscle.

The purpose of the studies described in this paper has been to characterize the ability of older adults to perform steady submaximal contractions and to determine the role of changes in motor unit size on the observed impairments in performance. The outcome variable in these studies has been fluctuations in the force and acceleration (steadiness) during isometric and anisometric contractions performed by hand and arm muscles.

Decline in steadiness

To characterize the ability of older adults to perform fine motor tasks, we measured the steadiness of the force exerted during isometric contractions (Galganski et al., 1993; Keen et al., 1994; Spiegel et al., 1996; Burnett et al., 1998; Graves et al., 1999), the linearity of the displacement achieved during target-directed, anisometric contractions (Laidlaw et al., 1996, 1997, 1999), and the steadiness of acceleration during constant-velocity anisometric contractions (Burnett et al., 1998; Graves et al., 1999). For the isometric contractions, subjects were instructed to exert a constant force for about 20 s. For the anisometric contractions, subjects were instructed to smoothly raise and lower a constant load in about 12 s. Each task was performed at several levels of intensity; that is, with various target forces and loads.

We compared the performance of young (20–30 yrs) and old (60–90 yrs) adults when they performed tasks with either the first dorsal interosseus muscle or the elbow flexor muscles. For the experiments on the first dorsal interosseus muscle, the subjects were required to exert an abduction force with the index finger of the left hand. Subjects sat with the left arm abducted so that the forearm and hand rested on a platform in a pronated position at about mid-chest level. The forearm was restrained to isolate the mechanical action of the first dorsal interosseus muscle on the index finger. For the experiments on the elbow flexor muscles, subjects were required to exert a force at the wrist in the direction of elbow flexion. Subjects sat with the left arm slightly abducted, the elbow resting on a padded support, and the forearm horizontal in a position midway in the supination-pronation range of motion.

Constant-force contractions

Subjects were asked to perform an isometric contraction so that the force exerted by the index finger would match one of several target forces (range: 2.5 to 75% of the maximum voluntary contraction [MVC] force) displayed on an oscilloscope and to sustain a steady force for about 20 s. The force exerted by the index finger was sensed with a button transducer located at the level of the first interphalangeal joint of the index finger. For the elbow flexor muscles, the force exerted at the wrist was measured with a transducer that was capable of measuring the forces in three directions and the torques about three axes. Steadiness was quantified as the absolute (standard deviation) and normalized (coefficient of variation) fluctuations of the force exerted by the subject about the target value.

For both the young and old subjects, the standard deviation of the fluctuations in the force exerted by the index finger and at the wrist increased as a function of the target force (Galganski et al., 1993; Keen et al., 1994; Burnett et al., 1998; Graves et al., 1999). For example, the standard deviations for young adults ranged from 0.03 N at a target force of 2.5% MVC to 0.61 N at 75% MVC for the index finger and from 0.25 N at a target force of 5%

MVC to 5.89 N at 65% MVC for the wrist. When normalized relative to the target force, however, the relationship between the fluctuations and the target force was different for the index finger and the wrist (Fig. 1). For the index finger, the normalized fluctuations *decreased* as a function of the target force and were generally greater for the older adults, especially at the lower forces. At a target force of 5% MVC, the coefficient of variation (standard deviation/mean) was 4.3% for the young subjects and 10.2% for the old subjects, which decreased to 2.6% and 3.5% for the young and old subjects, respectively, at the 75% MVC target force. For the wrist, the normalized fluctuations *increased* as a function of target force. At a target force of 5% MVC, the coefficient of variation was 1.4% for the young subjects and 1.7% for the old subjects, which increased to 3.2% and 2.6% for the young and old subjects, respectively, at the 65% MVC target force. These findings indicate that the normalized fluctuations were greater for the index finger of the older adults, especially at the low forces, but the fluctuations were less and not different due to age for the wrist.

Constant-load contractions

Subjects raised and lowered a load (range: 2.5 to 75% of the maximum load that could be lifted once) that pulled on the index finger in the adduction direction or on the wrist in the direction of elbow extension. When the load was raised, the test muscles (first dorsal interosseus and the elbow flexor muscles) performed a shortening (concentric) contraction. When the load was lowered, the muscles performed a lengthening (eccentric) contraction. The angular displacement of the metacarpophalangeal joint or the elbow joint was monitored with an electrogoniometer. A triangular template was displayed on an oscilloscope and the subjects were required to match the angular displacement of the joint to the template; the requirement, therefore, was to perform constant-velocity shortening and lengthening contractions. The range of motion about the metacarpophalangeal joint was about 0.35 rad and for the elbow joint it was about 0.52 rad. The subjects were instructed to raise the load steadily within a 6-s

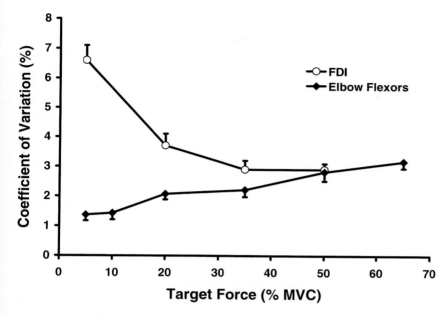

Fig. 1. Normalized force fluctuations (coefficient of variation) for the index finger (first dorsal interosseus muscle: FDI) and the wrist (elbow flexor muscles) during constant-force contractions as a function of target force for young adults.

interval and to lower it steadily in the subsequent 6 s.

For the constant-load contractions, steadiness was quantified as the standard deviation of the fluctuations in the acceleration-time record. For these measurements, an accelerometer was attached to the radial surface of the index finger over the proximal interphalangeal joint or to the radial surface of the wrist. For comparison across subjects, loads, and tasks, acceleration was normalized to the load that was lifted (ms^{-2}/kg). When the index finger was used to raise and lower a load, the standard deviation of the normalized acceleration declined as a function of load for both the young and old subjects, and also for both the shortening and lengthening contractions (Table 1). At the lesser loads (2.5, 5, and 20% of maximum), the fluctuations were greater for the old adults and for the lengthening contractions compared with the shortening contractions.

A similar pattern was observed when the load was lifted with the elbow flexor muscles. The standard deviation of the normalized acceleration declined as a function of load for both the shortening and lengthening contractions. The slope

of the decline in the relationship was greater for the old adults, which was mainly due to greater standard deviations at the lightest loads (10 and 15% of the maximum load). Because of differences in the load that was lifted, the standard deviation of

TABLE 1

Mean ± SE of the standard deviation of the normalized acceleration (ms^{-2}/kg) during the raising (shortening contraction) and lowering (lengthening contraction) phases of a constant-load task

	Young	Old
Index finger		
2.5% Load		
Shortening	2.322 ± 0.256	4.472 ± 1.082
Lengthening	2.704 ± 0.313	7.281 ± 1.217
75% Load		
Shortening	0.105 ± 0.012	0.103 ± 0.013
Lengthening	0.073 ± 0.013	0.127 ± 0.027
Wrist		
10% Load		
Shortening	0.064 ± 0.007	0.090 ± 0.017
Lengthening	0.084 ± 0.009	0.113 ± 0.011
35% Load		
Shortening	0.044 ± 0.007	0.037 ± 0.003
Lengthening	0.037 ± 0.006	0.042 ± 0.005

392

the normalized acceleration was less for the wrist compared with the index finger.

Muscle activity patterns

To determine the mechanisms responsible for differences in steadiness across tasks, we measured the electromyographic (EMG) activity of the agonist and antagonist muscles. For the index finger tasks, the EMG of the agonist muscle (first dorsal interosseus) was measured with surface electrodes (4 mm diameter, interelectrode distance ~ 10 mm) while the EMG of the antagonist muscle (second palmar interosseus) was measured with intramuscular fine wire electrodes (50 and 100 μm diameter).

For the constant-force contractions, the average EMG for first dorsal interosseus increased linearly as a function of target force for the young subjects. For the old adults, however, average EMG increased linearly across the lowest forces (2.5, 5, 20, and 50% of maximum) but was less than expected (~58%) at the greatest target force (75%). Both the young and old subjects coactivated

the agonist and antagonist muscles when the index finger exerted a constant force (isometric contraction). However, the level of EMG for the antagonist muscle was generally greater for the old adults (see also, Spiegel et al., 1996). At the 75% MVC target force, for example, the average EMG for second palmar interosseus was 35% of maximum for the old adults compared with 17% for the young adults. Despite these differences in the average EMG for first dorsal interosseus and second palmar interosseus at the greatest target force, there was no difference between the two groups of subjects in either the absolute (standard deviation) or normalized (coefficient of variation) force fluctuations at this force.

For the constant-load task, the average EMG for first dorsal interosseus increased more-or-less linearly during the shortening contraction (Fig. 2). The peak average EMG, which occurred at the end of the shortening contraction, increased as a function of the load that was lifted. There was no difference in the peak value of the average EMG between the two groups of subjects at the greatest loads (20, 50, and 75% of maximum). For the two

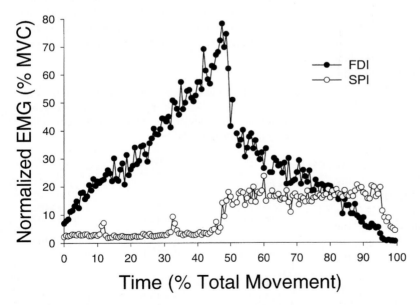

Fig. 2. Average EMG of the first dorsal interosseus (FDI) and second palmar interosseus (SPI) muscles during a single trial of the constant-load task. The EMG is normalized relative to the value recorded during an isometric MVC with each data point representing the average EMG for ~ 100 ms. The load (% of maximum) was raised (shortening contraction of FDI) for the first half of the task (~ 6 s) and lowered (lengthening contraction of FDI) for the second half of the task.

lightest loads (2.5 and 5%), however, the peak EMG was greater for the old adults. While some subjects (both young and old; ~23%) did not coactivate the antagonist muscle during the constant-load contractions, most subjects did choose to coactivate second palmar interosseus when raising and lowering a load. The most typical pattern involved greater coactivation during the lengthening contraction (Fig. 2). Nonetheless, we did not observe alternating activation of the agonist and antagonist muscles that might explain the fluctuations in the kinematics of the movement (Vallbo and Wessberg, 1993). Furthermore, there were no systematic differences between the two groups of subjects in the prevalence or magnitude of coactiva-

tion that might explain the difference in steadiness.

For the tasks involving the elbow flexor muscles, the EMG of brachialis was recorded with intramuscular fine wire electrodes (100 μm) while the EMG of the other muscles (short and long heads of biceps brachii, brachioradialis, and the lateral head of triceps brachii) was recorded with surface electrodes (8 mm diameter). For the constant-force contractions, the average EMG increased as a function of target force for both the young and old subjects. The relationships between EMG and force were similar for the two groups of subjects for the short and long heads of biceps brachii and brachioradialis. Conversely, the EMG for brachialis was

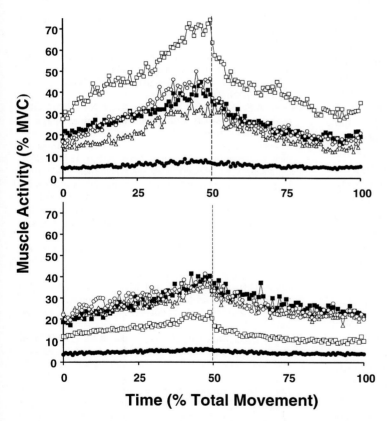

Fig. 3. Average EMG of the agonist and antagonist muscles during a constant-load task in which a load was raised and lowered with the wrist. The EMG is normalized relative to the value recorded during an isometric MVC with each data point representing the average EMG for 100 ms. The load, which was 35% of maximum, was raised for the first half of the task (~ 6 s) and lowered for the second half. The EMG values, which are averages for young subjects (upper panel) and old subjects (lower panel), are for the short head of biceps brachii (filled squares), the long head of biceps brachii (open triangles), brachioradialis (open circles), brachialis (open squares), and triceps brachii (filled circles).

slightly greater for the young adults and lower for the old adults at most target forces. EMG in the antagonist muscle (triceps brachii) was modest and increased linearly for both groups of subjects as a function of target force. The EMG in triceps brachii reached a maximum of ~10% for both groups at the 65% target force.

For the constant-load contractions with the elbow flexor muscles, the EMG increased during the shortening contraction and decreased during the lengthening contraction (Fig. 3). As others have shown, the EMG for all muscles was less during the lengthening contraction. For example, note the reduction in EMG in the upper panel of Fig. 3 at the transition from the shortening to the lengthening contraction (50% time). The greatest difference between the young and old subjects across the four loads (10%, 15%, 25%, and 35% of maximum) was the relative use of the brachialis muscle. Both groups of subjects activated the short and long head of biceps brachii and brachioradialis to similar levels in each task. However, the brachialis EMG was much greater for the young subjects and much less for the old subjects. When lifting a load that was 35% of maximum, for example, the peak value of the average EMG in brachialis was ~70% for the young subjects and ~20% for the old subjects (Fig. 3). Despite this difference, no bursting activity was observed in the EMG of either the agonist or antagonist muscles for either group of subjects. As with the constant-force contractions, the amount of EMG in the antagonist muscle (triceps brachii) was minimal for both groups and reached maximum values of ~10% with the greatest load.

Conclusion

When performing submaximal muscle contractions, old adults are less steady than young adults. This impairment can be observed by greater fluctuations in the force or acceleration records associated with the task. These differences are most pronounced when old subjects are asked to exert low forces, to lift light loads, or to perform lengthening contractions. Although there were differences due to age in the average EMG of the agonist and antagonist muscles for the various tasks, these did not appear to explain the differences in steadiness.

Acknowledgement

The work described in this chapter was supported by NIH award AG 09000.

References

Anniansson, A., Grimby, G. and Hedberg, M. (1992) Compensatory muscle fiber hypertrophy. *J. Appl. Physiol.*, 73: 812–816.

Binder, M.D. and Mendell, L.M. (1990) *The Segmental Motor System*. Oxford University Press, New York.

Burnett, R.A., Laidlaw. D.H. and Enoka, R.M. (1998) Less steady lengthening contractions are not associated with changes in coactivation patterns. *Satellite Symp. Ann. Mtg Soc. Neurosci.*, Tucson, AZ, November 4–6, p. 58.

Campbell, M.J., McComas, A. J. and Petito, F. (1973) Physiological changes in ageing muscles. *J. Neurol. Neurosurg. Psychiatry.*, 36: 174–182.

Cope, T.C. and Pinter, M.J. (1995) The Size Principle: still working after all these years. *News Physiol. Sci.*, 10: 280–286.

Galganski, M.E., Fuglevand, A.J. and Enoka, R.M. (1993) Reduced control of motor output in a human hand muscle of elderly subjects during submaximal contractions. *J. Neurophysiol.*, 69: 2108–2115.

Graves, A.E., Kornatz, K.W. and Enoka, R.M. (1999). Older adults are less steady with submaximal contractions of the elbow flexors. *Med. Sci. Sports Exerc.*, 31: S206.

Henneman, E. (1957) Relation between size of neurons and their susceptibility to discharge. *Science*, 126: 1345–1347.

Kadhiresan, V.A., Hassett, C.A. and Faulkner, J.A. (1996) Properties of single motor units in medial gastrocnemius muscles of adult and old rats. *J. Physiol.*, 493: 543–552.

Kanda, K. and Hashizume, K. (1989) Changes in the properties of the medial gastrocnemius motor units in aging rats. *J. Neurophysiol.*, 89: 737–746.

Keen, D.A., Yue, G.H. and Enoka, R.M. (1994) Training-related enhancement in the control of motor output in elderly humans. *J. Appl. Physiol.*, 77: 2648–2658.

Laidlaw, D.H., Bilodeau, M. and Enoka, R.M. (1996) Slow finger movements are less steady in elderly adults. *Proc. 20th Ann. Meeting Amer. Soc. Biomech.*, Atlanta, GA, October 18–19.

Laidlaw, D.H., Bilodeau, M. and Enoka, R.M. (1997) Motor unit discharge rate is more variable in older adults performing slow finger movements. *Med. Sci. Sports Exerc.*, 29: S22.

Laidlaw, D.H., Kornatz, K.W., Keen, D.A., Suzuki, S. and Enoka, R.M. (1999) Strength training improves the steadiness of slow eccentric contractions in older adults. *J. Appl. Physiol.*, 87: 1786–1795.

Lexell, J., Taylor, C.C. and Sjöstrom, M. (1988) What is the cause of ageing atrophy? Total number, size and proportion of different fiber types studied in whole vastus lateralis muscle from 15- to 83-year-old men. *J Neurol Sci.*, 84: 275–294.

Masakado, Y., Noda, Y., Nagata, M., Kimure, A., Chino, N. and Akaboshi, K. (1994) Macro-EMG and motor unit recruitment threshold: differences between the young and the aged. *Neurosci. Lett.*, 179: 1–4.

Narici, M.V., Bordini, M. and Cerretelli, P. (1991) Effect of aging on human adductor pollicis muscle function. *J. Appl. Physiol.* 71: 1277–1281.

Spiegel, K.M., Stratton, J., Burke, J.R., Glendinning, D.S. and Enoka, R.M. (1996) The influence of age on the assessment of motor unit activation in a human hand muscle. *Exp. Physiol.*, 81: 805–819.

Tomlinson, B.E. and Irving, D. (1977) The number of limb motor neurons in the human lumbosacral cord throughout life. *J. Neurol. Sci.*, 34: 213–219.

Vallbo, Å.B. and Wessberg, J. (1993) Organization of motor output in slow finger movements in man. *J. Physiol.*, 469: 673–691.

M.D. Binder (Ed.)
Progress in Brain Research, Vol 123
© 1999 Elsevier Science BV. All rights reserved.

CHAPTER 35

Mechanical actions of compartments of the cat hamstring muscle, biceps femoris

Dario I. Carrasco and Arthur W. English*

Department of Cell Biology, Emory University School of Medicine, Atlanta, GA 303022, USA

Introduction

Movement is produced as a result of an interaction of circuits in the central nervous system and elements of the musculoskeletal system. The elements of the musculoskeletal system with which spinal circuits interact are usually described as muscles. Individual muscles have distinct morphologies and well-documented bony attachments. They receive exclusive innervation from groups of motoneurons whose axons are fasciculated to form distinct muscle nerves, and they have distinct mechanical actions. These attributes form much of the rationale for thinking of muscles as output elements, the targets for interaction with neuronal circuits.

Evidence from study of human muscles exists for a subdivision of the actions of single muscles. Different actions are attributed to different anatomical portions of the human deltoid (Buneo et al., 1997; Bolhuis et al., 1998), biceps brachii (ter Haar Romeny et al., 1982), other elbow joint muscles (van Zuylen et al., 1988), pectoralis major (Inman et al., 1944), and the first dorsal interosseous muscle (Desmedt and Godaux, 1979; Masquelet et al., 1986, but cf. Thomas et al., 1986). Motor units in different portions of these muscles are activated differently. An anatomical basis for these observations may exist, since a number of muscles in

different species are partitioned anatomically. These neuromuscular compartments have many of the same attributes as muscles. They have distinctive attachments and morphology and they receive exclusive innervation by motoneurons whose axons fasciculate into *branches* of muscle nerves (English et al., 1993). Smaller portions of these compartments lack this exclusive innervation – their muscle fibers share innervation with other muscle partitions. Thus, neuromuscular compartments are, at least anatomically, elements in that they are the smallest subdivision of the musculoskeletal system above the level of individual motor units.

In order for a neuromuscular compartment to be an output element, it ought to have a distinct mechanical action. More precisely, different compartments within a muscle ought to exert different mechanical actions on the skeletal structures to which they attach. If different compartments produce the same mechanical action, then their role as output elements would be more difficult to support.

We have investigated the mechanical actions of the cat biceps femoris (BF) muscle. This muscle is subdivided into different compartments by branches of its nerves (English and Weeks, 1987; Chanaud et al., 1991), and they are arranged roughly in parallel, from anterior or rostral to posterior or caudal. During the application of postural perturbations, a rostral to caudal gradient of activation of different compartments was found as the direction of the perturbation was changed

*Corresponding author. Tel.: 404-727-6250; Fax: 404-727-3677; e-mail: art@cellbio.emory.edu

(Chanaud and Macpherson, 1991). Thus, motor units in different parts of this single muscle were activated independently. It s not known whether the different compartments of BF, as defined both anatomically and functionally, produce unique mechanical actions, as would be expected of elements of the musculoskeletal system with which neuronal circuits interact. In this chapter we report the results of experiments aimed at testing this hypothesis. We find that different compartments of BF produce different mechanical actions.

Material and methods

The cat BF muscle can exert effects about the hip, knee, and ankle joints. As a measure of the mechanical actions of BF compartments, we determined the torque produced by different compartments about each of these joints. A multi axis force-moment sensor (ATI Gamma 65/5) was attached to the limb segment (femur, tibia, or foot) just distal to the joint being studied, and was used to measure a three dimensional reaction force vector elicited by tetanic suprathreshold activation of each compartment through its muscle nerve branch. The cross product of this vector and a three dimensional position vector from the center of the joint to the center of the transducer face resulted in the determination of a single torque vector about that joint for each BF compartment. Limb segments proximal to the joint under study were clamped to mechanical ground. Limb segments distal to the transducer were mechanically immobilized to prevent their movement during recordings, but they were not grounded, so as to isolate the action of the stimulated compartment to a singe joint. All measurements were made at the same position in different cats unless specified. The femur was fixed in a vertical position relative to the transducer in both transverse and sagittal planes. The knee and ankle angles were held at 90°. The transducer was carefully positioned to lie in the same position, relative to the limb, in all experiements and when studying different joints. The vertical and transverse axes of the transducer were oriented parallel and perpendicular to the femur, respectively. Data were analyzed using a two-way ANOVA. The Tukey post-hoc procedure was used for planned comparisons. A significance level of 0.05 was used throughout.

Results

There is a partitioning of mechanical action of BF compartments about the three joints. In Fig. 1A, each bar represents the resultant of the torque vector produced by different BF compartments about the hip, knee, and ankle joints. The anterior-most partitions (BFa, BFm1) produce their main effect about the hip joint; more caudal compartments (BFm2, BFp) produce smaller effects. At the knee, BFm2 and BFp produce strong torques and BFm1 a lesser torque. The BFp compartment exerts a strong effect about the ankle and the BFm1 and BFm2 compartments produce much smaller torques. Wicke and Zajac (1981) showed that the mechanical action of BF about the ankle is a consequence of the attachments of its caudal compartments to the superficial layer of deep fascia of the leg, the crural fascia. After carefully removing the attachments of this crural fascia to the calcaneus, approximately half of the torque produced by BFm2 and BFp, but not BFm1 is lost. If we cut the tendo calcaneus (Fig. 1B), the torque produced about the ankle by all three compartments is eliminated, suggesting that these compartments exert some of their mechanical action about the ankle by pressure on the trceps surae muscles via tensing the crural fascia.

None of the compartments produce purely sagittal torques. Each torque vector has three components: pitch, roll, and yaw. These mechanical terms were chosen to help differentiate torques from movements. In Fig. 2 the magnitudes of these three components of the torques are plotted against each other for each of the three joints studied. In each plot, the length of the line represents the magnitude of the torque and the displacement off of vertical represents the direction of the torque. At all three joints, compartments of BF produce mainly pitch, which is the component of the torque vector associated with flexion-extension movements. However, each compartment also produces significant yaw (abduction–adduction) and roll (axial rotation) components. At the hip, the magnitude of the yaw component (abduction) is relatively small, but the magnitude of the roll component (lateral rotation or eversion) can be substantial. At the knee and ankle joints, the opposite is true. The yaw component (adduction at the knee, abduction at the ankle) is usually greater than the roll component (internal rotation or inversion at the knee, eversion at the ankle).

The directions of torques at the different joints produced by BF compartments are significantly different from one another. To compare these different directions, we normalized the magnitude of the compartment torques by dividing each component by the resultant. This produces an adjusted vector whose magnitude is one, but whose

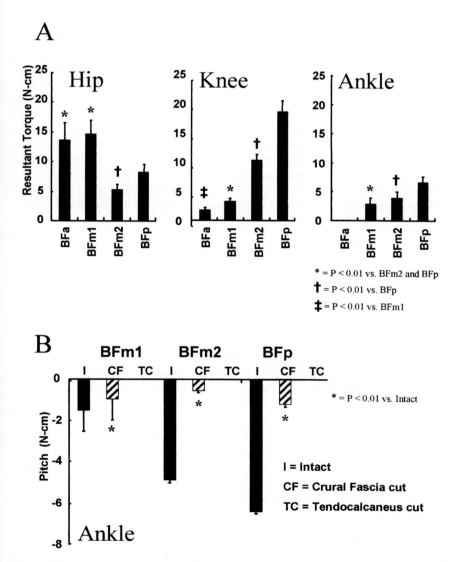

Fig. 1. BF compartment torque magnitudes are partitioned about the different joints of the hindlimb. A. In each plot, the mean magnitude ($\pm$ SEM) of the resultant torque produced by the different compartments of BF in six different cats is represented. B. The magnitude of the torque generated about the ankle joint by the BFm1, BFm2, and BFp compartments is shown for intact muscles (solid bar), after carefully removing the crural fascia from its attachment to the calcaneus (CF, hatched bars), and after removing both the crural fascia and cutting the tendocalcaneus (TC).

direction is the same as its unadjusted vector. We then used ANOVA to evaluate the significance of differences in the three rectilinear components of these adjusted vectors for different compartments. At the hip and knee joints, each of the BF compartments generates torques with a significantly different trajectory. At the ankle, both the BFm2 and BFp compartments produce torques with similar trajectories, but different from that of BFm1. Thus, based on both the magnitude and directions of the torques they produce, each of the compartments of BF produces a different mechanical action. These findings are consistent with the hypothesis that the compartments of the cat BF muscle can act as an element of the musculoskeletal system with which neuronal circuits interact to produce movement.

To evaluate the extent to which the mechanical actions of compartments of BF might be context dependent, we determined the torques produced about the hip at different limb positions throughout the range available to the cat. The ability of these compartments to generate force might be different at different positions, as may their architectural relationship to the axes about which the torques were measured. Using the method described by Giszter et al. (1993), we then constructed torque fields to demonstrate the torques produced throughout the animal's workspace. Examples of this analysis are shown in Figs 3 and 4.

In each panel of Fig. 3, two components of the projected torque vector produced by a single compartment (BFa) are shown as two-dimensional vectors (arrows) at several different positions of the femur in the workspace of the animal's hindlimb. The length of each arrow represents the magnitude of this vector and its orientation represents its direction. In different panels, pitch vs. roll (A), pitch vs. yaw (B), or roll vs. yaw (C) are plotted. Although the magnitude of the pitch-roll vectors varies at different positions, the direction of this torque vector remains remarkably constant through

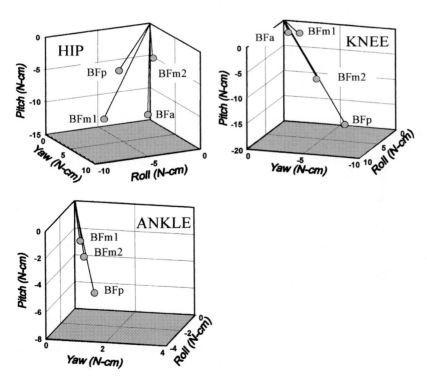

Fig. 2. Directions of torques produced by BF compartments. In each three-dimensional graph, the magnitude of the pitch, yaw, and roll components of the torque vectors produced by each BF compartment are plotted to show the trajectories of the different vectors.

401

the animal's workspace (Fig. 3A). In contrast, both the magnitude and the direction of the pitch-yaw vectors change dramatically (Fig. 3B), and tend to converge on a region near the transverse center of the workspace. Deviations from this region in the direction of abduction move the limb to a position where the magnitude of the adduction torque increases, and vice-versa. A similar observation has been made for muscles crossing the cat ankle joint (Young et al., 1992). The plots of yaw-roll components of the torque vectors reflect both the relatively consistent roll and changing yaw components (Fig. 3C).

In Fig. 4, torque field plots are shown for the pitch and yaw components of the torques about the hip produced by different BF compartments. For all of the compartments, these fields represent a

convergent relationship to limb position, but the exact nature of that relationship varies considerably from one compartment to another. We feel that these torque fields offer a novel way of assessing the mechanical actions of compartments of BF and they offer similar novelty in the assay of the action of compartments of all the muscles.

Discussion

The main finding of this study is that different compartments of a single muscle produce different mechanical effects on the skeletal structures to which they attach. In addition, we report here that the nature of these effects, at least at the hip joint, may be dependent on the position of the limb in space. The magnitude of the torques produced by

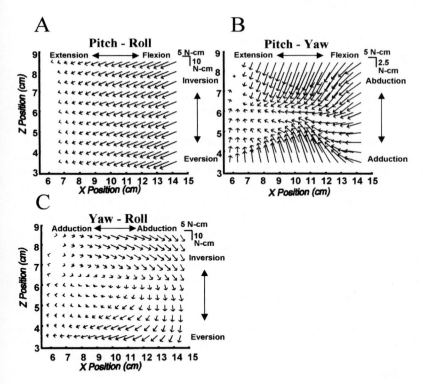

Fig. 3. Torque fields associated with the BFa compartments. In each panel, two components of the projected hip torque vector for BFa are shown at number of positions of the femur in the workspace of the animal. This workspace can be visualized as if looking at the left hindlimb of a cat from above. The positions at which the limb is fully flexed are shown at the right of each panel, full extension is shown to the left. At the top of each panel are positions of maximal abduction of the hip joint, at the bottom, maximal adduction. The actual coordinates in each panel indicate the position of the transducer used to determine the torques and are given in cm. Each arrow plots the two components of the projected torque vector at that position. Scale bars for these arrows are given at the upper right of each panel.

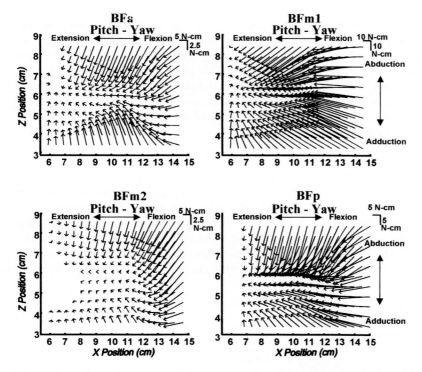

Fig. 4. Torque fields of different BF compartments. In each panel the pitch and yaw components of the projected torques at different positions in the workspace of the cat are plotted for a different BF compartment. The format is the same as in Fig. 3.

different BF compartments is partitioned about the joints crossed. Anterior compartments produce their largest effects about the hip joint, while more caudal compartments exert their largest effect about the knee and ankle joints. The directions of these compartment torques are also different. Each compartment produces a torque with significant off-sagittal components, and the relative magnitudes of these components determine their trajectories. As predicted by others (Chanaud et al., 1991), all of the BF compartments produce abduction and eversion (lateral rotation) torque components about the hip, in addition to a sizeable extension component. The magnitude of these off sagittal components varies in different compartments. In BFm1 and BFp, for example, the off-sagittal components are 3–5 time those produced by BFa and BFm2. The same is true for compartment torques about the knee joint. All BF compartments produce some knee flexion torque (although the magnitude of the BFa compartment is almost negligible), and it was predicted that

inversion and adduction would be produced by these compartments (Chanaud et al., 1991). However, BFm2 and BFp produce off-sagittal torque components nearly twice or four times greater, respectively, than those produced by BFm1.

We think that the significance of these findings is that these compartments could act as output elements of the musculoskeletal system with which neural circuits interact to generate movement. Each of these compartments is innervated by a distinct group of motoneurons. During both posture (Chanaud and Macpherson, 1991) and locomotion (English and Weeks, 1987), there is strong evidence that motoneurons innervating the different BF compartments are not activated uniformly as a common pool, but are selected for participation according to the behavioral demands imposed upon the animal. Given our finding that the mechanical actions produced by the different compartments are quite different, such a differential activation could be used to produce different mechanical effects on the limb. Since it is unlikely that different compartments of BF will be activated in total isolation, the different mechanical effects may be subtle, as other compartments of other limb muscles might also be differentially activated.

The elements of the musculoskeletal system with which neuronal circuits interact to produce movement have been thought of as being muscles. The evidence is now accumulating that these elements are smaller than whole muscles and they might be neuromuscular compartments. In some muscles, such as the cat sartorius (Hoffer et al., 1987a, b), the compartmental organization of motor units and their functional partitioning is less clear than in others. In muscles, such as BF, where the compartmental organization is clear, neuromuscular compartments may be thought of as output elements.

Acknowledgements

This work was completed with support from grant HD32571 from the USPHS. William Goolsby provided the software for the torque field analysis. We are grateful to Drs. Thomas Abaleew, Timothy Cope, Eleanor Feingold, T. Richard Nichols, and Richard Segal for helpful discussions and suggestions for data analysis.

References

Bolhuis, B.M., Gielen, C.C. and van Ingen Schenau, G.J. (1998) Activation patterns of mono- and bi-articular arm muscles as a function of force and movement direction of the wrist in humans. *J. Physiol (Lond.)*, 508: 313–324.

Buneo, C.A., Soechting, J.F. and Flanders, M. (1997) Postural dependence of muscle actions: implications for neural control. *J. Neurosci.*, 17: 2128–2142.

Chanaud, C.M. and Macpherson, J.M. (1991) Functionally complex muscles of the cat hindlimb. III. Differential activation within biceps femoris during postural perturbations. *Exp. Brain Res.*, 85: 271–280.

Chanaud, C.M., Pratt, C.A. and Loeb, G.E. (1991) Functionally complex muscles of the cat hindlimb. II. Mechanical and architectural heterogenity within the biceps femoris. *Exp. Brain Res.*, 85: 257–270.

Desmedt, J.E. and Godaux, E. (1979) Voluntary motor commands in human ballistic movements. *Ann. Neurol.*, 5: 415–421.

English, A.W. and Weeks, O.I. (1987) An anatomical and functional analysis of cat biceps femoris and semitendinosus muscles. *J. Morphol.*, 191: 161–175.

English, A.W., Wolf, S.L. and Segal, R.L. (1993) Compartmentalization of muscles and their motor nuclei: the partitioning hypothesis. *Phys. Ther.*, 73: 857–867.

Giszter, S.F., Mussa-Ivaldi, F.A. and Bizzi, E. (1993) Convergent force fields organized in the frog's spinal cord. *J. Neurosci.*, 13: 467–491.

Hoffer, J.A., Loeb, G.E., Sugano, N., Marks, W.B., O'Donovan, M.J. and Pratt, C.A. (1987a) Cat hindlimb motoneurons during locomotion. III. Functional segregation in sartorius. *J. Neurophysiol.*, 57: 554–562.

Hoffer, J.A., Sugano, N., Loeb, G.E., Marks, W.B., O'Donovan, M.J. and Pratt, C.A. (1987b) Cat hindlimb motoneurons during locomotion. II. Normal activity patterns. *J. Neurophysiol.*, 57: 530–553.

Inman, V., Saunders, J.dM. and Abbott, L. (1944) Observations on the function of the shoulder joint. *J. Bone Joint Surg.*, 26: 1–30.

Masquelet, A.C., Salama, J., Outrequin, G., Serrault, M. and Chevrel, J.P. (1986) Morphology and functional anatomy of the first dorsal interosseous muscle of the hand. *Surg. Radiol. Anat.*, 8: 19–28.

ter Haar Romeny, B.M., Denier van der Gon, J.J. and Gielen, C.C. (1982) Changes in recruitment order of motor units in the human biceps muscle. *Exp. Neurol.*, 78: 360–368.

Thomas, C.K., Ross, B.H. and Stein, R.B. (1986) Motor-unit recruitment in human first dorsal interosseous muscle for static contractions in three different directions. *J. Neurophysiol.*, 55: 1017–1029.

van Zuylen, E.J., Gielen, C.C. and Denier van der Gon, J.J. (1988) Coordination and inhomogeneous activation of human arm muscles during isometric torques. *J. Neurophysiol.*, 60: 1523–1548.

Wicke, R.W. and Zajac, F.E. (1981) Isometric torque produced by the cat hamstrings muscle about the ankle as a function of hindlimb position. Soc. Neurosc., Abstr. 7: 684.

Young, R.P., Scott, S.H. and Loeb, G.E. (1992) An intrinsic mechanism to stabilize posture-joint-angle-dependent moment arms of the feline ankle muscles. *Neurosci. Lett.*, 145: 137–140.

M.D. Binder (Ed.)
Progress in Brain Research, Vol 123
© 1999 Elsevier Science BV. All rights reserved.

CHAPTER 36

What might the brain know about muscles, limbs and spinal circuits?

Gerald E. Loeb*

Department of Biomedical Engineering, University of Southern California, Los Angeles, CA90089, USA

System identification and feedforward control

Engineers divide control into feedback and feedforward systems. Feedback systems use online information from sensors to adjust command signals incrementally in order to achieve a target condition as represented by those sensor signals. Feedback control is useful for controlling systems whose dynamic properties may be largely unknown but it may converge only slowly to the desired state or become frankly unstable in the face of loop delays. Neuromuscular systems have particularly long delays in the conduction of action potentials, transmission through oligosynaptic circuits, and electromechanical activation within muscle.

Survival often depends on making rapid and accurate movements, so it is likely that the brain depends heavily on feedforward control as well. Feedforward systems rely on an internal model of the system to be controlled. The controller computes or selects command signals that are expected to reach the desired target without modification by feedback from sensors. This raises the question of how the internal model is learned and represented. In biological systems this presumably requires sensory information, particularly from the complex and numerous proprioceptors in skeletal muscles. This discussion considers three of the problems that

_____
*Corresponding author. Tel.: 213–821–1112; Fax: 213-821-1120; e-mail: gloeb@bmsr.usc.edu

the brain must solve in implementing feedforward control for musculoskeletal tasks.

Engineers designing feedforward controllers for robots usually have the luxury of specifying actuators, sensors and communications systems that simplify the nature of the internal model. The muscles, proprioceptors and spinal circuits of biological systems evolved long before higher brain functions such as eye-hand coordination, so the brain must have evolved ways of dealing with rather than specifying the properties of the periphery. The properties discussed here are particularly complex and dissimilar to their counterparts in robotic systems, so they might be expected to constrain the evolution of the brain toward solutions that may be unlike those familiar to robotics engineers.

Examples of biological problems

Coping with post-activation potentiation in muscle

Physiologists have long known that the contractile force generated by a muscle depends on the history of activation of the muscle as well as kinematic factors such as length and velocity of the contractile elements. One such dependency is post-activation potentiation (PAP, also known as post-tetanic potentiation), in which fast-twitch muscle increases its twitch force for several minutes following vigorous (e.g. tetanic) activation. The molecular mechanism appears to be related to phosphorylation of the myosin light chains, per-haps acting through a change in the stereochemical position of myosin heads with respect to actin binding sites (Sweeney et al., 1993). Recent studies of this phenomenon in the homogeneous fast-twitch feline muscle caudofemoralis have demonstrated that the effect can be quite large at physiological muscle lengths around L_0 (about 400% for single twitches and 200% for 43 pps trains). Furthermore, PAP occurs rapidly and maximally following patterns of activation that are well within the normal physiological range for simple, repetitive tasks such as locomotion (Brown and Loeb, 1998). Thus, PAP is not just a laboratory curiosity. Indeed, near-maximal potentiation may be the normal operating state of many muscles, with the dispotentiated state representing an atyp-ical condition despite its more common use in muscle physiology studies.

Consider the problem of designing an open-loop (feed-forward) controller for an actuator subject to PAP. The internal model would have to include a way to anticipate and compensate for changes that depend on the whole integrated history of muscle use. Alternatively, the nervous system may use 'higher level' strategies in order to assure that the muscle is always in a stable and predictable state. By 'warming up' the muscle with several practice repetitions of the required task, the CNS can use the saturated PAP state that tends to persist for minutes after such activation. Athletes and their coaches are certainly familiar with such warm-up strategies, but they are not usually explained on this basis.

Both approaches – an internal model of the rise, fall and consequences of PAP or a work-around that avoids the dispotentiated state – constitute 'knowl-edge' that the brain might be said to have about muscle. Yet they are entirely different in their implications for the way in which such knowledge is represented computationally and used in motor control.

Representing limb motion from proprioceptive information

Information about starting position is required to plan a movement. Information about trajectory and final position is required to judge the execution of a movement. In a biological limb, such information is provided primarily by spindle receptors located within individual muscles. The lengths of these muscles are not independent variables because they are attached to a common skeleton that constrains their motion to anatomically realizable postures. The length of a sensor within a given muscle is not simply proportional to the length of the whole muscle (from bony origin to insertion of the muscle) because many muscles include substantial series elasticity in tendons and aponeuroses (Scott and Loeb, 1995). Thus, the natural coordinate system for the sensors is a non-orthogonal space with no simple computational relationship to the coordinates of other sensors related to motor planning, such as the retinotopic space of vision in which targets for hand movement are often pre-sented (Scott and Loeb, 1994). Furthermore, these sensors are under the control of a complex system of intrafusal muscle fibers and their fusimotor neurons, which produce large changes in the absolute and relative sensitivity of the sensors to length and velocity within the muscle. This fusimo-tor activity is modulated complexly and differently for various motor tasks (Loeb, 1984; Prochazka, 1996); see also A. Taylor et al., Chapter 10 and Prochazka, Chapter 11, this volume).

At some point the brain must be able to convert raw proprioceptive information into a sense of body position that can be reconciled with other natural coordinate systems for the same information, such as retinotopic space. One way to do so is to make use of an intermediate coordinate frame imposed by the skeletal linkage, i.e. joint angles. While such an approach is common in robotics, there is actually little evidence that it is used in biological control. Psychophysical studies reveal large errors when subjects are asked to perform tasks in this coordinate space, suggesting that estimation of joint angles requires additional computation beyond that naturally performed by the CNS (Soechting and Ross, 1984). Various illusory distor-tions of body shape and posture arise when the natural coherence of proprioceptive information is distorted experimentally, e.g. by vibrating one muscle (Lackner and Taublieb, 1983, 1984) or by introducing discordant tactile information (Craske et al., 1984). No such distortions seem to occur when similar modulations of spindle activity are self-generated by fusimotor activity (Vallbo, 1970).

All of the above suggests that the brain does not have an explicit representation of the geometry of the skeletal linkage, despite the constancy and supposed computational utility of that constraint. Thus, it could be said that the brain 'knows' a large set of valid relationships between proprioceptive signals and body posture, but it does not 'know' that limbs are composed of rigid bones and joints.

Controlling reflex responses of the spinal cord

To a controller residing in the brain, the rest of the neuromusculoskeletal system (the 'periphery') might appear to be something of a black box. Most of the output signals from the controller are sent to spinal interneurons rather than individual motoneurons or motor pools (Schomburg, 1990; Pierrot-Deseilligny, 1996). A single output line thus contributes to the excitation and inhibition of many different muscles with different mechanical actions on the skeleton. The actual contribution is contingent on other input to these spinal interneurons, which generally receive descending commands from many parts of the brain as well as input from many different somatosensory neurons (McCrea, 1986). Sensory feedback to the controller tends to be pooled from sensors representing many different modalities and anatomical locations, with only the most general anatomical relationship to the portion of the musculature affected by that particular control signal.

Consider the brain's view of a mechanical perturbation applied to a limb during a movement that the brain has commanded in feedforward mode. The perturbation gives rise to a time-varying pattern of sensory signals, different from the pattern expected when the movement proceeds without perturbation. The actual pattern depends on the mechanical impedance of the limb, which in turn depends on the level of activity of the muscles and their intrinsic mechanical properties (e.g. the steep, nonlinear relationship between active muscle force and sarcomere velocity). It also depends on the segmental reflex responses generated by the spinal cord and perhaps on other reflex generators acting downstream from the higher motor centers. Those reflex responses depend on the pattern of hyper- and depolarization of the various interneurons and motoneurons that potentially contribute to the reflex. All of these musculoskeletal and reflex responses are thus 'under the control' of the brain, but there is no way for the brain to separate its command signals into components required for the feedforward command to the muscles and components that modulate the segmental response to perturbations (Loeb et al., 1990, 1999). That is to say, the brain 'knows' how to get the rest of the motor plant, including the spinal cord, to perform a task successfully and even robustly in the face of perturbations, but it probably doesn't 'know' that there are motor nuclei or particular classes of spinal interneurons.

In such a distributed system, it is difficult to see how the brain might develop a model that makes use of the traditional coordinates employed by biomechanists and neurophysiologists. These tend to be based on the geometry of linked skeletal segments (e.g. joint angles, segment orientations or end-point locations in extrapersonal space) or on the anatomical identity of individual actuators (e.g. individual muscles or groups of synergists and antagonists). If anything, the brain seems more likely to become organized according to patterns of coherence that it detects in the somatosensory information that it receives, as is theorized to occur in self-organizing neural network models of sensory and associative cortical areas.

We can identify at least three different classes of input and output signals to and from a structure like motor cortex (Loeb et al., 1990), each with its own natural coordinate frame (Fig. 1):

(1) Command input, possibly in extrapersonal space coordinates.
(2) Command output, mostly in spinal interneuron coordinates.
(3) Sensory feedback, mostly in muscle-based proprioceptive coordinates.

A simple goal or condition such as a position of the hand in space can be expressed in each of these coordinate frames (although often not uniquely because the spaces are overcomplete or non-orthogonal). Thus, it is not surprising that post hoc analyses of psychophysical data on motor or perceptual error or of neurophysiological data from individual cortical neurons have produced correlations with any or all such coordinate frames. Such

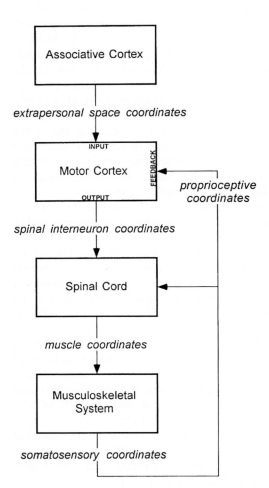

Fig. 1. Two of the three main input/output systems with which motor cortex must interact have natural coordinate frames that are well-known: descending commands from motor cortex project largely to spinal interneurons; somatosensory feedback tends to be dominated by proprioceptive signals that originate in individual muscles. Inputs to motor cortex that specify motor targets tend to originate in exteroceptive senses such as vision and hearing. It is possible but not necessary that the brain creates a non-specific coordinate system in extrapersonal space, whose origin might correspond to a body segment such as the trunk or a focus of attention such as gaze. (Simplified from concepts discussed more completely in Loeb et al., 1990, and Loeb et al., 1999)

correlations do not tell us what the brain 'knows' about the periphery. *We know* that the brain must contain an excellent model of the overall properties of the periphery, but *we know* this simply from the brain's ability to use feedforward control to perform motor tasks successfully. It seems unlikely that the brain 'knows' about the periphery in the same coordinates that biomechanists and neurophysiologists use to study and describe muscles, limbs and spinal circuits or even that it decomposes the periphery into such constituent entities.

An evolutionary perspective

Instead of trying to reverse engineer a highly evolved neuromusculoskeletal system, it might be useful to think about design constraints that result from its evolution in the first place. As Partridge (Partridge, 1982) pointed out, "evolution is not engineering".

First there were muscles; many of the nonlinear properties of muscle that biomechanists find so vexing have been around since the invention of contractile myofilaments. Many others were added to improve specialized performance in primitive organisms with extremely simple nervous systems (e.g. catch-locking of bivalve shells, self-oscillation of insect flight muscles). Properties such as the nonlinear force-velocity relationship continue to be useful in higher organisms because they respond to perturbations by producing stabilizing changes in force output that are instantaneous, avoiding loop delays in neural transduction, conduction, transmission and muscle activation (Brown and Loeb, 1999).

Next there were sensory feedback loops. Many of the mammalian proprioceptors and spinal circuits have obvious counterparts in invertebrate somatosensors and ganglionic circuits. Such circuits are useful because they permit perturbations of one part of a limb, affecting certain muscles directly, to give rise to corrective responses distributed to many muscles, including those not initially perturbed.

Next there were central pattern generators. Complex sequences of muscle activation needed for important tasks such as locomotion were built into self-oscillating neural circuits. Genetically specified pattern generators were retained and refined in higher animals because they avoid the long training time associated with trial-and-error learning in general neural networks.

Finally there were brains. By and large, the output circuits of the brain do not bypass the intervening circuitry or cancel the nonlinearities of muscles and sensors in order to implement computational approaches to motor control based on joint torques (see contribution by Strausfeld, Chapter 24, in this volume). To do so would deprive the brain of hundreds of millions of years of evolution directed at producing rapid, stable movements without brains. Physiologists who study the peripheral neuromusculoskeletal apparatus have an obligation to keep reminding robotics engineers and cortical neurophysiologists of its properties and of the power of those properties.

References

Brown, I.E. and Loeb, G.E. (1998) Post-activation potentiation – A clue for simplifying models of muscle dynamics. *Am. Zool.*, 38: 743–754.

Brown, I.E. and Loeb, G.E. (1999) A reductionist approach to creating and using neuromusculoskeletal models. In: J. Winters and P. Crago (Ed.), *Neuro-control of posture and movement.* (in press).

Craske, B., Kenny, F.T. and Keith, D. (1984) Modifying an underlying component of perceived arm length: adaptation of tactile location induced by spatial discordance. *J. Exp. Psych.: Hum. Percept. Perform.*, 10: 301–317.

Lackner, J.R. and Taublieb, A.B. (1983) Reciprocal interactions between the position sense representations of the two forearms. *J. Neurosci.*, 3: 2280–2285.

Lackner, J.R. and Taublieb, A.B. (1984) Influence of vision on vibration-induced illusions of limb movement. *Exp. Neurol.*, 85: 97–106.

Loeb, G.E. (1984) The control and responses of mammalian muscle spindles during normally executed motor tasks. *Exerc. Sport Sci. Rev.*, 12: 157–204.

Loeb, G.E., Brown, I.E. and Cheng, E. (1999) A hierarchical foundation for models of sensorimotor control. *Exp. Brain Res.*, 126: 1–18.

Loeb, G.E., Levine, W.S. and He, J. (1990) Understanding sensorimotor feedback through optimal control. *Cold Spring Harbor Symposia on Quantitative Biology*, 55: 791–803.

McCrea, D.A. (1986) Spinal cord circuitry and motor reflexes. *Exerc. Sport Sci. Rev.*, 14: 105–141.

Partridge, L.D. (1982) The good enough calculi of evolving control systems: evolution is not engineering. *Am. J. Physiol.*, 242: R173–R177.

Pierrot-Deseilligny, E. (1996) Transmission of the cortical command for human voluntary movement through cervical propriospinal premotoneurons. *Prog. Neurobiol.*, 48: 489–517.

Prochazka, A. (1996) Proprioceptive feedback and movement regulation. In: L.G. Rowell and J.T. Sheperd JT (Eds), *Handbook of Physiology. Section 12. Exercise: Regulation and Integration of Multiple Systems. 3*, American Physiological Assoc, New York: pp. 89–127.

Schomburg, E.D. (1990) Spinal sensorimotor systems and their supraspinal control. *Neurosci. Res.*, 7: 265–340.

Scott, S.H. and Loeb, G.E. (1994) The computation of position sense from spindles in mono-and multiarticular muscles. *J. Neurosci.*, 14: 7529–7540.

Scott, S.H. and Loeb, G.E. (1995) The mechanical properties of the aponeurosis and tendon of the cat soleus muscle during whole-muscle isometeric contractions. *J. Morphol.*, 224: 73–86.

Soechting, J.F. and Ross, B. (1984) Psychophysical determination of coordinate representation of human arm orientation. *Neurosci.*, 13: 595–604.

Sweeney, H.L., Bowman, B.F. and Stull, J.T. (1993) Myosin light chain phosphorylation in vertebrate striated muscle: regulation and function. *Am. Physiol. Soc.*, 264: 1085–1095.

Vallbo, A.B. (1970) Discharge patterns in human muscle spindle afferents during isometric contractions. *Acta Physiol. Scand.*, 80: 552–566.

M.D. Binder (Ed.)
Progress in Brain Research, Vol 123
© 1999 Elsevier Science BV. All rights reserved.

CHAPTER 37

Animal models of motor systems: cautionary tales from studies of head movement

Frances J.R. Richmond*, Brian D. Corneil and K. Singh

MRC Group in Sensory-Motor Neuroscience, Queen's University, Kingston, ON K7L 3N6, Canada

Historical perspective

Studies of motor systems have always depended in large measure on the use of cats as experimental animals. Those of the head-movement system are no different. As early as the nineteenth century, experiments on decerebrate cats gave us insight into the basic reflexes and pathways responsible for the control of head movement (e.g. Sherrington, 1897; Magnus, 1926). Cats later became the animals of choice for most anatomical and electrophysiological studies of neural pathways (e.g. Wilson and Peterson, 1988; Brink, 1988), and for electromyographic studies of neck-muscle activities during head movements of different types and directions (e.g. Richmond et al., 1992; Thomson et al., 1994). However, cats are not little people. In the early 1970s, many researchers expressed concerns about the applicability of results from quadrupeds, which they believed to have horizontally oriented necks, to humans, who clearly held their heads on top of a vertically oriented cervical spinal column. It was with great relief to some that fluoroscopic studies in the early 1980s identified as misconception the view that the feline neck was oriented horizontally. Sitting and standing cats were found instead to hold their heads on a vertically-oriented upper cervical column in much the same way as

*Corresponding author. Tel.: (613) 545-2806; Fax: (613) 545-6840; e-mail: fjr@biomed.queensu.ca

human bipeds (Vidal et al., 1986). Instead, differences were found to be present more caudally, at the cervicothoracic junction, where the vertebral column bends nearly 90 degrees, and the thoracic cord adopts a horizontal orientation (Fig. 1).

Was the new information suggesting similarities in human and feline cervical posture sufficient to allay concerns about cats as experimental models for head movement? Two problems were still to be faced. First were the obvious differences in behaviors for which the feline head appears to be adapted. The cat relies on its jaws for a diversity of tasks including fighting, killing, tearing food and carrying objects – tasks for which most humans generally use their hands. Specializations of feline neck muscles and more generally of head-movement control might be expected to enhance the performance of necessary behaviors without which the cat would be unlikely to survive. In addition, the cat is a quadruped, whose head is borne on a shoulder and forelimb system very different from that in man. As long as one believed that the head-movement system was confined to the upper cervical region, it was possible to ignore the differences below. However, we now know from EMG studies that muscles with attachments to the shoulder girdle are active during many head movements (Richmond et al., 1992; Thomson et al., 1994). We are drawn into the problem eventually faced by most motor physiologists, of where 'our' motor system ends and that of 'everyone else' begins.

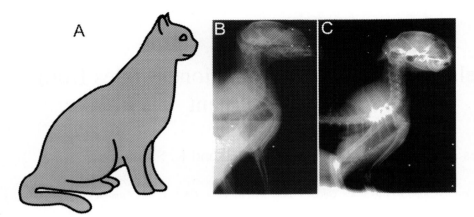

Fig. 1. Vertebral configuration of the feline neck. The outward appearance of the neck (A) belies the sharply curved cervico-thoracic region, shown in stereo X-rays (B and C). White dots in the X-rays are markers associated with a calibration device. Adapted with permission from Runciman and Richmond, 1997.

The neck-bone's connected to the shoulder-bone

In order to understand the coupling from forelimb to neck through the shoulder, it is necessary to know the position of the feline clavicle and scapula with respect to the joints of the neck. These positions and centers of rotation determine the moment-generating capacity of several key muscles as well as the transmission of forces through the bones and ligaments of the joints themselves. To answer this question, a fluoroscopic study was carried out to identify shoulder-girdle position when the feline head and neck were held in different postures. Furthermore, by posing cats on force plates when stereo X-rays were taken (e.g. Fig. 1), data could also be used for a three-dimensional static analysis of the effects of ground reaction forces from the limbs through the various joints of the forelimb and shoulder (Runciman and Richmond, 1997). It was perhaps not surprising to find that loading on the scapula in these cursorial animals was confined primarily to the sagittal plane. What was unexpected was the rather large size of the moment in this plane that tended to rotate the vertebral border of the scapula caudoven-trally with respect to the head of the humerus (counterclockwise in Fig. 2). How then can the cat sit immobile? The loading forces must be counter-balanced by a force directed cranially; we postulated this might be transmitted by muscles linking the skull to the scapula. One candidate muscle, rhomboideus capitis (also called occipito-scapularis), is known to be active tonically when the animal adopts quietly sitting or standing postures (Richmond et al., 1992). This suggests that nature may use the weight of the head as an efficient way to counterbalance the loading forces transmitted from the paws. Does this biomechanical arrangement change the control of head movement so significantly that results from the cat cannot be used to understand human head movement?

The feline head-neck control system

In cats, much of the research done to date has been concerned with the coordination of head and eye movements. The work suggests the presence of at least two separate brainstem systems controlling the vertical and horizontal components of combined head and eye movements in such diverse species as cats, owls and man (e.g. Hess, 1954; Isa and Sasaki, 1988; Masino and Knudsen, 1992). It also suggests substantial task-related specificity among the neck muscles. Vertical movements appear to be produced by recruiting extensor muscles containing high proportions of slow fibers. Particularly important seem to be the biventer cervicis (Fig. 3) and occipitoscapularis, which are active tonically when the head is raised or held stationary in most postures, and which even show activity, albeit reduced activity, as the head is lowered in a controlled way from a high-held to a low-held position (Richmond et al., 1992). Muscles associated with horizontal movements, in contrast, tend to have high proportions of fast fibers (Richmond and Vidal, 1988).

However, feline head movements are important for more than watching prey; they often must also subdue it. The need for large forces, such as those employed when a cat shakes and tears prey, appears to be reflected in the adaptations of the first and second cervical vertebrae, whose dorsal and lateral processes are much larger than those typical of man (Reighard and Jennings, 1963; Selbie et al., 1993)

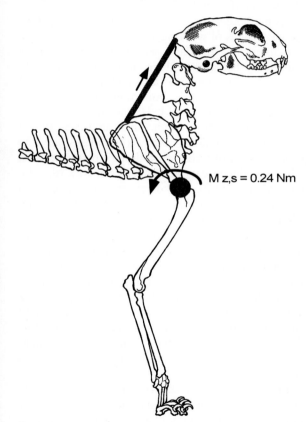

Fig. 2. Loading of the feline scapula from ground reaction forces in the sitting cat. A caudoventrally directed moment, M_{zs}, around the glenohumeral joint may be resisted by rostrally-directed forces generated in part through a muscular tether to the head. One possible tether is the muscle, occipitoscapularis, illustrated by the line joining the scapula and the skull.

(Fig. 4), and whose attached muscles have larger cross-sectional areas than allometric scaling would predict (Richmond et al., 1998). It is not yet clear whether these behaviors are controlled by the same central pathways that are responsible for the head movements in gaze. However, it is likely that their control strategies may be different from those in humans, where the head has been freed by the hands carrying out many functions for which the head must be used in carnivores.

Non-human primates: not just scaled-up cats

The differences that seem to separate cats from humans might be avoided in experimental studies by choosing a more appropriate species, and monkeys are the most obvious candidates. Monkeys have been used extensively to investigate

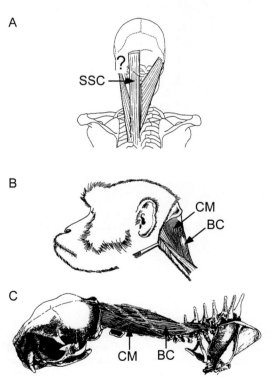

Fig. 3. Comparison of long dorsal extensors in human (A), rhesus monkey (B) and domestic cat (C). Humans have a single muscle, semispinalis cervicis (SSC), and lack a homologue to complexus (CM) (usual location marked by a question mark). Monkeys and cats have two muscles complexus (CM) and biventer cervicis (BC).

414

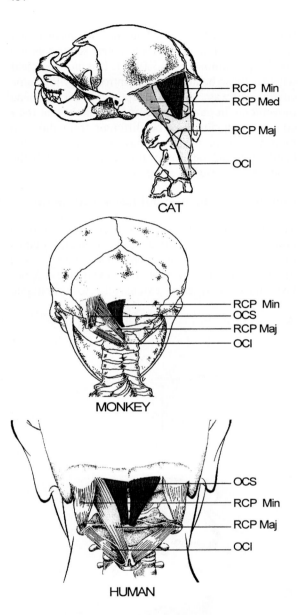

Fig. 4. Comparisons of suboccipital muscles in humans, monkeys and cats. Note the similar morphology of upper cervical vertebrae and similar relationships of suboccipital extensors in humans and monkeys. Cats have longer C1 and C2 vertebrae and a more longitudinal orientation of muscles linking the skull to C1. Adapted with permission from Kamibayashi and Richmond, 1998; Selbie et al., 1993. RCP: rectus capitis posterior; Min: minor; Med: medius; Maj: major; OCI: obliquus capitis inferior; OCS: obliquus capitis superior.

neural activity in motor systems responsible for limb and eye movements. The delays in adopting monkeys as experimental models of choice for studies of head movement may be attributed, at least in part, to the relatively poor information available about the musculoskeletal organization of the monkey neck. Further, electrophysiological studies of neural strategies are complicated by the challenges of freeing the head during recording sessions in a species not inclined to sit docilely on a platform. Head movements can interfere with microelectrode recordings from the brain and can be difficult to monitor without highly specialized equipment such as large search coils (e.g. Freedman and Sparks, 1997) or videofluoroscopy (e.g. Keshner et al., 1997).

As methods are developed to address the technical challenges of working with head-free monkeys, it is likely that monkeys will be used much more commonly because of their closer resemblence to man. Before monkeys are embraced as ideal models, however, it is important to ask whether monkeys, like cats, will be found to have specializations that may limit the applicability of experimental findings. Rhesus monkeys are the products of a different evolutionary path from that which produced cats and other carnivora (e.g. Le Gros Clark, 1962). The divergence is reflected in the bones and muscles of the neck and shoulder. Monkeys, like humans, have a shoulder girdle whose strut-like clavicle pushes the acromion of the scapula laterally and changes the sites available for attachment of the trapezius and sternomastoid muscles. Its vertebrae are also configured in ways that seem more similar to patterns in man. The C2 vertebra, for example, has a much shorter body and smaller spine than that in the cat, and this difference is associated with more human-like patterns of suboccipital muscle attachments (Fig. 4).

Between the most superficial and deep muscle layers in the monkey neck, however, there are muscles whose structures are strongly reminiscent of those observed previously in the cat. Simian dorsal extensors, for example, are relatively large and similarly structured to feline homologues. Some of this similarity may relate to the similar locomotor styles of rhesus monkeys and cats. Both are terrestrial quadrupeds that must hold the rostrally-cantilevered head and neck in a stable position against gravitational forces. But simian muscles are not identical to those in cats either. Extensor muscles in monkeys have smaller proportions of slow fibers than homologous feline muscles, even though most other simian neck muscles have similar or higher proportions of slow fibers than feline homologues (Fig. 5). The reduced slow-fiber content may reflect the fact that monkeys walk like other quadrupeds, but sit like bipeds; their necks and backs are often held in a 'human-like' vertical orientation, in which the weight of the head is borne largely by compressive forces onto the stacked vertebrae. Regular use of such postures may reduce the need for large, tonic extensor forces and therefore may shorten the daily 'duty-cycle' of extensor muscles.

Quadrupeds vs. brachiators

Most anthropological texts appear to share a common view that old-world monkeys such as macaques are not the direct antecedents of man but rather represent a different branch of the simian tree from which the hominids evolved. Although little is known about the comparative anatomy of their neck musculature, we might predict that the neck and shoulder anatomy of arboreal monkeys and humans will show substantial differentiation from that of macaques. Among the differences that

we might expect in man are reductions in the relative cross-sectional areas of extensor muscles in the neck and increases in the cross-sectional areas of muscles that lift and retract the shoulder.

Human primates: not just scaled-up monkeys

At least two features of head-neck biomechanics sets humans apart from quadrupedal monkeys such as macaques. First, the center of mass of the skull is located almost directly over the cervical vertebral column rather than in front of it. Thus relatively modest forces are needed to balance the head on top of the cervical vertebral column. Second, the scapulae lie in the frontal plane. This orientation increases the range of arm movements and changes the biomechanical relationships of many muscles. The biomechanical changes are reflected in the organization of neck muscles, especially extensor muscles. For example, two differentiable muscles in the simian neck, biventer cervicis and complexus, are replaced by a single muscle in man called semispinalis capitis (Fig. 3). Further, the rhomboideus capitis muscle, which runs from the skull to the scapula in the monkey as in the cat, is no longer present in man (Kamibayashi and Richmond, 1998).

When human necks are compared to simian or feline necks, the general impression is one of structural regression. Perhaps such 'backward' change should not be too surprising. In man, head

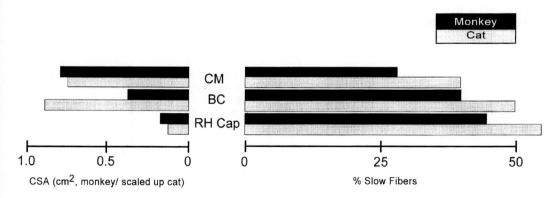

Fig. 5. Comparison of CSA and fiber-type distribution in three cat and monkey extensors, complexus (CM), biventer cervicis (BC) and rhomboideus capitis (Rhcap). To compare CSAs of extensors across species, feline muscles were scaled up by a factor of body mass$^{2/3}$ (1.8 × actual values). Note the relatively higher density of slow fibers in all cat muscles and the larger CSA of the chief extensor, BC. Data from Richmond and Vidal, 1988; Richmond, unpublished observations.

movements are generally used for a narrower range of purposes, to extend the visual range and orient the other sensory structures mounted on the head. Human head movements are also used expressively to convey an added dimension to the spoken word. However, all of these purposes can be achieved with relatively low levels of muscle force. The relatively low demands on the neck musculature presumably contribute to its gradual reduction in strength and complexity. This may predispose the human neck to damage and dysfunction in situations for which the neck was never adapted. Differences between the necks of humans and other animals may limit the usefulness of animal models, especially when trying to interpret the pathophysiology of common neck disorders. An understanding of the nature and extent of differences in the biomechanics of head movement may clarify both the homologies and differences in neural mechanisms for head-movement control in different species that must be used for experimental studies that cannot be carried out in man.

Acknowledgements

This work was supported by the MRC of Canada. Thanks to J. Creasy, C. Evans, and S. Overington for help with illustrations and experiments.

References

Brink, E.E. (1988) Segmental organization of the upper cervical cord. In: B.W. Peterson and F.J. Richmond (Eds), *Control of Head Movement*. Oxford University Press, New York, pp. 76–89.

Freedman, E.G. and Sparks, D.L. (1997) Eye-head coordination during head-unrestrained gaze shifts in rhesus monkeys. *J. Neurophysiol.*, 77: 2328–2348.

Hess, W.R. (1954) Diencephalon: Autonomic and extrapyramidal functions. *Monographs in Biology and Medicine*. Grune and Stratton, New York 25: 3.

Isa, T. and Sasaki, S. (1988) Effects of lesion of paramedian pontomedullary reticular formation by kainic acid injection on the visually triggered horizontal orienting movements in the cat. *Neurosci. Lett.*, 87: 233–239.

Kamibayashi, L.K. and Richmond, F.J.R. (1998) Morphometry of human neck muscles. *Spine*, 23: 1314–1323.

Keshner, E.A., Statler, K.D. and Delp, S.L. (1997) Kinematics of the freely moving head and neck in the alert cat. *Exp. Brain Res.*, 115: 257–266.

Le Gros Clark, W.E. (1962) *The Antecedents of Man: An Introduction to the Evolution of the Primates*. Edinburgh: Edinburgh University Press.

Magnus, R. (1926) Some results of studies in the physiology of posture (Cameron Prize lectures). *Lancet*, 211: 531–536, 585–588 (2 parts).

Masino, T. and Knudsen, E.I. (1992) Anatomical pathways from the optic tectum to the spinal cord subserving orienting movements in the barn owl. *Exp. Brain Res.*, 92: 194–208.

Reighard, J. and Jennings, H.S. (1963) *Anatomy of the Cat*. New York: Holt, Rinehart and Winston.

Richmond, F.J.R., Singh, K. and Corneil, B.D. (1998) Morphometric and histochemical differences between primate and feline neck muscles. *Soc. Neurosci*, 24: 1672 (abstract)

Richmond, F.J.R., Thomson, D.B. and Loeb, G.E. (1992) Electromyographic studies of neck muscles in the intact cat. I. Patterns of recruitment underlying posture and movement during natural behaviors. *Exp. Brain Res.*, 88: 41–58.

Richmond, F.J.R. and Vidal, P.P. (1988) The motor system: joints and muscles of the neck. In: B.W. Peterson and F.J.R. Richmond (Eds), *Control of Head Movement*, Oxford University Press, New York, pp. 1–21.

Runciman, R.J. and Richmond, F.J.R. (1997) Shoulder and forelimb orientation and loading in sitting cats: implications for head and shoulder movement. *J. Biomech.*, 30: 911–919.

Selbie, W.S., Thomson, D.B. and Richmond, F.J.R. (1993) Suboccipital muscles in the cat neck: morphometry and histochemistry of the rectus capitis muscle complex. *J. Morphol.*, 216: 47–63.

Sherrington, C.S. (1897). Decerebrate rigidity and reflex coordination of movements. *J. Physiol.*, 22: 319–332.

Thomson, D.B., Loeb, G.E. and Richmond, F.J.R. (1994) Effect of neck posture on the activation of feline neck muscles during voluntary head turns. *J. Neurophysiol.*, 72: 2004–2014.

Vidal, P.P., Graf, W. and Berthoz, A. (1986) The orientation of the cervical vertebral column in unrestrained awake animals. I. Resting position. *Exp. Brain Res.*, 61: 549–559.

Wilson, V.J. and Peterson, B.W. (1988) Vestibular and reticular projections to the neck. In: B.W. Peterson and F.J.R. Richmond (Eds), *Control of Head Movement*, Oxford University Press, New York, pp. 129–140.

SECTION IX

Control of movement
studied in man

M.D. Binder (Ed.)
Progress in Brain Research, Vol 123

CHAPTER 38

The sharing principle

J.A. Stephens,* L.M. Harrison, M.J. Mayston, L.J. Carr and J. Gibbs

Department of Physiology, University College London, Gower Street, London WC1E 6BT, UK

Introduction

Even the simplest movements require the co-contraction of many different muscles acting around different joints. Making a fist, for example, involves flexion at the inter-phalangeal and met-acarpo-phalangeal joints, combined with extension at the wrist: co-contraction of the intrinsic hand muscles and forearm finger flexor muscles is combined with the co-contraction of forearm wrist extensor muscles. Another example might be touching the tip of the shoulder with the index finger. Here flexion at the wrist is combined with flexion at the elbow. Contraction of the forearm wrist flexor muscles is combined with contraction of elbow flexor muscles.

How are patterns of muscle co-contraction brought about?

Our approach to this problem has been to study the distribution of common synaptic input shared between motoneurones innervating the different muscles (Bremner et al., 1991a, b; Carr et al., 1994; Gibbs et al., 1995a). The presence of such shared synaptic input activity is indicated by a peak in the cross-correlogram constructed from the times of occurrence of motor unit spikes recorded from the different coactive muscles (Moore et al, 1970;

Sears and Stagg, 1976; Kirkwood and Sears, 1978; Kirkwood et al, 1982; Kirkwood and Sears, 1991).

A typical experiment

Figure 1 shows the results of a typical experiment. The subject is asked to carry out a number of different tasks while recording simultaneously multi-unit surface EMG signals from a number of different muscle pairs. The subject is provided with an RMS voltmeter and asked to maintain steady EMG activity at 10–20% of maximum.

Figure 1A, shows a cross-correlogram constructed from the times of occurrence of motor unit spikes recorded from first dorsal interosseous (1DI) in the hand and extensor indicis in the forearm while the subject raised a straightened index finger, with the rest of his hand and forearm resting on a table. The correlogram contains a central peak. These two motoneurone pools are receiving shared common synaptic input. In Fig. 1B, recordings were made from the radial and ulnar wrist flexor muscles while the subject flexed his wrist. Again the cross-correlogram contains a central peak. These two motoneurone pools are also receiving shared common synaptic input.

But the results in Fig. 1C and 1D are different. The cross-correlograms are flat. Co-contraction of the radial wrist extensor and index finger flexor during fist clenching is accomplished in the absence of synaptic input shared between the two motoneurone pools. The same is true for the co-contraction of the radial wrist flexor and biceps as the subject flexed the wrist and elbow.

*Corresponding author. Tel.: (0) (+44) 171 209 6085;
Fax: (0) (+44) 171 387 6368;
e-mail: j.stephens@ucl.ac.uk

420

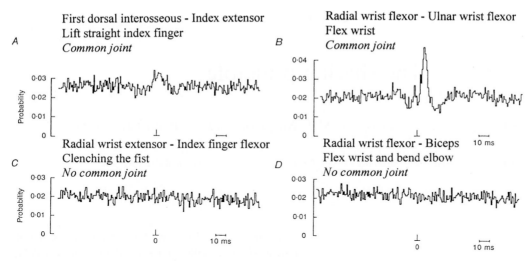

Fig. 1. Cross-correlograms constructed from multi-unit surface EMG recordings obtained from different co-contracting muscle pairs. Correlograms constructed from approximately 5000 spikes, selected from each recording using a level detector circuit. The ordinate gives the probability of finding a spike in the 'event' muscle (the second muscle in the pair) in a 1 ms bin at times before and after a spike occurring at time 0 (indicated on the figure) in the 'trigger' muscle (the first muscle of the pair). Recordings made during voluntary sustained isometric contractions at 10–20% of that achieved during a maximum voluntary contraction (from Gibbs et al., 1995a).

The sharing principle

The results of these experiments raise the question as to whether there might be a simple principle governing the distribution of synaptic input shared between different motoneurone pools. The simplest would be that motoneurones innervating muscles that share a common mechanical action share a common synaptic input.

The data in Fig. 1 conform to this idea. In Fig. 1A and 1B the muscle pairs are acting at a common joint and cross-correlograms contain a central peak. But in Fig. 1C and 1D the muscle pairs do not and the correlograms are flat.

We have now recorded from many different muscle pairs (see Table 1). In every case, muscle pairs that share action about a common joint share common pre-synaptic input. The converse is also true – motoneurones innervating co-contracting muscles that do not share a common action about a common joint do not share a common input (see Table 2). We call this the sharing principle (Gibbs et al, 1995a, b).

But does there have to be a common joint? No, not in the simple anatomical sense. The sharing principle has more general application.

Cross-correlogram peaks have been found for bilateral homologous muscle pairs such as left and right masseter, diaphragm, rectus abdominis and erector spinae. In every case, however, shared mechanical action is accompanied by activity in shared synaptic input. The masseter muscles co-contract to lift the jaw symmetrically about an axis through the temporomandibular joints and the two halves of diaphragm co-contract to draw the central tendon of insertion downwards and forwards in the mid-line. Rectus abdominis and the erector spinae also act symmetrically along a central common mid-line axis to compress the abdominal cavity and extend the vertebral column respectively.

Is input sharing obligatory?

Is the sharing of common synaptic input between motoneurone pools sharing a common mechanical action obligatory? No. It appears not! (Gibbs et al., 1995a).

Gastrocnemius and medial hamstring become active together during standing with the trunk flexed forward and the cross-correlogram recorded under these conditions contains a central peak.

They also become active when the subject is lying prone and asked to point the toes and extend the knees and hip. But in this situation the correlogram is flat! Gastrocnemius and the hamstrings share a common action about a common joint, they flex the knee joint. But they also act at separate joints, gastrocnemius to extend the ankle and the hamstrings to flex the hip. In the postural task, when the two muscle combine to play a common support role, common synaptic inputs are active. But when the subject carries out a task directed towards independent action around the separate joints, common synaptic inputs are inactive. The common action of the two muscles at the knee remains, but the associated common synaptic input activity is absent.

TABLE 1

Muscles that share a mechanical action share common pre-synaptic input

Muscles	Movement (shared mechanical axis)	Shared common pre-synaptic input (central cross-correlogram peak)
Radial wrist extensor ulnar wrist extensor	wrist extension (wrist joint)	yes
Gastrocnemius soleus	ankle plantar flexion (ankle joint)	yes
Gastrocnemius medial hamstring	knee flexion (knee joint)	yes
Left masseter right masseter	clench teeth (axis through temporo-mandibular joints)	yes
Left–right diaphragm	breathe in (central tendon of insertion)	yes
Left–right rectus abdominis	forced expiration (homologous bilateral attachments to ribs and pubis)	yes
Left–right erector spinae	back extension (homologous bilateral attachments to sacrum and lumbar and thoracic vertebrae)	yes

TABLE 2

Muscles that do not share a mechanical action do not share common pre-synaptic input

Muscles	Movement (shared mechanical axis)	Shared common pre-synaptic input (central cross-correlogram peak)
Wrist extensor index flexor	make fist (no : separate joints)	no
Wrist flexor biceps brachii	wrist and elbow flexion (no : separate joints)	no
Tibialis anterior quadriceps	ankle dorsiflexion and knee extension (no : separate joints)	no
Soleus medial hamstring	ankle plantar flexion and knee flexion (no : separate joints)	no

Another interesting example of the sharing principle at work can be found recording from left and right gastrocnemius and left and right tibialis anterior muscles (Gibbs et al., 1995a). If the subject is asked to co-contract these homologous muscle pairs while lying prone either by simultaneously pointing the toes (for gastrocnemius), or flexing the two ankles (for tibialis anterior), the cross-correlograms are flat. In this situation the common mechanical actions of these homologous muscle pairs in the different legs is controlled by independent presynaptic input activity. But, if recordings are made during standing, the cross-correlograms contain a central peak (see Fig. 2). In this situation, there is a common mechanical action, which is to control rotation around a horizontal axis through the two ankle joints. The sharing principle applies. Co-contracting muscles sharing a common mechanical action share common synaptic input.

Henneman and the sharing principle

The sharing principle extends to the control of different motoneurone pools the mechanism envisaged by Henneman to be responsible for the coherent action of motoneurones within a single pool: the sharing of synaptic input.

Spike triggered averaging in cat had shown that individual Group Ia muscle spindle afferent fibres produced excitatory post synaptic potentials in

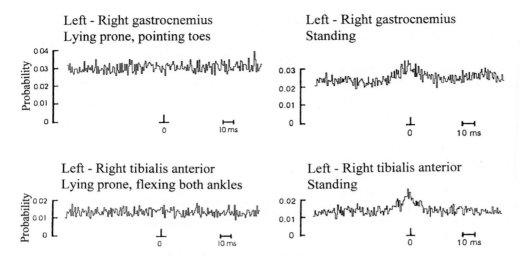

Fig. 2. Cross-correlograms constructed from multi-unit surface EMG recordings obtained from left and right gastrocnemius and left and right tibialis anterior muscles during standing, and during simultaneously pointing the toes (for gastrocnemius) or flexing the two ankles (for tibialis anterior) while lying prone. Correlograms constructed from approximately 5000 spikes, selected from each recording using a level detector circuit. The ordinate gives the probability of finding a spike in the 'event' muscle (the second muscle in the pair) in a 1 ms bin at times before and after a spike occurring at time 0 (indicated on the figure) in the 'trigger' muscle (the first muscle of the pair) (from Gibbs et al., 1995a).

almost all homonymous medial gastrocnemius motoneurones. Individual Group II muscle afferents also produced widespread effects. From this and other evidence, Henneman put forward the generalisation that motoneurones in the same pool share the same synaptic input. The coherent action of a motoneurone pool was ensured by the distribution of synaptic input to its members through activity in the branched connections of presynaptic input fibres innervating many motoneurones within the pool (Henneman, 1985). Such activity, from whatever source, can be expected to produce a central cross-correlogram peak between motoneurone discharges (Sears and Stagg, 1976). This has now been observed in a wide variety of different motoneurone pools including those supplying cat and human respiratory muscles (Sears and Stagg, 1976; Kirkwood and Sears, 1978; Kirkwood, et al., 1982) and human upper and lower limb muscles and jaw muscles (for review see Farmer et al., 1997). No pool has yet been found that does not show this evidence of shared synaptic input between motoneurones.

Sharing of common pre-synaptic input within a motoneurone pool ensures that motor units sharing a common mechanical action operate as a functional entity. Sharing of common pre-synaptic input between motoneurone pools allows different combinations of muscles to operate as a different functional entities. The group of motoneurone pools sharing synaptic input in a particular task work as a functional unit.

Is the strength of shared synaptic input strong enough to determine the functional unit?

The proportion of synaptic input shared between motoneurone pools can be estimated from the size of the cross-correlogram peaks. These indicate that about 20% of the total synaptic drive to each motoneurone pool is shared (Tuck, 1977; Bremner et al., 1989; Bremner et al., 1991b). This is quite sufficient to be the deciding factor in determining which motoneurone pools become active.

Sources of shared synaptic input

One obvious source conveying motor commands to co-activate several different muscles during a voluntary contraction is the corticospinal tract which for monkey forelimb contains individual axons which branch to innervate up to four motor nuclei (Shinoda et al., 1981) and spike triggered averaging experiments have shown such neurones capable of producing post-spike facilitation of EMG activity in several different muscles (Fetz and Cheney, 1980; Cheney and Fetz, 1985; Buys et al; 1986). By their individual projection patterns to different motoneurone pools, each corticospinal neurone can be thought of specifying a movement unit. Rather as the term motor unit has been used to describe the indivisible final element of motor output for a particular muscle consisting of a motoneurone and the muscle fibres it innervates, so the term movement unit describes the corticospinal neurone and the motoneurone pools it innervates, each motoneurone pool receiving a different strength of projection. To use Hughling-Jackson's musical analogy, the cortex commands movements not muscles and each cortico-motoneuronal cell specifies cord not notes, each note receiving a different weight. A particular movement is produced by a combination of activity of different corticospinal neurones each specifying an indivisible element of the movement.

Other descending systems can also be expected to provide shared last order synaptic input specifying movement units. Extensive branching of reticulospinal neurones throughout the spinal cord in the opossum has been described (Martin, et al., 1981; Nathan et al., 1996). Multiple collaterals from vestibulospinal neurones have also been demonstrated within the spinal cord of the cat (Shinoda, et al.,1988). Fibres of both of these descending tracts have been shown to make monosynaptic connections with motoneurones (Lundberg, 1975; Cheney, et al., 1991) and some lateral vestibulospinal tract neurones are known to branch and innervate the ventral spinal grey matter bilaterally (Shinoda, et al., 1988). Activity in these fibres can be expected to contribute to the common synaptic input found to be active to the motoneurone pools innervating homologous left-right leg muscles during standing, leaning backwards and forwards.

Pre-synaptic synchronisation of neurones projecting to different motoneurone pools may also contribute to the generation of a common synaptic

drive (Kirkwood, et al., 1982; Kirkwood and Sears, 1991). Correlograms constructed from the firing of pairs of corticomotoneuronal cells projecting to the same motoneurone pools, for example, show a narrow central peak indicating that they receive a shared common pre-synaptic drive (Smith and Fetz, 1989; Fetz, et al., 1990; see also Allum, et al., 1982; Murphy, et al., 1985). Just as members of an individual lower motoneurone pool are co-ordinated in their action by activity in shared last order branched stem pre-synaptic input fibres so presumably are the members of an upper motoneurone pool selected to work together by the same mechanism to command a particular movement.

What happens when the sharing of common synaptic input is abnormal?

We have observed abnormal sharing of common synaptic input to motoneurone pools in three different clinical situations: Klippel-Feil syndrome (Farmer et al., 1990), hemiplegic cerebral palsy (Carr et al., 1993) and X-linked Kallmann's syndrome (Mayston, et al., 1997). In each the development of the corticospinal system is affected. Most interesting have been those individuals in which focal magnetic brain stimulation of the hand area of the motor cortex indicates the presence of fast conducting bilateral corticospinal projections. In these individuals, cross-correlation analysis of motor unit activity shows common synaptic input to be shared between left and right homologous muscle pairs in situations where there is none shared in normal subjects. Noticeably, where this type of abnormal common input has been found, subjects have exhibited mirror movements: involuntary movements of one side of the body that accompany and mirror intentional movements on the other side.

An example is shown in Fig. 3. In a normal subject, voluntary co-contraction of left and right first dorsal interosseous muscles is not accompanied by shared common synaptic input. The cross-correlogram of motor unit activity between the two muscles is flat. But in the patient with congenital hemi-plegia, there is a clear central peak. Common synaptic input is shared between the left and right homologous motoneurone pools.

Interestingly, the distribution of common synaptic drive is quite specific (see Fig. 4). The subject is asked to spread the fingers of both hands. The cross-correlograms between motor unit spikes recorded between left-right first dorsal interosseous muscles and left-right abductor digiti minimi muscles contain a central peak. The correlogram between spikes recorded from right first dorsal interosseous muscle and right abductor digiti minimi is flat. So is the correlogram between right first dorsal interosseous muscle and left abductor digiti minimi. The pattern of shared common synaptic input on one side has been mirrored on the other. It is presumably this mirroring of shared synaptic input that produces the shared mechanical output that results in mirroring.

The fact that abnormal sharing of synaptic input following abnormal corticospinal development produces a mirrored movement rather than a discordant co-contraction of muscles indicates that the innervation pattern of descending corticospinal fibres to different motoneurone pools is preserved,

to whichever side of the spinal cord it is directed. This reinforces the idea that it is sharing of common synaptic input from this source that allows combinations of muscles to operate as functional entities.

Conclusion

Cross-correlation analysis of simultaneously recorded multi-unit EMG signals has been used to study the distribution of common synaptic input shared between motoneurones innervating different muscles in man. From these experiments, a simple new generalisation emerged for the organisation of synaptic drive to motoneurones which we call the sharing principle – motoneurones innervating muscles that share a common mechanical action share a common presynaptic input. The converse is also true – motoneurones innervating co-contracting muscles that do not share a common action do not share a common input. The sharing principle extends to the control of different motoneurone

Left - Right first dorsal interosseous   Normal subject

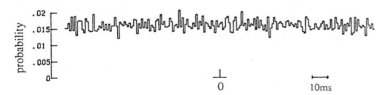

Left - Right first dorsal interosseous   Congenital hemi-plegia
(with mirror movements)

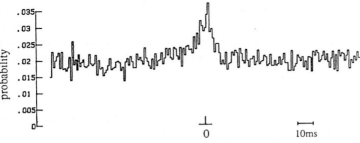

Fig. 3. Cross-correlograms constructed from multi-unit surface EMG signals recorded simultaneously from left and right first dorsal interosseous muscles. Correlograms constructed from approximately 3500 spikes, selected from each recording using a level detector circuit. The ordinate gives the probability of finding a spike in the 'event' muscle (the second muscle in the pair) in a 1 ms bin at times before and after a spike occurring at time 0 (indicated on the figure) in the 'trigger' muscle (the first muscle of the pair) (from Carr et al., 1993).

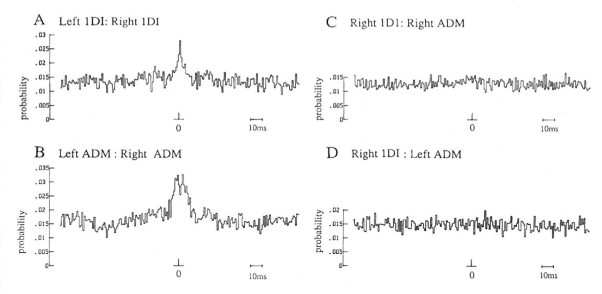

Fig. 4. Cross-correlograms constructed from multi-unit surface EMG signals recorded simultaneously from various intrinsic hand muscles in a subject with congenital hemi-plegia and mirror movements. Correlograms constructed from approximately 4500 spikes, selected from each recording using a level detector circuit. The ordinate gives the probability of finding a spike in the 'event' muscle (the second muscle in the pair) in a 1 ms bin at times before and after a spike occurring at time 0 (indicated on the figure) in the 'trigger' muscle (the first muscle of the pair). No central peaks are present when the correlograms are constructed from recordings obtained from non-homologous muscle pairs (from Carr et al., 1993).

pools the mechanism envisaged by Henneman to be responsible for the coherent action of motoneur-ones within a single pool: the sharing of synaptic input. Sharing of common synaptic input within a motoneurone pool ensures that motor units sharing a common mechanical action operate as a functional entity. Sharing of common pre-synaptic input between motoneurone pools allows different combinations of muscles to operate as different functional entities. The group of motoneurone pools sharing synaptic input in a particular task work as a functional unit.

Acknowledgements

This work was supported by Action Research Grant No. S/P/1893, the Scholl Trust and Wellcome Grant 044080/Z/95. L.J. Carr was supported by a MRC Training Fellowship and M.J. Mayston by a MRC PhD studentship. We also thank the staff at the Bobath Centre for the treatment of Children with Cerebral Palsy.

References

Allum, J.H., Hepp-Reymond, M.C. and Gysin, R. (1982) Cross-correlation analysis of interneuronal connectivity in the motor cortex of the monkey. *Brain Res.*, 231: 325–334.

Bremner, F.D., Datta, A.K. and Stephens, J.A. (1989) A mechanism for muscle synergy. In: H.D. Henatsh, U. Windhorst, Y. Laouris and Meyer-Lohmann (Eds), *Perspectives in Motor Control*, AIM Verlag, Gottingen, pp. 44–50.

Bremner, F.D., Baker, J.R. and Stephens, J.A. (1991a) Correlation between the discharges of motor units recorded from the same and from different finger muscles in man. *J. Physiol.*, 432: 355–380.

Bremner, F.D., Baker, J.R. and Stephens, J.A. (1991b) Variation in the degree of synchronization exhibited by motor units lying in different finger muscles in man. *J. Physiol.*, 432: 381–399.

Buys, E.J., Lemon, R.N., Mantel, G.W.H. and Muir, R.B. (1986) Selective facilitation of different hand muscles by single corticospinal neurones in the conscious monkey. *J. Physiol.*, 381: 529–549.

Carr, L.J., Harrison, A.L., Evans, A.L. and Stephens, J.A. (1993) Patterns of central motor reorganization in hemiplegic cerebral palsy. *Brain*, 116: 1223–1247.

Carr, L.J., Harrison, L.M. and Stephens, J.A. (1994) Evidence for bilateral innervation of certain homologous motoneurone pools in man. *J. Physiol.*, 475: 217–227.

426

Cheney, P.D. and Fetz, E.E. (1985) Comparable patterns of muscle facilitation evoked by individual corticomotoneuronal (CM) cells and by single intracortical microstimuli in primates: evidence for functional groups of CM cells. *J. Neurophysiol.*, 53: 786–804.

Cheney, P.D., Fetz, E.E. and Mewes, K. (1991) Neural mechanisms underlying corticospinal and rubrospinal control of limb movements. In: G. Holstege (Ed.), *Progress in Brain Research*, Vol. 87. Elsevier, Amsterdam. pp. 213–252.

Farmer, S.F., Ingram. D.A. and Stephens, J.A. (1990) Mirror movements studied in a patient with Klippel-Feil syndrome. *J. Physiol.*, 428: 467–484.

Farmer, S.F., Halliday, D.M., Conway, B.A., Stephens, J.A. and Rosenberg, J.R. (1997) A review of recent applications of cross-correlation methodologies to human motor unit recording. *J. Neurosci. Meth.*, 74: 175–187.

Fetz, E.E. and Cheney, P.D. (1980) Postspike facilitation of forelimb muscle activity by primate corticomotoneuronal cells. *J. Neurophysiol.*, 44: 751–772.

Fetz, E.E., Toyama, K. and Smith, W.L. (1990) Synaptic interactions between cortical neurons. In: E.G. Jones and A. Peters (Eds), *Cerebral Cortex*, Vol 9. Plenum Press, New York. pp. 1–47.

Gibbs, J., Harrison, L.M. and Stephens, J.A. (1995a) Organization of inputs to motoneurone pools in man. *J. Physiol.*, 485: 245–256.

Gibbs, J., Harrison, L.M., Mayston, M.J. and Stephens, J.A. (1995b) Mechanisms underlying muscle synergy studied in man In: A. Taylor, M.H. Gladden and R. Durbaba (Eds), *Alpha and gamma motor systems*. Plenum Press, New York. pp. 466–468.

Henneman, E. (1985) The size-principle: a deterministic output emerges from a set of probabilistic connections. *J. Exp. Biol.*, 115: 105–112.

Kirkwood, P.A. and Sears, T.A. (1978) The synaptic connexions to intercostal motoneurones as revealed by the average common excitation potential. *J. Physiol.* 275: 103–134.

Kirkwood, P.A., Sears, T.A., Tuck, D.L and Westgaard, R.H. (1982) Variations in the time course of the synchronization of intercostal motoneurones in the cat. *J. Physiol.*, 327: 105–135.

Kirkwood, P.A. and Sears, T.A. (1991) Cross-correlation analyses of motoneurone inputs in a coordinated motor act. In: J. Kruger (Ed.), *Neuronal Cooperativity.* Springer-Verlag, Berlin, pp. 225–248.

Lundberg, A. (1975) The control of spinal mechanisms from the brain. In: D.B. Tower (Ed.), *The Basic Neurosciences*, Vol. 1, *The Nervous System*. Raven Press, New York. pp 253 –265.

Martin, G.F., Cabana, T. and Humbertson, A.O. (1981) Evidence for collateral innervation of the cervical and lumbar enlargements of the spinal cord by single reticular and raphe neurons. Studies using fluorescent markers in double-labelling experiments on the North American opossum. *Neurosci. Lett.*, 24: 1–6.

Mayston, M.J., Harrison, L.M., Quinton, R., Stephens, J.A., Krams, M. and Bouloux, P.-M. G. (1997) *Brain*, 120: 1199–1216.

Moore, G.P., Segundo, J.P., Perkel, D.H. and Levitan, H. (1970) Statistical signs of synaptic interaction in neurons. *Biophys. J.*, 10: 876–900.

Murphy, J.T., Kwan, H.C. and Wong, Y.C. (1985) Cross correlation studies in primate motor cortex: synaptic interaction and shared input. *Can. J. Neurol. Sci.*, 12: 11–23.

Nathan, P.W., Smith, M. and Deacon, P. (1996) Vestibulospinal, reticulospinal and descending propriospinal nerve fibres in man. *Brain*, 119: 1809–1833.

Sears, T.A. and Stagg, D. (1976) Short-term synchronization of intercostal motoneurone activity. *J. Physiol.*, 263: 357–381.

Shinoda, Y., Yokota, J. and Futami, T. (1981) Divergent projection of individual corticospinal axons to motoneurones of multiple muscles in the monkey. *Neurosci. Lett.*, 23: 7–12.

Shinoda, Y., Ohgaki, T., Futami, T. and Sugiuchi, Y. (1988) Vestibular projections to the spinal cord: the morphology of single vestibulospinal axons. In: O. Pompeiano and J.H. Allum (Eds), *Progress in Brain Research*, Vol. 79, Elsevier, Amsterdam. pp. 17–27.

Smith, W.S. and Fetz, E.E. (1989) Effects of synchrony between primate corticomotoneuronal cells on post-spike facilitation of muscles and motor units. *Neurosci. Lett.*, 96: 76–81.

Tuck, D.L. (1977) Investigation of intercostal neuronal intra-cellular processes and connectivity by signal analysis and computer simulation. PhD Thesis, University of London.

M.D. Binder (Ed.)
Progress in Brain Research, Vol 123

CHAPTER 39

Properties of human peripheral nerves: implications for studies of human motor control

David Burke and S.C. Gandevia*

Prince of Wales Medical Research Institute, Department of Neurology, Prince of Wales Hospital and University of New South Wales, Sydney, Australia

Introduction

In neurophysiological studies on human subjects considerable reliance is placed on the data previously obtained from studies in animals. This translation has been extremely fruitful for both groups of neurophysiologists with, for example, development of methods to record and stimulate single human axons (microneurography) and to stimulate the cortex non-invasively (transcranial electrical and magnetic stimulation). However, in many cases those studying human subjects have assumed that what is known from animal studies can be applied without reservation to the more problematic world of human physiology and, more importantly, pathophysiology. In this review we address some issues involving peripheral nerve function and draw implications for studies of motor control in human subjects.

Activity-dependent changes in axonal excitability

When an axon carries an impulse train, whether short or long, its excitability decreases because it hyperpolarizes (Gasser, 1935). There are at least two mechanisms for this. Activation of a slow K^+

*Corresponding author. Tel.: Int +61 2 9382 2677; Fax: Int +61 2 9382 2724; e-mail: S.Gandevia@unsw.edu.au

conductance is probably the major cause with brief impulse trains containing 10–20 discharges (Bergmans, 1970; Baker et al., 1987). Activation of the electrogenic Na^+/K^+ pump appears to be the major cause of hyperpolarization following long impulse trains (Bergmans, 1970; Bostock and Grafe, 1985; Gordon et al., 1990; Morita et al., 1993). In human afferent axons, the activity-dependent hyperpolarization that follows brief impulse trains increases threshold by 30–40% (Lin et al., 1999) but subsides over 100–120 ms (Taylor et al., 1992; Miller et al., 1995). Long trains of impulses increase threshold by a similar amount, and this decays over many minutes, dependent on train length, such that normal excitability may not be restored for > 10–20 min after tetanic stimulation at 200 Hz for a couple of minutes (Kiernan et al., 1997). Because of biophysical differences between human afferent and motor axons (see Burke et al., 1997; Bostock et al., 1998), the hyperpolarization produced by long impulse trains seems to be greater in motor axons than sensory axons (Vagg et al., 1998).

That intense activity can have profound effects on axonal excitability is well known in the motor control literature. It is the rationale for the method developed by Coppin et al. (1970) to use tendon vibration to decrease the excitability of group Ia afferents so that electrical stimulation at group I strength excites only group Ib afferents. This method has been used to study autogenetic inhibition from Ia afferents and convergence between group Ia and Ib afferents (respectively, Fetz et al., 1979; Jankowska and McCrea, 1983). It has also produced the expected results in human studies (Heckman et al., 1984; Hayward et al., 1986; Cavallari and Katz, 1989; Rossi et al., 1991). However, caution is required when using the technique in human subjects because it is difficult to drive human muscle spindles with transversely applied tendon vibration without also stimulating some Golgi tendon organs (e.g. Burke et al., 1976; Cordo et al., 1993). The success of the technique depends on the fact that the axonal hyperpolarization does not significantly interfere with translation of the spindle's receptor potential into an impulse train in the Ia afferent axon. For some studies the conclusions rely critically on the assumption that the final afferent volley contains no Ia component.

That activity will decrease axonal excitability and, thereby, reduce the neural volley produced by a submaximal stimulus of fixed amplitude has not been considered in many motor control studies in animals and man. This phenonemon has a number of consequences and concerns.

• Afferent volleys evoked before, during and after a voluntary contraction may not be the same even if the stimulus intensity is identical and the electrode orientation to the nerve has not changed. The voluntary contraction will, of course, produce activity in motor axons, and their thresholds will increase (by 20–30% after a 1-min contraction, subsiding over 10–15 min; Vagg et al., 1998; Fig. 1). However, the contraction will also be associated with enhanced activity in group Ia and Ib axons, and consequently their thresholds will also increase, but by an unknown and unpredictable amount. An example of the activity-dependent changes in axonal threshold produced by voluntary contractions of different duration is shown in Fig. 1. An important assumption with much testing of muscles using twitch (or tetanic) stimulation before, during and after exercise, is that the efferent volley remains the same: this is unlikely to be the case unless precautions are taken to ensure that the volleys are supramaximal. One area in which this is of particular concern is the suggestion that human inspiratory muscles

fatigue readily in healthy subjects, even for example, during unloaded repetitive breathing tasks (e.g. Hamnegard et al., 1996). By contrast, using supramaximal phrenic nerve stimulation to assess twitch properties and voluntary activation with twitch interpolation, it has been found that the diaphragm does not fatigue during many minutes of voluntary contractions generating about 80% maximal inspiratory force (McKenzie et al., 1997). Not surpisingly, maximal voluntary inspiratory forces are unaltered by exercise or

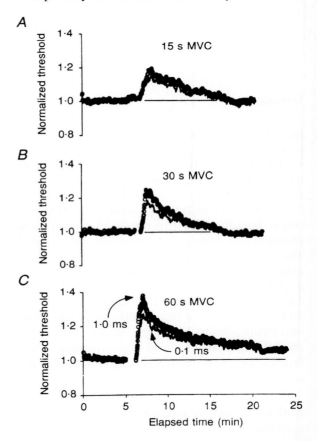

Fig. 1. Dependence of the decrease in excitability of human motor axons on the duration of a voluntary contraction. Threshold changes in human motor axons innervating thenar muscles measured using 1.0 and 0.1 ms test stimuli to the median nerve for maximal voluntary contractions lasting 15, 30 and 60 s. The increase in threshold (20–40%) results from hyperpolarization due to activation of the electrogenic Na^+/K^+ pump. Note that recovery after a contraction for only 15 s takes ~ 10 min. Each trace represents mean data for six subjects. Reproduced with permission from Vagg et al. (1998).

respiratory loading in normal subjects (Johnson et al., 1993).

- The biophysical properties of human sensory and motor axons differ. There appears to be a greater inwardly rectifying conductance and a greater persistent Na^+ conductance on sensory axons than motor axons (respectively, Bostock et al., 1994; Bostock and Rothwell, 1997), and their strength/duration properties differ (Panizza et al., 1994; Mogyoros et al., 1996). Human sensory axons have a longer strength-duration time constant and lower rheobase than motor axons (Mogyoros et al., 1996), and the lower rheobase (rather than axonal size) is probably the major reason why, with relatively wide stimuli, it is possible to activate group I afferents at lower stimulus intensities than motor axons. Largely due to these biophysical differences, the extent of activity-dependent hyperpolarization differs for sensory and motor axons (Burke et al., 1997; Vagg et al., 1998). As a result, matching the size of control and test M waves (the direct motor response) will not guarantee that the *afferent* volley is constant.

- If the motor axons contributing to the M wave produced by submaximal nerve or motor-point stimulation were active in a voluntary contraction, the stimulus intensity would need to be increased to produce an identical M wave. If a submaximal contraction was used, the contraction might be restricted to low-threshold small motoneurones and, if the M wave was small, it would involve electrically low-threshold axons (i.e. those of larger size). However, the stronger the contraction the greater the chance that the electrically evoked volley will contain motor axons that have been active in the voluntary contraction. These complexities have repercussions for studies of the neurophysiological and biochemical accompaniments of muscle fatigue in human subjects. One approach is to stimulate the quadriceps muscle tetanically at submaximal levels (supramaximal levels being too painful) either to produce fatigue or to test for it. An obvious difficulty is that a test tetanus will not activate the same motor axons and hence the same muscle fibres throughout the exercise. If the tetani are used to produce the fatigue, then the motor units used will change. Similar difficulties arise when H-reflex amplitude is measured during voluntary tasks: the use of a small M-wave to 'calibrate' the recordings may not be adequate.

- With the twitch interpolation technique for studying levels of voluntary activation and the mechanisms of fatigue in voluntary exercise (Gandevia et al., 1995), the stimulus needs to be supramaximal, probably by ~40%, to ensure that all motor axons are recruited during and after a maximal voluntary contraction lasting 1 min (Burke and Gandevia, 1998). As raised by Awiszus et al. (1997) this stimulus intensity runs the risk of inadvertent cross-stimulation of motor axons in the antagonist, but their solution, namely to use *sub*maximal stimulation, would introduce problems due to variable axonal excitability. Perhaps the best approach would involve being aware of the potential for error, but then persisting with supramaximal stimulation, while taking care with stimulating electrodes to avoid cross-stimulation (and measuring from the antagonist to ensure that this was so).

- The activity-dependent hyperpolarization is accompanied by an increase in latency (e.g. Miller et al., 1995; Kiernan et al., 1996, 1997). This increase is longer the longer the conduction pathway because the latency increase is small at each node (only a few microseconds, Miller et al., 1995), but it occurs at every node along the axon, and could amount to ~1 ms over the length of a human nerve. Accordingly, a change in latency during or after a contraction would need to be interpreted with caution. Interestingly, although the motor responses to transcranial magnetic stimulation increase in size and area with fatigue, there is a small increase in the onset latency of the responses, with only part of the increase being due to slowing along the peripheral motor axons (Taylor et al., 1999).

- Finally, when an H reflex cannot be readily elicited at rest (e.g. in tibialis anterior or extensor digitorum communis), delivering two stimuli 5 ms apart is sometimes used to produce temporal summation of the afferent input at the motoneurone pool. However, there can be long-lasting effects of the first stimulus such that, even if the two stimuli are of identical strength, the second samples afferents not activated by the first.

H reflexes and PSTHs

In the cat, the conducting pathways are relatively short, the conduction velocities of group I afferents are fast (72–120 m/s for hindlimb group I afferents), and there is little dispersion of the afferent volley by the time it reaches the motoneurone pool. However, with this spread of group I conduction velocities, the slowest group I afferents from soleus would still reach the soleus motoneurone pool ~ 2 ms after the fastest, arriving after the fastest Ib afferent input even though the Ib input must traverse one interneurone. In their pioneering intracellular recordings of the compound group I EPSP in triceps surae motoneurones, Eccles et al. (1957) reversed the IPSP produced by the Ib input to reveal the full extent of the Ia EPSP, and thereby demonstrated that the duration of the Ia EPSP is curtailed by disynaptic inhibition.

The same situation probably occurs in human subjects. Pierrot-Deseilligny and colleagues (1981) found that there was no demonstrable excitatory projection from medial gastrocnemius group I afferents to soleus motoneurones. The initial synaptic event was inhibition, beginning 2 ms after the expected onset of any group Ia excitation. This inhibition was considered to represent group Ib inhibition.

PSTHs are now extensively used in human subjects to document synaptic connectivity and, in these studies, the excitatory peak to tibial nerve stimulation in soleus motoneurones is taken to represent group Ia excitation. The duration of that peak in individual motoneurones is 1–2 ms. However, this implies a very narrow range of conduction velocities for human group Ia afferents (say 65–72 m/s), and it is likely that the true duration of the group Ia input to the motoneurone pool is much longer than this. A more plausible explanation is that something prevents the later arriving components of the Ia volley from contributing to motoneurone discharge. A likely candidate is Ib inhibition, which, much as in the cat, reaches the motoneurone pool shortly after the onset of group Ia excitation and is thus likely to curtail the EPSP by disynaptic inhibition (Pierrot-Deseilligny et al., 1981). The range of arrival times at the motoneurone pool is remarkably large in human studies, as much as several ms. For example, with a 1-m conduction path and a group I conduction velocity range of say 60–80 m/s, the difference in arrival times is 4.2 ms.

If this is so, regardless of whether there are any di- or oligosynaptic excitatory inputs from the tibial nerve to soleus, the size of the H reflex of soleus is determined by the balance between relatively synchronized inputs traversing monosynaptic excitatory and disynaptic inhibitory pathways. The H reflex could be increased in size by anything that altered this balance, whether it be increased monosynaptic excitation or reduced disynaptic inhibition. Ib inhibition is not the only candidate for this role: any disynaptic inhibitory pathway active within 1 ms of the arrival of the afferent volley could curtail the duration of the Ia excitation. Recurrent inhibition probably contributes to the prolonged suppression of activity seen in PSTHs after the initial short-latency excitatory peak (see Meunier et al., 1990, 1994), and it too could reduce the duration of the Ia excitation.

The afferent volley for the tendon jerk is more dispersed than that for the H reflex (Burke et al., 1983, 1984), and its afferent composition differs (Burke et al., 1983). An example of the dispersion and composition of the tendon-jerk volley is shown in Fig. 2. Furthermore, the spindle afferent contribution contains more than one impulse in individual axons, so that the frequency dependence of transmitter release and EPSP generation will be an additional complicating factor (e.g. Collins et al., 1986; Koeber et al., 1991). As argued elsewhere, the human motor control literature has long been too convinced that the H reflex and tendon jerk are simple reflexes that differ only in that the H reflex bypasses the receptor and is therefore not dependent on the level of fusimotor drive.

In a PSTH, the duration of the increased probability of firing may reflect the duration of the compound EPSP produced by the afferent volley but, as discussed above, that does not equate to the duration of group Ia excitation. Few would deny that the onset of the compound EPSP must

431

represent the fastest group Ia monosynaptic input, and this will be so until disynaptic inputs can reach the motoneurone pool. Using this rationale, Hultborn et al. (1987) examined the changes in the first 0.5 ms of the increased probability to a group I input, on the grounds that over this restricted time frame the only input could be monosynaptic Ia excitation. There are two caveats: first, the onset of the excitation must be defined accurately, and second, excitation reaching the pool over that first 0.5 ms is only a small fraction of the total monosynaptic Ia excitation. Hence there is an implicit, but untested, assumption that the initial component is representative of the total excitatory input.

PSTHs require that the neurone studied is rhythmically active and, in human studies, this means voluntarily active. Immediately, there is potential for the results from studies using PSTHs to be different from those using the H reflex,

particularly when the H reflex is elicited at rest. The PSTH technique requires that the subject's attention be focused on a specific motoneurone and that neural circuitry be set to keep that motoneurone firing steadily and other motoneurones quiescent. Usually only the lowest threshold motoneurones in the pool can be studied using PSTHs. In a PSTH, the strength of the synaptic effect is defined by a change in probability of discharge of the active motoneurone, whereas with the H reflex it is signalled by a change in the number of motoneurones recruited into the reflex. With the H reflex, the lowest-threshold motoneurones will be recruited in the control reflex, and the test manoeuvre does not alter whether they discharge reflexly or not: the reflex is facilitated or inhibited by altering whether or not higher-threshold motoneurones are recruited. These are the motoneurones most susceptible to anything that curtails the compound group I EPSP: if they are recruited, they will be so 1–2 ms after

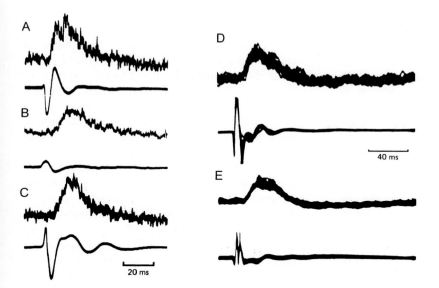

Fig. 2. Afferent volleys evoked by tendon percussion. Left panels: Muscle afferent response to percussion on the Achilles tendon. A and B, response of afferents from soleus, percussion being adequate (A) and subthreshold (B) for the Achilles tendon jerk. C, response of afferents from abductor hallucis in the same subject. Upper traces: the averaged full-wave rectified muscle afferent response (using sixteen, sixty-four and thirty-two sweeps in A, B and C, respectively); lower traces: output of an accelerometer on the Achilles tendon. The three neural and the three accelerometer traces are each at equivalent gains; the traces are aligned at the first deflexion of the appropriate acceleration wave. Right panels: Responses of muscle mechanoreceptors in abductor hallucis (D) and of cutaneous mechanoreceptors in the skin of the hallux and medial aspect of the sole (E) to weak percussion on the Achilles tendon. Percussion was above threshold for the tendon jerk. The limb was supported to avoid direct muscle stretch and skin contact. In D and E, the upper traces are neural activity (rectified and smoothed, time constant 10 ms): the lower traces, accelerometer outputs. Ten responses superimposed. Reproduced with permission from Burke et al. (1983).

the onset of group Ia excitation in the pool. In addition, the mental set of a subject who is trying to relax the test muscle is the opposite of that in a PSTH experiment requiring voluntary activation of a motoneurone. Differences in mental set can alter spinal reflexes, such as the H reflex, and there may be circumstances when this would produce differences in the behaviour of motoneurones in a PSTH and in the H reflex.

A well-recognized aspect of these sorts of studies is the need to control the motoneurone firing rate. Almost paradoxically, the 'responsiveness' of the motoneurone to the same excitatory input (measured as the peak in the PSTH) is greater when the firing rate is low and the membrane potential exponentially approaches threshold (Olivier et al., 1995; Jones and Bawa, 1997). Under such circumstances, particularly at low firing rates, the properties of the on-going synaptic noise will influence the PSTHs (e.g. Matthews, 1996). An additional issue here is the way that the PSTHs are 'constructed': one or more units can be sampled from a multi-unit recording with the stimulus delivered at random or a single unit can be sampled with the stimulus delivered non-randomly to 'test' the latter part of the after-hyperpolarization. Both methods have advantages, but with either it is crucial that sufficient counts are acquired to define the onset of the initial effect. A discussion of the interpretation of the peaks in PSTHs is beyond the scope of this chapter and is covered elsewhere: suffice to say that the size of the initial effect, the extent of background noise as well as the auto-correlation function for the unit need to be considered.

Dispersion of neural volleys

As mentioned above, neural volleys will be dispersed by the time they reach the motoneurone pool, whether they come from supraspinal centres or from peripheral sources. This is rarely recognised when 'central' conduction times are calculated. The degree of dispersion of the volley will depend on many factors:

- *The nature of the stimulus.* Neural volleys set up by mechanical stimuli are inevitably more dispersed than those set up by brief electrical

stimuli. For example, the afferent volley set up by percussion on the Achilles tendon lasts 35 ms at the popliteal fossa (Burke et al., 1983) and presumably much more by the time it reaches the motoneurone pool. The rise-time of the compound EPSP produced in soleus motoneurones by percussion on the Achilles tendon lasts >10 ms (Burke et al., 1984). The dampening effect of muscle and tendon results in distortion of the applied stretch so that even 'quick stretch' will last >6 ms at muscle spindle level. Latencies are, of necessity, measured from the onset of the imposed stretch but that is not when receptors are activated. For stimuli designed to activate muscle spindle afferents in a reproducible way, another critical factor is the state or 'history' of the muscle. The thixotropic properties (particularly) of intrafusal fibres mean that the history of fusimotor outflow to a muscle, and consequently whether 'slack' has been removed from the muscle spindle, will affect the afferent volley produced by muscle stretch (Proske, 1993; Gregory et al., 1999).

- *The duration of the stimulus.* A number of studies have compared PSTHs produced in the same motoneurones by transcranial magnetic or electrical stimuli with those produced by peripheral nerve stimuli, supposedly activating largely Ia afferents (however, see above). The duration of the peripheral nerve stimulus is usually 1 ms, as in conventional H reflex studies, and, because of their different strength-duration properties (discussed above), this is the optimal stimulus duration if one wishes to activate group I afferents at lower threshold than α motor axons. However, with a submaximal stimulus of 1-ms duration, few axons, if any, are activated at the onset of the stimulus and only the last-recruited axons are activated at the end of the 1-ms stimulus. In other words, the longer the stimulus the more dispersed will be the afferent volley, an effect beginning at the site of initiation of the stimulus. This factor is significant, given that the increased probability of firing produced by the afferent volley in single motoneurones lasts only 1–2 ms. In addition, the latency of H reflexes elicited by 1-ms stimuli is longer than that of those using shorter stimuli, 0.2–0.5 ms in duration (Mogyoros et al., 1997). With transcranial stimulation the stimulus waveform is very different: with electrical stimulation, it usually consists of a capacitively coupled pulse with a time constant of 50 μs or 100 μs, and with magnetic stimulation, it is commonly not monophasic.

- *The spread of conduction velocities for the afferent volley.* While the fastest conduction velocities have been documented for human corticospinal and peripheral nerve axons, there are, unfortunately, no good data on the range of conduction velocities for different populations of human axons, afferent or efferent. Over the last decade, different studies have invoked group II muscle afferents as the cause of synchronised EMG responses of relatively long latency (e.g. Schiepatti et al., 1997). Intuitively, this seems unlikely: if mechanically evoked group Ia volleys are significantly dispersed by the time they reach the motoneurone pool, there will be much greater dispersion in a population of afferents with slower conduction velocities. Such a dispersed input could produce a background facilitation or inhibition of the motoneurone pool, but how it could generate a synchronised EMG potential has not been adequately considered.
- *The length of the pathway to the target motoneurones.* Conduction pathways are obviously much longer for human subjects than for the cat, and in humans they are usually shorter for corticospinal volleys than for peripheral volleys. Other things being equal, there is greater opportunity for dispersion with the peripheral volley.
- *The existence of interneurones in the pathway.* The possibility that disynaptic inhibition (group Ib, recurrent) limits the duration of the compound EPSP produced by peripheral nerve stimuli has been addressed above. With descending corticospinal volleys, there is evidence that some of the descending drive reaches the motoneurone pool through an interneurone (Burke et al., 1994), possibly the pre-motoneurones of the putative 'propriospinal' system (Pierrot-Deseilligny, 1996).
- *The excitability of the responding neurones.* Dependent on the rise-time of the compound EPSP, significant changes in latency occur when an initially non-contracting muscle is contracted, so raising the excitability of the responding motoneurone pool. For example, when subjects perform weak voluntary contractions of soleus and reflex amplitudes are carefully matched, the latency of the Achilles tendon jerk shortens by ~2 ms but the latency of the soleus H reflex shortens by 0.2–0.3 ms (Uysal et al., 1999). One factor likely to contribute to this effect is the difference in rise-time of the appropriate compound EPSPs (see above). Presumably, significant delays can occur at each neurone in a reflex arc (including the α motoneurone), with the delays being greater the more dispersed the excitatory input.

Acknowledgements

The authors are supported by the National Health and Medical Research Council of Australia.

References

Awiszus, F., Wahl, B. and Meinecke, I. (1997) Influence of stimulus cross talk on results of the twitch-interpolation technique at the biceps brchii muscle. *Muscle Nerve*, 20: 1187–1190.

Baker, M., Bostock, H., Grafe, P. and Martius, P. (1987) Function and distribution of three types of rectifying channel in rat spinal rot myelinated exons. *J. Physiol. (Lond.)*, 383: 45–76.

Bergmans, J. (1970) *The Physiology of Single Human Nerve Fibres.* Vander, Louvain, Belgium.

Bostock, H., Burke, D. and Hales, J.P. (1994) Differences in behaviour of sensory and motor axons following release of ischaemia. *Brain*, 117: 225–234.

Bostock, H., Cikurel, K. and Burke, D. (1998) Threshold tracking techniques in the study of human peripheral nerve. *Muscle Nerve*, 21: 137–158.

Bostock, H. and Grafe, P. (1985) Activity-dependent excitability changes in normal and demyelinated rat spinal root axons. *J. Physiol. (Lond.)*, 365: 239–257.

Bostock, H. and Rothwell, J.C. (1997) Latent addition in motor and sensory fibres of human peripheral nerve. *J. Physiol. (Lond.)*, 498: 277–294.

Burke, D. and Gandevia, S.C. (1998) Influences of stimulus cross-talk on results of twitch-interpolation technique at the biceps brachii muscle. *Muscle Nerve*, 21: 970.

Burke, D., Hagbarth, K.-E., Löfstedt, L. and Wallin, B.G. (1976) The responses of human muscle spindle endings to vibration during isometric contraction. *J. Physiol. (Lond.)*, 261: 695–711.

Burke, D., Gandevia, S.C. and McKeon, B. (1983) The afferent volleys responsible for spinal proprioceptive reflexes in man. *J. Physiol. (Lond.)*, 339: 535–552.

Burke, D., Gandevia, S.C. and McKeon, B. (1984) Monosynaptic and oligosynaptic contributions to the human ankle jerk and H reflex. *J. Neurophysiol.*, 52: 435–448.

Burke, D., Gracies, J.M., Mazevet, D., Meunier, S. and Pierrot-Deseilligny, E. (1994) Non-monosynaptic transmission of the cortical command for voluntary movement in man. *J. Physiol. (Lond.)*, 480: 191–202.

Burke, D., Kiernan, M.C., Mogyoros, I. and Bostock, H. (1997) Susceptibility to conduction block: differences in the biophysical properties of cutaneous afferents and motor axons. In: J. Kimura and R. Kaji (Eds), *Physiology of ALS and Related Diseases*, Elsevier, Amsterdam, pp. 43–53.

Cavallari, P. and Katz, R. (1989) Pattern of projections of group I afferents from forearm muscles to motoneurones supplying biceps and triceps muscles in man. *Exp. Brain Res.*, 78: 465–478.

Collins, W.F., Davis, B.M. and Mendell, L.M. (1986) Amplitude modulation of EPSPs in motoneurones in response to a frequency-modulated train in single Ia afferent fibers. *J. Neurosci.* 6: 1463–1468.

Coppin , C.M.L., Jack, J.J.B. and MacLennan, C.R. (1970) A method for the selective electrical activation of tendon organ afferent fibres from the cat soleus muscle. *J. Physiol. (Lond.)*, 210:18P–20P.

Cordo, P., Gandevia, S.C., Hales, J.P., Burke, D. and Laird, G. (1993) Force and displacement-controlled tendon vibration in humans. *Electroenceph. clin Neurophysiol.*, 89: 45–53.

Eccles, J.C., Eccles, R.M. and Lundberg, A. (1957) Synaptic actions on motoneurones caused by impulses in Golgi tendon organ afferents. *J. Physiol. (Lond.)*, 138: 227–252.

Fetz, E.E., Jankowska, E., Johannisson, T. and Lipski, J. (1979) Autogenetic inhibition of motoneurones by impulses in group Ia muscle spindle afferents. *J. Physiol. (Lond.)*, 293: 173–195.

Gandevia, S.C., Allen, G.M. and McKenzie, D.K. (1995) Central fatigue: critical issues, quantification and practical implications. In S.C. Gandevia, R.M. Enoka, A.J. McComas, D.G. Stuart and C.K. Thomas (Eds) *Fatigue: Neural and Muscular Mechanisms*, Plenum, New York, pp. 281–294.

Gasser, H.S. (1935) Changes in nerve-potentials produced by rapidly repeated stimuli and their relation to the responsiveness of nerve to stimulation. *Am. J. Physiol.*, 111: 35–50.

Gordon, T.R., Kocsis, J.D. and Waxman, S.G. (1990) Electrogenic pump activity in rat optic nerve. *Neuroscience*, 37: 829–837.

Gregory, J.E., Wise, A.K., Wood, S.A., Prochazka, A. and Proske, U. (1999) Muscle history, fusimotor activity and the human stretch reflex. *J. Physiol. (Lond.)*, 513: 927–934.

Hamnegard, C.H., Wragg, S., Kyroussis, D., Mills, G.H., Polkey, M.I., Moran, J., Road, J., Bake, B., Green, M. and Moxham, J. (1996) Diaphragm fatigue following maximal ventilation in man. *Eur. Resp. J.*, 9: 241–247.

Hayward, L.F., Nielsen, R.P., Heckman, C.J. and Hutton, R.S. (1986) Tendon vibration-induced inhibition of human and cat triceps surae group I reflexes: evidence of selective Ib afferent fiber activation. *Exp. Neurol.*, 94: 333–347.

Heckman,, C.J., Condon, S.M., Hutton, R.S. and Enoka, R.M. (1984) Can Ib axons be selectively activated by electrical stimuli in human subjects? *Exp. Neurol.*, 86: 576–582.

Hultborn, H., Meunier, S., Morin, C. and Pierrot-Deseilligny, E. (1987) Assessing changes in presynaptic inhibition of Ia fibres: a study in man and the cat. *J. Physiol. (Lond.)*, 389: 729–756.

Jankowska, E. and McCrea, D. (1983) Shared reflex pathways from Ib tendon organ afferents and Ia muscle spindle afferents in the cat. *J. Physiol. (Lond.)*, 338: 99–111.

Johnson, B.D., Babcock, M.A., Suman, O.E. and Dempsey, J.A. (1993) Exercise-induced diaphragmatic fatigue in healthy humans. *J. Physiol. (Lond.)*, 460: 385–405.

Jones, K.E. and Bawa, P. (1997) Computer stimulation of the responses of human motoneurons to composite 1a EPSPs: effects of background firing rate. *J. Neurophysiol.*, 77: 405–420.

Kiernan, M.C., Mogyoros, I. and Burke, D. (1996) Differences in the recovery of excitabiity in sensory and motor axons of human median nerve. *Brain*, 119: 1099–1105.

Kiernan, M.C., Mogyoros, I., Hales, J.P., Gracies, J.-M. and Burke, D. (1997) Excitability changes in human cutaneous afferents induced by prolonged repetitive axonal activity. *J. Physiol. (Lond.)*, 500: 255–264.

Koeber, H.R. and Mendell, L.M. (1991) Modulation of synaptic transmission at Ia-afferent connections on motoneurons during high-frequency afferent stimulation: dependence on motor task. *J. Neurophysiol.*, 65: 1313–1320.

Lin, C., Mogyoros, I., Dowla, S. and Burke, D. (1999) Differences in the properties of cutaneous afferents in median and sural nerves. *Electroenceph. clin Neurophysiol.*, in press.

Matthews, P.B.C. (1996) Relationship of firing intervals of human motor units to the trajectory of post-spike afterhyperpolarization and synaptic noise. *J. Physiol. (Lond.)*, 492: 597–628.

McKenzie, D.K., Allen, G.M., Butler, J.E. and Gandevia, S.C. (1997) Task failure with lack of diaphragm fatigue during inspiratory resistive loading in human subjects. *J. Appl Physiol.*, 82: 2011–2019.

Meunier, S., Penicaud, A., Pierrot-Deseilligny, E. and Rossi, A. (1990) Monosynaptic Ia excitation and recurrent inhibition from quadriceps to ankle flexors and extensors in man. *J. Physiol. (Lond.)*, 423: 661–675.

Meunier, S., Pierrot-Deseilligny, E. and Simonetta-Moreau, M. (1994) Pattern of heteronymous recurrent inhibition in the human lower limb. *Exp. Brain Res.*, 102: 149–159.

Miller, T.A., Kiernan, M.C., Mogyoros, I. and Burke, D. (1995) Activity-dependent changes in impulse conduction in normal human cutaneous axons. *Brain*, 118: 1217–1224.

Mogyoros, I., Kiernan, M.C. and Burke, D. (1996) Strength-duration properties of human peripheral nerve. *Brain*, 119: 439–447.

Mogyoros, I., Kiernan, M.C., Burke, D. and Bostock, H. (1997) Excitability changes in human sensory and motor axons during hyperventilation and ischaemia. *Brain*, 120:, 317–325.

Morita, K., David, G., Barrett, J.N. and Barrett, E.F. (1993) Posttetanic hyperpolarisation produced by electrogenic Na^+–K^+ pump in lizard axons impaled near their motor terminals. *J. Neurophysiol.*, 70: 1874–1884.

Olivier, E., Bawa, P. and Lemon, R.M. (1995) Excitability of human upper limb motoneurones during rhythmic discharge tested with transcranial magnetic stimulation. *J. Physiol. (Lond.)*, 485: 257–269.

Panizza, M., Nilsson, J., Roth, B.J., Rothwell, J. and Hallett, M. (1994) The time constants of motor and sensory peripheral nerve fibers measured with the method of latent addition. *Electroenceph. clin. Neurophysiol.*, 93: 147–154.

Pierrot-Deseilligny, E., Morin, C., Bergego, C. and Tankov, N. (1981) Pattern of goup I fibre projections from ankle flexor and extensor muscles in man. *Exp. Brain Res.*, 42: 337–350.

Pierrot-Deseilligny, E. (1996) Transmission of the cortical command for human voluntary movement through cervical propriospinal premotoneurons. *Prog. Neurobiol.*, 48: 489–517.

Proske, U., Morgan, D.L. and Gregory, J.E. (1993) Thixotropy in skeletal muscle and in muscle spindles: a review. *Prog. Neurobiol.*, 41: 705–721.

Rossi, A., Mazzocchio, R. and Parlanti, S. (1991) Cortical projection of putative group Ib afferent fibres from the human forearm. *Brain Res.*, 547: 62–68.

Schiepatti, M. and Nardone, A. (1997) Medium-latency stretch reflexes of foot and leg muscles analysed by cooling the lower limb in standing humans. *J. Physiol. (Lond.)*, 503: 691–698.

Taylor, J.L., Burke, D. and Heywood, J. (1992) Physiological evidence for a slow K^+ conductance in human cutaneous afferents. *J. Physiol. (Lond.)*, 453: 575–589.

Taylor, J.L., Butler, J.E. and Gandevia, S.C. (1999). Responses of human elbow flexors to peripheral and cortical stimulation during a sustained maximal voluntary contraction, *Exp. Brain Res.*, in press.

Uysal, H., Mogyoros, I. and Burke, D. (1999). Reproducibility of tendon jerk reflexes during a voluntary contraction, *Clin. Neurophysiol.*, 110: 1481–1487.

Vagg, R., Mogyoros, I., Kiernan, M.C. and Burke, D. (1998) Activity-dependent hyperpolarization of motor axons produced by natural activity. *J. Physiol. (Lond.)*, 507: 919–925.

M.D. Binder (Ed.)
Progress in Brain Research, Vol 123
© 1999 Elsevier Science BV. All rights reserved.

CHAPTER 40

Rhythmic cortical activity and its relation to the neurogenic components of normal and pathological tremors

B.A. Conway,[1] D.M. Halliday and J.R. Rosenberg*

[1]*Bioengineering Unit, University of Strathclyde, Glasgow, G4 0NW and Division of Neuroscience and Biomedical Systems, University of Glasgow, Glasgow G12 8QQ, Scotland UK*

Introduction

The work of Stiles and Randall (1967) and that of Elble and Randall (1976) established that the spectrum of a tremor signal consists of two components: an inertial load dependent component and a neurogenic component. The former is a property of the structure exhibiting the tremor, and shifts toward lower frequencies with increased inertial loading (Stiles and Randall, 1967). The neurogenic component is load independent and was first attributed to central descending processes in the frequency range 8–12 Hz (Elble and Koller, 1990). During a maintained postural task an additional 15–30 Hz neurogenic component of tremor was identified and associated with motor unit synchronisation (Halliday et al., 1995, 1999). Farmer et al. (1993) inferred, on the basis of indirect evidence, that the common drive to the synchronised motor units was of descending origin. Conway et al. (1995), using magnetoencephalographic (MEG) techniques, and Halliday et al. (1998), with conventional electroencephalographic (EEG) techniques, demonstrated a correlation between localised cortical activity in the 15–30 Hz frequency band and the neurogenic component of

tremor associated with motor unit synchronisation. These results imply that the localised rhythmic cortical activity in the 15–30 Hz frequency band, that occurs during maintained postural tasks, accounts for the 15–30 Hz component of neurogenic tremor, which in turn is a consequence of motor unit synchronisation. The analysis of the correlation between the 15–30 Hz rhythmic cortical oscillations and the neurogenic component of tremor is equivalent to an investigation of the descending drive that synchronises motor units during maintained postural tasks.

The application of spectral and coherence analyses (Halliday et al., 1995; Rosenberg et al., 1998) therefore provides a powerful procedure for characterising the central drive associated with rhythmic cortical activity and motor unit synchrony in normal and pathological tremors. The application of these analytical methods will be seen to reveal significant differences in the correlation between cortical drive and tremor in normal subjects with that observed in cases of essential tremor and Parkinsonian tremor. Preliminary reports of aspects of this work has appeared elsewhere (Halliday et al., 1997; Conway et al., 1998).

Methods

Experimental procedures – Electrophysiological recordings were obtained with ethical committee

*Corresponding author. Tel.: 0141–330–6589; Fax: 0141–330–4100; e-mail: gpaa07@udcf.gla.ac.uk

approval from five healthy adult subjects, six subjects with essential tremor, and one subject with Parkinson's Disease subsequent to a left pallidotomy. Cortical activity was recorded with either a single channel MEG system or conventional bipolar EEG electrodes. Surface EMGs were recorded from the extensor digitorum communis (EDC) muscle or the first dorsal interosseous muscle (1 DI). The postural task for each subject consisted of repeated periods of wrist extension/flexion or finger abduction. Coherence and spectral analyses were based on 120 s of data sampled at 1 ms intervals. The surface EMG was rectified prior to analysis.

Details of the experimental protocols are given in Conway et al. (1995) and Halliday et al. (1998).

Analytical methods – The recorded signals were assumed to be realisations of stationary zero-mean time series. Two time series parameters, the auto-spectrum and the coherence, formed the basis for the analysis. The auto-spectrum may be interpreted as the distribution of power in the signal as a function of frequency. The spectra of the recorded signals were estimated by the method of disjoint sections, which is equivalent to applying a data window to the entire record (Bloomfield, 1976; Halliday et al., 1995), and has the advantage of resulting in simple expressions for confidence intervals for spectral estimates. The complete record, denoted by R, is divided into L non-overlapping sections each of length T so that R = LT. The periodogram of each section is formed from the estimated finite Fourier transform of the section (Rosenberg et al., 1989; Halliday et al., 1995). The estimated auto-spectrum is then taken as the periodogram averaged over all of the sections. The logarithm of this estimate of the spectrum will have variance independent of frequency, taking the simple form $(\log_{10}(e))^2 L^{-1}$ where L is the number of disjoint sections. A 95% confidence interval based on this expression is shown as a vertical line in the upper left hand corner of each graph of the logarithm of the estimated auto-spectrum. Details of setting the confidence interval, with many examples are given in Halliday et al. (1995). The coherence between two time series $x(t)$ and $y(t)$ is a bounded linear measure of association between these processes, and necessarily takes on values between zero and one, where zero occurs when the two processes are independent. The coherence is analogous to the correlation coefficient squared for ordinary random variables and gives a measure of correlation between these signals at each frequency (Rosenberg et al., 1998). Details of the procedure for estimating coherences may be found, with many examples, in Halliday et al. (1995) and Rosenberg et al. (1989). If the component spectra of the coherence are formed by the method of disjoint sections, then under the assumption that the two processes are independent an approximate upper level of the 100%α confidence limit for the coherence is given as $1 - (1 - \alpha)^{1/(1-L)}$, where L, the number of disjoint sections, is the same for each record. In each coherence graph the upper level of the 95% confidence interval under the assumption that the two processes are independent is represented by a dashed horizontal line. Values of the coherence at each frequency exceeding this level are assumed to be significant.

Results

The relation between rhythmic cortical activity and the neurogenic component of tremor in normal subjects

Figure 1 illustrates, in a healthy adult subject, the spectral and coherence analysis of the relation between the EEG recorded over the sensorimotor cortex of the dominant hemisphere and the rectified surface EMG from the contralatal EDC muscle during a maintained postural contraction. Although the EEG spectrum has most of its power concentrated below 10 Hz, there is a distinct and significant peak centred about ~20 Hz (Fig.1, upper panel). The spectrum of the rectified EMG (Fig. 1, center panel) is dominated by two distinct peaks; one centred about 10 Hz and the other spanning the range 15–35 Hz. The latter represents the neurogenic component of tremor (Halliday et al., 1995, 1999) attributable to motor unit synchronisation. The coherence between the cortical

Healthy Subject - EEG Spectrum

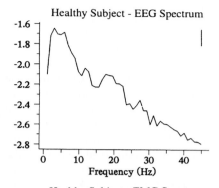

Healthy Subject - EMG Spectrum

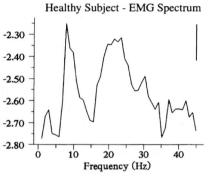

Healthy Subject
EEG-EMG Coherence

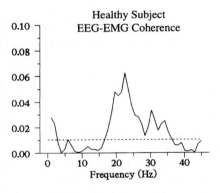

Fig. 1. A spectral and coherence analysis of the relation between cortical activity and rectified surface EMG in a normal subject. Upper panel: $\log_{10}$ auto-spectrum of the EEG recorded over the sensorimotor cortex. Middle panel: $\log_{10}$ auto-spectrum of the rectified surface EMG recorded from the EDC muscle on the side contralaleral to the EEG recording. Lower panel: Coherence between EEG and EMG. The vertical line in each of $\log_{10}$ auto-spectrum graphs represents an approximate 95% confidence interval for the estimated spectrum, and can used as a guide to significant features in the spectrum. The horizontal dashed line in the graph of the estimated coherence represents the upper level of an approximate 95% confidence interval for the estimate under the assumption that the two processes are independent. Spectra and coherence estimates are based on 120 s of data sampled at 1ms intervals.

activity and the rectified surface EMG is significant over the frequency band corresponding to the neurogenic component of the tremor, and therefore illustrates the common rhythmic drive to the motor pool. Although most of the power in the EEG is below 10 Hz (Fig. 1, upper panel), and the EMG also has a significant peak centered about this frequency (Fig. 1, middle panel), the coherence between these signals is not significant at these lower frequencies (Fig. 1, lower panel). Consequently during a maintained postural contraction the coherence analysis demonstrates rhythmic cortical activity in the 15–30 Hz directly related to motor unit synchronisation.

The relation between rhythmic cortical activity and the neurogenic component of tremor in subjects with essential tremor

Figure 2 illustrates, in a subject with essential tremor, the relation between the MEG recorded over the sensorimotor cortex of the dominant hemisphere and the rectified surface EMG from the contralateral 1 DI muscle during a maintained contraction.

The dominant spectral components of cortical activity in subjects with essential tremor (Fig. 2, upper panel) is very similar to that observed in normal subjects – most of the power is concentrated in the frequency band below 10 Hz, with a significant spectral contribution over the range 12–25 Hz. The spectrum of the rectified surface EMG in these subjects (Fig. 2, middle panel) shows a sharp peak at the characteristic frequencies associated with essential tremor (4–8 Hz, Elble and Koller, 1990). The coherence between the cortical activity and the rectified surface EMG in subjects with essential tremor is not significant at the characteristic 4–8 Hz essential tremor frequencies. The coherence in these subjects is similar to that observed in normal subjects (Fig. 1., lower panel). This observation is consistent with the inference that the correlation between rhythmic cortical activity recorded over the motor cortex associated with motor unit synchronisation is normal in subjects with essential tremor during maintained postural tasks (Halliday et al., 1997)

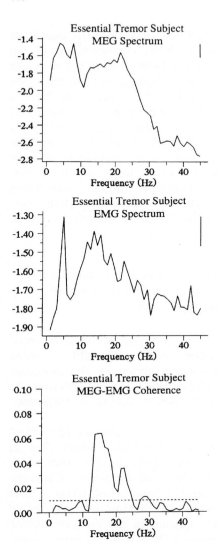

Fig. 2. A spectral and coherence analysis of the relation between cortical activity and rectified surface EMG in a subject with essential tremor. Upper panel: $\log_{10}$ auto-spectrum of the EEG recorded over the sensorimotor cortex. Middle panel: $\log_{10}$ auto-spectrum of the rectified surface EMG recorded from the 1 DI muscle on the side contralaleral to the EEG recording. Lower panel: Coherence between EEG and EMG. The vertical line in each of $\log_{10}$ auto-spectrum graphs represents an approximate 95% confidence interval for the estimated spectrum, and can used as a guide to significant features in the spectrum. The horizontal dashed line in the graph of the estimated coherence represents the upper level of an approximate 95% confidence interval for the estimate under the assumption that the two processes are independent. Spectra and coherence estimates are based on 120 s of data sampled at 1ms intervals.

The relation between rhythmic cortical activity and the neurogenic component of tremor in subjects with Parkinsonian tremor

The left-hand column in Fig. 3 illustrates the spectral and coherence analysis of cortical rhythmicity and the neurogenic component of tremor on the untreated side of a subject with Parkinson's disease. The spectrum of the EEG recorded over the motor cortex is dominated by a sharp peak spanning the range of frequencies associated with the Parkinsonian tremor (3–5 Hz, Elble and Koller, 1990; Volkman et al., 1996) (Fig. 3, left column, upper panel). In addition, there is a small, but significant peak in the range 15–30 Hz associated with motor unit synchronisation. The spectrum of the rectified surface EMG from the contralateral EDC muscle is strongly dominated by the Parkinsonian tremor and multiples of its frequencies (Fig. 3, left column, middle panel). The coherence between the EEG and the EMG is significant only at the tremor frequency and its first harmonic – there is no significant coherence at the frequencies corresponding to the neurogenic component of tremor – suggesting the absence of the normal 15–30 Hz common drive synchronising motor units during maintained postural tasks.

The right hand column in Fig. 3 illustrates the spectral and coherence analysis of cortical rhythmicity and the neurogenic component of tremor on the treated side. By contrast with the results on the untreated side, the spectrum of the EEG associated with the treated side is no longer dominated by the tremor rhythm, and exhibits a significant increase, compared with the untreated side, in the 15–30 Hz frequency band associated with motor unit synchronisation. In addition, the spectrum of the rectified surface EMG from the EDC muscle associated with the treated side is no longer dominated by the Parkinsonian tremor and higher harmonics, but shows a large and significant peak centered about the frequencies attributed to the neurogenic component of tremor observed in normal subjects (Fig. 3, right column, middle panel compared with Fig. 1 middle panel). The most striking feature on the treated side is the coherence between the cortical and electromyographic activity (Fig. 3, right column, lower panel). There is a

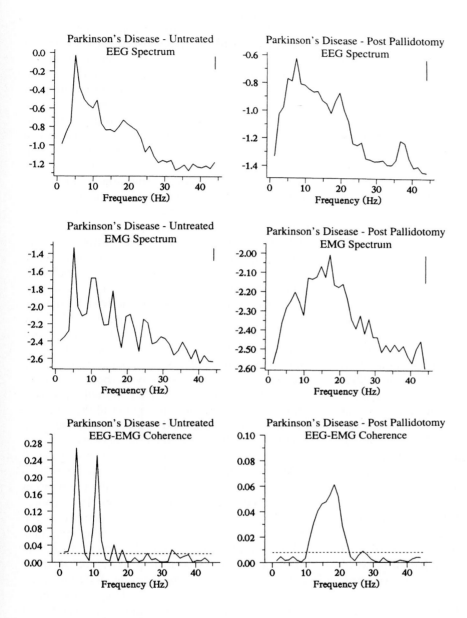

Fig. 3. A spectral and coherence analysis of the relation between cortical activity and rectified surface EMG in a subject with Parkinson's disease following a left pallidotomy. The left column shows the spectral and coherence analysis on the untreated side, whereas the right column shows the same analysis on the treated side. In each column the upper panel shows the $\log_{10}$ of the auto-spectrum of the EEG, the middle panel the $\log_{10}$ of the auto-spectrum of the EMG on the side contralateral to the EEG recording, and the lower panel the coherence between EEG and EMG. The vertical line in each of $\log_{10}$ auto-spectrum graphs represents an approximate 95% confidence interval for the estimated spectrum, and can used as a guide to significant features in the spectrum. The horizontal dashed line in the graphs of the estimated coherences represent the upper level of an approximate 95% confidence interval for the estimate under the assumption that the two processes are independent. Spectra and coherence estimates are based on 120 s of data sampled at 1ms intervals.

complete absence of correlation between motor cortex and rectified surface EMG of the contralateral EDC motor pool at the Parkinsonian tremor frequencies. This coherence is significant only over the frequency range 10–23 Hz, corresponding to the neurogenic component of tremor – suggesting the return of a normal common drive to the motor pool subsequent to pallidotomy. On the untreated side the patients motor performance remained poor and was accompanied by a large low frequency tremor. On the treated side, however, there was a considerable improvement in motor performance in which the patient could maintain postural contractions.

Discussion

The spectral and coherence analyses of the relation between rhythmic cortical activity and the EMG during a maintained postural contraction establishes a relation between a localised 15–30 Hz cortical rhythm and motor unit synchronisation (Fig. 1) during these tasks (Conway et al., 1995; Halliday et al., 1995, 1998, 1999). The characteristics of the spectrum of the cortical signal and that of the rectified surface EMG, together with the presence of a significant 15–30 Hz peak in the coherence between motor cortex and muscle activity can be taken as a reference against which aspects of pathological tremors may be assessed, and provide some insight into the neuronal mechanisms underlying these tremors during postural tasks. On the basis of a spectral and coherence analysis the two pathological tremors investigated in our study reveal quite different relations between rhythmic cortical activity and motor unit synchronisation.

In the case of essential tremor (Fig. 2) the spectrum of the cortical activity is very similar to that observed in normal subjects (Fig. 1), whereas the spectrum of the rectified surface EMG has a strong peak at the frequencies associated with essential tremor (Fig. 2), as well as significant power over a broad frequency range associated with motor unit synchronisation in healthy subjects. The presence of a normal pattern of coherence between cortical activity and EMG in subjects with essential tremor (Fig. 2, lower panel) is consistent with the hypothesis that the pyramidal system does not play a significant role in the transmission or generation of the essential tremor rhythm, and that the motor unit synchronisation, of motor cortical origin, may be normal in these subjects. The normal coherence observed in subjects with essential tremor during a maintained postural task further suggests that an independent oscillatory drive at the tremor frequencies, of non-pyramidal origin, becomes superimposed upon the motor output during attempted movements.

The Parkinsonian patient who had undergone unilateral (left) palliodtomy for treatment of tremor and drug induced dyskinesia demonstrated a beneficial and clear functional improvement as a consequence of this procedure. The rationale behind this operative procedure is that a lesion of the globus pallidus normalises activity within the thalamacortical pathway by disrupting the low frequency rhythmic oscillations from the basal ganglia to the thalamus (e.g. see Obeso et al., 1997, and references therein). A comparison of the spectral and coherence analyses between motor cortex and EMG on the treated and untreated side provides strong evidence in support of the rationale for this procedure, and further illustrates the manner in which the relation between cortical activity and motor output becomes re-organised following pallidotomy. The analysis of the behaviour of the untreated side confirms the observation by Volkmann et al. (1996) of a significant coherence between cortical and muscle activity at the tremor frequency. The consequence of the unilateral pallidotomy is clearly revealed in the coherence between cortical activity and rectified surface EMG on the treated side. Subsequent to pallidotomy the normal cortical drive associated with motor unit synchronisation is re-established (Fig. 3, right column, lower panel). The reduction in tremor and dyskinesia may therefore, in part, be attributed to re-establishing an effective common cortical drive to the motor pool.

The structure of the EMG spectrum and the coherence between the cortical activity and EMG raises a number of issues concerned with the nature of the oscillatory generators associated with Parkinson's disease. The presence of harmonics of the basic Parkinsonian rhythm that appear in both the EMG spectrum and in the coherence may be the result of different mechanisms not distinguishable by the spectrum or coherence. The harmonics may represent oscillations from independent processes that occur at multiples of the basic Parkinsonian rhythm, that is, the 5 Hz and 10 Hz components of the spectrum and the coherence result from independent processes. This interpretation is consistent with the results of a recent study by Hurtado et al., (1999, see their Fig. 5). Alternatively, since the recorded signals represent the results of the interactions of a number of different processes, separate oscillators, at multiples of a common frequency, may be phased locked and give rise to harmonics in the spectra or coherences. In either case, the presence of independent or coupled oscillators cannot be distinguished by the ordinary power spectrum or coherence, but requires a higher-order analysis of the relation between the recorded signals (e.g. see Raghuveer, 1990; Brillinger, 1994; Halliday et al., 1995).

A combined auto-spectral and coherence analysis of the relation between cortical and electromyographic activity is seen to provide a new approach to understanding the role that rhythmic cortical activity may have in shaping motor output. In a clinical context this analysis has demonstrated a clear difference in the relation between rhythmic cortical activity and tremor in patients with essential and Parkinsonian tremor, and in the latter illustrated that a clinical procedure re-established a normal pattern of correlation between cortical activity and motor output. These results suggest that such analyses may prove to be of clinical value.

Acknowledgements

This work was supported in part by a grant from the Wellcome Trust (Grant 048128). We also thank Dr. A. Russell and Dr. A.I. Weir of the Wellcome Biomagnetism Unit, Department of Neurophysiology, The Southern General Hospital NHS Trust, Glasgow, Scotland for making available the essential tremor subjects, and Professor I. R. Whittle of the Department of Clinical Neuroscience, University of Edinburgh for making available the Parkinsons disease patient.

References

Bloomfield, P. (1976) *Fourier Analysis of Time Series: An Introduction*. John Wiley and Sons, New York.

Brillinger, D.R. (1994) Some basic aspects and uses of higher-order spectra. *Signal Process.*, 36: 239–249.

Conway, B.A., Halliday, D.M., Farmer, S.F., Shahani, U., Maas, P., Weir, A.I. and Rosenberg, J.R. (1995) Synchronization between motor cortex and spinal motoneuronal pool during the performance of a maintained postural task in man. *J. Physiol.*, 489: 917–924.

Conway, B.A., Halliday, D.M., Hooper, J., Whittle, I.R. and Rosenberg, J.R. (1998) Restoration of normal coupling between cortical activity and motor output following neurosurgery for Parkinson's disease. *Soc. Neurosci. Abs.* 24: 1717.

Elble, R.J. and Koller, W.C. (1990) *Tremor*. Johns Hopkins University Press, Maryland.

Elble, R.J. and Randall, J.E. (1976) Motor-unit activity responsible for 8–12 Hz component of human physiological finger tremor. *J. Neurophysiol.*, 39: 370–383.

Farmer, S.F., Bremner, F.D., Halliday, D.M., Rosenberg, J.R. and Stephens, J.A. (1993) The frequency content of common synaptic inputs to motoneurones studied during voluntary isometric contractions. *J. Physiol.*, 470: 127–155.

Halliday, D.M., Conway, B.A., Farmer, S.F. and Rosenberg, J.R. (1998) Using electroencephalography to study functional coupling between cortical activity and electromyograms during voluntary contractions in humans. *Neurosci. Lett.*, 241: 5–8.

Halliday,D.M., Conway, B.A., Farmer, S.F. and Rosenberg, J.R. (1999) Load independent contributions from motor unit synchronization to human physiological tremor. *J. Neurophysiol.*, 82: 664–675.

Halliday, D.M., Conway, B.A., Shahani, U., Russell, A., Farmer, S.F., Wier, A.I. and Rosenberg, J.R. (1997) Coherence estimates between cortical activity and motor output in subjects with essential tremor. *J. Physiol.*, 501: 38P.

Halliday, D.M., Rosenberg, J.R., Amjad, A.M., Breeze, P., Conway, B.A. and Farmer, S.F. (1995) A framework for the analysis of mixed time/series point process data – theory and application to the study of physiological tremor, single motor unit discharges and electromyograms. *Prog. Biophys. Molec. Biol.*, 64: 237–278.

Hurtado, J.M., Gray, C.M., Tamas, L.B. and Sigvardt, K.A. (1999) Dynamics of tremor-related oscillations in the human globus pallidus: a single case study. *Proc. Nat. Acad. Sci. USA*, 96: 1674–1679.

Obeso, J.A., Guridi, J. and DeLong, M. (1997) Surgery for Parkinson's disease. *J. Neurol. Neurosurg. Psychiatry*, 62: 2–8.

Raghuveer, M.R. (1990) Time-domain approaches to quadratic phase coupling estimation. *IEEE Trans. Auto. Cont.*, 35: 48–56.

Rosenberg, J.R., Amjad, A.M., Breeze, P., Brillinger, D.R and Halliday, D.M. (1989) The Fourier approach to the identification of functional coupling between neuronal spike trains. *Prog. Biophys. Molec. Biol.*, 53: 1–31.

Rosenberg, J.R., Halliday, D.M., Breeze, P. and Conway, B.A. (1998) Identification of patterns of neuronal connectivity – partial spectra, partial coherence and neuronal interactions. *J.*

Neurosci. Methods, 83: 57–72.

Stiles, R.N. and Randall, J.E. (1967) Mechanical factors in human tremor frequency. *J. Appl. Physiol.*, 23(3): 324–330.

Volkmann, J., Joliot, M., Mogilner, A., Ionnides, A.A., Lado, F., Fazzini, E., Ribary, V. and Llinás, R. (1996) Central motor loop oscilations in Parkinsonian resting tremor revealed by magnetoencephalography. *Neurology*, 46: 1359–1370.

M.D. Binder (Ed.)
Progress in Brain Research, Vol 123

CHAPTER 41

Stopping and turning during human walking

Richard B. Stein* and Kimitaka Hase[1]

Division of Neuroscience, University of Alberta, Edmonton AB, T6G 2S2, Canada

Introduction

Walking is one of the most common of human activities and many studies have examined a range of physiological and pathological features. However, most studies of walking have treated steady-state conditions. Fewer have considered the initiation and even fewer the termination of walking or other modifications such as turning. These latter topics form the subject of this chapter. One of the few studies comparing the initiation and termination of walking is the biomechanical study of Jian et al. (1993). Figure 1 combines two figures from that study. In part A subjects stood quietly with their feet on two force plates (FP2 and FP3) and started walking by lifting their right foot and placing it onto a third force plate (FP1). The solid points give the trajectory of the body's center of mass as the subject begins to move forward and the weight is shifted first to the left and them to the right. The open circles show the center of pressure and the arrows show the direction of the forces exerted by the center of pressure on the center of mass to move it laterally and forward. The meaning of the other notations is given in the original paper. Here, we merely want to compare the trajectory during initiation of walking with that during its termination (Fig. 1B). At first glance the data appear almost identical, except that the directions are reversed (see the arrows indicating walking

direction at the top of each part). The subject was walking from right to left and took his last step on FP1 before coming to rest, as requested, with the weight balanced between FP2 and FP3. Jian et al. (1993) concluded that, biomechanically, termination was approximately the mirror image of the initiation of walking. They also calculated the velocity profiles of the center of mass and found that subjects reached or ended their steady-state walking speed within little more than one step. Again, the profiles for starting and stopping walking seemed to be mirror images.

Two qualifications must be raised to these simple conclusions. First, the muscles in the front and the back of the body are quite different in size, orientation and composition, so the physiological mechanisms underlying the biomechanical events must be asymmetric. Second, Jaeger and Vanitchatchavan (1992) found that if subjects were asked to stop quickly, rather than in a controlled fashion on force plates, they almost always ended with one foot in front of the other, rather than with the feet side by side. We obtained similar results and decided to study the mechanisms further by measuring electromyograms (EMG) from several muscles, as well as joint angles and forces under the feet. We also wished to see how these mechanisms varied during the course of the step cycle. For this purpose, we applied a stimulus (one or two pulses) to the superficial peroneal nerve. This nerve innervates the dorsum (top) of the foot, so the sensation is as if an object hit the top of the foot. This was quite a natural cue for the subjects to use to stop or turn, as required in different

---

*Corresponding author. Tel.: (780) 492-1618; Fax: (780) 492-1617; e-mail: richard.stein@Ualberta.ca
[1] Current address: Department of Rehabilitation Medicine, Keio University, Tokyo, Japan.

446

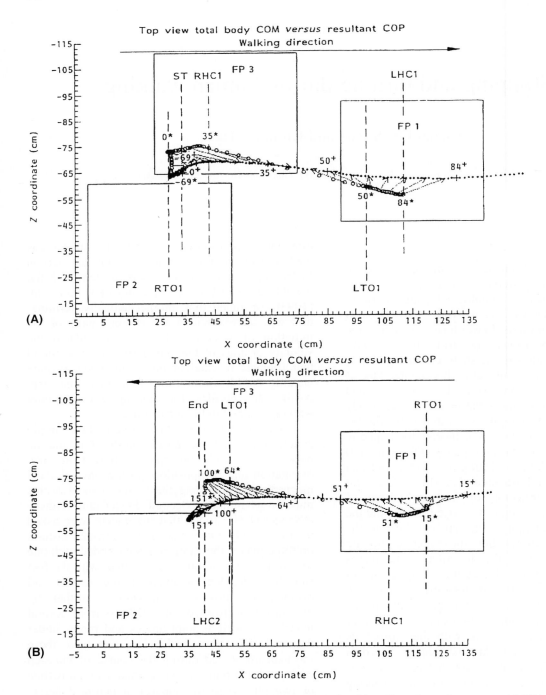

Fig. 1. Comparison of (A) initiating and (B) terminating a period of walking. Three force plates were used (FP1, FP2 and FP3) and the trajectories of the center of mass (COM, ●) and center of pressure (COP, ○) were computed. The direction of walking is indicated by arrows at the top and was reversed for initiating and terminating the gait. The arrows connecting the points for the COM and COP indicate the direction of the net forces moving the body. Modified from Jian et al. (1993). Further explanation in the text and in the original article.

experiments. The stimulation was not intense enough to produce reflex responses (Zehr et al., 1997), but was easily and quickly perceived by the subjects. Further details of the methods can be found in Hase and Stein (1998).

Stopping

Figure 2A shows the forces measured under the right heel using a force-sensitive resistor (Zehr et al., 1995) in a typical experiment. The solid lines in the figure give averages of the responses to cues that occurred in different parts of the step cycle. The cycle was divided into 16 equal parts, starting with heel strike, and part 1 gives all those that occurred close to heel strike. In each successive part the cues occurred progressively later in the cycle, until in part 16 the cues occurred just prior to the next heel strike. The dotted lines show the corresponding values for control steps, when no cues were applied. In part 1, for example, the force profile is not changed initially, but a second heel strike is absent from the trace at the time when it would normally have occurred. In fact, the subject stopped with his left leg in front of the right and any weight that remained on the right foot was concentrated on the ball (Figure 2B), rather than the heel of that foot.

Later in the cycle (parts 7–12) the time of heel strike was actually earlier than it would have occurred without cues. Thus, although the cue was to stop walking, the step cycle was actually speeded up in the sense that the right foot was placed on the ground sooner than it would have been. The force came off of the heel and onto the ball of the foot much sooner. At the end of the traces force was again observed on the heel of the right foot, as the subject stopped with his right foot on the ground in front of the body.

Figure 3A shows data for a number of muscles (rectified and smoothed EMGs) from part 4 of the step cycle. At this time in the step cycle the right foot is on the ground and just beginning the push-off phase in which the body is propelled up and forward. Much of the torque required comes from the ankle extensors (Winter, 1991) and the dotted line in the soleus (SOL) EMG shows the normal increase in the ankle extensor activity during push-off. However, 150–200 ms after the cue is applied,

this increase in EMG activity is quickly reversed and the muscle turns off. In contrast, ankle (tibialis anterior, TA) and knee (biceps femoris, BF) flexors show a large burst of activity that can be several times the peak amplitude of the normal burst during walking (compare the solid lines with the dotted lines for control cycles). Increased activity is also seen in the hip (gluteus medius, GM) and spine (erector spinae, ES), again occurring after only 150–200 ms. We will refer to this pattern as *a flexor synergy* (see Fig. 4 below) in what becomes the trailing leg (the leg behind the center of mass) as walking is terminated.

Results for part 12 (swing phase) are shown for comparison in Figure 3B. Now there is a large and early burst in the ankle extensors (soleus, SOL) and the knee extensors (vastus lateralis, VL). Early activity is also seen in hip extensors (Gluteus medius, GM) and the spine (erector spinae, ES). Although there were variations when the cues were applied in different parts of the step cycle, two basic patterns could be observed in the legs that ended up in front (leading leg) or behind the body (trailing leg), when the walking stopped. The first, which we refer to as the *extensor synergy* (Fig. 4A), occurs in the leading leg and was described above in relation to Fig. 3B. The large burst in soleus muscle will bring the foot down flat on the ground and bring the shank of the leg back. This activity, combined with that in VL will straighten the knee. Similarly, the activity in GM will extend the hip and that in ES will straighten the back. All this activity is required to brake the forward movement of the body and keep the center of mass behind the leading leg. In contrast, Fig. 4B shows the flexor synergy that is found in the trailing leg. As described in relation to Fig. 3A this leg is normally propelling the body up and forward, but activity in the ankle extensor muscles such as soleus quickly ceases. Instead, a burst is seen in TA that will bring the body down with the foot flat on the ground. Activity in BF, GM and ES will act to bring the body backwards while extending the hip and spine. All these actions will counter the forward mementum of the body.

Which legs are trailing and leading depends on when in the step cycle the cues occur. Clearly, a decision must be made and parts 5–6 and parts

13–14 were transitional in that sometimes an extra step was taken and sometimes not. These correspond to the mid-stance portions of the step cycle for the right and left legs respectively. When the cues were applied in these parts, the stance phase was completed and the other leg began its stance phase. Fig. 4C shows that as the next mid-stance phase is reached, the kinetic energy of the body is converted to potential energy as the center of mass rises over the stance foot. If the conversion is complete before the highest point is reached no further step is needed. However, if there is a slight

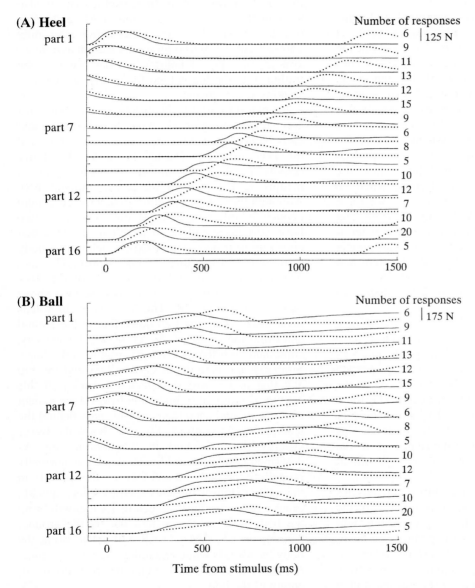

Fig. 2. Average forces (solid lines) under (A) the heel and (B) the ball of the right foot before and after a cue was given ($t = 0$). The step cycle, beginning at the time the right heel contacted the ground, was divided into 16 equal parts. The cues were given randomly and the numbers that were applied at each part of the step cycle are shown on the right. The dotted lines show the corresponding averages for control steps in which no cue were given. From Hase and Stain (1998).

excess of kinetic energy, the body will continue moving forward. An extra step will be needed, although it may be shortened. Clearly, the decisions are complex concerning which foot will end up in front and how much EMG is required in all the muscles of the body to stop effectively and safely. Yet, as we showed above, EMG activity is modified in 150–200 ms, which is the time generally seen for a simple reaction time to the presence or absence of cues.

Turning

We next examined the mechanisms underlying turning using the same cues. Subjects were now asked to turn quickly and continue back toward the starting point when the cue was felt. Does one stop

(A) Flexor Synergy in Trailing Leg

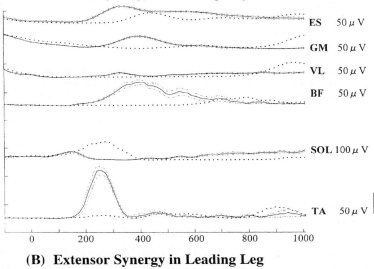

(B) Extensor Synergy in Leading Leg

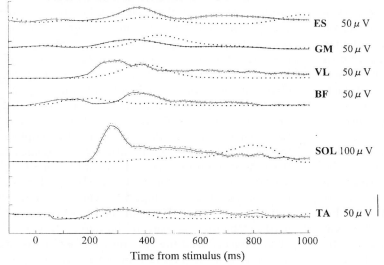

Fig. 3. Average rectified and filtered EMGs in the right leg when the cues were applied at (A) part 4 or (B) part 12 of the step cycle. Again, average values after a cue (solid lines) are compared to control steps (dotted lines). Standard errors (dashed lines) are also shown for the averages. Modified from Hase and Stein (1998).

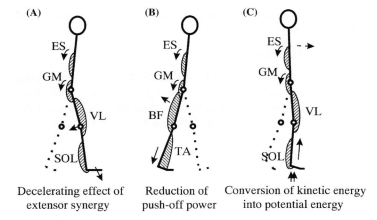

(A) Decelerating effect of extensor synergy

(B) Reduction of push-off power

(C) Conversion of kinetic energy into potential energy

Fig. 4. Schematic diagram of decelerating mechanisms during rapid stopping. (A) the activation of extensor muscles for the knee and ankle bring the foot flat on the ground and straighten the knee. Muscles at the hip and spine prevent the trunk from bending forward. (B) activation of ankle flexors and inhibition of ankle extensors will flex the ankle. Together with the activity of muscles at the knee, hip and spine, the body lowers and remains behind the forward leg. (C) As the center of mass rises during mid-stance, kinetic energy is converted into potential energy. Note that the leg from the opposite side of the body is shown in (B), compared to (A) and (C). SOL = soleus, TA = tibialis anterior, VL = vastus lateralis, BF = biceps femoris, GM = gluteus medius, ES = erector spinae. From Hase and Stain (1998).

and then turn or do the two actions meld into a smooth sequence? Are there distinct mechanisms for turning, depending on when the cue occurred in the step cycle? These questions motivated our study. Figure 5A shows the sequence observed when the cue was applied at about the time the left heel contacted the ground. The average data when the cues were present (solid lines) are again compared to control steps (dotted lines). Complex force changes are observed, not only at the heels of the two feet, but also at the lateral (near the fifth metatarsal) and the medial (near the first met-atarsal) surfaces of the ball of the foot. Above are diagrams of the two feet at different times during a 1.5 s period after the cues were applied. After left heel contact the right foot is raised off the ground (indicated by a dashed symbol) and lands on the ball of the foot. This is indicated as strong forces on the right medial and lateral traces, but not on the right heel traces between 400 and 500 ms. This subject made the full turn by spinning on the right foot until eventually the left foot was placed on the ground going back toward the starting point. At the end of the trace the pressure came off the ball of the right foot and it began a normal swing phase. We refer to this sequence as a *spin turn*, since the

subject completed the whole turn by spinning on the ball of the right foot about a single axis (indicated by a horizontal dotted line).

When the cue occurred at the time of the right heel strike (Figure 5B) and the subject was asked to turn to the right, a different pattern emerged. Some turning occurred on the right foot, but the left foot was placed in front at an angle. Further turning occurred while the right foot was placed at an angle to the new line of movement, but it was not until the left foot was again placed on the ground that the direction was fully back toward the original position. We refer to this as a *step turn*, since more than one step, involving more than one axis (horizontal dotted lines), was required to complete the turn. The step turn can also be distinguished from the spin turn in that it does not have the long period of pressure maintained on the ball of the foot (see top two traces in Fig. 5A) while the subject completes the spin. Three of ten subjects studied used a step turn in all parts of the step cycle, but the other subjects used the spin turn in some parts of the cycle and the step turn in others, as shown in Figure 5. Why some normal subjects chose one strategy and others chose another strategy is unknown.

One final point is illustrated in Fig. 6. This shows the forces on the ball of the foot on a longer time scale for two subjects. Cues were applied in all parts of the cycle and a diagonal line is drawn that goes roughly through the peaks of the force records. This same diagonal line has been redrawn

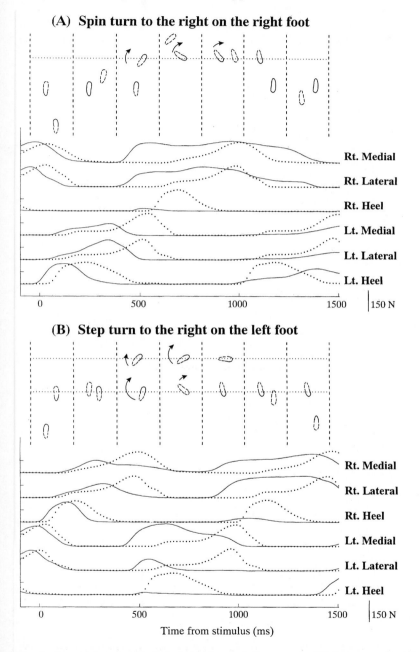

(A) Spin turn to the right on the right foot

Rt. Medial
Rt. Lateral
Rt. Heel
Lt. Medial
Lt. Lateral
Lt. Heel

0   500   1000   1500 |150 N

(B) Step turn to the right on the left foot

Rt. Medial
Rt. Lateral
Rt. Heel
Lt. Medial
Lt. Lateral
Lt. Heel

0   500   1000   1500 |150 N

Time from stimulus (ms)

Fig. 5. Average forces under both feet before and after a cue in (A) late stance (part 8) and (B) late swing (part 16) phases. Typical patterns of foot placements are shown above, together with horizontal dotted lines indicating the axes of rotation for pivoting during the turns. The toe and the heel of each foot are shown as solid lines when on the ground and as dashed lines when in the air.

after shifting it along the time axis by the duration of 1, 2 and 3 step cycles. Following the cue at $t = 0$, a spin turn or a step turn was completed, depending on when the cue occurred in the step cycle. Yet, after 3 step cycles (2–3 s) the diagonal line in Fig. 6A still passes through the force peaks in nearly all parts of the cycle. This suggests that all the mechanisms needed to turn the body were super-imposed on a basic walking rhythm that continued to run.

The same analysis for a second subject is shown in Fig. 6B. Now the diagonal line after several steps

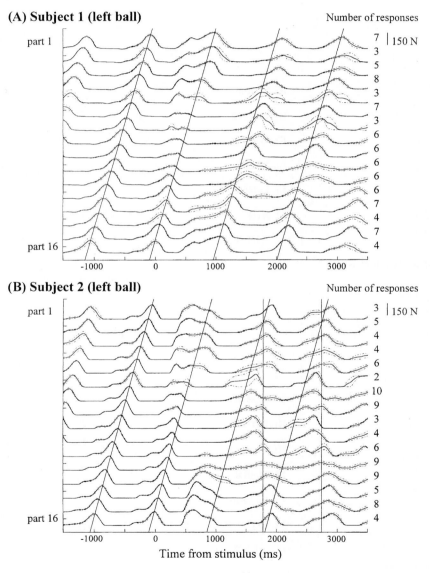

(A) Subject 1 (left ball)

Number of responses

part 1

7 | 150 N
3
5
8
3
7
3
6
6
6
6
6
7
4
7

part 16

4

-1000   0   1000   2000   3000

(B) Subject 2 (left ball)

Number of responses

part 1

3 | 150 N
5
4
4
6
2
10
9
3
4
6
9
9
5
8

part 16

4

-1000   0   1000   2000   3000

Time from stimulus (ms)

Fig. 6. Average forces (with standard errors, dashed lines) under the ball of the left foot for two subjects (A) and (B) who used both spin and step turns, depending on when the cue was applied in different parts of the step cycle. Diagonal lines indicate the timing of the peak force predicted from the average cycle time of control steps (no resetting). The vertical lines in (B) would result if the walking rhythm was reset by the stimulus. Further details in the text.

does not pass through the force peaks. It occurs during the stance phase in some parts and the swing phase in others. The vertical line does somewhat better in that it always passes through the part of the stance phase when force is being exerted on the ball of the foot. This suggests that the basic walking rhythm has been reset during the turn. Peaks occur close to a fixed time with respect to the cues, not to the part of the cycle when they occurred prior to the cues. Both subjects in Fig. 6 used a mixture of spin turns and step turns. The same difference, between those who reset or did not reset the rhythm, could be seen in subjects who only used step turns. Again, we do not know why some normal subjects chose one strategy and others chose a different strategy.

Conclusion

The mechanisms underlying stopping and turning in human walking are complex. The subjects initiate changes in a large number of muscles within 150–200 ms of receiving a cue and make the complex, strategic decisions necessary within what is usually considered to be the time required for a simple reaction time. When the subjects are asked to turn rather than stop, they again quickly make strategic decisions about what type of turn to use (step or spin turn) and initiate EMG activity so that the turn is carried out smoothly and efficiently. Different subjects make different choices about whether to use a spin turn or not. They may also reset the basic walking rhythm or not, but the strategies chosen are carried out fluently. It remains to be seen how these mechanisms are affected by disease processes that lead to subjects falling frequently, when they try to react quickly to environmental cues.

Acknowledgements

The original research described in this paper was supported by the Medical Research Council of Canada.

References

Hase, K. and Stein, R.B. (1998) Analysis of rapid stopping during human walking. *J. Neurophysiol.*, 80: 255–261.

Jaeger, R.J. and Vanitchatchavan, P. (1992) Ground reaction forces during termination of human gait. *J. Biomech.*, 25: 1233–1236.

Jian, Y., Winter, D.A. Ishac, M.G. and Gilchrist, L. (1993) Trajectory of the body COG and COP during initiation and termination of gait. *Gait Post.*, 1: 9–22.

Winter, D.A. (1991) *The Biomechanics and Motor Control of Human Gait: Normal, Elderly and Pathological*, 2nd edn. University of Waterloo Press, Waterloo, Canada.

Zehr, E.P., Komiyama, T. and Stein, R.B. (1997) Cutaneous reflexes during human gait: electromyographic and kinematic responses to electrical stimulation. *J. Neurophysiol.*, 77: 3311–3325.

Zehr, E.P., Stein, R.B., Komiyama, T. and Kenwell, Z. (1995) Linearization of force sensing resistors (FSRs) for force measurement during gait. *IEEE Eng. Med. Biol. Soc.*, 16: 1571–1572.

M.D. Binder (Ed.)
Progress in Brain Research, Vol 123
© 1999 Elsevier Science BV. All rights reserved.

CHAPTER 42

Disturbances of voluntary movement coordination in stroke: problems of planning or execution?

Randall Beer, Jules Dewald and Zev Rymer*

Sensory Motor Performance Program, Rehabilitation Institute of Chicago, Northwestern University Medical School, Chicago, IL 60611, USA

Introduction

Thrombotic or embolic stroke in the middle cerebral artery territory of the brain in man results in a complex set of clinical signs on the contralateral side of the body, including spasticity (defined primarily as an increase in muscle tone), weakness for voluntary movement, and impaired motor coordination (Twitchell, 1951; Wing et al., 1990; Roby-Brami et al., 1997). These three factors are not independent in their etiology, because for example, both spasticity and weakness may contribute to impaired movement coordination. However, we now believe that incoordination is mediated primarily by a loss of appropriate control signals to limb muscles, and it is often expressed even when weakness and spasticity are not severe. In the present discussion, we will focus largely on this third factor, which is impaired motor coordination. With the exception of Levin (1996), there has been virtually no description of limb kinematics in the impaired upper extremity of the hemiparetic subject

There are a large number of neural mechanisms that could potentially contribute to the impairment in motor coordination in human stroke syndromes. For example, based on controlled lesion studies in non-human primates there is increasing informa-

tion about the functional roles and connectivity of many of the cortical areas that are presumably affected by stroke lesions in man. Although the anatomical and functional features are not identical, the broad flow of information from visual areas through parietal lobes to prefrontal areas and to the motor cortex and supplementary motor areas appears to be closely comparable in human and many non-human primates. As a result of these similarities, we are now in a position to assess how several potentially important neural systems and pathways could contribute to the impairment in motor coordination.

We will briefly consider four mechanisms for the incoordination:

1 Spastic muscular restraint

Here we mean that an antagonist muscle, which should normally be silent or at best minimally active, is inappropriately excited during stretch because of the presence of an hyper-excitable stretch reflex arc.

2 Abnormal coupling between muscles acting at different joints (muscle synergies)

These stereotypic coupling patterns or muscle 'synergies' have been recognized for many years, and have been separated precisely by Brunnstom (Brunnstrom, 1970) into clear flexor and extensor

*Corresponding author. Tel.: (312) 908–3919; Fax: (312) 908–2208; e-mail: w-rymer@nwu.edu

patterns. In the context of impaired coordination, these abnormal muscle synergies restrict choices for independent muscle activity (and therefore independent joint control), thereby imposing significant constraints on voluntary motion. These synergies have been characterized largely under static or postural conditions (e.g. Dewald et al., 1995) and it remains to be determined whether they cause similar restrictions on muscle activation during voluntary movement.

3 Disruption of spatial coordinate frameworks

While middle cerebral artery lesions do not routinely damage the posterior parietal lobe, we know that there is extensive convergence of connecting fibers from parietal and then pre- motor and motor areas onto motor cortex and the supplementary motor area. Many of these connecting fibers would (presumably) be involved in transforming desired spatial movement commands into specific patterns of muscle activity, and these fibers traverse regions which are frequently at risk in thrombotic or hemorrhagic stroke. It follows that lesions of white matter or of connecting fibers could produce systematic distortions in the spatial profiles of voluntary movement, especially if the reference coordinate framework was lost or degraded. Under these conditions, we might expect to see systematic distortions of limb movement trajectory orientation, accompanying a distorted perception of the workspace.

4 Degradation of internal models of limb performance

Because of damage to connecting fibers and to cortical neurons, stroke patients may (at least hypothetically) lose the ability to synthesize an accurate picture of limb behavior in the course of rapid motion. This degradation may result in impaired movement control especially during ballistic motion, when limb segment inertia and inter segmental coupling torques become especially important. We refer to such an outcome as a loss of the capacity to develop an accurate internal model of the limb, which could impact the subject's ability to predict limb behavior for a given set of

neural commands and initial conditions (see Flanagan and Wing, 1997).

To address these possibilities, we have examined planar movements of the impaired and contralateral limbs of our six hemiparetic subjects, to see whether we could distinguish these four possibilities.

Experimental methods

Three normal adults and six patients with unilateral hemispheric lesions resulting primarily from stroke participated in this study. Patients with significant sensory, speech and cognitive disturbances were excluded.

Subjects were seated in front of a table, with the trunk stabilized, and with the wrist and finger joints immobilized by a fiberglass cast. Support of the limb was provided by a light platform, which functioned as an air bearing, allowing the forearm to slide virtually without resistance across the table top. An OPTOTRAK/3010 motion analysis system was used to track the position of infrared-emitting diodes located on the upper limb. EMGs were recorded from as many as 13 shoulder and elbow muscles using surface electrodes. We compared voluntary movements in the horizontal plane using a supported arm protocol in which subjects alternately moved impaired or the contralateral or unimpaired limb (for normal controls) over the table-top. The whole arm was held as close to horizontal as possible, although shoulder abduction and flexion movement constraints often limited the extent to which the upper arm could approach the horizontal.

Subjects completed the protocol with the right and left limbs in separate sessions. For each trial, the initial direction of movement was determined as the direction of the vector between the starting point and the position on the hand path after 1/4 of the movement was completed. An inverse dynamics analysis was then used to calculate joint torques. The spatial tuning of the initial joint torques was characterized by estimating torque transition angles (defined as those target directions for which the sign of the initial joint torque was as equally likely to be flexion as extension).

Results

Normal controls: comparison between dominant and non-dominant limbs

For the three control subjects, statistically significant differences in the initial direction of movement were found between dominant and non-dominant limbs. These differences were confined to targets requiring either shoulder flexion and elbow extension (i.e. reaching movements) or shoulder extension and elbow flexion (i.e. retraction movements). These differences in initial trajectory were also accompanied by systematic deviations in the path of hand motion, by greater trial to trial variability in the hand trajectory, and by greater errors in target acquisition. These differences are important, because our protocol compares the behavior of the impaired limb with that of the contralateral limb.

Figure 1(a) shows the characteristic hand trajectories in the dominant limb of normal control subjects. This figure illustrates that even normal limbs display systematic trajectory deviations from straight-line behavior in the course of the movement, and these deviations are most evident in two regions of the work space. For example, the paths

with the least initial curvature, the smallest amount of overshoot in position, and the smallest variance about the mean trajectory were in the 45° and the 225° directions (which are in the first and third quadrants of the workspace respectively). (The zero angle corresponds to the right axis 0° plane, and the angular directions are labeled using a counter-clockwise rotation.) In each of these cases, the movement is generated primarily by motion at the elbow and there is relatively limited movement at the shoulder. As a consequence, there is a reduced need for precise coordination of elbow and shoulder torques and kinematics in these directions. These deviations from linear trajectory were evident in the dominant limb of our normal control subjects, but they were even more prominent in the contralateral (non-dominant limb) of our normal controls.

Hemiparetic subjects: comparison between impaired and contralateral limbs

In the hemiparetic population, we found that there were systematic errors in movement trajectories in the paretic upper limb in all six of our subjects. Movements performed with the paretic limb exhibited errors in the initial direction of movement, and

Hand Trajectories in Normal and Paretic Limbs

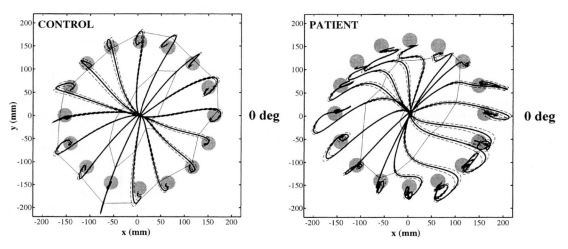

Fig. 1. Mean ± 1 SEM (standard error of the mean) hand paths for all target directions for the dominant (right) limb of a control subject (left panel) and the paretic (right, dominant) limb of a patient TW (right panel). Targets are indicated (to scale) by the shaded circles. Also shown are contour lines that indicate the mean hand position at 100 and 200 ms after movement onset.

these errors also varied systematically with target location, and were most prominent for reaching and retraction movements (at 135° and 225°). In joint coordinates, these 'errors' were associated with an excessive rotation of the elbow with respect to the shoulder.

These altered spatial patterns are shown in the target directed hand movements of the stroke subject depicted in Fig. 1(b). Here, the errors are now very much larger in magnitude than occurred in our control population (for either dominant or non dominant limb). There are again systematic deviations from the target in the initial direction of motion, in the straightness of the movement trajectory, in the pattern of velocity change with time and distance, and finally in the trajectory approaching capture of the target.

Kinetic analysis

An analysis of movement kinetics revealed two primary disturbances in the spatio-temporal organization of joint torques. First, in comparison to the contralateral limb, the elbow torque transition angles were increased in the prevailing direction of elbow rotation, indicating a failure to appropriately compensate for the dynamics of the upper limb. Second, there was a directionally dependent reversal in the normal proximal to distal sequence of torque onsets.

Forward dynamics simulations were conducted to evaluate the hypothesis that the misdirections had their basis in a failure to fully compensate for segmental interaction torques. These simulations predicted the observed shifts in elbow torque transition angles but not the reversal of torque onsets. It appears that the abnormal movement patterns are a result of systematic disruptions in the central control signal to limb muscles, and are not attributable simply to abnormal synergies, to spasticity or to muscle weakness.

Role of abnormal muscle synergies:

A qualitative examination of EMG spatial tuning indicated that the kinematic and kinetic abnormalities described above could not be directly attributed to abnormal muscle synergies, in that there was no evidence of a stereotypic relation between EMG magnitudes in muscles that were activated at the same time. While many subjects did show stereotypic coupling of EMG activities during isometric contractions of upper extremity muscles (e.g. Dewald et al, 1995), these isometric contraction patterns did not relate in any straight-forward manner to the movement trajectory disturbances, and the movement errors were also not correlated with the occurrence of any clear disturbances in spatial tuning of muscle activity.

(Perhaps this lack of evidence for 'synergies' was linked to our subject selection criteria, in that subjects who were able to perform at least rudimentary goal directed movements may have been those with little or no evidence for synergic limitations.)

Disturbances of spatial coordinate framework:

There were also no consistent spatial features of the movement incoordination that could be attributed to disruption or distortion of a spatial coordinate framework for the voluntary movement. If spatial coordinate disturbances were responsible, we would expect to see systematic errors in EMG tuning direction which would extend over particular geographical areas of the work space, not necessarily confined to regions in which two joint movements predominate. This distortion was not a feature of the recorded trajectory errors.

Role of spastic restraint:

In most instances, it did not appear that the errors in trajectory were due to 'spastic restraint'. To ascribe trajectory problems of this type to spasticity, we would need to demonstrate the occurrence of inappropriate activation of an antagonist muscle at the point of the trajectory where the antagonist is being rapidly stretched, *after beginning in a passive state*. Both conditions are obligatory for this mechanism to be plausible. In our experience, this sequence was rarely evident and the trajectory errors cannot therefore be readily be attributed to this mechanism. While this notion of spastic restraint is probably not a useful way to characterize the disturbances of movements such as those depicted in figure 1, there are some instances where spasticity appears to play a significant role.

Figure 2 illustrates such an example, in which there are marked mid-course deviations of movement trajectory, which appear in movement directions where the key elbow flexors are subjected to substantial and rapid length changes. These trajectory errors were sometimes most severe during forward reaching movements, in which elbow muscles would be stretched, although this is not unique to this particular direction. In many such cases the elbow flexors such as the brachialis and biceps begin in a quiescent state, since limb motion is initiated by shoulder flexors and elbow extensors. The ensuing limb motion relies primarily on intersegmental coupling in which momentum is transferred from the proximal limb segment to the forearm and hand.

It appears that in some patients, they may have hyperexcitable motoneurons innervating muscle such as the brachioradialis, which is being stretched, yet which begins in an initially passive or quiescent state. The differences in BRD EMG activity in this series of movements is quite striking, as shown in Fig. 2, with unexpected EMG activity in the 45–135° angular directions (right panel). These conditions are ideal for generating inappropriate reflex activation, which may account for the mid-course trajectory errors. This set of conditions is relatively uncommon as pointed out earlier, and it does not appear likely that much of the movement disturbance can be ascribed to spastic restraint.

Role of internal models

The final option, which we favor, is that the cortical damage which occurs as part of the stroke or the brain injury impairs the brain's ability to assemble the appropriate spatial and temporal command sequence to muscles. Expressed somewhat differently, the brain may be unable to synthesize information derived from visual, vestibular and proprioceptive cues to generate an internal model of how the limb would behave under conditions of

ROLE OF FLEXOR SPASTICITY

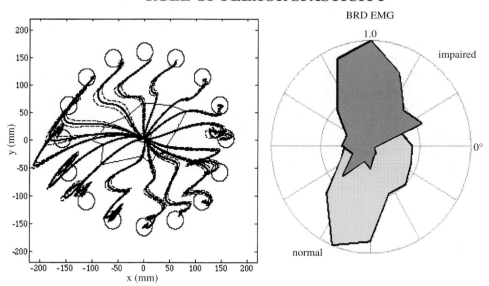

Fig. 2. The subject (RC, age 55) was right-handed with a lesion of the left hemisphere. Her Fugl-Meyer was 17/66 and Modified Ashworth score 5/5. Left Panel: Mean ± SEM for the right (dominant) arm of a hemiparetic subject, with significant motor weakness and spasticity (Ashworth 3/4 in elbow flexor muscles). Note the severe distortions of hand trajectory, with particular disorganization in the forward reaching movements. Right panel: This represents the integrated EMG response of the brachioradialis muscle, recorded over the full range of motion for each movement direction in both paretic and the contralateral limbs of the same subject.

voluntary movement. This problem could underlie many of the observed errors in initial direction in the path of voluntary motion, and it could also account for errors in target capture, which may arise because braking of the limb is inaccurate.

Discussion

When we examine the hand trajectory for goal-directed motion to a visible target in hemiparetic subjects, there are consistent differences between the hand paths taken by the impaired limb as compared with either the contralateral or normal control limbs. There are trajectory curvatures evident in the trajectory of normal limbs, and there may also be overshoot in position as the normal limb approaches the target, however, these features are greatly exaggerated in the paretic limb. Furthermore, the trajectory errors are most evident in hand paths that involve coordinated motion of the shoulder and elbow i.e. where intersegmental coordination of proximal and distal segments is most needed.

The mechanisms of these changes in hand path in hemispheric lesions are not yet understood, but they do not appear to be caused by weakness, by spasticity, or by abnormal muscle coupling (synergies) in most instances. It appears that the deficit may be of a more synthetic origin, in that the brain cannot assemble an appropriate internal model, or (in other words), a prediction of the impact of a given set of neural commands on limb motion.

Finally, it is helpful to reassess the movement disturbances in light of the potential lesion impact on the sequence of information flow as a signal travels from visual areas to the motor cortex. There do not appear to be grounds to label these movement errors as arising from connecting pathways from parietal cortex to prefrontal and motor areas, nor are they attributable to cortical outflow pathways, in that there is no marked weakness, spasticity or evidence of abnormal synergies. If follows that the problem is best sited at the movement planning stage, in which some form of prediction of limb motion is being assembled

Acknowledgements

This research was supported by NIH grants NS19331 (WZR) and 1T32HD07418 (RFB), NIDRR stroke center grant H133B30024 (JPD) and the Ralph and Marion C Falk Trust.

References

Brunnstrom, S. (1970) *Movement Therapy in Hemiplegia.* New York: Harper and Row.

Dewald, J.P.A., Pope, P.S., Given, J.D., Buchanan, T.S. and Rymer, W.Z. (1995) Abnormal muscle coactivation patterns during isometric torque generation at the elbow and shoulder in hemiparetic subjects. *Brain*, 118: 495–510.

Flanagan, J.R. and Wing, A.M. (1997) The role of internal models in motion planning and control: evidence from grip force adjustments during movements of hand-held loads. *J. Neurosci.*, 17: 1519–1528.

Levin, M.F. (1996) Interjoint coordination during pointing movements is disrupted in spastic hemiparesis. *Brain*, 119: 281–293.

Roby-Brami, A., Fuchs, S., Mokhtari, M. and Bussel, B. (1997) Reaching and grasping strategies in hemiparetic patients. *Mot. Cont.*, 1: 72–91.

Twitchell, T.E. (1951) The restoration of motor function following hemiplegia in man. *Brain*, 74: 443–480.

Wing, A.M., Lough, S., Turton, A., Fraser, C. and Jenner, J.R. (1990) Recovery of elbow function in voluntary positioning of the hand following hemiplegia due to stroke. *J. Neur. Neurosurg. Psychiatry*, 53: 126–134.

M.D. Binder (Ed.)
Progress in Brain Research, Vol 123

CHAPTER 43

Group II spindle afferent fibers in humans: their possible role in the reflex control of stance

Marco Schieppati[1,2,*] and Antonio Nardone[2]

[1]*Section of Human Physiology, Department of Experimental Medicine, University of Genoa, Genoa, Italy*
[2]*Posture and Movement Laboratory, Fondazione Salvatore Maugeri, Medical Center of Veruno (NO), Italy*

Introduction

Since the first description by Ruffini of primary and secondary spindle endings, it has been tacitly assumed that they subserve different reflex functions. Whilst everybody agrees on the role played in the monosynaptic response by group Ia afferents originating from the primary endings, some textbooks attribute to the small diameter myelinated group II afferent fibers, originating from the secondary endings, a role in producing flexor reflex effects. Accordingly, these fibers are classified as flexor reflex afferents together with high-threshold skin and joint afferents. Back in his preface to a 1972 Monograph of the Physiological Society, however, Matthews presented the notion that spindle group II fibers from secondary endings played a part in reflexly producing the hypertonia of the decerebrate preparation instead of merely contributing to a generalized flexor reflex (Matthews, 1972).

Group Ia and Group II afferent fibers in the cat

Group II afferent fibers that innervate muscle spindles discharge in response to muscle stretch as well as Ia fibers, and are subjected to similar

*Corresponding author. Tel.: +39 010 3538190; Fax: +39 010 3538194; e-mail: schieppa@csita.unige.it

gamma (Bessou et al., 1986) and descending effects (see Schomburg, 1990). Group II fibers can make both monosynaptic (Kirkwood and Sears, 1974; Stauffer et al., 1976; Munson et al., 1980) and oligosynaptic connections with homonymous and synergist hindlimb alpha motoneurons (Lundberg et al., 1987; Jankowska, 1992). A large number of spindle group II afferent fibers exists in the cat (Hunt, 1954); and these fibers are roughly the same in number as the Ia fibers in all muscles in which they have been counted (Barker, 1962). It is highly possible that the same is true also in humans, judging from the distribution of fibers of different diameter in the dorsal roots of human lumbar spinal cord (Dyck et al., 1993b).

Group II afferent fibers and the stretch reflex of human muscles

The hypothesis that we considered in a series of investigations was that the discharge along the group II fibers might play a major role in the medium-latency component of the human stretch reflex, and in particular in the reflex response of lower limb antigravity muscles, evoked by a perturbation of upright stance inducing body destabilization by upward rotation of a platform upon which the subject stands. A corollary of this hypothesis is that quiet, non-perturbed upright stance would also be contingent upon segmental control exerted by impulses originating, albeit non exclusively, in spindle secondaries.

Is the medium-latency response a segmental reflex or a long-loop?

This issue was addressed by several different experimental approaches. Our finding that the postural perturbation described above was able to induce both short- and medium latency responses (SLR and MLR respectively) to stretch of both the foot (flexor digitorum brevis muscle, FDB) and leg (soleus muscle, Sol) postural muscles was the condition for several of these approaches (Fig. 1). The SLR is the counterpart of the monosynaptic reflex, and its latency is in fact explained by the responsible impulses travelling along the fast spindle Ia fibers. The latency of the SLR is in fact slightly longer than that of the tendon (T) reflex, which in turn is slightly longer than the latency of the H reflex, both in the Sol and the FDB (Schieppati et al., 1995). There are hints that the MLRs in the leg muscles may also be a segmental

reflex, as has been shown for the proximal muscles of the upper limb (Thilmann et al., 1991), though the MLR in the case of the distal muscles of the upper limb has been shown to be mediated in humans by the Ia impulses travelling along a long-loop transcortical pathway (Matthews, 1989, 1992; see Schieppati, 1991). If this is the case, the MLR might be mediated either by a repetitive discharge of spindle Ia fibers, which would last for the entire duration of the stretch, or by a reverberating circuit at spinal level, or by a discharge along slowly conducting afferent fibers.

Changes in the delay of the medium-latency responses with subject height

On the basis of previous suggestions that group II afferent fibers might be responsible for the MLR (Dietz, 1992; Marque et al., 1996), we tested the last hypothesis (slowly conducting afferent fibers). If this were true, the latency of the MLR should

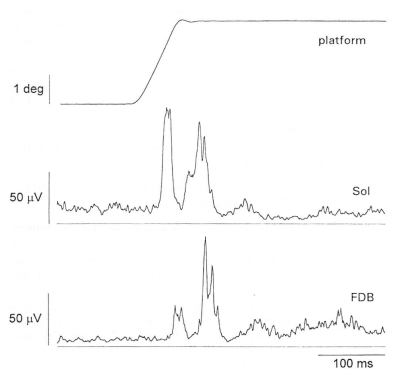

Fig. 1. Example of EMG recording obtained from soleus (Sol) and flexor digitorum brevis (FDB) muscle in a normal subject during a toe-up rotation of the supporting platform. In each trace, the early and late burst correspond respectively to the short- and medium-latency response. Full-wave rectified and filtered (time constant = 1 ms) EMG signals, averaged over thirty trials.

increase with subject's height more than the latency of the SLR. As a matter of fact, height produced a larger increase in latency of the MLR than SLR in all the subjects tested, both in the Sol and in the FDB (Nardone et al., 1996). The main finding is summarized in Fig. 2. The latency of the MLRs is plotted for a number of subjects of various heights against the latency of the corresponding SLR evoked in the same subjects by the same stimulus in both the Sol and FDB. It is notable that the slope of the best fit lines was steeper (significantly so) than the identity line for both muscles. On the contrary, the two lines best fitting the data points of both muscles are almost superimposable and not significantly different.

The fact that MLR increases in latency with height more than the SLR points to a longer time spent peripherally by travelling along slow fibers. A similar approach used in the case of upper limb muscles (Noth et al., 1991) showed an identical increase in latency of both SLR and MLR, with a

constant difference between the two responses, independent of height. The latter feature is what one would expect in the case of a long-loop pathway for the MLR, triggered peripherally by the same Ia input responsible for the SLR. Our finding points instead to a slower conduction velocity (CV) of the fibers responsible for the MLR, and also lessens the possibility of a prolonged receptor discharge or reverberating circuit. Furthermore, the fact that the two groups of data points (belonging to the proximal and distal muscle) lay on superimposable lines indicates a similar organization of the two spinal circuits mediating the SLR and MLR in each muscle, the only difference in their position in the plot being a function of the distance of the two muscles from the cord.

Peripheral origin of the medium-latency response

Whilst the Sol is subjected to an obvious stretch with the platform rotation centered about the ankle joint, the case is less clear for the FDB muscle. It is however remarkable that, as happens for the Sol, a tap on the metatarso-phalangeal joints evokes a T reflex in the FDB, with almost the same latency as the SLR in the same muscle (the difference being explained by a less direct application of the stimulus by the platform) (Schieppati et al., 1995). This indicates that the FDB is indeed the site of a stretch reflex, possibly produced by the platform thrust on the foot sole with foot arch flattening – and therefore flexor muscle stretching – against the mass of the overlying body. Moreover, in order to exclude that cutaneous stimulation could contribute to, if not produce the MLR, we cooled the feet by immersion in ice water until the disappearance of cutaneous sensation as tested by light stroke to the digit and sole skin. Under these conditions, no increase in latency or decrease in amplitude of the SLR or MLR were noted, either in the Sol or FDB muscles (Fig. 3). It had been shown previously that electrical stimulation of the digital nerves of the foot did not induce detectable changes in the ongoing EMG of Sol and FDB muscle at the latency compatible with either the SLR or MLR (Abbruzzese et al., 1996).

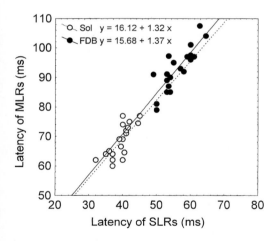

Fig. 2. The latency of both SLR and MLR is affected by height, both in the Sol and FDB muscles. Each subject ($n = 21$) is represented by one symbol for the Sol (open circles) and one symbol (closed circles) for the FDB muscle responses. The increase in latency of both responses in both muscles is due to the increase in subject height. However, the latency of the MLRs increases more than the latency of the corresponding SLRs. The solid line best fitting the filled circles alone ($R^2 = 0.70$) is not significantly different from the dotted line best fitting the open circles alone ($R^2 = 0.62$). Both lines are instead significantly different from the identity line ($y = x$). Two Sol points and one FDB point overlap points with equal coordinates.

464

Bilateral distribution of the medium-latency response

It is known from animal data that, whilst the response to Ia input is strictly autogenetic, the input along group II fibers can diverge and involve both ipsi- and contralateral motoneurons (Jankowska and Noga, 1990; Bajwa et al., 1992; see Jankowska, 1992 for a review). Therefore, we perturbed one limb in isolation, by having the subjects stand with one foot only on the platform, and recorded bilaterally from both Sol and FDB muscles. It turned out that, whilst contralaterally to the perturbed leg no SLR was present, the MLRs were present, though reduced in amplitude with respect

to those evoked by a bilateral perturbation (Corna et al., 1996). A summary of the main finding is reported in Fig. 4.

Effects of nerve cooling on the latency of the responses

Another approach has been to cool the nerve from the ankle to the groin by flowing cold water through a tube wrapped around the limb, with the

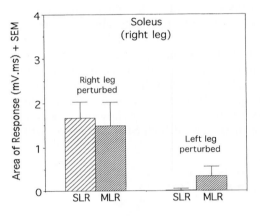

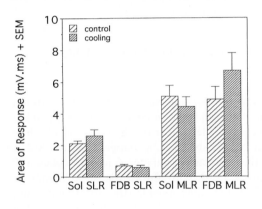

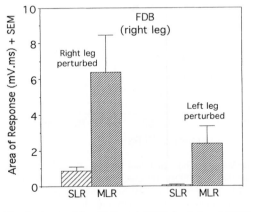

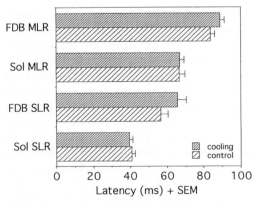

Fig. 3. Changes in area (upper graph) and latency of onset (lower graph) of SLR and MLR of Sol and FDB muscles after cooling of the foot sole. It appears that negligible effects are induced by cooling in either variable with respect to control condition. The bars are the average values of four subjects, whose feet were cooled by immersion in ice water until tactile perception was extinguished.

Fig. 4. Area of the SLR and MLR in Sol and FDB muscles when the right leg is perturbed alone by platform movement compared to when the same leg is off the platform and the left leg alone is perturbed. The leftmost bars represent the responses recorded in the perturbed right leg (control condition). The rightmost bars represent the responses recorded in the nonperturbed right leg. Under the latter condition the SLRs are absent, whilst the MLRs still occur albeit with a lesser amplitude than under control condition.

aim of decreasing the CV of the fibers. It is known that cooling decreases CV in constant proportion in both small and large diameter fibers (Paintal, 1965), therefore producing a larger absolute increase in transmission time in the slow conducting than fast conducting fibers. Such approach has been previously used by Matthews for the upper limb muscle stretch reflexes, and allowed him to prove a role for a long-loop transmission for the MLR of hand muscles (Matthews, 1989). In our experience, cooling of the leg produced a clear-cut delay in the latency of both SLR and MLR in both muscles tested, with a clear-cut larger slowing of the MLR than SLR in both muscles (Schieppati and Nardone, 1997). A summary of the main finding is reported in Fig. 5, where one may note that the increase in latency with cooling is larger for the MLR than for the SLR, both in the distal and proximal muscles.

Estimation of the group II conduction velocity (CV)

Having established, by means of the various approaches mentioned above, that the MLR are relayed by slow conduction spindle afferent fibers (see middle sketch of Fig. 6), it was now possible to address the issue of the group II CV (Nardone and Schieppati, 1998). To this end, we took advantage of the presence, in both the proximal and distal muscles of several subjects, of both SLR and MLR, concurrently evoked by the same stimulus. We reasoned that the delay of the distal muscle SLR with respect to the latency of the proximal muscle SLR would be due to the time needed to travel the distance between the muscles along both the afferent and efferent pathway. In an analogous way, the delay of the distal muscle MLR was due to the time to travel the same distance between muscles along both the afferent (now slower) and the efferent pathway (common to both the SLR and MLR). In a more formal way, one can state that:

a (ms) = latency of FDB-SLR − latency of
    Sol-SLR.
b (ms) = latency of FDB-MLR − latency of
    Sol-MLR

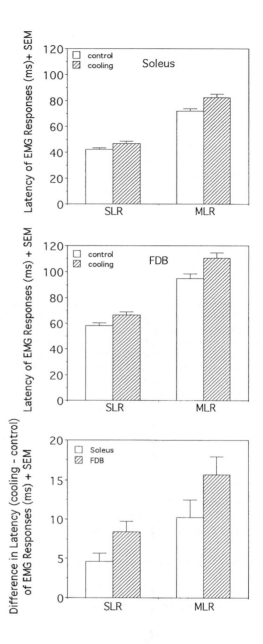

Fig. 5. Effect of cooling of the lower limb on the latency of onset of SLR and MLR of Sol (upper graph) and FDB (middle graph) muscles. For each response, a significant increase in latency appears after cooling with respect to the control value. A significantly larger increase in the latency of MLR than SLR is present in both muscles. Lower graph. With cooling, the latency of the MLRs of both Sol and FDB increases to a larger extent than that of the SLRs. Mean values + standard error of the mean (SEM) from nine subjects.

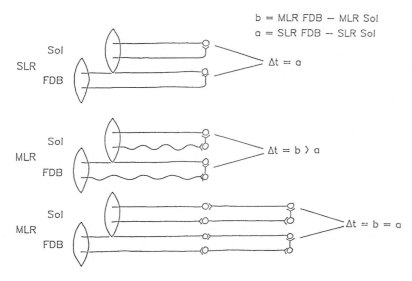

$$b = \text{MLR FDB} - \text{MLR Sol}$$
$$a = \text{SLR FDB} - \text{SLR Sol}$$

Fig. 6. Sketches of the possible pathways mediating the SLR and the MLR in both Sol and FDB muscles. The top sketch points to the monosynaptic reflex pathways fed by spindle Ia afferent fibers and producing the SLRs in both muscles. The sketches below present two alternative hypotheses considered for the origin of MLRs: in the middle sketch, the slow group II fibers are drawn winding to indicate slow transmission, whilst in the bottom sketch the delay of the MLRs has been attributed to a long-loop fed by Ia fibers. The latency difference between the two MLRs of the Sol and FDB muscle (*b*) would be longer than the latency difference between the SLRs in the group II hypothesis, but would be equal in the long-loop hypothesis. From the value of (*b* − *a*), the distance between FDB and Sol muscle, and the conduction velocity (CV) of the Ia fibers one can estimate the CV of the fibers responsible for the MLR of the FDB muscle (see text).

Therefore,

a = afferent time of FDB-SLR (from FDB to Sol)
+ efferent time of FDB-SLR (from Sol to FDB)
b = afferent time of FDB-MLR (from FDB to Sol)
+ efferent time of FDB-MLR (from Sol to FDB)

Since the same motor fibers convey both responses in each muscle,

efferent time of FDB-MLR = efferent time of FDB-SLR,
b − a = afferent time of FDB-MLR (from FDB to Sol) − afferent time of FDB-SLR (from FDB to Sol)

therefore,

afferent time of FDB-MLR (from FDB to Sol) = (b − a) + afferent time of FDB-SLR (from FDB to Sol)

One may note in passing that, in the long-loop hypothesis, the time interval (b − a) would be equal to zero, as shown in the bottom sketch of Fig. 6. Given that (b − a) can be directly measured, and that the afferent time of the SLR can be calculated on the basis of the CV of the Ia fibers of the FDB, then the afferent time of the FDB-MLR can be easily calculated. CV of the group II fibers can therefore be estimated by dividing the distance between the FDB and Sol muscle by the time thus calculated (Fig. 7). On average, this CV was 21 m/s, i.e. less than half the value of Ia fibers (51 m/s). These figures are in keeping with data in the cat showing that the CV of group II fibers is about half that of group Ia (Boyd and Kalu, 1979).

The assumptions implicit in this procedure are that the spinal organizations of group Ia or group II reflexes are similar (Shefner and Logigian, 1994) in both muscles, and that the CV of the FDB nerve fibers is similar along both the distal and proximal parts of the nerve. These assumptions appear

467

reasonable in the light of Fig. 2, and of data in the literature on the differences in CV between the various segments of a nerve (see Liveson and Ma, 1992). It is also notable that, in spite of these assumptions, the estimated CVs of all the subjects studied appear to fall within a relatively narrow range. It should be emphasized that these velocities do not necessarily correspond to the maximal velocities of the fiber group, as happens instead for the motor and group Ia fibers, which are calculated on the basis of the electrical stimulation that activates preferentially the fastest fibers.

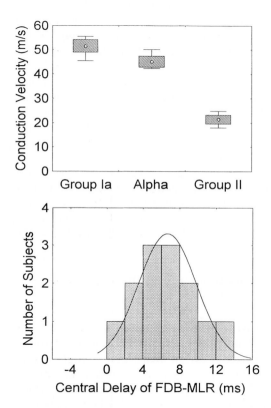

Fig. 7. Mean CV of group II fibers and mean central delay of the MLR fed by group II afferent fibers. Upper graph. Comparison of the CV of group Ia spindle afferent fibers, alpha motor fibers and group II spindle fibers. In each type of fiber, the circle represents the mean value of the CV, the box is ± 1 standard deviation, and the whisker shows the maximum and minimum estimated velocity (data from 13 subjects). It appears that group II fibers conduct at a velocity around half the value of group Ia and alpha fibers. Lower graph. The estimated value of the central delay of the FDB-MLR is about 7 ms, on average (same subjects as in the upper graph).

Central delay of the medium-latency response

Once having estimated the CV of the group II spindle afferents, one can try to estimate the central delay of the responses mediated by these fibers. Basically, this estimate implies the calculation of the afferent time and of the efferent time of the MLR, on the basis of the distance of the FDB from the cord and the respective conduction velocities of the secondary spindle afferents and of the motor fibers. The formula used is indicated below:

Central delay of FDB-MLR (ms) =

	latency of FDB-MLR (ms)
—time for excitation	*(SLR-T) (ms)*
of spindles by the	
platform rotation	
—afferent	*FDB muscle to Th12 (m)*
conduction time	*group II CV (m/s)*
—efferent	*Th12 to FDB muscle (m)*
conduction time	*alpha MN CV (m/s)*
—neuromuscular	*1 ms*
junction	

In this way, the central delay of the FDB-MLR proved to be about 7 ms, on average (Fig. 7B). Such a relatively long delay, for a reflex which has been shown in the cat to be oligosynaptic, can be explained by the very low CV of the axons of the spinal interneurons relaying the response (Fu and Schomburg, 1974; Stauffer et al., 1976), by their location at not necessarily the same level as the motoneurons (Jankowska, 1992), and by the fact that the afferent input is a desynchronized one, therefore not liable to immediately drive to the threshold the spinal neurons along the spinal pathway. On the contrary, it seems unlikely that such a delay of the FDB-MLR may be accounted for by a transcerebellar loop (Eccles et al., 1961). An analogous calculation, made with the CV of the Ia fibers, gave an average central delay of the SLR close to 1 ms. This is an indication of the validity of the method, since that is the delay one would expect for a mostly monosynaptic reflex. Such organization of the MLR reflex pahway is not dissimilar to that found in the cat for the spindle secondary reflexes by Jankowska (1992) and in the rat by Riddell and Hadian (1995).

Modulation of the synaptic transmission from group II afferents by monoamines

It should be recalled at this point that the excitability of the interneurons relaying this group II effect onto the motoneurons is modulated by descending monoaminergic pathways, very much as happens in the cat. In fact, we have shown that an α_2-adrenergic agonist agent is capable of inducing a sizeable decrease in the amplitude of the MLRs without affecting their latency (Corna et al., 1995). Figure 8 compares the effect of tizanidine with that of stance stabilization: both the administration of the adrenergic substance and the change in 'postural set' (Nardone et al., 1990; Schieppati and Nardone, 1995) produce a significant depression in the size of the FDB MLR, without affecting its latency. It might be entertained that the depression in reflex excitability occurring on stabilizing stance in normal subjects (but not in Parkinsonian

patients, see Schieppati and Nardone, 1991) are mediated by descending pathways from brain stem monoaminergic nuclei (Noga et al., 1992).

The medium-latency response is preserved in the absence of the short-latency response

There is an hereditary motor and sensory neuropathy, called Charcot-Marie-Tooth type 1A (CMT1A or HMSN type 1), which represents a natural model (Dyck et al., 1993a; Sereda et al., 1996) of predominant axonal demyelination and loss of the largest-diameter myelinated nerve fibers (Fig. 9). When these patients are subjected to a perturbation stretching the leg and foot muscles, the SLRs are typically absent in both muscles. It is also almost impossible to elicit an H reflex or T response in the FDB, pointing to a real functional loss of the fibers from the spindle primary terminations. Very interestingly, however, in a group of CMT1A patients studied in this laboratory, the MLRs were preserved. Further, their latency increase was explained by the diminished CV of the efferent motor fibers, which proved to be 22 m/s on average ($n = 10$) (Nardone et al., 1997). This indicates that in these patients the CV of the anatomically preserved group II afferent fibers, responsible for their MLR, is hardly affected by the disease.

Quiet stance is not affected by loss of Ia afferent fibers

These patients were also studied under conditions of quiet unperturbed upright stance, with the aim of detecting any effect on their stability connected to the absence of primary afferent fibers. As a matter of fact, the stabilogram of these patients, which measures the oscillations of the body center of pressure and the efforts to correct these oscillations, and is an indirect measure of their ability to maintain equilibrium, was within normal limits (Fig. 10), contrary to other forms of polyneuropathy (e.g. diabetic) (Bergin et al., 1995; Nardone et al., 1998) that may preferentially affect fibers of smaller diameter (Brown and Asbury, 1984).

Therefore, both the virtual absence of primary afferent fibers and the great reduction of CV of the

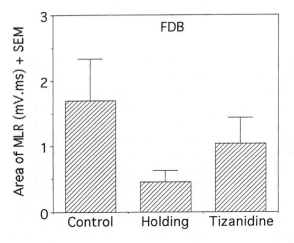

Fig. 8. The excitability of the spinal pathway mediating the MLR is decreased by administration of tizanidine, an α_2-adrenergic agonist agent. The graph shows the average size of the FDB-MLR evoked by foot dorsiflexion of the supporting platform, in six normal subjects, during normal free stance (left bar), stance stabilization obtained by holding onto a stable frame during the perturbation (middle bar), and free stance after administration of tizanidine, at the peak of its action (right bar). Both manoeuvres appear to significantly decrease the excitability of the interneuronal pathways mediating the response. The monosynaptic reflex pathway mediating the SLR is not affected, since the size of the SLR is not changed by the tizanidine. The latency of both the SLR and of the MLR is not changed, either.

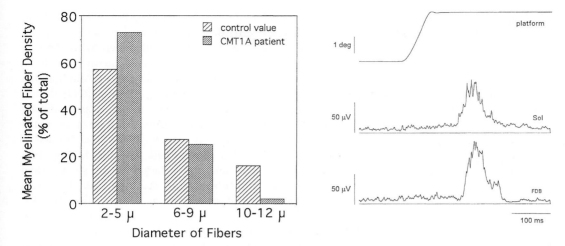

Fig. 9. The CMT1A patients have a loss of the largest myelinated afferent fibers, and lack SLRs from stretched muscles. Left panel. The graph shows the distribution of the myelinated fibers of the sural nerve of normal controls and of a CMT1A patient, within three classes of fiber diameter. Comparison with the normal data shows a striking reduction in the percent content of fibers within the largest diameter class, and a preserved content within the intermediate diameter class. No anatomical data are available for the tibial nerve, in this or in other patients, but there are indications in the literature (Dyck et al., 1993a) that the disease affects almost evenly all the nerves of both the lower and upper limb. Right panel. The EMG recordings from the stretched Sol and FDB muscles show complete absence of the SLRs and delayed but present MLRs. The increase in latency of the latter is explained by the increased efferent time, due to the decrease in the CV of the relevant motor fibers (23 m/s in this patient).

motor fibers are not detrimental to the control of quiet upright stance. This control can be posited, by exclusion, to rely mostly on the afferent input from the secondaries. It is noteworthy that the absence of the short-latency reflex in these patients does not lead to postural instability, as if the mechanical counterpart of this response plays a negligible role in the correction of body oscillations during normal stance.

Conclusions

1. Group II spindle afferent fibers have a CV about half that of the Ia fibers. In this connection, one should be warned that the comparison is between the *fastest* Ia fibers, as tested by the usual electrical stimulation methods, and the group II fibers responsible for the stretch reflex, which are not necessarily the fastest ones (Sypert et al., 1980). The method used here, rather than estimating the maximal CV of the group II fibers, gives an estimate of the velocity of the functional fibers activated by a stretch. It is notable that the range of CV of primaries and secondaries of the cat is

respectively 55–120 m/s and 20–65 m/s (see Jankowska, 1992). Other things being equal, therefore, group II mean CV would be about half the mean CV of Ia fibers, but less than half the maximal CV of Ia. Further attention should be paid to the fact that these are the CV values estimated for the fibers originating in the FDB and running through the tibial nerve; since Ia fibers in more proximal muscles may be faster than the Ia of the distal ones (see Liveson and Ma, 1992), one would expect the CV of group II to increase slightly for the proximal muscles of the lower limb.

2. Group II spindle afferent fibers are responsible for the late part of the stretch reflex in the lower limb postural muscles. In this connection, one may note that the size of this response is of the same order of magnitude as that elicited by Ia afferent input. In the case of the FDB muscle, the response is even larger than that of the monosynaptic, and creates a background torque anchoring the foot to the platform, a torque which creates a firm basis upon which the responses of the Sol are superimposed. This relatively larger size of the MLR with respect to the SLR may be at variance with the

470

cat data, where group II postsynaptic effects on the motoneurons have been shown to be smaller that the Ia EPSPs (Munson, 1990; Heckman and Binder, 1990).

3. Group II spindle afferent fibers impinge on a spinal circuit with few intercalated interneurons, whose localization may be slightly displaced with respect to the neuromeres where motoneurons are located, very much as happens in the cat (Edgley and Jankowska, 1987). Furthermore, the transmission through the interneurons intercalated in this pathway is modulated by descending noradrenergic pathways, in man as in the cat (Bras et al., 1989, 1990).

4. The functional loss of group Ia spindle afferent fibers may be complete in CMT1A, as witnessed by the absence of the SLRs to stretch (as well as of the T response and H reflex), both in the

Sol and FDB. This notwithstanding, the MLR to stretch is fully developed in these patients, pointing to the unlikelyhood of a Ia-mediated MLR through long-loops or segmental mechanisms, or to a continuous discharge of the Ia fibers throughout the muscle stretch. Most notably, these patients do not appear to undergo balance problems, since during the platform rotations nobody fell over or made steps in order to stay erect in spite of the absence of the SLR. Also unexpected was the finding that patients did not show larger body sways than normal subjects, when standing quietly on a dynamometric platform, as instead happens for other types of polyneuropathic patients where the disease affects both large and small-diameter fibers and where postural ataxia is a more common finding. This would point to a minor role of spindle primaries, and to a major role of spindle secondaries in the segmental control of quiet stance.

Acknowledgements

The financial support of Telethon, Italy (Grant no. 1071C) and Italian Ministry of Health (Grant Ricerca Corrente) is gratefully acknowledged.

References

Abbruzzese, M., Rubino, V. and Schieppati, M. (1996) Task-dependent effects evoked by foot muscle afferents on leg muscle activity in humans. *Electroenceph. clin. Neurophysiol.*, 101: 339–348.

Bajwa, S., Edgley, S.A. and Harrison, P.J. (1992) Crossed actions on group II-activated interneurons in the midlumbar segments of the cat spinal cord. *J. Physiol. (Lond.)*, 455: 205–217.

Barker, D. (1962) The structure and distribution of muscle spindle receptors. In: D. Barker (Ed.), *Symposium on Muscle Receptors*, Hong-Kong University Press, Hong-Kong, pp. 227–240.

Bergin, P.S., Bronstein, A.M., Murray, N.M.F., Sancovic, S. and Zeppenfeld, K. (1995) Body sway and vibration perception thresholds in normal aging and in patients with polyneuropathy. *J. Neurol. Neurosurg. Psychiatry*, 58: 335–340.

Bessou, P., Cabelguen J.-M., Joffroy, M., Montoya, R. and Pagès, B. (1986) Efferent and afferent activity in a gastrocnemius nerve branch during locomotion in the thalamic cat. *Exp. Brain Res.*, 82: 191–198.

Boyd, I.A. and Kalu, K.U. (1979) Scaling factor relating conduction velocity and diameter for myelinated afferent nerve fibers in the cat hind limb. *J. Physiol. (Lond.)*, 289: 277–297.

Bras, H., Cavallari, P., Jankowska, E. and Noga B.R. (1989) Comparison of effects of monoamines on transmission in

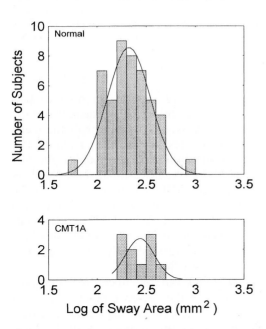

Fig. 10. The body sway, as measured by a stabilometric platform upon which subjects stood quietly with eyes open, is within normal limits in CMT1A patients. The CMT1A histogram indicates the distribution of the sway area values within the population of patients ($n = 10$), and is to be compared with the normal subjects ($n = 49$) distribution: all the data of the CMT1A patients fall within two standard deviations of the expected bell-shaped distribution of the normal subjects, and their mean value is not significantly different from the normal subjects' mean value.

spinal pathways from group I and group II muscle afferents in the cat. *Exp. Brain Res.*, 76: 27–37.

Bras, H., Jankowska, E., Noga, B.R. and Skoog, B. (1990) Comparison of effects of various types of NA and 5-HT agonists on transmission from group II muscle afferents in the cat. *Eur. J. Neurosci.*, 2: 1029–1039.

Brown, M.J. and Asbury, A.K. (1984) Diabetic neuropathy. *Ann. Neurol.*, 15: 2–12.

Corna, S., Galante, M., Grasso, M., Nardone, A. and Schieppati, M. (1996) Unilateral displacement of lower limb evokes bilateral EMG responses in leg and foot muscles in standing humans. *Exp. Brain Res.*, 109: 83–91.

Corna, S., Grasso, M., Nardone, A. and Schieppati, M. (1995) Selective depression of medium-latency leg and foot muscle responses to stretch by an α_2-agonist in humans. *J. Physiol. (Lond.)*, 484: 803–809.

Dietz, V. (1992) Human neuronal control of automatic functional movements: intercation between central programs and afferent input. *Physiol. Rev.*, 72: 33–69.

Dyck, P.J., Chance, P., Lebo, R. and Carney J.A. (1993a) Hereditary motor and sensory neuropathies. In: P.J. Dyck and P.K. Thomas (Eds), *Peripheral Neuropathy*, W.B. Saunders Company, Philadelphia, pp. 1094–1136.

Dyck, P.J., Giannini, C. and Lais, A. (1993b) Pathologic alterations of nerves. In: P.J. Dyck and P.K. Thomas (Eds), *Peripheral Neuropathy*, W.B. Saunders Company, Philadelphia, pp. 514–595.

Eccles, J.C., Oscarsson, O. and Willis, W.D. (1961) Synaptic action of group I and II afferent fibers of muscle on the cells of the dorsal spinocerebellar tract. *J. Physiol. (Lond.)*, 158: 517–543.

Edgley, S.A. and Jankowska, E. (1987) Field potentials generated by group II muscle afferents in the middle lumbar segments of the cat spinal cord. *J. Physiol. (Lond.)*, 385: 393–413.

Fu, T.C. and Schomburg, E.D. (1974) Electrophysiological investigation of the projection of secondary muscle spindle afferents in the cat spinal cord. *Acta Physiol. Scand.*, 91: 314–329.

Heckman, C.J. and Binder, M.D. (1990) Neural mechanisms underlying the orderly recruitment of motoneurons. In: M.D. Binder and L.M. Mendell (Eds), *The Segmental Motor System*, Oxford University Press, Oxford, pp. 182–204.

Hunt, C.C. (1954) Relation of function to diameter in afferent fibers of muscle nerves. *J. Gen. Physiol.*, 38: 117–131.

Jankowska, E. (1992) Interneuronal relay in spinal pathway from proprioceptors. *Progr. Neurobiol.*, 38: 335–378.

Jankowska, E. and Noga, B.R. (1990) Contralaterally projecting lamina VIII interneurons in middle lumbar segments in the cat. *Brain Res.*, 535: 327–330.

Kirkwood, P.A. and Sears, T.A. (1974) Monosynaptic excitation of motoneurons from secondary endings of muscle spindles. *Nature*, 252: 243–244.

Liveson, J.A. and Ma, D.M. (1992) *Laboratory Reference for Clinical Neurophysiology*, F.A. Davis Company, Philadelphia.

Lundberg, A., Malmgren, K. and Schomburg, E.D. (1987) Reflex pathways from group II muscle afferents. 1. Distribution and linkage of reflex actions to alpha-motoneurons. *Exp. Brain Res.*, 65: 271–281.

Marque, P., Pierrot-Deseilligny, E. and Simonetta-Moreau, M. (1996) Evidence for excitation of the human lower limb motoneurons by group II muscle afferents. *Exp. Brain Res.*, 109: 357–360.

Matthews, P.B.C. (1972) *Mammalian Muscle Receptors and their Central Actions*. Edward Arnold (Publishers) Ltd, London.

Matthews, P.B.C. (1989) Analysis of human long-latency reflexes by cooling the peripheral conduction pathway; which afferents are involved? In: J.H.J. Allum and M. Hulliger (Eds) *Afferent Control of Posture and Locomotion, Progress in Brain Research*, Vol. 80, Elsevier Science Publishers B.V., Amsterdam, pp. 103–112.

Matthews, P.B.C. (1992) Human studies in the analysis of the stretch reflex: an essay. In: L. Jami, E. Pierrot-Desilligny and D. Zytnicki (Eds) *Muscle Afferents and Spinal Control of Movement*. Pergamon Press, Oxford, pp. 401–413.

Munson, J.B. (1990) Synaptic inputs to type-identified motor units. In: M.D. Binder and L.M. Mendell (Eds), *The Segmental Motor System*, Oxford University Press, Oxford, pp. 291–307.

Munson, J.B., Fleshman, J.W. and Sypert, G.W. (1980) Properties of single fiber spindle group II EPSPs in triceps surae motoneurons. *J. Neurophysiol.*, 44: 713–725.

Nardone, A., Giordano, A., Corrà, T. and Schieppati, M. (1990) Responses of leg muscles in humans displaced while standing. Effects of types of perturbation and of postural set. *Brain*, 113: 65–84.

Nardone, A., Grasso, M., Giordano, A. and Schieppati, M. (1996) Different effect of height on latency of leg and foot short- and medium-latency EMG responses to perturbation of stance in humans. *Neurosci. Lett.*, 206: 89–92.

Nardone, A., Miscio, G., Pisano, F. and Schieppati, M. (1998) Sensory ataxia in polyneuropathy is connected to dysfunction of group II afferent fibers. *J. Peripher. Nerv. Syst.*, 3: 151.

Nardone, A., Pisano, F., Miscio, G. and Azan, G. (1997) Demyelinating neuropathy affects to a different extent the short- and medium-latency responses of lower limb muscles to stance perturbation. *J. Peripher. Nerv. Syst.*, 2: 99.

Nardone, A. and Schieppati, M. (1998) Medium-latency response to muscle stretch in human lower limb: estimation of conduction velocity of group II fibers and central delay. *Neurosci. Lett.*, 249: 29–32.

Noga, B.R., Bras, H. and Jankowska, E. (1992) Transmission from group II muscle afferents is depressed by stimulation of locus coeruleus/subcoeruleus, Kölliker-Fuse and raphe nuclei in the cat. *Exp. Brain Res.*, 88: 502–516.

Noth, J., Schwarz, M., Podoll, K. and Motamedi, F. (1991) Evidence that low-threshold muscle afferents evoke long-latency reflexes in human hand muscles. *J. Neurophysiol.*, 65: 1089–1097.

472

Paintal, A.S. (1965) Block of conduction in mammalian myelinated nerve fibers by low temperatures. *J. Physiol. (Lond.)*, 180: 1–19.

Riddel, J.S. and Hadian, M.R. (1995) Topographical organization of neurons in group II reflex pathways of the rat spinal cord. In: A. Taylor, M. Gladden and R. Durbaba (Eds), *Alpha and Gamma Motor Systems*, Plenum Press, London, pp. 384–386.

Schieppati, M. (1991) Motor unit reflex activity, normal and pathological. *Curr. Opin. Neurobiol.*, 4: 749–755.

Schieppati, M. and Nardone, A. (1991) Free and supported stance in Parkinson's disease. The effect of posture and postural set on leg muscle responses to perturbation, and its relation to the severity of the disease. *Brain*, 114: 1227–1244.

Schieppati, M. and Nardone, A. (1997) Medium-latency stretch reflexes of foot and leg muscles analysed by cooling the lower limb in standing humans. *J. Physiol. (Lond.)*, 503: 691–698.

Schieppati, M. and Nardone, A. (1995) Time-course of 'set'-related changes in muscle responses to stance perturbation in humans. *J. Physiol. (Lond.)*, 487: 787–796.

Schieppati, M., Nardone, A., Siliotto, R. and Grasso, M. (1995) Early and late stretch responses of human foot muscles induced by perturbation of stance. *Exp. Brain Res.*, 105: 411–422.

Schomburg, E.D. (1990) Spinal sensorimotor systems and their supraspinal control. *Neurosci. Res.*, 7: 265–340.

Sereda, M., Griffiths, I., Pühlofer, A., Stewart, H., Rossner, M.J., Zimmermann, F., Magyar, J.P., Schneider, A., Hund, E., Meinck, H.-M., Suter, U. and Nave, K.-A. (1996) A transgenic rat model of Charcot-Marie-Tooth disease. *Neuron*, 16:1049–1060.

Shefner, J.M. and Logigian, E. L. (1994) Conduction velocity in motor, cutaneous afferent, and muscle afferent fibers within the same mixed nerve. *Muscle Nerve*, 17: 773–778.

Stauffer, E.K., Watt, D.G., Taylor, A., Reinking, R.M. and Stuart, D.G. (1976) Analysis of muscle receptor connections by spike-triggered averaging. 2. Spindle group II afferents. *J. Neurophysiol.*, 39: 1393–1402.

Sypert, G.W., Fleshman, J.W. and Munson, J.B. (1980) Comparison of monosynaptic actions of medial gastrocnemius group Ia and group II muscle spindle afferents on triceps surae motoneurons. *J. Neurophysiol.*, 44: 726–738.

Thilmann, A.F., Schwarz, M., Töpper, R., Fellows, S.J. and Noth, J. (1991) Different mechanisms underlie the long-latency stretch reflex response of active human muscle at different joints. *J. Physiol. (Lond.)*, 444:631–643.

M.D. Binder (Ed.)
Progress in Brain Research, Vol 123
© 1999 Elsevier Science BV. All rights reserved.

CHAPTER 44

Indices of cortical motor function following severe brain injury in man

P.H. Ellaway,[1,*] S.H. Moosavi,[1] M.J. Stokes,[2] M. Catley[1] and N. Haque[2]

[1]*Department of Sensorimotor Systems, Division of Neuroscience and Psychological Medicine, Imperial College School of Medicine, Charing Cross Hospital, Fulham Palace Road, London W6 8RF, UK*
[2]*The Royal Hospital for Neuro-disability, London SW15 3SW, UK*

Introduction

The objective of this study was to assess the degree to which the function of the corticospinal tract and the motor cortex in man is affected by severe brain injury of a severity that results in a lack of purposeful movements and no apparent awareness of self or surroundings (Grossman and Hagel, 1996). Our subjects had suffered either anoxic or traumatic (possibly including anoxia) brain injury that resulted initially in an indefinite period of coma. On emergence from coma, a group of the subjects assumed sleep/wake cycles, with eyes open during the awake periods, but they exhibited no purposeful movements and showed no signs of awareness to a wide range of sensory stimuli. Such a condition is usually referred to as persistent vegetative state (Jennet and Plum, 1972) or apallic syndrome.

Previous studies have employed electrical or magnetic stimulation of the motor cortex (Ebner and Zentner, 1988; Facco et al., 1989, 1991; Netz and Homberg, 1992; Ying et al., 1992; Inghilleri et al., 1994; Bassetti et al., 1994; Kaneko, 1995) to assess the status of the corticospinal tract. In these studies the preservation of motor responses has been noted in a proportion of patients but none have

*Corresponding author. Tel.: 44(0) 181 846 7293; Fax: 44(0) 181 846 7338; e-mail: p.ellaway@ic.ac.uk

attempted to assess the excitability of the motor cortex in severely brain-damaged patients.

Certain attributes of transcranial magnetic stimulation (TMS), as a method for eliciting a corticospinal output from motor cortex, suggest that the technique may allow the level of excitability of the motor cortex to be assessed. TMS is thought to excite corticospinal neurons transsynaptically or, at least, at the initial segment (Day et al., 1989; Edgley et al., 1990; Burke et al., 1993). Only at higher strengths, well above threshold and at specific orientations of the magnetic coil (Nakamura et al., 1996), does direct stimulation of corticospinal axons occur. TMS also activates cortical inhibitory circuits (Davey et al., 1994). Thus, the stimulation of corticospinal neurons by TMS is likely to be influenced by concurrently active presynaptic inputs. Such a cortical basis is thought to account in large part for the facilitation by voluntary contraction of the motor evoked potential (MEP) response to TMS (Hess et al., 1987; Rothwell et al., 1987; Mazzocchio et al., 1994; Nielsen and Petersen, 1995). MEP responses to TMS are characterized by their inherent variability (Hess and Ludin, 1988; Amassian et al., 1989; Day et al., 1989; Kiers et al., 1993; Nielsen, 1996). It has been suggested that the variability may be caused by fluctuations in excitability at the level of the motor cortex and that such fluctuations might result from modulation of afferent input to the motor cortex or intrinsic rhythms (Steriade et al., 1990; Brouwer and Qiao, 1995; Ellaway et al., 1998). In a recent study we observed correlations in the amplitudes of MEPs of different muscles, including homologous muscles in opposite hands, to coincidental, bilateral stimulation of the two motor cortices (Ellaway et al., 1998). Between 20 and 25% of the variability in MEP amplitudes could be accounted for by the processes that correlated changes in excitability of corticospinal output to the different muscles, indicating that the variations in excitability were wide ranging and best explained by some common source of input. Preliminary accounts of this work have been published (Moosavi et al., 1997a, b).

Methods

The patients in this study had all suffered severe brain injury, from either anoxia or a combination of trauma and anoxia, that had resulted in a period of coma. The patients all recovered from coma and were studied, on average, 10 to 12 months after the original injury. They were placed in one of two categories according to the following criteria. When presented with simple verbal commands and multimodality sensory stimulation (Gill-Thwaites, 1997) some patients were consistently unresponsive (Category 1). Others were minimally responsive (Category 2) as revealed, for example, by reliable gaze directed selection of 'yes' or 'no' signs. However, no patient in either Category could make clear or repeatable, purposeful movements of limb muscles. The muscles we selected for study of their responses to TMS were the first dorsal interosseus (FDI) and the abductor digiti minimi (AbDM) of the hand. A magnetic stimulator (Magstim 200, MagStim Company Ltd., Dyfed, UK) connected to a 9 cm (average diameter) coil was employed with the centre of the coil placed over the vertex with the appropriate orientation to stimulate the left or right cortex (Day et al., 1990).

Threshold for a muscle was defined as the stimulus strength, to the nearest 5% of maximum stimulator output (MSO) that just produced a significant response in an average of twenty trials. Central motor conduction time was calculated by subtracting the peripheral conduction time, esti-

mated using the F-wave technique (Kimura, 1974), from the latency of the MEP.

Ethical approval for this study was obtained from Riverside Health Authority and Charing Cross and Westminster Medical School. Informed consent was obtained according to the declaration of Helsinki and following the procedures of the Royal Hospital for Neuro-disability.

Cortical motor evoked potentials

Figure 1 shows examples of typical MEP responses in FDI and AbDM muscles in a normal subject and in both Category 2 and Category 1 patients. The records in each instance are the responses to a strength of TMS 15%MSO above threshold. MEPs were observed frequently in Category 1 patients, only two of 11 patients failing to show a response to TMS. All Category 2 patients and normal subjects showed responses to TMS although in four of the eight Category 2 patients MEPs could not be elicited in all muscles. Discounting the non-responders, mean thresholds for MEPs in hand muscles were significantly greater than normal for Category 1 patients ($p < 0.01$, Mann-Whitney), but not for Category 2 patients.

The MEPs in the Category 1 patient in Fig. 1 are smaller, appear more polyphasic and are of slightly longer latency than those in either the normal subject or the Category 2 patient. Both the normal subject and the Category 2 patient had thresholds in the range 25 to 30%MSO whereas the lowest threshold for the Category 1 patient was 50%MSO. Thus, although a MEP response could be elicited by TMS in the Category 1 patient, the motor cortex appeared less excitable than either the normal subject or the Category 2 patient.

Recruitment of MEPs

In Fig. 2 the size of the MEP in hand muscles is plotted against the strength of TMS. The size of the MEP was taken as the area of the averaged, rectified response to twenty trials and expressed as a proportion of the maximum M-wave. The M-wave is the EMG response to electrical stimulation of the peripheral muscle nerve. Again, it is clear that thresholds for the normal subject and Category

2 patient are similar and are about half that of the Category 1 patient. In addition, in the Category 1 patient the recruitment of motor units occurs less steeply with increasing stimulus strength. Stimulation was not increased beyond 70%MSO (1.4 times threshold) for the Category 1 patient. The recruit-

ment in terms of percentage of the M-wave is less than 5% at 1.4 times threshold for the Category 1 patient compared with an average of 15% for the normal and 40% for the Category 2 patient. The increase in size of the MEP with increasing TMS for the normal subject is well within the reported

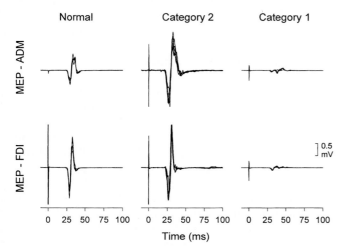

Fig. 1. Motor evoked potential responses of hand muscles to TMS of the contralateral motor cortex. Five consecutive responses, recorded using surface electromyography, are superimposed in each frame. Stimulation occurred at time zero and was at a strength 15% MSO above threshold. Threshold TMS was 30%MSO (AbDM) and 25%MSO (FDI) for the normal subject, 25%MSO (AbDM and FDI) for the category 2 patient and 50%MSO (AbDM and FDI) for the Category 1 patient.

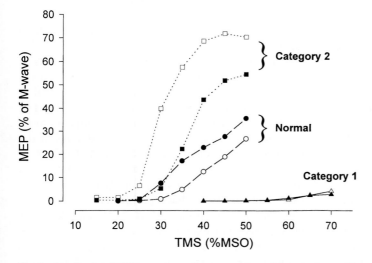

Fig. 2. Amplitude of MEPs, expressed as percentage of the maximum M-wave for that muscle, plotted against strength of TMS in percentage of %MSO. Symbols: circles, normal subject; squares, Category 2 patient; triangles, Category 1 patient; open symbols, FDI; filled symbols, AbDM.

range for the relaxed FDI muscle (Kiers et al., 1993). The greater size of the MEP for the Category 2 patient in Fig. 2 is also within the normal range during facilitation produced by voluntary contraction. Inspection of the individual records for the Category 2 patient revealed background EMG during the TMS trials. This can be observed in the superimposed records in Fig. 1. The fact that the FDI muscle of this patient was not relaxed during the recordings may account for the MEP responses being larger than those of the relaxed normal subject.

Central conduction time of sensory and motor pathways is frequently used to detect disorders of the CNS. None of our brain-injured subjects had suffered peripheral nerve damage. The distribution of central conduction times was significantly (Mann-Whitney $p < 0.005$) prolonged compared with normal subjects in both categories. However, in the large majority of patients central conduction time was within normal limits.

Variability of MEP amplitude

There is considerable variability in the response to TMS of uniform strength and we have attributed this principally to fluctuations in excitability at the level of the motor cortex rather than at spinal motoneurons (Ellaway et al., 1998). In this study, variability in MEP responses to TMS was expressed as the coefficient of variation in amplitude (area of the rectified MEP) of twenty trials at two standardized strengths (5 and 10%MSO) of TMS above threshold. Mean coefficients of variation at the two strengths of TMS were 0.72 and 0.74 for Category 1 and 0.81 and 0.62 for Category 2 patients. They were not significantly different from those of normal subjects (0.75 and 0.65). The result implies that brain-injured patients with cortically evoked responses show fluctuations in excitability of the motor cortex. The variability in normal individuals appears not to be limited to the cortical output to individual muscles (Ellaway et al., 1998; this was also the case in brain-injured patients. Significant positive correlations in amplitude of MEPs of FDI and AbDM muscles were observed in both categories of brain-injured patient, as well as in normal subjects. Correlation coeffi-

cients indicated that the proportion of the variance accounted for by the process responsible for producing a simultaneous change in excitability of the corticospinal pathways to both muscles was 49% for normal subjects, 51% for Category 2 patients and 46% for Category 1 patients. The similarity in these proportions suggests that the underlying mechanisms may not have been different in the brain-injured and normal groups.

H-reflex and MEP variability

The above analysis of differences in threshold to TMS and variability in MEP amplitude has used indirect reasoning to attribute the source of variation in excitability of the corticospinal pathway to the motor cortex. The H-reflex is used as a direct approach for testing the excitability of the motoneuron pool (Schieppati, 1987). However, the interpretation of H-reflexes has to be carried out with the same caution as MEP responses to TMS. If threshold or amplitude of the H-reflex and MEP vary to same degree then the variability in both responses might simply reflect fluctuations in excitability of corticospinal neurons transmitted on to the motoneurons. If the responses to the two test stimuli are different, separate mechanisms can only be deduced if the same type and group of motoneurons is involved. Some debate exists as to whether TMS and H-reflexes access the same motoneurons. Indirect reasoning suggests that they do. It is generally accepted (see Burke et al., 1994) that the sequence of recruitment of motor units is similar in voluntary contractions, stretch reflexes and H-reflexes (Milner-Brown et al., 1973; Buller et al., 1980; Henneman and Mendell, 1981). The recruitment order of motor units also appears to be the same for voluntary contraction and TMS of the motor cortex (Gandevia and Rothwell, 1987, Hess et al., 1987; Bawa and Lemon, 1993), However, these generalizations may not apply to all muscles. Morita et al. (1998) have preliminary evidence in one human arm muscle that TMS and H-reflex testing may not excite exactly the same group of motor units. H-reflexes and tendon jerks can be elicited rarely in the relaxed muscles of the hand and, in our study, H-reflexes were observed only infrequently in brain-injured patients (three in each category). The reflexes were observed independently of background EMG in the muscle (Schieppati, 1987) and were associated with high threshold for the MEP in that hand muscle. When it was possible to compare H-reflexes and MEPs (four instances, both Categories) the variability in size of the H-reflex was always less than for the MEP even when the mean size of each response was similar. Greater variability for MEPs than H-reflexes has been observed in normal man for leg (Day et al., 1991) and hand muscles (Kiers et al., 1993). If this can be interpreted as independent fluctuations in excitability of cortical neurons and motoneurons then our results suggest that the brain-injured patients have some functional connections of elements within the motor cortex that cause their variation in excitability. An argument against this interpretation might be that the greater variability of MEPs results from phase cancellation of EMG signals caused by fluctuations in latency of individual motor unit responses, these being greater for TMS than for the more synchronous H-reflex. Magistris et al. (1998) have used a collision routine to show, for example, that TMS does indeed excite all spinal motoneurons innervating a target muscle even though the motor evoked potential to TMS is smaller in size than the M-wave response to direct nerve stimulation, and they attribute this to phase cancellation. However, phase cancellation is unlikely to account for all the difference in variability between MEP and H-reflex responses. Burke et al. (1995) report variability in the size of the corticospinal volley itself, particularly the I-wave component, and suggest that even greater variability would be present in awake human subjects.

Conclusions

The aim of this study was to determine the functional integrity of the motor cortex and corticospinal tract in post-coma, severely brain-injured subjects. Given that TMS excites corticospinal neurons either presynaptically or at the level of the initial segment, the presence of MEPs in the majority of both Categories of patient indicated survival of populations of corticospinal neurons. This is consistent with the finding that Betz cells

are relatively resistant to hypoxic-ischaemic brain injury (Murayama et al., 1990). The variability in size of MEPs to constant TMS was not significantly different from normal in either category of brain-injured patient, and the variability of MEPs was consistently greater than that of H-reflexes. MEP amplitude was also correlated between muscles. Variability in the size of MEPs is likely to reflect fluctuations in the excitability of the motor cortex to afferent input or intrinsic oscillations. The observed variability of response to TMS may therefore be interpreted cautiously as an indication that corticospinal neurons have functional connections with presynaptic elements in brain-injured individuals with a severity that precludes consciousness and voluntary movement.

Acknowledgements

The Wellcome Trust and the Living Again Trust supported this project. We are grateful to patients and their relatives at the Royal Hospital for neurodisability for their participation.

Abbreviations

AbDM	Abductor digiti minimi
MEP	Motor evoked potential
FDI	First dorsal interosseus
MSO	Maximum stimulator output
TMS	Transcranial magnetic stimulation

References

Amassian, V.E., Cracco, R.Q. and Maccabee, P.J. (1989) Focal stimulation of human cerebral cortex with the magnetic coil: a comparison with electrical stimulation. *Electroenceph. clin. Neurophysiol.*, 74: 401–416.

Bassetti, C., Mathis, J. and Hess, C.W. (1994) Multimodal electrophysiological studies including motor evoked potentials in patients with locked-in syndrome: report of six patients. *J. Neurol. Neurosurg. Psychiatry.*, 57: 1403–1406.

Bawa, P. and Lemon, R. (1993) Recruitment of motor units in response to transcranial magnetic stimulation in man. *J. Physiol.* 471: 445–464.

Brouwer, B. and Qiao, J. (1995) Characteristics and variability of lower limb motoneurone responses to transcranial magnetic stimulation. *Electroenceph. clin. Neurophysiol.*, 97: 49–54.

Buller, N.P., Garnett, R. and Stephens, J.A. (1980) The reflex response of single motor units in human hand muscles

478

following muscle afferent stimulation. *J. Physiol.*, 303: 337–349.

Burke, D., Gracies, J.M., Mazevet, D., Meunier, S. and Pierrot-Deseilligny, E. (1994) Non-monosynaptic transmission of the cortical command for voluntary movement in man. *J. Physiol.*, 480: 191–202.

Burke, D., Hicks, R., Gandevia, S.C., Stephen, J., Woodforth, I. and Crawford, M. (1993) Direct comparison of corticospinal volleys in human subjects to transcranial magnetic and electrical stimulation. *J. Physiol.*, 470: 383–393.

Burke, D., Hicks, R., Stephen, J. Woodforth, I. and Crawford, M. (1995) Trial-to-trial variability of corticospinal volleys in human subjects. *Electroenceph. clin. Neurophysiol.*, 97: 231–237.

Davey, N.J., Romaiguère, P., Maskill, D.W. and Ellaway, P.H. (1994) Suppression of voluntary motor activity revealed using transcranial magnetic stimulation of the motor cortex in man. *J. Physiol.*, 477: 223–235.

Day, B.L., Dressler, D., Maertens de Noordhout, A., Marsden, C.D., Nakashima, K., Rothwell, J.C. and Thompson, P.D. (1989) Electric and magnetic stimulation of human motor cortex: surface EMG and single motor unit responses. *J. Physiol.*, 412: 449–473.

Day, B.L., Dressler, D., Hess, C.W., Maertens de Noordhout, A., Marsden, C.D., Mills, K., Murray, N.M.F., Nakashima, K., Rothwell, J.C. and Thompson, P.D. (1990) Direction of current in magnetic stimulating coils used for percutaneous activation of brain spinal cord and peripheral nerve. *J. Physiol.*, 430: 617.

Day, B.L., Riescher, H., Struppler, A., Rothwell, J.C. and Marsden, C.D. (1991) Changes in the response to magnetic and electrical stimulation of the motor cortex following muscle stretch in man. *J. Physiol.*, 433: 41–57.

Ebner, A. and Zentner, J. (1988) Prognostic value of somatosensory and motor evoked potentials in patients with severe head injury. In: P.M. Rossini, C.D. Marsden (Eds.). *Non-invasive Stimulation of Brain and Spinal Cord: Fundamental and Clinical Applications*. New York: Alan R. Liss, pp. 313–319.

Edgley, S.A., Eyre, J.A., Lemon, R.N. and Miller, S. (1990) Excitation of the corticospinal tract by electromagnetic and electrical stimulation of the scalp in the macaque monkey. *J. Physiol.*, 425: 301–320.

Ellaway, P.H., Davey, N.J., Maskill, D.W., Rawlinson, S.R., Lewis, H.S. and Anissimova, N.P. (1998) Variability in the amplitude of skeletal muscle responses to magnetic stimulation of the motor cortex in man. *Electroenceph. clin. Neurophysiol.*, 109: 104–113.

Facco, E., Baratto, F., Munari, M., Donà, B., Casartelli Liviero, M., Behr, A.U. and Giron, G.P. (1991) Sensorimotor central motor conduction time in comatose patients. *Electroenceph. clin. Neurophysiol.*, 80: 469–476.

Facco, E., Caputo, P., Fiore, D. and Giron, G.P. (1989) Sensorimotor and auditory central conduction time in locked-in syndrome. *Electroenceph. clin. Neurophysiol.*, 73: 552–556.

Gandevia, S.C. and Rothwell, J.C. (1987) Knowledge of motor commands and the recruitment of human motoneurones. *Brain*, 110: 117–1130.

Gill-Thwaites, H. (1997) The sensory modality assessment rehabilitation technique: a call for assessment and treatment of patients with severe brain injury in a vegetative state. *Brain Inj.*, 11: 723–734.

Grossman, P. and Hagel, K. (1996) Post-traumatic apallic syndrome following head injury. Part 1: Clinical characteristics. *Disabil. Rehabil.*, 18: 1–20.

Henneman, E. and Mendell, L.M. (1981) Functional organisation of motoneuron pool and its inputs. In: J.M. Brookhart and V.B. Mountcastle (Eds.), *Handbook of Physiology*, section 1, *The Nervous System*, Vol II, Motor Control, part 1, pp. 423–507. American Physiological Society, Bethesda, USA.

Hess, C.W., Mills, K.R. and Murray, N.M. (1987) Responses in small hand muscles from magnetic stimulation of the human brain. *J. Physiol.*, 388: 397–419.

Hess, C.W. and Ludin, H.P. (1988) Die transkranielle Kortex-stimulation mit Magnetfeldpulsen: methodische und physiologische Grundlagen. (Transcranial brain stimulation by magnetic pulses: methodological and physiological considerations.) EEG-EMG Zeitsch. Electroenzeph. Elektromyograph. Verwandte Gebiete, 19: 209–215.

Inghilleri, M., Formisano, R., Berardelli, A., Saltuari, L., Gerstenbrand, F. and Manfredi, M. (1994) Transcranial electrical stimulation in patients with apallic syndrome. *Acta. Neurol. Scand.*, 89: 15–17.

Jennett, B. and Plum, J. (1972) Persistent vegetative state after brain damage. *Lancet*, i: 734–737.

Kaneko, M. (1995) Prognostic evaluation of patients with severe head injury by motor evoked potentials induced by transcranial magnetic stimulation combined analysis with brain stem auditory evoked potentials. *No-To-Shinkei*, 47: 491–496.

Kiers, L., Cros, D., Chiappa, K.H. and Fang, J. (1993) Variability of motor potentials evoked by transcranial magnetic stimulation. *Electroenceph. clin. Neurophysiol.*, 89: 415–423.

Kimura, J. (1974) F-wave velocity in the central segment of the median and ulnar nerves. *Neurology*, 24: 539–546.

Magistris, M.R., Rosler, K.M., Truffert, A. and Myers, J.P. (1998) Transcranial stimulation excites virtually all motor neurons supplying the target muscle. A demonstration and a method improving the study of motor evoked potentials. *Brain*, 121, 437–450.

Mazzocchio, R., Rothwell, J.C., Day, B.L. and Thompson, P.D. (1994) Effect of tonic voluntary activity on the excitability of human motor cortex. *J. Physiol.*, 474: 261–267.

Milner-Brown, H.S., Stein, R.B. and Yemm, R. (1973) The orderly recruitment of human motor units during voluntary isometric contractions. *J. Physiol.*, 230: 359–370.

Moosavi, S.H., Catley, M., Ellaway, P.H., Stokes, M.J. and Bradley, J. (1997a) Compound motor evoked potentials elicited by transcranial magnetic stimulation after severe brain damage. *J. Physiol.*, 501: 44–45P.

Moosavi, S.H., Catley, M., Ellaway, P.H. and Stokes, M.J. (1997b) Motor evoked potentials and H-reflexes used in assessment of corticospinal function after severe brain damage in man. *Soc. Neurosci.*, Abstracts 23: 851.13.

Morita, H., Baumgarten, J., Christensen, L.O.D. and Nielsen, J. (1998) Recruitment of extensor carpi radialis motor units by corticospinal and Ia afferent input in human subjects. *J. Physiol.*, 509: 174P.

Murayama, S., Bouldin, T.W. and Suzuki, K. (1990) Selective sparing of Betz cells in primary motor area in hypoxic-ischemic encephalopathy. *Acta. Neuropathol. Berlin*, 80: 560–562.

Nakamura, H., Kitagawa, H., Kawaguchi, Y. and Tsuji, H. (1996) Direct and indirect activation of corticospinal neurons by transcranial magnetic and electrical stimulation. *Neurosci. Letts.*, 210: 45–48.

Netz, J. and Hömberg, V. (1992) Intact conduction of fastest corticospinal efferents is not sufficient for normal voluntary muscle strength: transcranial motor cortex stimulation in patients with tetraplegia. *Neurosci. Letts.*, 146: 29–32.

Nielsen, J. and Petersen, N. (1995) Changes in the effect of magnetic brain stimulation accompanying voluntary dynamic contraction in man. *J. Physiol.*, 484: 777–789.

Nielsen, J.F. (1996) Improvement of amplitude variability of motor evoked potentials in multiple sclerosis patients and in healthy subjects. *Electroenceph. clin. Neurophysiol.*, 101: 404–411.

Rothwell, J.C., Thompson, P.D., Day, B.L., Dick, J.P.R., Kachi, T., Cowan, J.M.A. and Marsden, C.D. (1987) Motor cortical stimulation in intact man. I. General characteristics of EMG responses in different muscles. *Brain*, 110: 1173–1190.

Schieppati, M. (1987) The Hoffman reflex: a means of assessing spinal reflex excitability and its descending control in man. *Prog. in Neurobiol.*, 28: 345–376.

Steriade, M., Gloor, P., Llinas, R.R., Lopes-de Silva, F.H. and Mesulam, M.M. (1990) Report of IFCN committee on basic mechanisms. Basic mechanisms of cerebral rhythmic activity. *Electroenceph. clin. Neurophysiol.*, 76: 481–508.

Ying, Z., Schmid, U.D. and Schmid, J. Hess. (1992) Motor and somatosensory evoked potentials in coma: analysis and relation to clinical status and outcome. *J. Neurol. Neurosurg. Psychiatry*, 55: 470–474.

Subject Index

Subjects listed are discussed in the chapters that start on pages referenced here